AF898533

ENVIRONMENT AND COMMUNITY HEALTH

Dr. Chebli Akli Islam

ALLIED
HEALTH
PRESS

Environment and Community Health

Author: **Dr. Chebli Akli Islam**

Allied Health Press
4164 Lakeshore Road
Burlington ON L7L 1A4
Canada
www.alliedhealthpress.com
Email: orders@arclereducation.com

© 2026 Allied Health Press
ISBN: 978-1-77956-788-8

This book contains information obtained from highly regarded resources. Reprinted material sources are indicated and copyright remains with the original owners. Copyright for images and other graphics remains with the original owners as indicated. A Wide variety of references are listed. Reasonable efforts have been made to publish reliable data. Authors or Editors or Publishers are not responsible for the accuracy of the information in the published chapters or consequences of their use. The publisher assumes no responsibility for any damage or grievance to the persons or property arising out of the use of any materials, instructions, methods or thoughts in the book. The authors or editors and the publisher have attempted to trace the copyright holders of all material reproduced in this publication and apologize to copyright holders if permission has not been obtained. If any copyright holder has not been acknowledged, please write to us so we may rectify.

General Disclaimer:

This book is a summation of information from different sources and encompasses a wide range of medical conditions, the latest therapy methods, principals and techniques that are used in current practice, at the time of publication. This book offers general information with educational purposes, it is not to be applied or relied on for any diagnostic or treatment purposes. Please do not use the data/matter as a substitute for professional diagnosis and treatment. Please consult your healthcare provider or a licensed physician before making any healthcare queries or treatment choices. The medical information and research findings presented in this book are for educational purposes only and should not be used for the treatment of specific individual patients, as individual cases may vary. The author(s), editors(s) and publisher cannot be held accountable and make no guarantees that the information provided in this book will apply to each and individual patient. This book is meant to serve as a basic guideline and other relevant literature sources should be used for more specific information. This text can be a vital resource for students, trainees, and practitioners, covering essential topics. This book encompasses a wide range of medical conditions and the latest therapy options used in current practice. Through the utilization of many different medical studies this book provides the basics of different medical conditions, which can be used as a basic guide from where medical students, trainees and practitioners can extract necessary information. Further, some of the books have graphic images to explain anatomy for medical/educational purposes only. Hence, the book is intended for students or teachers/staff or individuals with a mature outlook looking to learn or enhance their knowledge.

Notice: Registered trademark of products or corporate names are used only for explanation and identification without intent of infringement.

Allied Health Press publishes wide variety of books and eBooks. For more information about Allied Health Press and its products, visit our website at www.alliedhealthpress.com

ABOUT THE AUTHOR

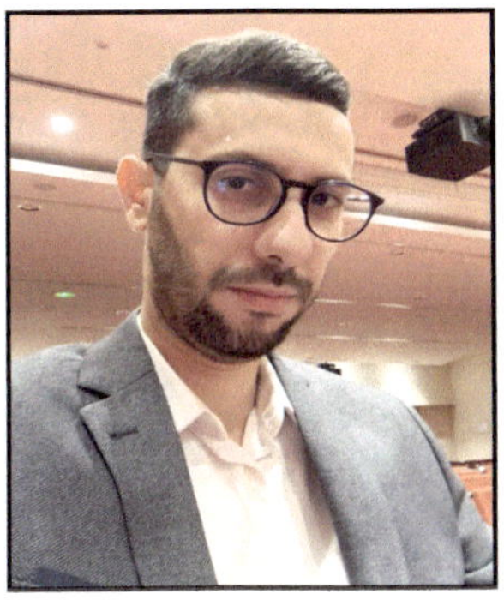

Dr. Chebli Akli Islam, PharmD, and holder of a PhD in Toxicology, epitomizes excellence in the field of hospital-university research. As a researcher at the University of Constantine, Faculty of Medicine, he passionately dedicates himself to studying various aspects of toxicology, including medicolegal, clinical, kinetic, food, and environmental toxicology. With over 10 years of experience, Dr. Chebli Akli Islam has cultivated expertise in a multitude of toxicological domains. His academic and professional career showcases an unwavering commitment to advancing knowledge in the field of toxicology. Dr. Chebli Akli Islam not only earned a pharmacy degree but also deepened his skills by pursuing a PhD in Toxicology, demonstrating his dedication to academic and scientific excellence. As a hospital-university researcher, Dr. Chebli Akli Islam tackles critical issues related to toxicology, such as toxic risk assessment in various contexts, identification of harmful substances in food and environmental products, and innovative solutions to mitigate the adverse effects of toxins on human health. His multidisciplinary expertise enables him to address the complex challenges of toxicology from different angles, ranging from clinical data analysis to the search for practical solutions to prevent poisonings and improve treatment protocols. Within the academic and scientific community, Dr. Chebli Akli Islam is recognized for his dedication to teaching and mentoring students, thereby inspiring future generations of researchers and healthcare professionals to pursue excellence in the field of toxicology. With his ambitious vision and unwavering commitment to scientific research, Dr. Chebli Akli Islam has become a prominent figure in the field of toxicology, making significant contributions to the safety and well-being of society.

Brief Table of Contents

Detailed Table of Contents

CHAPTER 3

Social Determinants of Health 71

CHAPTER 4

Sources of Community/Public Health Problems in Rural and Urban Areas of Less Developed Countries 105

CHAPTER 5

Environmental and Occupational Health 137

CHAPTER 6

Water Supply and Sanitation 171

LIST OF FIGURES

PREFACE

Environmental conditions and population health are core elements of public health practice. Air, water, waste management, and land use establish the physical setting where individuals reside, work, and play. Wherever these conditions are violated—by pollution, poor sanitation, or substandard housing—populations face heightened risks of disease and injury. Conversely, societies emphasizing clean air, stable water resources, and green areas facilitate lower disease burdens, improved mental health, and overall resilience. To protect and promote population well-being, it is important to understand how environmental exposures lead to community health outcomes.

Community health extends beyond separate care to encompass joint action targeting the conditions affecting health outcomes. Social cohesion, access to resources, cultural habits, and economic opportunities all have a bearing on communities' reactions to environmental risks. Where infrastructure is limited, the overlap of social determinants—education, income, and social support—has the potential to further exacerbate vulnerabilities when confronted with environmental risk. Unpacking these overlaps enables practitioners to craft interventions that not only mitigate hazards but also activate communities to be the drivers of their own health, ushering in the potential for long-term change.

This book, *Environment and Community Health*, offers a comprehensive discussion of the interplay between environmental processes and population health. It merges theoretical foundations, empirical data, and applied fixes to give readers an inclusive picture. From explaining the health impacts of climate change to analyzing legal frameworks that govern public health, this book offers an integrated framework that brings together academic studies and field practice. It aims to serve as a study guide for students and a blueprint for officials in government agencies, non-governmental organizations, and research institutions.

Chapter 1 provides an introduction to the elementary concepts of the relationship between environment and community health, including definitions of key terms and illustrations of the breadth of environmental health science. Chapter 2 deals with the multifaceted effects of climate change, detailing how shifts in temperature, rainfall, and storm patterns influence patterns of disease and community resilience. Chapter 3 moves on to social determinants of health, explaining how factors such as housing quality, food security, and education affect inequities in health across different populations. Chapter 4 presents rural and urban causes of health problems in less-developed countries, citing pollution, inadequate waste disposal, and inadequate access to medical care as primary causes.

Chapter 5 addresses environmental and occupational health, detailing workplace hazards, control measures, and the role of regulatory requirements as a method of employee protection.

Chapter 6 discusses water supply and sanitation, outlining technologies and management practices that deliver safe drinking water and proper sewage treatment, and the health impacts of system failure. Chapter 7 is concerned with community-based health care systems, identifying models of primary care integration, community health worker programs, and participatory planning processes. Chapter 8 explains epidemiology and public health research methods, providing study design tools, data analysis, and results translation into policy.

Chapter 9 addresses mental illness in community settings, considering how environmental stress, social isolation, and resource deficiencies are factors that cause psychological disorders, and mechanisms of community support. Chapter 10 provides nutrition interventions for public health enhancement, including school feeding interventions, micronutrient supplementation, and food policy programs to avoid malnutrition and obesity. Chapter 11 considers vector-borne diseases, the ecological determinants underpinning populations of mosquitoes, ticks, and other vectors, and control measures from habitat manipulation through to community education.

Chapter 12 deals with emergency response and disaster management, detailing the stages of disaster management in terms of preparedness, response, recovery, and mitigation using the framework of inter-agency coordination and community involvement. Chapter 13 addresses food safety and environmental hygiene, examining routes of contamination, inspection systems, and behavior change campaigns to restrict foodborne illness. Environmental and public health law is addressed in Chapter 14, such as international treaties, national legislation, and municipal regulations that govern pollution control, occupational health, and the availability of health services. Chapter 15, the final chapter, integrates sustainable development and environmental health concepts and outlines how governance, innovation, and public participation can build enduring health equity.

This book is aimed at undergraduate and postgraduate students of public health, environmental science, and allied health sciences. It will also be beneficial to community health practitioners, environmental protection officials, non-governmental organizations, and policy-making bodies. This book tries to help readers develop evidence-based interventions, plan good research studies, and develop policies to improve health outcomes at the level of the community by offering conceptual frameworks along with applied case studies.

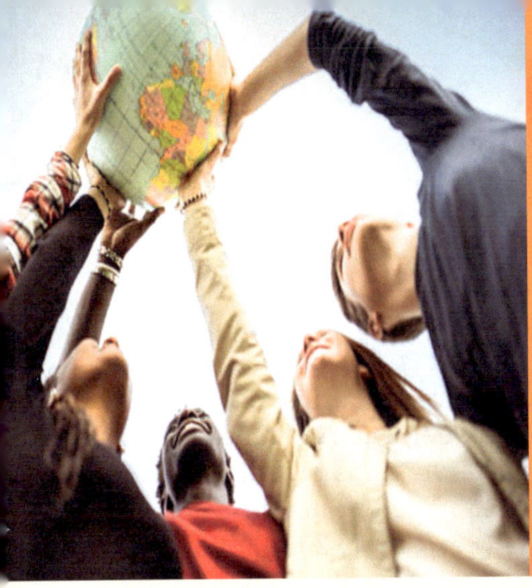

Chapter 1

INTRODUCTION TO ENVIRONMENT AND COMMUNITY HEALTH

Contents

Introduction

The interrelatedness of the environment and community health is a critical area of study that focuses on the multifaceted pathways through which ecological components shape public health. Various environmental physical, chemical, and biological components are all responsible for shaping individual and community health, illustrating to us that health is not merely the absence of disease but has powerful determinants based on our environment. Urbanization, pollution, and climate change are just a few of the environmental factors identified as affecting the prevalence of respiratory illnesses, cardiovascular disease, and psychiatric disorders. It is important to understand these processes so that interventions can be developed to reduce health disparities and promote health in communities. This holistic strategy requires collaboration between city planners, public health practitioners, and environmental scientists to create healthier living spaces, substantiating the argument that the community's health is intimately linked to the health of its setting. In writing about how important the setting is to the health of a community, one must consider the role that the microbiome plays as a new front for examining health outcomes. It has been demonstrated in studies that sophisticated microbial communities play an important role in human health, both in immune function and the stability of mental health. Notably, the research field in microbiomes has been receiving more attention, yet consistency in definitions and study methodology is lacking, which indicates the need for uniform methods within the field. This indicates the potential impact of microbiome studies on public health policies, particularly concerning anthropogenic drivers of microbial diversity. By integrating microbiome research into broader environmental health programs, communities have the ability to make responsive health interventions that are relevant to local environmental conditions, eventually building resilience and improved health outcomes for residents through targeted interventions based on individual needs (Berg et al., 2020). Moreover, technological advancements in environmental monitoring and assessment have initiated further realization of worldwide health impacts of climate change and other environmental changes. With the introduction of missions like Gaia by the European Space Agency, scientists now have unrivaled information about the Earth's systems and an opportunity to conduct a more detailed examination of environmental health intersections. The mission that is rooted in astrometry and mapping stellar objects is an example of how to use a larger science initiative that combines celestial observation with terrestrial interests. The lessons learned from ambitious initiatives can inform public health interventions and policies, yet again highlighting the need for cross-disciplinary understandings to address issues of environmental-borne health concerns. As the climate crisis becomes more stringent, this collaborative approach is crucial in building resilient societies able to adapt to the shifting landscape of health issues at local and global levels (Prusti et al., 2016) (Figure 1.1).

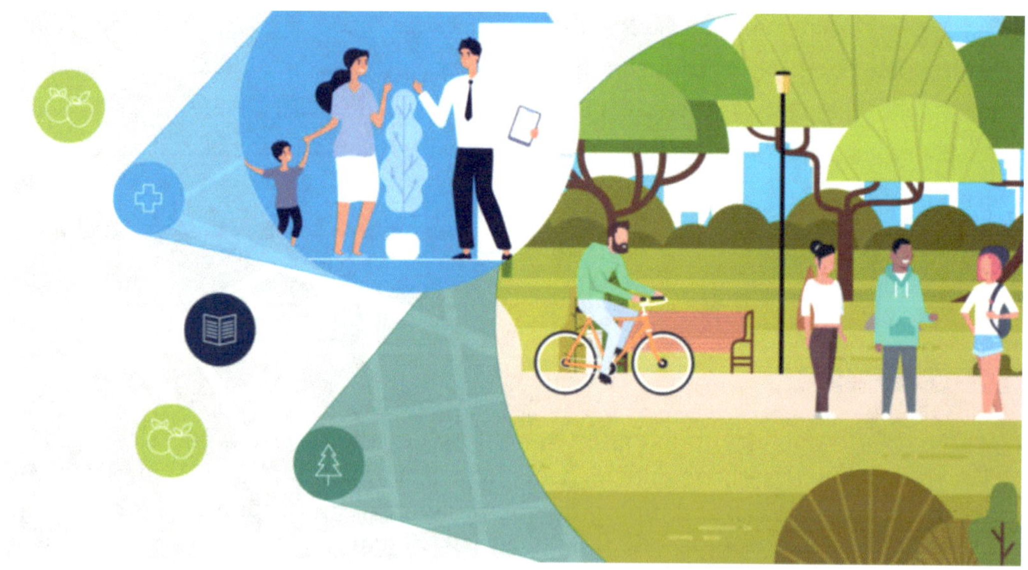

Figure 1.1. Environment and community health.

Source: https://external-content.duckduckgo.com/iu/?u=https%3A%2F%2Fwww.elmhurst.edu%2Fwp-content%2Fuploads%2F2020%2F02%2Fwhat-is-community-health-illustration-768x402.jpg&f=1&nofb=1&ipt=bcf2637f09ccb2aa184e506986294dbbcf176afe771925307bf3d06082f94f08.

Definition of Environment and Community Health

Understanding the appreciation of the health environment and community health is paramount to comprehending the interconnectedness of health systems and environmental settings. Environmental health is a field that looks into how environmental factors—physical and biological—impact human health and how health can be maximized through modifications in these factors. This encompasses a range of factors, including air quality and water quality, exposure to toxic substances, and the built environment. Community health, on the other hand, is about the outcomes of health specific to a group in a given area. It emphasizes not only the aggregate health of the population but also the determinants of social factors that influence access, equity, and outcomes for health. In putting these concepts together, we are better able to create a holistic framework for the design of public health interventions that elevate the community's quality of life. One of the fundamental dimensions of this discussion involves relating to industrialization and technological transformation implications on public health. As noted, the exponential growth driven by projects like Industry 4.0 and Made in China 2025 brings forward the extensive transformations in manufacturing technologies. The initiatives extrapolate an ongoing trend towards automation and productivity in manufacturing, but fuel underlying concerns with the degradation of the environment and occupational health risks. For instance, the industrial processes of manufacturing have a direct connection to adverse health implications through emissions of pollutants into water and air streams. Hence, it is critical to comprehend the mechanisms of interaction of modern industry with environmental health, as this will enable scientists and policy developers to devise measures that balance economic development with ensuring that community health is safeguarded against adverse impacts (Xu et al., 2018). Moreover, the oxidative stress theory provides a sophisticated explanation of the biology of environmental and community health issues. Oxidative stress occurs when there is an imbalance between the production of reactive species and the ability of the body to quench them, causing cellular damage. It describes how toxic substances in the environment can contribute to health issues through complex biochemical mechanisms. The dual nature of oxidative stress, where large amounts are toxic but physiological amounts are necessary to regulate the process of life, is reflective of the complexity of human health environments. This area of research interlaces biochemistry with community health, underscoring the need for environments that both reduce exposure to toxics and maximize biological processes important for human health, thereby advancing knowledge in the areas of environmental medicine and chemical redox signaling (Sies et al., 2017).

Importance of the Interconnection Between Environment and Health

Health outcomes and the environment's interaction is a central element of community health research that highlights the need for interdisciplinary approaches. Various social determinants, for instance, socioeconomic status, healthcare access, and environmental factors, have a significant influence on population health. For instance, populations with limited access to sports facilities may experience higher frequencies of related health issues, such as obesity and the attendant disease. The implications are important, as the most at-risk populations are often disproportionately affected by environmental hazards. Studies probing the link between county incarceration rates and stroke death examine the relationship between community environment and health, and conclude that rising rates of imprisonment are correlated with poorer health outcomes. Early awareness of such connections can lead to improved policy interventions with respect to environmental and health disparities with a view to achieving an enriched community health result (Sonderlund et al., 2025). Further, the constructed environment also has a direct impact on mental health, particularly in children. It has been found that exposure to adverse environmental factors during periods of development can have long-term effects on psychosocial outcomes. A complete understanding of these dynamics is significant to the development of education policy and public health policy. It is especially significant for urban regions where environmental stressors such as noise and pollution have the potential to exacerbate mental health issues. More recent special issue pieces have highlighted the significance of these relationships and have suggested rethinking urban planning priorities to make the environment more health-promoting. By keeping youth at the forefront of such a discussion, it is then possible to create strategies that diminish unwanted environmental consequences, demonstrating the pivotal importance of interrelations between environment and health (Wong et al., 2025). Finally, establishing interrelations between environment and health can make creating interventions easier to promote holistic well-being in the community. There is a requirement to tackle environmental issues, such as access to fresh air and clean water, to reduce health inequities between vulnerable groups. In addition, interventions addressing physical environments aim not only to resolve existing health problems but also to enhance the long-term resilience of the community. Studies have shown that enhancing access to healthy food sources and green spaces has a significant influence on population health in a positive direction. By using these environmental determinants in health interventions, communities are in a position to advance overall health equity better. This multifaceted approach acknowledges the reality that health cannot be divorced from the environment, once again highlighting the importance of collective efforts in environmental health and community health programs (Sonderlund et al., 2025) (Figure 1.2).

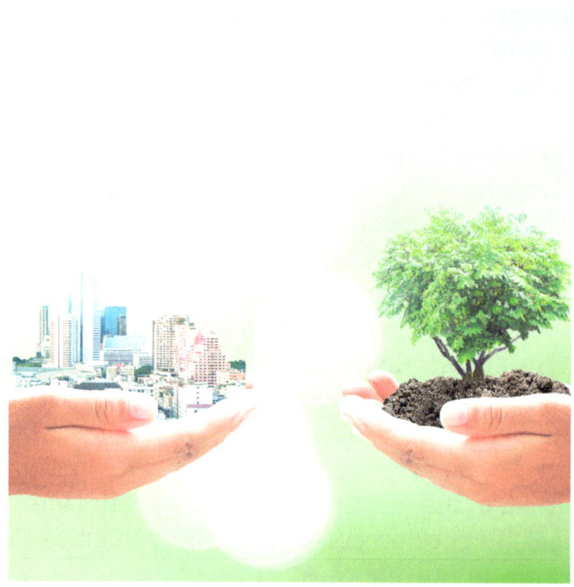

Figure 1.2. Environmental Health: the foundation of global public health.

Source: https://external-content.duckduckgo.com/iu/?u=https%3A%2F%2Fonline.umich.edu%2Fmedia%2FCityTree.png&f=1&nofb=1&ipt=ad3a725285l0a09 31631ee737a496a1399b53092eaf99d183f3299e7edc9f183.

Historical Context of Environmental Health Issues

Historically, environmental health issues have been most closely associated with political decisions and social justice, which underscores the way inequalities built into systems reinforce health risk to marginalized populations. Environmental health history is characterized by instances where public facilities were intentionally withheld from certain groups as a form of protest against desegregation, best exemplified in the case of public pools in Montgomery, Alabama. As Heather McGhee explains in her three-part investigation, the decision to cover the public spaces rather than include them is a perfect illustration of how natural resources end up being the arena for racial conflict. This occurrence highlights that environmental health is not a technical or scientific issue; it is socially one, where access and equity influence the entire population's health, demonstrating how previously public goods were employed to load non-dominant groups to finance racial stratification (Cohen, 2021). The relevance of this historical background goes beyond public infrastructure like swimming pools to encompass broader systemic failure, particularly in urban planning and infrastructure. Redlining and racist housing policies have had the long-term effect of localizing toxicants within largely people-of-color communities. These communities accumulate additive exposures to environmental toxins, leading to increased incidences of respiratory disease, toxic exposures, and poor overall health outcomes. In addition, economic development has traditionally outweighed environmental conservation in policy, with vulnerable population groups being made to endure the fruits of industrial pollution. The pattern reinforces the connection between environmental degradation and socioeconomic status, necessitating a critical examination of policy frameworks that continue to perpetuate these health inequities among populations (Rashid et al., 2020). Finally, being aware of the history of environmental health entails an appreciation of the growing recognition of community resilience amidst adversity. Environmental justice movements have emerged as a response to these disparities, mobilizing communities to challenge unequal access to clean air, water, and public resources. Grassroots movements have been key to raising awareness about environmental hazards and health advocacy for communities, building a sense of unity among otherwise fragmented populations with common experiences of structural marginalization. The intersection of environmental justice and health equity illustrates the power of social action to upend historic injustices and address emerging health inequities. Thus, the fight for environmental health justice remains both a moral imperative and a component of broader social justice movements, emphasizing the need for an inclusive model of community health that amplifies all voices and addresses systemic inequities (Cohen, 2021).

1.1. Key Environmental Factors Affecting Health

The interplay between the environment and public health is a key area of study in the field of community health. These are wide-ranging components such as air and water quality, access to pollution, and green spaces, and all have been proven to have substantial impacts on health outcomes. For instance, poor air quality due to industrial emissions can lead to respiratory ailments as well as exacerbate existing conditions in vulnerable populations such as children and the elderly. Further, water inequality may cause waterborne diseases, necessitating measures of integrated environmental management to end such health disparities. The mitigation of these environmental determinants takes a multi-faceted approach through public policy, community organization, and health education to build healthier communities and improve well-being. The social determinants of health, also entwined with environmental determinants, further elucidate the complexities of health impact within communities. Socio-economic status, level of education, and availability of resources in communities all influence people's access to healthcare and healthy environments. For example, poor community residents will be exposed more to environmental risk elements such as toxic waste and few green spaces. Subsequently, this exposure often results in higher rates of chronic disease, mental illness, and disability in general health. Community-level interventions like effective programs, such as the Friendship Bench in Zimbabwe, deploy local resources to provide culture-sensitive assistance, emphasizing the critical nature of community engagement in closing these gaps. An understanding of these determinants is necessary for the proper development of public health interventions. Additionally, some health issues, such as children's stunting, demonstrate the causal link between environmental determinants and health outcomes. Research conducted in the Cibodasari Puskesmas Community Health Center in Tangerang City demonstrates the contribution of maternal nutrition, socio-economic status, and accessibility of healthcare facilities to child health. The study found stunting to be prevalent among children, attributable to both environmental and household factors. This highlights the necessity for public health policy to leverage multi-sectoral interventions addressing environmental health, emphasizing the necessity for comprehensive methods addressing the root causes. These not only address stunting rates but also improve overall health and development among children, emphasizing the potential of improved living conditions to impact widespread health benefits for generations ahead, as seen in research (Ilham et al., 2024) (Figure 1.3).

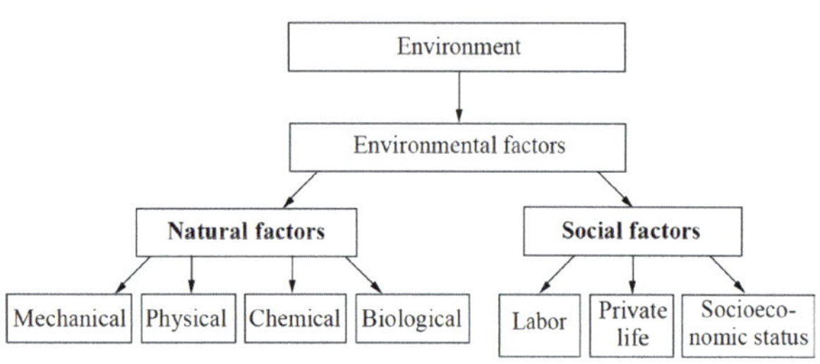

Figure 1.3. Environmental factors affecting health.

Source: https://www.researchgate.net/profile/Yuri_Vorokhta/publication/200029521/figure/fig1/AS:669533517926410@1536640638387/Main-Environmental-Factors-Influencing-Human-Health.png.

1.1.1. Air Quality and Respiratory Health

Air quality contributes enormously to the health of the respiratory system, particularly in urban settings, because of manufacturing activities and vehicle emissions. Air pollutants such as particulate matter and ozone are a significant component of harmful airborne agents that individuals are continually exposed to. A thorough body of literature has established a robust association between exposure to poor air and increased respiratory disease, such as asthma and chronic obstructive pulmonary disease (COPD). The health consequences extend beyond brief discomfort, as long-term exposure can lead to life-threatening chronic diseases and higher mortality. These risks are minimized by a multipronged effort involving public awareness campaigns along with educational initiatives to mark the dangers of air pollution and demand cleaner industry methods, and thereby contribute to better results in community health. Efforts to ensure monitoring and regulation of air quality have included installing technologies designed to detect airborne particles and determine their concentration in various environments. An instance is a community service project addressing the briquette manufacturing industry, which successfully installed an air particle detection system, sensitizing people to the harmful effects of air pollutants on the respiratory system. Such computerized systems play a crucial role in identifying sources of pollution and giving the required interventions. By monitoring the air quality index (AQI), stakeholders can measure the impact of the measures instituted and make necessary adjustments to achieve improved atmospheric conditions. Training and socialization exercises played a significant role in increasing factory workers' awareness about environmental health, highlighting proactive measures to control air quality and confirming the community's responsibility for maintaining a healthy breathing environment (Faridah et al.,

2024). The injurious effect of air pollution on lung function is not merely directly associated with momentary discomfort but is also associated with aggravating chronic conditions and making people more vulnerable to severe illness, i.e., lung cancer. Epidemiologic and clinical studies substantiate the link between lower air quality and heightened respiratory disease, and this is therefore an emergent public health problem. As the lung is a central interface with the environment and foreign pollutants, the impact of pollutants cannot be overstated. Socioeconomic factors further complicate this link, for vulnerable populations may not be able to cut down exposure to toxins in a meaningful way. Thus, comprehensive strategies involving community mobilization, effective health education, and political activism are required to reverse this alarming trend, such that air quality enhancement realizes improved respiratory well-being for all (Cacciottolo et al., 2013) (Figure 1.4).

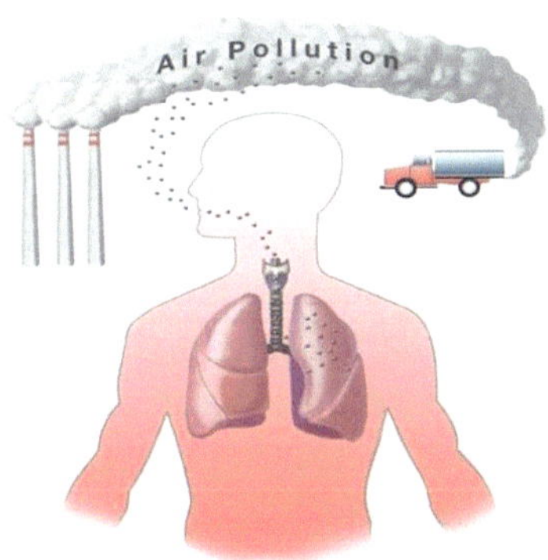

Figure 1.4. Air quality and respiratory health.

Source: https://external-content.duckduckgo.com/iu/?u= https%3A%2F%2Fwww.the-pool.com%2Fwp-content%2Fuploads%2F2022%2F02%2FLung-damage.jpg&f= 1&nofb=1&ipt= 59808797d698cd883a26294d9c8 d95f926785e6b6af3304267c94b2071fc6f61.

1.1.2. Water Quality and Its Impact on Public Health

An important aspect of public health that is not always taken into account is the quality of water. Water, as a fundamental human need, is instrumental in sustaining well-being and health but has serious health implications when it is contaminated. Pathogens, heavy metals, and chemical pollutants in water sources are public health hazards of concern. For instance, contaminated drinking water is associated with waterborne diseases such as cholera, dysentery, and typhoid fever that disproportionately affect vulnerable populations in developing and developed countries. The pathogenicity of these diseases has the ability to overwhelm healthcare systems, highlighting the powerful nexus between water quality and public health consequences. By making clean and safe water available, communities are able to reduce these diseases to a massive extent, illustrating the importance of good water management practices and policy interventions with a view to sustaining the quality of water. By considering how water quality interacts with public health, it becomes increasingly apparent that the role of the community is central. Public perception is an integral part of the measurement and maintenance of public utility performance, particularly for water services. It has been shown through evidence that public satisfaction with the quality of water not only represents the service provided by households but is also influenced by comparisons with the experience of neighbours and broader community attributes, according to Deichmann and Lall. Knowledge of these dynamics can be used to inform more responsive and effective governance approaches that, in the long run, lead to improved community health outcomes. Moreover, when communities get involved in monitoring and assessing their water services, they become change agents who can be responsible for advocating for improvements. Civic participation thus enhances the validity of appraisal in relation to water quality and enables a more nuanced approach in public health. To properly deal with water quality problems and their consequence on public health, education programs and policy recommendations must be developed. Emphasized in introductory environmental health courses, knowledge of the relationship among people, communities, and environmental agents is essential in preventing the health hazards of poor water quality. These courses equip the students with key information regarding environmental agents, including those affecting water, and their respective regulatory regimes. An interdisciplinary training of environmental epidemiology, toxicology, and policy is critical to developing effective interventions. Emphasis on these educational areas can lead to a learned populace that pressures for better environmental health policies. In the end, it will take a collaborative effort on the part of all stakeholders, including educators, policymakers, and community members, to guarantee sustained and equitable access to safe water.

1.1.3. Soil Contamination and Food Safety

Soil contamination is a key hazard to food safety and human health as it directly affects the farm food system that sustains humankind. Heavy metals, pesticides, and industrial effluents can readily accumulate in soil and have adverse consequences on crop quality. The application of pesticides, despite being necessary for controlling pests and producing greater yields of the crops, poses chemical residue threats that may seep into the earth and continue to infiltrate the food chain, impacting human health. It is suggested that crop yield would experience a disastrous loss between 32% and 78% for various crops in the absence of pesticide use. Hence, as pesticides are a part of ensuring food security, their potential for environmental and soil pollution calls for a scrupulous analysis of their use and handling within agricultural systems, emphasizing the fine line between farm productivity and ecosystem well-being (Tudi et al., 2021). Additionally, the occurrence of heavy metals in soil increases the complexity of the food safety arena. These toxic substances, such as mercury, arsenic, lead, cadmium, and chromium, are capable of disrupting human metabolism and leading to serious health issues, even loss of life. The pathways of these contaminants often involve the discharge of industrial effluent, clandestine dumping, and atmospheric deposition, all of which lead to the ingestion of hazardous materials by crop plants. Thus, this leads to contaminated crops that are hazardous for human consumption. Recent studies highlight the need for heightened awareness and regulatory measures to mitigate the consequences of heavy metal accumulation in agricultural production. The danger of such contaminants entering the food supply necessitates ongoing discourse on soil management practices that strike a balance between human health and environmental conservation (Kumar et al., 2019). To fulfill these functions, adopting sustainable agricultural practices is essential for going green. Practices such as crop rotation, organic farming, and integrated pest management not only reduce reliance on chemical inputs but also enhance soil quality, thereby increasing food safety outcomes. Additionally, ongoing monitoring of soil quality and the level of contamination is a prerequisite for ensuring public health protection. Farmers' training and education about the environmental impacts of soil contaminants can instill a culture of sustainability in farming practice. By emphasizing the interdependencies among food crop quality, soil quality, and human health, it is evident that there should be integrated measures to effectively address soil pollution. In this way, societies can work towards maintaining food safety, promoting healthier food systems, and ultimately developing a resilient environment (Tudi et al., 2021; Kumar et al., 2019) (Figure 1.5).

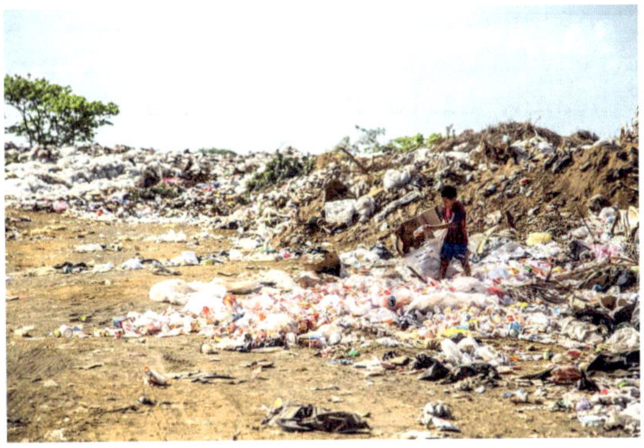

Figure 1.5. Increased soil contamination threatens food security.

Source: https://archive.siasat.com/wp-content/uploads/2018/12/Soil-Pollution-FLICKR.jpg.

1.2. Social Determinants of Health

Social determinants of health (SDOH) are the places where individuals are born, grow, live, work, and age. They are central to the understanding and influencing of health outcomes and health disparities. Disparities in health outcomes can usually be seen most clearly in vulnerable populations with issues of socioeconomic, systemic racism, or environmental exposures. For instance, air pollution combined with climate change has given specific research attention because both elements proportionally affect vulnerable populations, exacerbating pre-existing conditions such as asthma. More recent studies indicate that exposure to pollution not only has a correlation with worsening pre-existing illnesses but also induces new diseases. Thus, it is necessary to deal with such inequalities through enhanced understanding of SDOH towards enhancing the health outcomes of the public in communities, particularly those that have long been underserved due to systematic disparities (Felicia et al., 2024). Community coalitions are a significant means of reacting to SDOH at the community level, inducing health activity by leveraging the combined assets and knowledge. Such coalitions are formalized structures comprising varied stakeholders, including healthcare providers, residents, and community organizations. Success is often contingent on particular characteristics such as structural stability, resource management, and community engagement. Numerous studies show that coalitions can influence proximal and distal outcomes on health through activities with a focus on SDOH, for example, health equity, nutrition, and physical activity. By establishing alliances among various organizations, coalitions can implement policy shifts and enhance readiness in the community, ultimately resulting in improved health outcomes. The variety of effective coalition traits contributes to recognizing the importance of examining and understanding these elements to further strengthen participants' focus on people-centered health promotion programs (Nagorcka-Smith et al., 2022). Despite growing recognition of the social determinants of health, ongoing research is required to understand their implications within environmental as well as community health contexts. More research must investigate the interaction between SDOH and environmental determinants like climate resilience and air quality, with a focus on the following implications for health in susceptible groups of people. In addition, interdisciplinary models that integrate environmental science, public health, and social justice thinking are needed in developing solutions that are integrated. Understanding what specific interventions are optimally effective in mitigating the adverse impact of social determinants not only will alleviate the burden of disparities but also will guide policymakers on optimal resource allocation. In doing so, concerted action towards the resolution of SDOH through bold research and community initiatives has vast opportunities for advancing public health equity and healthy communities (Felicia et al., 2024) (Figure 1.6).

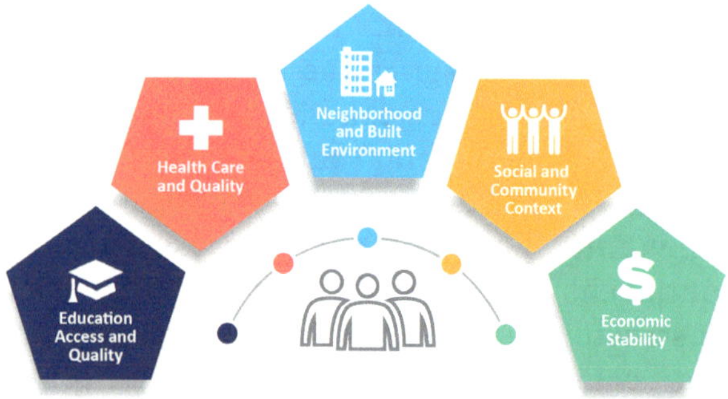

Figure 1.6. Social determinants of health (SDOH).

Source: https://www.cdc.gov/public-health-gateway/media/images/images/sdoh/SDOH-icons.png.

1.2.1. Socioeconomic Status and Health Disparities

The interaction between socioeconomic status (SES) and health inequality is a key area of focus in community health. Those who have lower SES tend to have poorer health, something that can be explained by a variety of social determinants such as healthcare access, education, and resources. The evidence has demonstrated that SES is an important predictor of mental health and that environmental views and social relationships act as mediators. For instance, a study illustrated the influence of neighborhood interactions and environmental perception within the community on health differences between social classes. To this end, lower SES participants recorded lower mental health indices, resulting in an emergent need for such differences to be addressed through interventions that facilitate greater community participation and ecological governance (Lei et al., 2025). Other than mental health, socioeconomic determinants characterize children's overall health through diet quality and physical activity levels. A powerful cross-sectional study in the Canary Islands showed how children from families with higher SES build healthier habits and therefore replicated the vast impact of SES on physical activity and diet. The positive relationship between SES and healthy habits illustrates that economic conditions have a powerful role in children's food habits and physical activity. Interestingly, the spatial dimension of these inequalities is low, suggesting that local and individual SES have strong effects on health behavior. Children living in neighborhoods where more households earn less than a certain income had lower scores for healthy behaviors, thereby underscoring the role of public health interventions in enhancing healthier behaviors among economically downtrodden populations (Rodr et al., 2024). Socioeconomic differences in health must be addressed through a multidimensional intervention. Interventions in public health must target not only quality improvement in access to healthcare services but also quality improvement in the environmental setting to promote social interaction among the inhabitants. Prioritizing quality improvement in the environment and establishing community participation, healthcare professionals can bridge the gap in the pattern of health outcomes between different socioeconomic groups. Moreover, knowledge of urban-rural health heterogeneity in health disparities informs tailored interventions that respond to the particular needs of various populations. Rural residents, for instance, will be very responsive to changes in their environment, whereas urban dwellers may require interventions aimed at promoting social contact. Ultimately, addressing socioeconomic factors within community health systems is critical in developing health equity and improving population health outcomes generally (Lei et al., 2025).

1.2.2. Access to Healthcare Services

Access to healthcare services is a central aspect of community health that affects the well-being and resilience of the entire population. Quality and accessibility of healthcare services generally rely on numerous interconnected factors that encompass geographical position, socioeconomic status, and social determinants. Urban populations may be more likely to have access to health care facilities, but not always, because the cities themselves can be subject to health care deserts that exclude marginalized groups. Insurance is also important to a person's ability to seek and receive care, particularly in lower-income settings where expense can prevent needed medical care. It is pertinent to understand these complexities for formulating people-centered policies towards improving accessibility of healthcare for everyone, especially for economically underdeveloped regions that are severely affected by economic inequality. Second, the international health context reflects alarming trends toward healthcare access, namely, in the development of growing antimicrobial resistance (AMR). Challenges in accessing care within low-resource settings aggravate the impact of AMR, both in terms of treatment and mortality. Estimated research attributes about 4.95 million deaths in 2019 to bacterial AMR, underlining the weakness of populations that lack access to effective and timely healthcare interventions (Christopher et al., 2022). Populations with poor access to essential antibiotics and fragile infection prevention interventions are most vulnerable. A twin emphasis on increasing access to healthcare services, along with pushing back against the problems caused by antimicrobial resistance, is needed to prevent negative health consequences. This requires system-level efforts, which include the strengthening of local health infrastructures and enhanced public awareness on the significance of infection control and antibiotic stewardship. Apart from enhancing access to healthcare, the promotion of physical activity as part of the core of community health has been given increased prominence in recent approaches. The new WHO guidelines put high priority on physical activity among every age group to lower risks of chronic diseases, thus the indirect impact on access to healthcare through healthier lifestyles (Bull et al., 2020). Physical activity interventions can be highly vital in countries with limited healthcare resources, as they avert cases of chronic illness that otherwise would have required a lot of medical treatment. More focus on healthcare access and active living can lead to healthier communities, which in turn will lower the demand on the healthcare system and have improved outcomes for citizens. These intertwined arenas highlight the importance of an integrated model of community health in realizing that access, prevention, and lifestyle modifications are closely intertwined in ensuring a healthier populace (Figure 1.7).

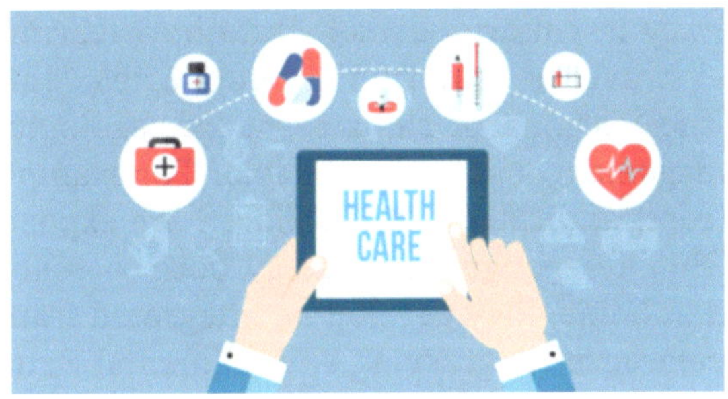

Figure 1.7. Access to healthcare services.

Source: https://images.yourstory.com/cs/wordpress/2016/06/ Healthcare- 01.jpg?mode=crop&crop= faces&ar= 2%3A1&format=auto&w=1920&q=75.

1.2.3. Education and Health Literacy

The intersection of health literacy and education is fundamental to shaping community health outcomes. In an attempt to successfully navigate through health information and make good decisions, one must possess a level of literacy that encompasses not only reading and understanding abilities but also the ability to apply this knowledge in real-life situations. Education offers the origin for building this ability, with it inculcating a continuous interest in issues concerning health. While there are extreme disparities in access to learning, particularly in developing countries, inadequate education commonly stifles health literacy capability. If children leave school with poor literacy skills, they are not able to advance their own, as well as that of their family's, health, and thereby perpetuate patterns of illness and illiteracy. This emphasizes the imperative for change within educational structures, projecting the need to incorporate health literacy into curricula that build sustainable futures (Howes et al., 2006). Additionally, carbon literacy presents a new way in which education and health literacy can be connected by means of environmental awareness. As climate change becomes a further factor affecting public health, the capability to read and respond to environmental information is essential. Initiatives in cultivating carbon literacy in children demonstrate how learning may traverse traditional boundaries, such as the learning of climate change, ecological management, and health behavior. For example, research indicates that if children are exposed to climate change terminology both in school and at home, they develop an integrated frame of reference for grasping environmental issues that informs their health behavior (Satchwell et al., 2013). Thus, by adopting a multidimensional education policy that integrates theoretical knowledge and practical skills, communities can foster healthy individuals who are not only health-literate but also green, addressing community health in a world with climate change. The role of nonformal education in health and environmental literacy must also not be overlooked. Compared with formal education, nonformal training tends to focus on the practical skills that can directly respond to the community's needs, particularly for poorer communities. By providing complementary learning experiences focused on health and sustainability, such programs offer channels for people to acquire essential insight that will not be available through education. Through community initiatives, individuals can learn about sanitation, nutrition, and environmental stewardship in an inspiring setting that recognizes the urgency of these issues. This participatory approach not only enhances health literacy but also helps community members become active in their own well-being and environmental concerns. Therefore, the integration of nonformal education strategies into the already established hierarchy of education can facilitate more extensive change and facilitate healthier and better-educated communities in the long run, ultimately contributing to sustainability and outcomes in health (Howes et al., 2006).

1.3. Environmental Policies and Regulations

In the field of environmental laws and policies, the role of governance frameworks is increasingly important for the purpose of public safety and well-being. Policies of the European Union (EU) have been at the forefront in regulating food value chain issues, both sustainability-related and food integrity-related. Food systems in nature call for a robust regulatory system intended to balance the interests of farmers, consumers, and the environment. The increasing focus on unfair trading practices and having a better share of profits in such chains highlights the role of ethical regulation to enhance not only economic stability but also community health outcomes. Governments are increasingly coming to appreciate that policies must go beyond economic metrics to encompass health and safety considerations, an approach in line with current evidence within EU regulatory frameworks emphasizing the interdependence of food integrity and consumer well-being (Barling et al., 2019). Health impact assessments (HIAs) are a critical means of environmental policies to integrate health considerations into sectors such as transportation, energy, and agriculture. The governing framework for HIAs has evolved to facilitate their incorporation into decision-making, thereby ensuring a holistic understanding of community health. Legislation that encourages the application of HIAs in environmental decision-making facilitates the creation of health vulnerabilities due to pollution and degradation of natural resources. The ability of stakeholders to perform HIAs guarantees accountability and openness in environmental planning since communities are best suited to understand the implications of various policies. Regulations for maximizing the authority and application of HIAs in different sectors indicate a growing recognition of the importance of taking into account not only the short-term economic benefit but also long-term health gains to local communities (Corbett et al., 2012). In addition, free debate around equality and transparency in environmental management is at the core of ensuring equal health outcomes among different populations. Since policies are created to respond to environmental risks, engaging stakeholders from local communities has become imperative in crafting effective policies.

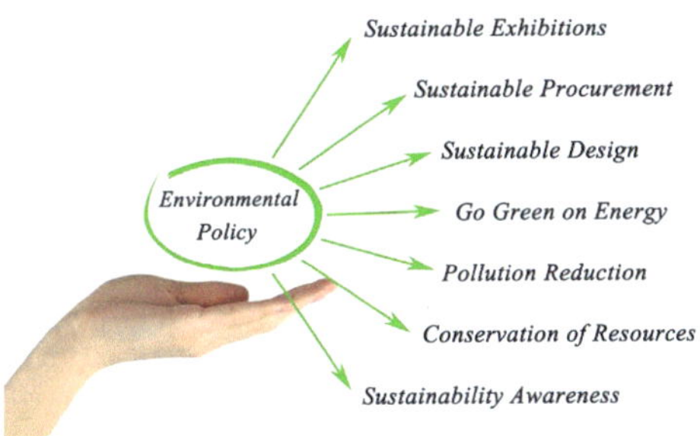
Environmental Policy
Sustainable Exhibitions
Sustainable Procurement
Sustainable Design
Go Green on Energy
Pollution Reduction
Conservation of Resources
Sustainability Awareness

Figure 1.8. Environmental policies and regulations.

Source: https://www.tutorialspoint.com/environmental_studies/images/environmental_policy.jpg.

The dynamic nature of food value chains necessitates policy frameworks that are stakeholder-attentive, particularly in health and safety. With the incorporation of inputs from various sectors like agriculture and waste management, policymakers can craft a more holistic framework addressing the root causes of environmental health disparities. The findings from community stakeholder surveys indicate a consensus among stakeholders on the necessity to align regulatory interventions with community health priorities, leading to more effective and efficient governance that enhances overall public health in such communities (Corbett et al., 2012; Barling et al., 2019) (Figure 1.8).

1.3.1. Overview of Major Environmental Health Legislation

The foundation of environmental health law in the US is based on the existence of several significant statutes aimed at safeguarding public health and the environment. The National Environmental Policy Act (NEPA) of 1969 established a framework that compels federal agencies to assess the environmental and public health impacts of their actions prior to decision-making. NEPA's passage gave prominence to the role of educated public involvement and established an example for environmental considerations within government decision-making. Subsequent legislation, such as the Clean Air Act and the Clean Water Act, supplemented these fundamental principles but specifically targeted air and water quality. These laws empower the regulatory agencies to determine standards for managing pollution, thereby not only improving the environment but also mitigating public health risk from exposure to toxic contaminants. From these pieces of legislation, an integrated approach to the preservation of the public's health has been formulated, demonstrating the synergistic relationship between environmental status and public health. With the evolving structure of environmental health legislation, the Toxic Substances Control Act of 1976 is an important one in the context of regulating chemicals in commerce. The TSCA gives the Environmental Protection Agency (EPA) the authority to review and regulate chemicals that can pose an unreasonable risk to human health or the environment. This legislation is particularly pertinent to increasing the complexity of chemical exposure in consumer goods, from building supplies to household cleaners. More recent legislation, the Frank R. Lautenberg

Chemical Safety for the 21st Century Act of 2016, tightened the EPA's authority to screen currently approved chemicals and conduct more transparent public health assessments. The present reform of TSCA mirrors the shift towards a more proactive stance in addressing potential chemical threats, thus protecting communities from hazardous exposures leading to long-term illnesses and ecological contamination. The interaction between legislation and public health is also highlighted through the emergence of sustainability and resilience models as depicted in the case of the U.S. Army Corps of Engineers' programs (Katherine et al., 2019). These standards reflect a higher sense of the importance of ecological solutions to environmental health that address both short- and long-term issues. Through an emphasis on sustainable actions and increased resilience in populations, recent policy aims to counter the complexity of environmental health challenges in socio-ecological systems. This shift reflects a growing understanding of the interconnectedness of human well-being, environmental conditions, and responses of systems to disturbances, consistent with the mandates articulated in earlier legislative efforts. In anticipation of developing environmental challenges, ongoing policy evolution and the incorporation of sustainability principles will be critical to the promotion of well-being and the delivery of responsible stewardship of our natural resources (Gulliver, 2024).

1.3.2. Role of Government Agencies in Protecting Public Health

Government agencies play a crucial role in maintaining public health through regulation, monitoring environmental conditions, and enforcing adherence to health standards. Through various federal and state programs, these agencies develop standards for the safeguarding of communities from environmental pollutants that may inflict harmful effects on health. For instance, the Environmental Protection Agency (EPA) regulates pollutants and ensures that everyone has access to clean air and water. By implementing environmental regulations and promoting environmentally sustainable practices, these agencies also promote public health while promoting responsible environmental stewardship. By taking proactive measures, they reduce exposure to harmful substances, thereby improving community well-being and resilience to health crises. One of the most pertinent examples of effective government intervention lies in medical waste disposal, based on case histories of toxic wastes such as those discussed in Law Number 32 of 2009. Where potentially toxic wastes, e.g., HIV blood bags, find their way to be disposed of in the wrong manner, the role of government agencies is implicated. Local health institutions and environmental enforcement authorities collaborate to investigate the incidents, undertake remedial measures, and promote community awareness about safe waste disposal. The policy of regulation instills responsibility among healthcare providers to ensure compliance with safety measures for the protection of public health. This holistic approach addresses both short-term health risks and promotes a culture of environmental conservation, ultimately transforming community health outcomes. In addition to this, the fight against industrial pollution is also one area where governmental institutions significantly affect public health. The marble industry, for instance, has environmental concerns that impact water and soil quality, as documented in most studies, such as those conducted in Tehsil Shabqadar, Khyber Pakhtunkhwa. If left untreated, industrial effluents released into the environment can lead to augmented levels of heavy metals and other pollutants, which play a tremendous role in human health as well as ecosystems. Government intervention is very crucial here because agencies must implement rules that allow proper treatment of the waste and implement sustainable processes in industries. Through enabling monitoring and supplementing efforts towards environmental health, government agencies can neutralize the detrimental effects of industrial processes and thus ensure a healthier environment for current and future generations (Figure 1.9).

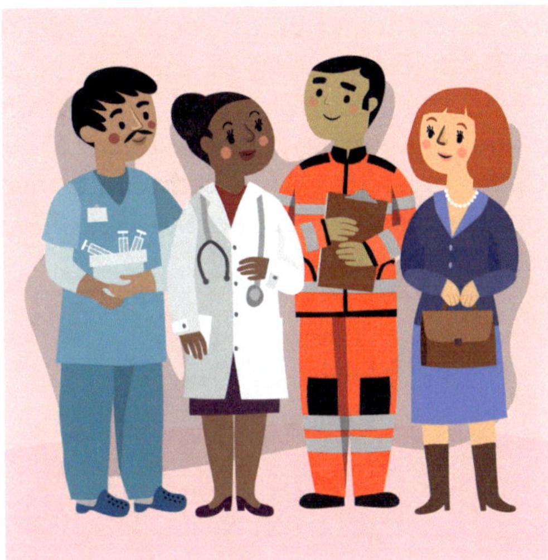

Figure 1.9. The role of government in supporting health.

Source: https://cdn.who.int/media/images/default-source/initiatives/uhc-advice/who-cards-08-healthy-world-02.jpg?sfvrsn=39f001b5_7.

1.3.3. Impact of Policy on Community Health Outcomes

The intersection of policy and community health outcomes is essentially characterized by social determinants of health (SDoH), which cover numerous factors like economic security, education, and housing. Public health policies that tackle the determinants well are able to minimize risk factors for various illnesses, particularly cardiovascular illnesses. However, existing frameworks fail to account for the intricate pathways through which determinants affect outcomes. For instance, cardiovascular morbidity and mortality are strongly influenced by SDoH, but not much research has been done to investigate this relationship. Redefining the health policies to recognize and reduce the disparities in SDoH can facilitate certain interventions, thereby improving the health status of the population. Improved insight into the biological mechanisms connecting SDoH and health outcomes will allow policymakers to make more impactful steps that will contribute to reducing health inequities, ultimately leading to better community health outcomes (Tiffany et al., 2022). There is another very important policy influence on community health outcomes that can be illustrated through the lens of eye health. Limited access to affordable eye care services results in uncontrolled vision impairment, particularly among the populations of low- and middle-income countries. Vision loss has a detrimental impact on educational achievement and productivity and drastically limits economic potential. Policy approaches that bring together comprehensive health policies for strategic prioritization of universal access to eye care have the potential to alter lives by minimizing economic and social costs of vision loss. Furthermore, studies reveal that investment in eye health yields considerable rewards as sound interventions are among the most cost-effective interventions within health care (Matthew et al., 2021). By approaching eye health as a development and medical concern, policy can enhance overall community health levels and enhance quality of life, especially for the poor and marginalized. Lastly, the effectiveness of health policies also hinges on their ability to facilitate intersectoral action. Involving a range of stakeholders, including government, NGOs, and the private sector, is critical to arguing for health equity and effective outcomes. Policies that integrate health services with school, work, and housing programs can facilitate planning integrative environments that benefit community well-being. In addition, community-based participatory approaches involving the people in policy-making ensure that interventions are not only equitable but also culturally relevant. Building a robust platform for addressing the SDoH, along with ensuring universal access to primary health care, will significantly enhance performance at the grassroots level. By considering and solving complex policy–environment–community health interactions, we can be at the forefront of innovations that reshape public health landscapes in a sustainable manner (Tiffany et al., 2022; Matthew et al., 2021).

1.4. Community Health Assessment

A community health assessment (CHA) is a valuable tool in understanding the multiple health needs of the population, specifically focusing on how environmental factors relate to population well-being. By going through the process of gathering and examining data in an orderly fashion on health status, resources, and socio-economic conditions, a CHA enables public health officials and stakeholders to identify health disparities and make recommendations for priority intervention areas. This is community empowerment and participation, where the residents can be part of planning health initiatives that directly impact them. Additionally, addressing the social determinants of health, like economic stability, education, and access to health care, is crucial in coming up with effective plans that provide health equity in the community. Thus, a thorough CHA informs policy decisions that can potentially improve health outcomes and ensure equitable access to necessary resources among all residents of the community (Karos et al., 2020). The success of community health assessments depends significantly on the integration of both qualitative and quantitative data. While quantitative data provides statistical proof of patterns and trends in health, qualitative data, such as community voice and experience, enhances the understanding of health issues. Employment of diverse community voices via the focus group, interviews, and surveys enhances the assessment with hints to hidden social and environmental determinants that may lead to health disparities. This dual-pronged approach, in addition to facilitating accurate problem identification, constructs public trust and interphase collaboration between people and health officials empowered to facilitate effective implementation of the intervention. Moreover, the adaptability of a CHA allows continuous monitoring and adjustment of health programs as needs in the community evolve, keeping programs as supportive and effective (Kenneth et al., 2019).

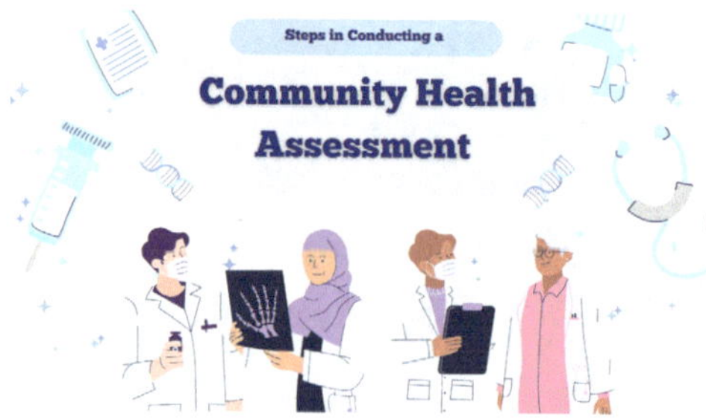

Figure 1.10. Community health assessment.

Source: https://blogger.googleusercontent.com/img/b/R29vZ2xl/AVvXsEhZ9p_cYZsRhKLIX5f7miIA4EoM0C-AHYVx507jPwLZL4Yta-neA8C7JFNwr-Z8xCzcJc6pciMJAFVW_yrb45-06LlUz9-sXnRp1_7ToxC36VUAseQj7Cj_gQvWoRjrzqikNDK_pnmvFG9vykWdMCI2rO7AXH23wo5tqZFTh 0EpoRJnzqBs5ZJD3X3K7aj6/s1920/ Community%20Health%20Assessment.jpg.

Lastly, the importance of community health assessments lies in contributing to public health initiatives by bridging resources to determinants of need. Through the facilitation of the acquisition of comprehensive health data, CHAs allow for the delivery of population-tailored strategies in resolving unique attributes and challenges of specific populations. This renders interventions evidence-based and culture-responsive, thus enhancing the likelihood of accomplishment and sustainability. As communities grapple with the ongoing impact of social determinants on health, data collected by CHAs can be utilized as the foundation for advocacy, resource planning, and policy formulation to drive improved health outcomes. By doing so, CHAs not only solve the short-term health situation but also drive long-term structural change that enhances the resilience and overall health of populations (Karos et al., 2020) (Figure 1.10).

1.4.1. Methods for Assessing Community Health Needs

Assessment of community health needs provides the foundation for the creation of successful public health policy. This is usually undertaken by the collection of quantitative and qualitative data in an effort to establish priority health issues in a community. Surveys, screening for health, and demographic evaluation supply a basis for measurable health indicators, while forums, focus groups, and interviews supply knowledge and comprehension of the community's specific health issues. By applying mixed-methodologies, the health workers and researchers can obtain a general overview of health needs in communities, with intervention strategies targeting both short- and long-term health concerns. Moreover, stakeholder engagement, including input from organizations at the local level, health professionals, and community members, enhances the findings' appropriateness and effectiveness to ensure cultural sensitivity and widespread acceptance by the population (Brenda, 2020). Another essential method of analyzing health needs in the community is reviewing existing health data obtained from public health information bases and health informatics systems. Health departments usually collect vast quantities of data on disease trends, access to care, and social determinants of health. Using this data can help identify trends and disparities that must be targeted, such as higher rates of chronic diseases among specific populations. Geographic information systems (GIS) can also support this assessment through mapping the health information to community assets, allowing public health professionals to identify areas that require increased efforts. Further, partnerships between academic institutions and health agencies can allow for data sharing and collaborative research activities, significantly enriching the evaluation process. This extensive examination of data not only educates targeted health interventions but also facilitates ongoing observation of program effectiveness (Rashid et al., 2020). Community health needs assessments (CHNAs) serve to play a key function in establishing the baseline for health programs and influencing policy results. By conducting a CHNA, stakeholders get to develop strategic plans for resource allocation effectively after establishing the needs for health. The results of these assessments can then be utilized for informing local health plans and guiding health policy, with a focus on the populations that have the widest health disparities. Further, the intersection of social media platforms and technology offers new avenues for participation from communities and data collection with immediate feedback on responses and demands for health. Periodic reassessment is unavoidable with a shifting social context while responding to developing health concerns with an adaptive approach. Lastly, methods of ascertaining community health needs play a very critical role in developing healthy environments that can adapt in a manner associated with changing community dynamics (Brenda, 2020).

1.4.2. Importance of Community Engagement in Health Assessments

Community participation is essential to health evaluation, particularly in promoting health equity and the specific needs of populations with diverse groups. Through the incorporation of perspectives and knowledge of community members, health workers can create assessments that are sensitive to the specific health concerns and cultural contexts of the population. This helps to empower individuals, win their trust, and assure them that they have a stake in health intervention. In addition, community engagement offers a chance to determine appropriate determinants of health such that measures capture a complete image of community health dynamics. As observed in the case of the COVID-19 pandemic, communities where there was greater community participation in health screening were better able to adapt their responses to the requirements of their populations, proving that inclusive action can produce better health outcomes and compliance with public health advice (Geoffrey et al., 2020). In addition, community involvement increases the effectiveness of health screenings by making it easier to collect data through culturally appropriate means and to involve more people. Engaging community members not only assists researchers in collecting qualitative information but also assists in the identification of factors hindering access to health services, including transportation, lack of knowledge, or economic limitations. With this knowledge, health screenings can integrate interventions aimed at addressing them, leading to more effective health policy. Furthermore, when communities engage in the process of assessment, they are sensitized towards health promotion and prevention of disease activities. This brings awareness, which acts as a feedback mechanism to ensure constant dialogue between health professionals and the people within the community, hence encouraging collective work towards improved public health outcomes (Brenda, 2020).

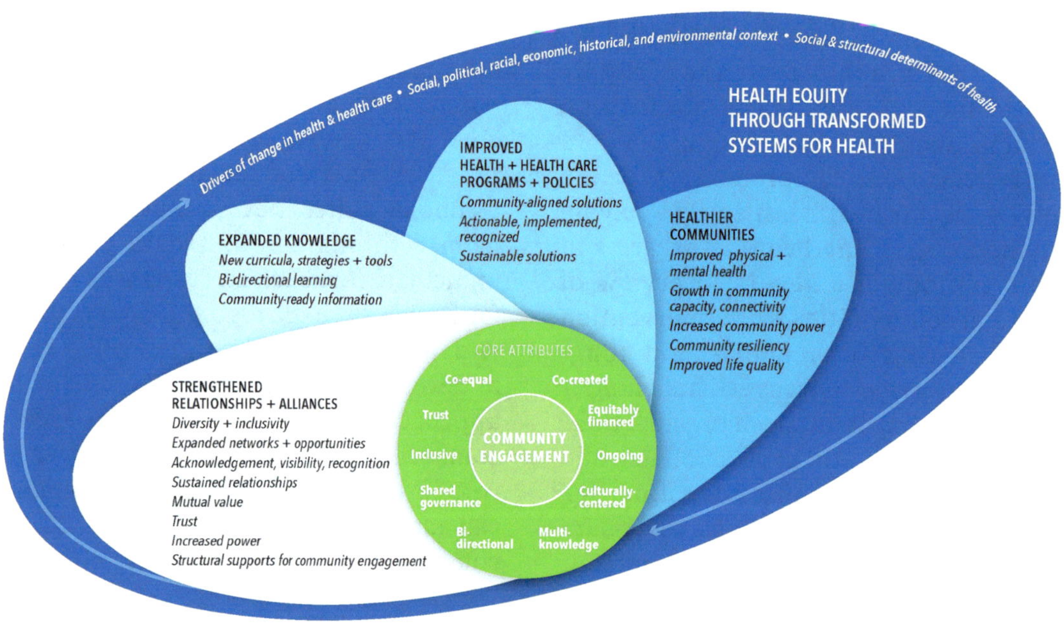

Figure 1.11. Achieving health equity and systems transformation through community engagement.

Source: https://nam.edu/wp-content/uploads/2023/03/v2-p1.png.

Finally, the sustainability of health assessments largely depends on consistent involvement by communities. Successful health interventions leverage neighborhood assets, networks, and champions to drive health-related change that is beyond a single round of assessment. Community engagement in longitudinal health evaluation encourages a sense of ownership and leads individuals to be active participants in continuous processes of health enhancement. When dynamics change in the health landscape, repeated involvement of the community ensures that continuous evaluations remain pertinent and responsive to new needs. When communities are encouraged to take an active role in health assessments, they foster resilience and adaptability, helping to strengthen the overall public health infrastructure. Ultimately, integrating community engagement into the fabric of health assessments not only enhances their accuracy and effectiveness but also builds healthier communities that are better equipped to address future challenges (Geoffrey et al., 2020) (Figure 1.11).

1.4.3. Utilizing Data to Inform Health Interventions

The integration of health data is imperative in the development of effective public health interventions that respond to the needs of communities. As health professionals grapple with rising differences in health outcomes, using authoritative sources of data helps in better understanding how determinants of the environment influence health. For instance, data can be applied in health impact assessments (HIAs) for the identification of certain urban inequities. These assessments not only quantify the distribution of environmental health risks but also identify risk groups that are disproportionately affected by these risks.

Through systematic analysis of information collected using both quantitative and qualitative approaches, HIAs are capable of offering targeted suggestions for preventing adverse health outcomes in risk groups. These data-driven interventions are significant in supporting an equitable distribution of health resources, addressing the broader consequences of social determinants of health, and enhancing the overall health effects for marginalized groups (Properzi et al., 2025). Further, the application of data supports an inclusive health intervention culture, particularly when faced with a diversifying population. As environmental health professionals increasingly work with issues of diversity, equity, and inclusion (DEI), it is imperative to understand and respond to differential perceptions of the need for health. Data from stakeholders such as the Public Health Workforce Interests and Needs Survey show stark disparities within the environmental health workforce itself. The study reveals Black, Indigenous, and People of Color (BIPOC) employees experience systemic inequities in job roles and organizational dedication to DEI perceptions. Organizations can use this information to chart gaps in equity and align legislative and organizational changes to address workplace diversity to the advantage of public health interventions. Identifying and acting on these disparities not only enhances the effectiveness of health initiatives but also contributes to establishing confidence in underserved populations (Maurica et al., 2025). Finally, employing data-driven approaches in informing health interventions encourages the development of targeted policies that directly respond to established health inequities. Recurring review of community-level data permits the health messaging and interventions, which are adjusted to be appealing to particular demographic populations. For example, when interventions are guided by demographic data that include socioeconomic status, health beliefs, and local disease patterns, they are in a stronger position to gain community acceptance and adherence. The application of geographic information systems (GIS) mapping in this instance can provide key visual information on spatial inequalities in health, guiding effective resource planning and allocation. As communities evolve and issues shift, ongoing exploration of health data is essential to ensure that interventions remain relevant and beneficial. This responsive strategy eventually creates healthier settings that are responsive to the specific needs of diverse populations (Properzi et al., 2025).

1.5. Public Health Interventions and Strategies

Public health interventions are crucial in remediating and mitigating health inequities among communities since they can significantly improve health outcomes and quality of life. Interventions can range from promoting preventive practices such as immunization and sanitation to enhancing education campaigns on nutrition and exercise. Community-based interventions are crucial in ensuring interventions are respectful of local culture and tailored to meet targeted needs. For instance, the treatment of disadvantaged groups will help alleviate the health access gap that these groups face. This is particularly observed in the field of eye care, where the utilization of cost-effective interventions like cataract surgery can heavily improve the health of millions of individuals. Eye care directly relates to the attainment of the Sustainable Development Goals (SDGs), demonstrating the role that intervention approaches can play in setting the stage for larger public health growth (Matthew et al., 2021). Also, technology deployment continues to become increasingly critical within public health efforts. Telemedicine and digital health platforms synergize to enhance access and efficiency of service delivery, especially in remote areas. With the COVID-19 pandemic, telehealth services, for instance, became in high demand as a solution to ensure patient care, illustrating the strength of digital solutions to bridge gaps in healthcare access. Telehealth utilization backs how innovation is essential to public health interventions; through developing new tools and methods, healthcare professionals can deliver comprehensive care more effectively. These innovations not only improve health outcomes but also demonstrate marked cost-effectiveness within the healthcare system. This adoption of technology is in accordance with the push towards universal health coverage, stressing the point that access to health care is essential for all, particularly for vulnerable populations (Rashid et al., 2020). Lastly, intersectoral collaboration among education, health, and social services is essential in developing integrated public health programs. Intersectoral partnerships can increase the strength of health interventions by addressing social determinants of health, including environment, economic stability, and education. Through this intersectoral approach, public health programs are able to address the root causes of health issues rather than treating them. Through collaboration, all stakeholders can create holistic interventions that address not only prevalent health concerns but also overall well-being. These are effective strategies in building healthy communities that can cope with and withstand health challenges. Lastly, effective public health interventions are characterized by their ability to bring together innovative solutions, technology, and collective engagement to make substantial contributions to community health gains and build sustainable change (Matthew et al., 2021) (Figure 1.12).

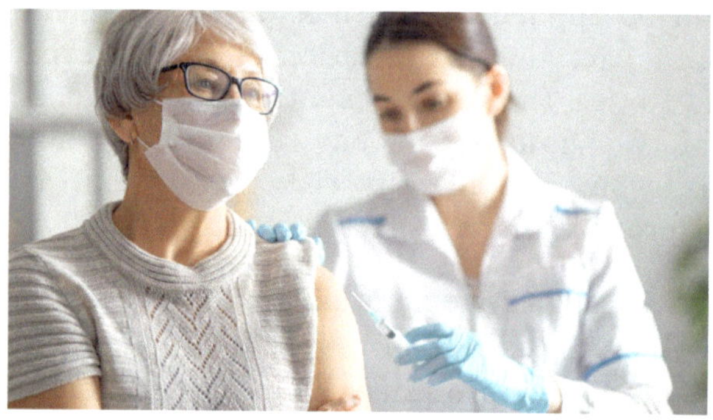

Figure 1.12. Five public health interventions.

Source: https://assets.everspringpartners.com/dims4/default/f003974/2147483647/strip/true/crop/889x500+350+0/resize/1200x675!/quality/90/?url=http%3A%2F%2Feverspring-brightspot.s3.us-east-1.amazonaws.com%2Fa4%2F51%2F0386cc084cf4b19618293f56670f%2Fkent-mph-epi-blog-2024-alookatpublichealthintervention-headerimage.jpg.

1.5.1. Preventive Measures for Environmental Health Risks

The growing recognition of environmental health risks has necessitated the development of meaningful prevention strategies that encompass individuals and populations. One aspect of these prevention strategies is raising awareness about environmental determinants of health and how pollution, chemical exposure, and other environment-induced factors cause chronic conditions. By focusing on training programs that equip citizens with knowledge of potential dangers, regional health authorities can encourage active health habits. These programs not only create personal responsibility but also collective resilience against environmental threats. Furthermore, integrating such knowledge into school curricula can reinforce early training in health-environmental associations, eventually leading to an improved and healthier generation. Thus, effective education outreach becomes a key preventive measure, and people are strengthened to overcome health risks in their surroundings. Aside from education, laws have also come a long way in addressing environmental health risks. The government can issue policies to regulate harmful emissions from industries, require clean water and air, and promote the use of environmentally friendly materials. These rules have the key function of setting up better living standards as well as reducing cases of disease caused by the environment. For instance, initiatives that provide for frequent inspections and adherence can effectively restrict contact with toxic products in communities. In the same way, zoning laws can serve to prevent the establishment of pollution-emitting industries near residential parts of an area in order to safeguard susceptible groups. The success of such measures, nevertheless, hinges on collaboration between policymakers, healthcare professionals, and civil society activists ensuring that controls are rigorous as well as sensitive to emerging environmental health risks (Hubbard, 2009). Finally, bottom-up action and community involvement are important aspects of preventive action against environmental health risks. By involving local individuals in environmental monitoring, advocacy, and response, societies can take ownership of their own health outcomes. Public health agencies can involve individuals within the communities to act on priority concerns such as waste management, water safety, and air quality. The direct involvement encourages not only accountability from the stakeholders but also increased community-led actions to reduce environmental hazards. In addition, addressing social determinants of health through collective interventions—such as green space development and public transport—can prevent adverse environmental health conditions. Finally, a comprehensive approach with educational, regulatory, and community-based initiatives offers a good foundation for the prevention of environmental health risks and promotion of overall well-being in the community (Pollack et al., 2001).

1.5.2. Community-Based Health Programs

Community-based health programs are a central component in the eradication of health inequities among various groups, particularly among marginalized populations. They usually engage the local populace to varying degrees in the detection and resolution of health issues peculiar to their specific locations. Utilizing a Community-Based Participatory Research (CBPR) paradigm, such programs empower participants by actively involving them in the design, implementation, and assessment of health interventions. For instance, a research project in Malmö, Sweden, showed how young people, accompanied by their caregivers and leaders within their communities, developed an environment of health to foster their development. This participatory strategy not only establishes ownership among members but also enhances the efficacy of health interventions by ensuring that they are responsive to community-level dynamics and cultural contexts, which could potentially lead to improved health outcomes as emphasized in community health studies (Ramji et al., 2024). Furthermore, community-based health interventions are particularly vital for addressing the special needs of marginalized communities, such as migrant populations. Research has shown that social determinants like language and socio-economic status often discourage migrant women from accessing health promotion programs. A community-academic partnership that employed participatory research methods provided a platform for such women to become more engaged in health programs. Through networking and the employment of local facilitators, participants enhanced their health literacy and subsequently bridged their knowledge into functional health-promoting practices. This collaborative effort highlighted the significance of culturally appropriate interventions in the design of health programs that effectively engage marginalized groups and provide a favorable environment for health promotion (Lindsjö et al., 2023). Beyond building individuals, community-based health programs achieve long-term health benefits by fostering collaboration among stakeholders. Through their incorporation of participant feedback and input from prominent community leaders, these programs, over time, have the capacity to respond to changing health needs. The cyclical nature of participatory involvement works to ensure that health projects remain both effective and relevant, strengthening community bonds and fostering shared responsibility for health. For instance, the construction and piloting of the Socioculturally Aligned Survey Instrument for Children applied in Malmö demonstrates the importance of community opinion in guiding health interventions. This dynamic approach not only reinforces data collection on health need but also re-establishes community commitment within health programs, ultimately creating a culture of health promotion extending beyond isolated programs and toward an enhanced appreciation of community welfare (Ramji et al., 2024) (Figure 1.13).

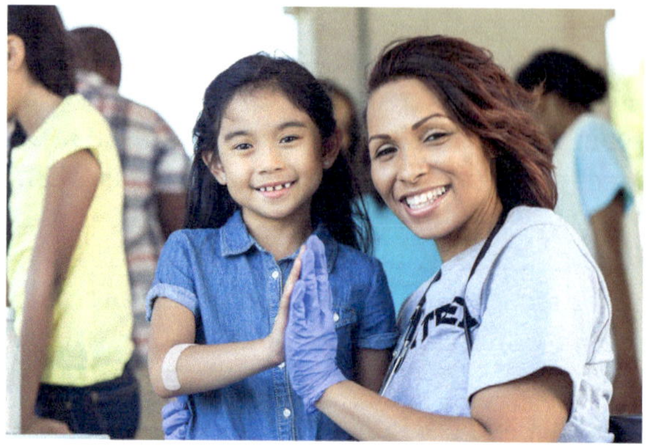

Figure 1.13. Community-based health programs.

Source: https://ostrowonline.usc.edu/wp-content/uploads/2021/11/public-health-pyramid-and-community-oral-health-program-planning-feature.jpg.

1.5.3. Role of Non-Governmental Organizations in Health Promotion

Non-Governmental Organizations (NGOs) have emerged as key players in the realm of health promotion, exercising significant impact on public health policy and practice. With their unique stand, NGOs can act as a bridge between community engagement and mitigating health disparities through prevention and education. Through the implementation of evidence-based interventions, NGOs tackle an extensive array of health issues, such as non-communicable and infectious diseases, and increasing health literacy. The broad scope of their work usually involves collaborating with government agencies and other stakeholders, which enhances their capacity for providing programs targeting social determinants of health. As emphasized by the Shanghai Declaration on Promoting Health in the 2030 Agenda for Sustainable Development, NGOs need to not only engage in working on health outcomes but also on political and social determinants leading to health inequities, thus making efforts to promote equitable and effective health outcomes (Kilibarda, 2024). In addition to traditional health programs, NGOs also have the duty to mobilize communities in order to struggle for their health and rights. Community empowerment is imperative for the construction of a sustainable health culture, and NGOs usually play the role of catalysts in this regard. With methods embracing community voices in decision-making, NGOs become more efficient and transferable across various contexts. As global awareness of the right to health continues to grow, citizen engagement has emerged as a strong force that can shape health policies and build just health systems. This is in tandem with the World Health Organization's focus on social participation in health policy decisions to foster collaborative efforts aimed at improving overall public health (Madhusudhana, 2021). Therefore, NGOs not only take a proactive role in directly contributing towards work in health promotion but also shape the world of health governance and policy-making. Moreover, the future of health promotion will need innovative solutions that appeal to rapidly changing global health trends. As long as issues such as climate change, pandemics, and social inequality continue to exist and impact health systems, NGOs will be forced to establish flexible strategies that emphasize sustainability and resilience. These kinds of organizations are able to leverage local resources and expertise to tackle increasingly complicated health issues. By operating through intersectoral partnerships and the application of a Health in All Policies approach, NGOs are actually able to operate across sectors to encourage overall health initiatives. As expressed in paradigm debates on health promotion, integrating health into broader social policies not only solves immediate health problems but also enhances long-term public welfare (Kilibarda, 2024). In the future, the role played by NGOs in health promotion will be instrumental in building healthier communities and responding to emerging health challenges (Figure 1.14).

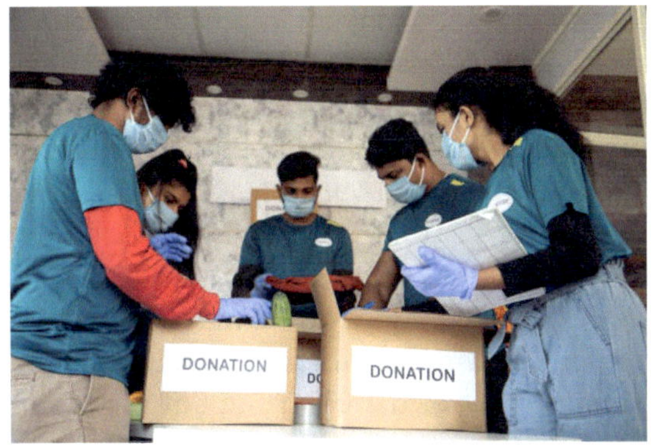

Figure 1.14. Role of NGO in providing healthcare facilities.

Source: https://miro.medium.com/v2/resize:fit:612/1*M7uNg2mEmFke_qQ8RjlhQg.jpeg.

1.6. Emerging Issues in Environment and Community Health

The intersection of environmental issues and public health becomes increasingly pertinent as urbanization accelerates and global warming escalates the risk of exposure to vulnerabilities. Emerging trends indicate that communities are confronted with complex issues tied to pollution, resource depletion, and population shifts. For instance, industrial pollutants and ineffective waste management practices have a tendency to contribute to intensified air and water pollution within urban areas. This increase in pollution has a direct implication for the public's health, leading to chronic respiratory diseases, waterborne illnesses, and mental health issues among people living in these areas. Solving these interrelated problems involves multi-faceted strategies that synchronize environmental policies with community health efforts so that vulnerable groups of people receive proper assistance and resources to curb health threats from environmental degradation. Mental health problems are becoming an important area of community health, particularly regarding environmental changes. When there is a significant change in communities, such as changes in education, they tend to feel isolated and insecure, which exacerbates mental health issues. In studies, emerging adults have been found to experience heightened emotional distress in periods of educational transitions based on variables such as social network changes and heightened learning pressures. These shifts require facilitating environments to promote resilience in young people. Effective interventions must include community action and development of resources to allow people to cope with change and minimize feelings of isolation. Improving the experience of transition can produce a more cohesive social fabric and promote mental health. Waste management is an important part of the environment and community health umbrella, and matters of scale emanate from open dumps, which are prevalent in Sub-Saharan Africa. Dumps like Olusosun in Nigeria and Dandora in Kenya are concerns to public health and environmental quality by virtue of causing air and water pollution, soil pollution, and disease transmission among the residents. Current evaluations emphasize the need to improve waste management practices, placing growing emphasis on preventive measures such as waste segregation and recycling measures, among others. In addition, community-based interventions can be encouraged so as to empower local communities to address the adverse effects of dumpsites. By emphasizing sustainable waste management practices and community involvement, public health objectives can be encouraged while simultaneously minimizing environmental vulnerability, culminating in healthier societies throughout the region (Figure 1.15).

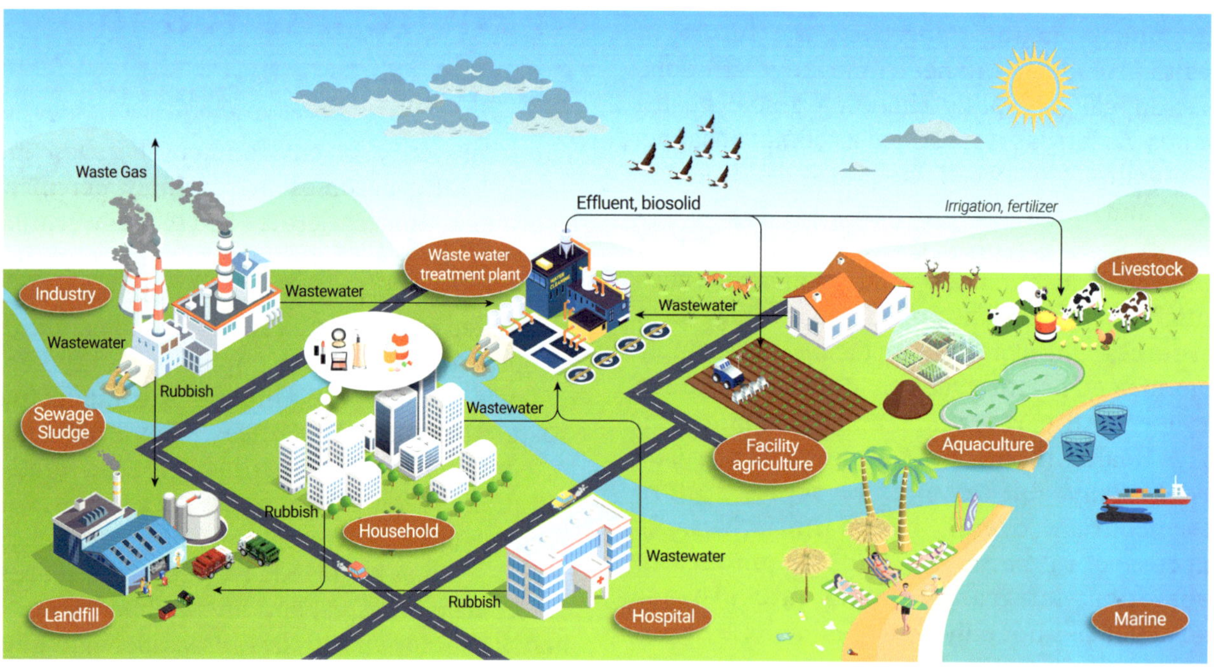

Figure 1.15. Emerging contaminants: A one health perspective.

Source: https://www.cell.com/cms/10.1016/j.xinn.2024.100612/asset/04841d64-20db-4aa2-b893-19c68ae3a650/main.assets/gr2_lrg.jpg.

1.6.1. Climate Change and Its Health Implications

The intricate relationship between climate change and public health has drawn greater attention to environmental health researchers. Rising global temperatures, altered precipitation patterns, and extreme weather events have far-reaching implications for many determinants of health. The prevalence and distribution of infectious diseases are likely to shift as climates shift due to the fact that they are controlled by many ecological variables.

For instance, alterations in environmental factors impact vectors such as ticks and mosquitoes that impact rates of disease transmission for infections such as malaria and Lyme disease. As stipulated in current research, climatic factors' impact on the host, the pathogen, and the epidemiologic dynamics call for immediate consideration of public health measures as well as readiness interventions, particularly in vulnerable populations (McFarlane et al., 2020). Besides, the confluence of advances in technology, such as the sustainable health Internet of Things (IoT), has tremendous potential in mitigating health impacts emanating from climate change. This new platform can offer improved monitoring and sensing of health risks across populations, thereby facilitating an integrated environmental health strategy. By integrating systems in various fields of health, IoT provides valuable knowledge that can aid in sustainable healthcare programs in the era of climatic uncertainty. These programs are particularly vital for populations exposed to amplified health inequalities as a result of socioeconomic conditions heightened by environmental variability.

To this end, the development and deployment of an integrated health IoT not only guarantees enhanced sustainability outcomes but also fosters resilience in community health programs addressing the intricate character of challenges presented by climate change (McFarlane et al., 2020). Additionally, the long-term consequences of climate-related public health hazards include zoonotic diseases that reveal a multifaceted and disquieting nexus with environmental changes. The majority of zoonotic infectious diseases are climate-sensitive due to their dependence on the ecological and biological characteristics of hosts and vectors. For example, understanding the dynamics of Ebola would involve taking note of how habitat changes might affect species interactions and human contact with reservoirs. As climatic factors impact the behavior and populations of wildlife, the danger of zoonoses spilling over to human populations is heightened, thus the need for robust health systems. The inclusion of dependable climatic data into health policy is essential for the preventive management of dangers that result from emergent infectious diseases, on which agreement must be reached through the One-Health approach, emphasizing the interconnectedness among human, animal, and environmental health (Bourgarel et al., 2015).

1.6.2. Urbanization and Public Health Challenges

As urbanization continues at a fast pace, the relationships between public health concerns and urbanization have become more pronounced. Urban migration generates a wide range of social and environmental stressors that impact health outcomes. Overcrowding, which is generally a consequence of urbanization, promotes the spread of infectious diseases and increases health inequalities among vulnerable populations. Moreover, the dilapidated infrastructure and congested healthcare systems in fast-developing urban centers struggle to accommodate the growing demand for services, rendering residents of cities extremely susceptible to health crises. The urban dynamics require comprehensive public health strategies that address not only immediate health concerns but also the causative factors of urban health disparities, as seen in a number of reports regarding global risks and urban planning measures (N/A, 2015). The twin punch of zoonotic diseases—like the Lassa virus and the COVID-19 pandemic—on urban health underscores the need for a comprehensive approach to health governance. In countries like Nigeria, the intersection of these diseases demonstrates how unchecked urban expansion accelerates health fragilities, piling environmental degradation together with social causes like poverty and food insecurity. These pandemics widen existing inequalities that affect marginalized groups that are generally denied proper healthcare and nutrition. This condition underscores the urgency for One Health, integrating human, animal, and environmental health into an integrated paradigm for local and global response (Akanwa et al., 2022). Refinement of community health infrastructure remains important in a bid to reverse the adverse effects of urbanization and facilitate resilience to emerging public health risks. In a bid to reverse the public health challenges of urbanization, interdisciplinary collaboration and innovative policy measures are necessary. By comprehending that health, urbanization, and environment are interdependent, actors can facilitate inclusive measures that attain equal health results. This entails not only expanding access to care in cities but also investing in sustainable urban development that enhances biodiversity and supports ecosystem services. Further, community engagement is a vital element in designing particular interventions that match the particular needs of urban communities. As urban areas grow, the emergence of partnerships among government, civil society, and people will become a critical component in managing the public health challenges brought about by urbanization while serving to ensure the highest prospects for enhanced health for everyone (N/A, 2015) (Figure 1.16).

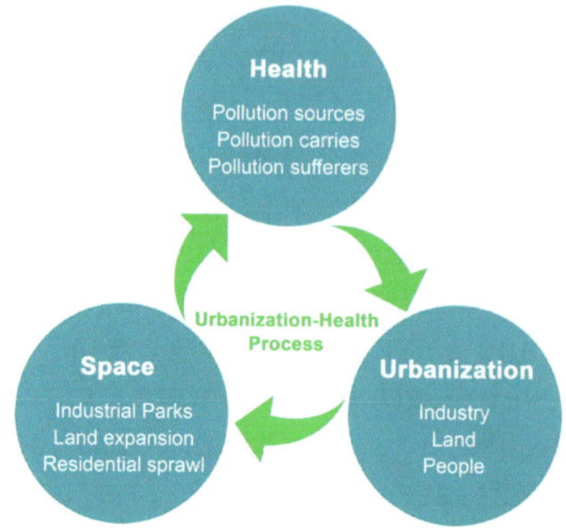

Figure 1.16. Urbanization health process.

Source: https://www.researchgate.net/publication/360694247/figure/fig1/AS:11431281079706670@1660822060514/Interactions-between-urbanization-and-public-health-with-spatiotemporal-scales.jpg.

1.6.3. Technological Advances in Environmental Health Monitoring

The advent of technological innovations has revolutionized the field of environmental health monitoring, with unparalleled opportunities for enhancing community health gains. Emerging technologies such as remote sensing, geographic information systems (GIS), and mobile health apps have redesigned the steps involved in collecting, analyzing, and utilizing environmental data. For instance, remote sensing technologies allow for instant monitoring of environmental factors such as air quality and water contamination levels, providing critical information to practitioners as well as policymakers. In addition, GIS integration allows for spatial analysis of the environmental hazards, allowing for specialized interventions among risk-exposed communities. These advancements not only raise the quality of information but also enhance public education and engagement in monitoring activities, ultimately culminating in a more informed and active response to environmental health concerns. Emerging technologies applied to environmental health monitoring also involve predictive analytics and artificial intelligence (AI) that significantly increase the capacity to identify and prevent health threats. Through the utilization of huge quantities of environmental data, predictive models are able to accurately predict potential health effects, for example, respiratory diseases due to air pollution or waterborne diseases due to contaminated water sources. These AI models give public health authorities the capability to predict problems early enough before they can be catastrophic, thus eventually leading to early interventions. Further, technology supports the creation of portable monitoring instruments, which offer immediate feedback to people on environmental pollutants and toxins. This movement has significant implications for the everyday health of people and communities since it encourages proactive action toward environmental health concerns and empowers individuals to assume responsibility for making informed decisions regarding their environment. Furthermore, technology-enabled collaboration platforms enable more stakeholders to participate in environmental health monitoring. Initiatives that integrate citizen science and high-tech monitoring technologies enhance community engagement in data collection and analysis. For example, apps allow citizens to report environmental hazards, therefore creating ownership and responsibility in society. Additionally, networks between scientists, healthcare professionals, and community members offer an inclusive approach to environmental health since more targeted and efficient interventions are facilitated. The emphasis on partnership is key in the context of growing environmental risk complexity, as highlighted through studies on ocean preservation and climate resilience (N/A, 2015; N/A, 2016). In the end, such technological advances represent a step forward towards an integrative and participatory model of environmental health monitoring, and this will have significantly improved community health in the long run.

CLOSER LOOK

IMPROVING OUR ENVIRONMENTAL HEALTH

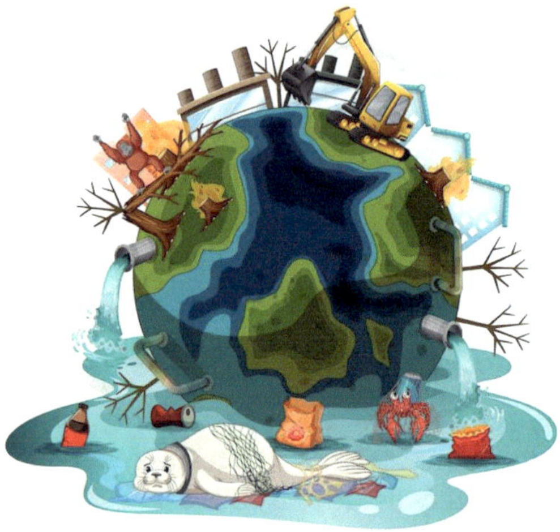

Figure 1.17. Illustration depicting global environmental pollution and its impact on marine life.

Source: https://releaf.in/wp-content/uploads/2023/08/environmental-sanitation.jpg.

Improving our environmental health is crucial in a bid to sustain life on our planet and the well-being of future generations. The environment directly affects human health through the air we breathe, the water we drink, and the food we eat. Improving environmental health calls for personal and community efforts. Pollution, particularly air and water pollution, is one of the most effective ways to reduce it. This comprises stricter controls on industrial discharges, the promotion of cleaner modes of transport such as electric vehicles and public transit, and the reduction of the application of harmful chemicals in agriculture and industry. Waste control is also crucial; preventing single-use plastic, recycling materials, and proper disposal of toxic waste can significantly minimize pollution. Conservation of natural resources like forests, wetlands, and oceans is important in promoting biodiversity and environmental stability. Protection of these areas not only conserves wildlife habitats but also regulates the climate and purifies natural resources. The public can participate in this by adopting sustainable practices like energy conservation, the use of eco-products, and support for green businesses. Governments and institutions must invest in renewable energy resources like solar and wind power to reduce their reliance on fossil fuels. Additionally, environmental education at all levels is required to sensitize people to the necessity of a healthy environment and allow them to make the right choices. Urban planning also helps a great deal in environmental health by designing greener cities with greater gardens and parks, efficient waste disposal systems, and green infrastructure. It is needed to fight climate change both globally and at the local level because global warming exacerbates environmental problems such as extreme weather, sea-level rise, and disease spread. Overall, it requires a multi-pronged approach that includes policy, innovation, education, and everyday action to promote environmental health. Through environmental ownership and prioritization of sustainability, we can create healthier communities and a more resilient planet.

SUMMARY

Inclusion of the environmental determinants into community health is of critical significance in improving overall public health outcomes. As this essay provides, understanding the intricate interdependencies that exist between the environmental determinants and community health is imperative in advising effective public policy on healthcare. Through the recognition of the complexity of health-focused issues, the stakeholders are able to point out more targeted interventions that meet the unique conditions of different communities. It is a method that supports better comprehension of how the environment influences health and enables communities to collaborate in resolving challenges. Identification of such associations is instrumental in shaping sustainable health promotion practice and the formation of resilient communities, particularly in the face of environmental adversity. Apart from that, the role technology plays in facilitating community health cannot be quantified. Innovation with technology provides new technologies that have the potential to significantly improve access to health care resources and quality of life among residents. As mentioned, older people, who prefer most to age in place, benefit from those technologies that promote independence, safety, and social support (Micha et al., 2015). Through technology use, health workers and decision makers are able to effectively promote significant inequalities, maximizing older adults' and other vulnerable populations' health. It is consequently desirable that new research addresses the development and application of easy-to-use technology tailored to the specific needs of various population groups in various community environments. Lastly, synergistic development between environmental health and community health is of utmost importance for the achievement of healthier societies. Strategies emphasizing the interconnected interaction of these spheres will not only advance public health initiatives but will also promote environmental protection among members. Training and sensitization programs are required to empower the population, encouraging them to take responsibility for their health as well as their environment. Further, the incorporation of preventive interventions, such as the use of probiotics among vulnerable populations, has been shown to reduce morbidity and improve healthcare outcomes (Dermyshi et al., 2017). By incorporating an integrated approach focusing on these interdependent factors, communities are better able to manage the complexity of health promotion while concurrently building more sustainable, resilient environments.

In exploring the relationship between environment and community health, core issues that are controversial relate to the need for models of integrated care that consider ecological factors as well as social determinants of health. Current trends of debate focus on how fragmented knowledge and training hinder the implementation of effective integrated care models. Policymakers and professionals are likely to be operating in silos, focusing on specific competencies that are relevant only in their context. This gap undermines the global goal of health equity and justice for everyone. Workshops as a tool for promoting collective wisdom offer rich opportunities for community actors, health practitioners, and policymakers to engage in meaningful discussions, which results in their comprehensive understanding of the principles of integrated care and facilitating long-term community health change, per (Stein et al., 2023). One important topic that emerges in addressing resource distribution and its impact on the health of communities, particularly in the context of microbiomes that impact health outcomes in environmental settings, is that microbial communities are of vital importance to ecosystems, impacting plant health, and therefore the production of agriculture. Understanding the dynamic interaction between these microorganisms and their hosts can be employed in creating strategies for building resilience in natural and community health systems. The integration of synthetic community experiments and computer simulations provides valuable insights into interspecies interactions within these biota. By studying the development of different bacterial strains on different carbon sources, scientists are able to make more accurate predictions about the consequences of these interactions, which expose key metabolic interactions that can improve knowledge of community assembly and health consequences, showing how critical resource availability is in health and environmental situations, as depicted in Schäfer et al. (2023). Lastly, conversations stress the importance of considering performance and outcome measures for coordinated care programs. The absence of gaps in current measurements frequently results in unsuccessful implementations, and therefore, putting high priority on thorough evaluation strategies that address both health and environmental variables is crucial. Involving a wider range of stakeholders, such as those with lived experience across health and social care, helps ensure that all perspectives are used in developing effective interventions. Furthermore, closing these gaps enables not just healthcare access equity but also fostering the culture of ongoing learning and adaptability in health systems. Defining clearly the formats to measure the success of integrated care models enables societies to better pursue health justice and align resources to meet the heterogeneity of their populations, as stipulated in the proposed workshops' initiatives in Stein et al. (2023).

REFERENCES

1. Asimullah, S., Khan, F., Afridi, J., & Hayat, S. (2025). Environmental impacts of marble industrial effluents on water and soil in Tehsil Shabqadar, Khyber Pakhtunkhwa. Indus Journal of Bioscience Research. https://www.semanticscholar.org/paper/7e713ad60ed6fcc3359333b6c928a90dd9a9d2da (accessed on 11th June 2025).
2. Asokan, N. (2023). Community dermatology: Current status and the way forward. Indian Dermatology Online Journal, 14, 762–768. https://www.semanticscholar.org/paper/a55c7ef0d0a978498df191776f935cefb9d3df18 (accessed on 11th June 2025).
3. Barling, D., Gresham, J., Mylona, K., et al. (2019). *Characterization Framework of Key Policy, Regulatory and Governance Dynamics and Impacts Upon European Food Value Chains: Fairer Trading Practices, Food Integrity, And Sustainability Collaborations* (VALUMICS project "Understanding Food Value Chains and Network Dynamics" funded by EU Horizon 2020 G.A. No 727243. Deliverable D3.3). https://core.ac.uk/download/287582350.pdf (accessed on 11th June 2025).
4. Bashshur, R. L., Doarn, C. R., Frenk, J., Kvedar, J. C., & Woolliscroft, J. O. (2020). Telemedicine and the COVID-19 pandemic, lessons for the future. Telemedicine Journal and e-Health, 26, 571–573. https://doi.org/10.1089/tmj.2020.29040.rb.
5. Berg, G., Rybakova, D., Fischer, D., Cernava, T., Champomier Vergès, M. C., Charles, T. C., Chen, X., et al. (2020). Microbiome definition re-visited: Old concepts and new challenges. *Microbiome, 8*. https://doi.org/10.1186/s40168-020-00875-0.
6. Bourgarel, M., Kassie, D., & Roger, F. (2015). Climate change and Ebola outbreaks: Are they connected? https://agritrop.cirad.fr/577071/7/ID577071p.pdf (accessed on 11th June 2025).
7. Bull, F., Al-Ansari, S. S., Biddle, S., Borodulin, K., Buman, M. P., Cardon, G., Carty, C., et al. (2020). World Health Organization 2020 guidelines on physical activity and sedentary behavior. *British Journal of Sports Medicine, 54*, 1451–1462. https://doi.org/10.1136/bjsports-2020-102955.
8. Burton, M. J., Ramke, J., Marques, A. P., Bourne, R., Congdon, N., Jones, I., Ah Tong, B. A. M., et al. (2021). The Lancet Global Health Commission on global eye health: Vision beyond 2020. The Lancet Global Health, 9, e489–e551. https://doi.org/10.1016/s2214-109x(20)30488-5.
9. Bynum, M. D., Kearney, G. D., Jilcott Pitts, S. B., Greer, A. G., & Imai, S. (2025). Assessing diversity, equity, and inclusion in the US environmental health workforce: Challenges and opportunities. Journal of Public Health Management and Practice: JPHMP. https://www.semanticscholar.org/paper/384bc7cade6ed6c911ccfb5381599cc9712250e9 (accessed on 11th June 2025).
10. Cacciottolo, J. (2013). *Lung Health and Outdoor Air Pollution: A Review*. https://core.ac.uk/download/83019957.pdf (accessed on 11th June 2025).
11. Canaday, F. T., Georas, S. N., & Croft, D. P. (2024). Examining the impact of air pollution, climate change, and social determinants of health on asthma and environmental justice. *Current Opinion in Pulmonary Medicine, 30*, 276–280. https://www.semanticscholar.org/paper/63552bcbff7b16a5b9b553948d4cf8efba294c20 (accessed on 11th June 2025).
12. Chambers, K., Baker, A., McKay, S., & Morgan, H. (2019). *Retrospective Sustainability and Resilience: Complementary Concepts for Managing Systems*. https://www.semanticscholar.org/paper/a2c0c6323929b47dd8289f654c1bd7e7f93962a7 (accessed on 11th June 2025).

13. Cohen, M. H. (2021). The sum of us: What racism costs everyone and how we can prosper together. Harvard Educational Review, 91, 540–543. https://doi.org/10.17763/1943-5045-91.4.540.

14. Corbett, A., Fuse, E., Hodge, J., & Scanlon, M. (2012). *Legal Review Concerning the Use of Health Impact Assessments in Non-Health Sectors.* https://core.ac.uk/download/71358594.pdf (accessed on 11th June 2025).

15. Craig, K. D., Holmes, C., Hudspith, M., Moor, G., Moosa-Mitha, M., Varcoe, C., & Wallace, B. (2019). Pain in persons who are marginalized by social conditions. *Pain, 161*, 261–265. https://doi.org/10.1097/j.pain.0000000000001719.

16. Deichmann, U., & Lall, S. V. (2025). *Are You Satisfied? Citizen Feedback and Delivery of Urban Services.* https://core.ac.uk/download/pdf/6373687.pdf (accessed on 11th June 2025).

17. Dermyshi, E., Wang, Y., Yan, C., Hong, W., Qiu, G., Gong, X., & Zhang, T. (2017). The "Golden Age" of probiotics: A systematic review and meta-analysis of randomized and observational studies in preterm infants. *Neonatology, 112*, 9–23. https://doi.org/10.1159/000454668.

18. Faridah, L., Hiron, N., & Rahayu, A. U. (2024). *Air Quality Monitoring in Briquette Industrial Environments Through Air Particle Detection Systems.* https://core.ac.uk/download/622061617.pdf (accessed on 11th June 2025).

19. Folorunsho, I., Harry, N. M., & Anugwom, G. (2024). Mitigating the negative impact of social and environmental factors on mental well-being through community-based interventions. *Journal of Advances in Medicine and Medical Research.* https://www.semanticscholar.org/paper/d4b7b6af59ca9765225a572418255059f1a548e8 (accessed on 11th June 2025).

20. Gulliver, R. (2024). The fossil fuel façade. M/C Journal. https://www.semanticscholar.org/paper/da403185cf6dfc91901f882f54d7cd430836bf08 (accessed on 11th June 2025).

21. Hill, T. (2015). *PUBH 3136 A–Principles of Environmental Health.* https://core.ac.uk/download/229147365.pdf (accessed on 11th June 2025).

22. Howes, A. J., & Shohel, M. M. C. (2006). *Nonformal Education for Sustainable Development: A Bangladeshi Perspective.*

23. Hubbard, T. (2009). Healthy People in A Healthy Economy: A Blueprint for Action in Massachusetts. https://core.ac.uk/download/71346659.pdf (accessed on 11th June 2025).

24. Ilham, M., & Amelia, R. (2024). Analysis of risk factors for stunting among toddlers aged 24–59 months in the working area of Cibodasari Puskesmas Community Health Center, Tangerang City. International Journal on ObGyn and Health Sciences. https://www.semanticscholar.org/paper/4b9c01e81a6ba78045d41ba65f5c9884756b8ddb (accessed on 11th June 2025).

25. Kadariya, S., Ball, L., Chua, D., Ryding, H. G., Hobby, J., Marsh, J. K., Bartrim, K., et al. (2023). Community organizing frameworks, models, and processes to improve health: A systematic scoping review. International Journal of Environmental Research and Public Health, 20. https://www.semanticscholar.org/paper/5aa32532b80b704e609991fcde87a4fbeaae24ea (accessed on 11th June 2025).

26. Karos, K., McParland, J., Bunzli, S., Devan, H., Hirsh, A. T., Kapos, F. P., Keogh, E., et al. (2020). The social threats of COVID-19 for people with chronic pain. *Pain, 161*, 2229–2235. https://doi.org/10.1097/j.pain.0000000000002004.

27. Kilibarda, B. (2024). Global challenges and opportunities in health promotion. *Proceedings of the International Congress Public Health–Achievements and Challenges–Zbornik Radova.* https://www.semanticscholar.org/paper/bce0d1aea33eb6a60140ae55c6a164aab5840c49 (accessed on 11th June 2025).

28. Kumar, P., Lee, S. S., Zhang, M., Tsang, Y. F., & Kim, K. H. (2019). Heavy metals in food crops: Health risks, fate, mechanisms, and management. Environment International, 125, 365–385. https://doi.org/10.1016/j.envint.2019.01.067.

29. Lei, K., Yang, J., & Ke, X. (2025). The impact of neighborhood environment on mental health: Evidence from China. *Frontiers in Public Health, 12.* https://www.semanticscholar.org/paper/e17dfd93f015f066ae954bf228cebf55c5ca44ef (accessed on 11th June 2025).

30. Lindsjö, C., Sjögren Forss, K., Kumlien, C., Kottorp, A., & Rämgård, M. (2023). Migrant women's engagement in health-promotive activities through a women's health collaboration. *Frontiers in Public Health, 11.* https://www.semanticscholar.org/paper/eb7341f240fc13c17c4e2a559ea7ae25a67992d5 (accessed on 11th June 2025).

31. Madhusudhana, K. (2021). *Role of Information and Promotional Strategies for Indian Pharmaceutical Firms in The Age of Digital Marketing.* https://www.semanticscholar.org/paper/b582f823aafb6a153cdd689f9cbcd94cc9d43277 (accessed on 11th June 2025).

32. McFarlane, A. C., Crimmins, A., Rappold, A. G., Hansen, A., Kumar, A., Dewan, A. M., Markandya, A., et al. (2020). *Internet of Things for Sustainable Human Health.* https://core.ac.uk/download/286368298.pdf (accessed on 11th June 2025).

33. Murray, C. J. L., Ikuta, K. S., Sharara, F., Swetschinski, L. R., Robles Aguilar, G., Gray, A. P., Han, C., et al. (2022). Global burden of bacterial antimicrobial resistance in 2019: A systematic analysis. *The Lancet, 399,* 629–655. https://doi.org/10.1016/s0140-6736(21)02724-0.

34. Nagorcka-Smith, P., Bolton, K., Dam, J. L., Nichols, M., Alston, L., Johnstone, M., & Allender, S. (2022). The impact of coalition characteristics on outcomes in community-based initiatives targeting the social determinants of health: A systematic review. BMC Public Health, 22. https://www.semanticscholar.org/paper/fdc4e1299194d91d8535e0311d506ecd1e2284b0 (accessed on 11th June 2025).

35. Omokaro, G. O., Michael, I., & Evgenievich, P. V. (2024). Assessing the environmental and health implications of waste disposal: A case study of Africa's largest dumping site. *Journal of Geography, Environment and Earth Science International.* https://www.semanticscholar.org/paper/d6d8e446a8e7fdcfb59cf946d551b9af576d2321 (accessed on 11th June 2025).

36. Peek, S. T. M., Luijkx, K., Rijnaard, M. D., Nieboer, M., van der Voort, C. S., Aarts, S., van Hoof, J., et al. (2015). Older adults' reasons for using technology while aging in place. Gerontology, 62, 226–237. https://doi.org/10.1159/000430949.

37. Pollack, R. (2001). Gene Maps Lead Medicine Down the Wrong Road. https://core.ac.uk/download/617171184.pdf (accessed on 11th June 2025).

38. Powell-Wiley, T. M., Baumer, Y., Baah, F. O., Baez, A. S., Farmer, N., Mahlobo, C. T., Pita, M. A., et al. (2022). Social determinants of cardiovascular disease. Circulation Research, 130, 782–799. https://doi.org/10.1161/circresaha.121.319811.

39. Properzi, S., Coa, A. A., Fiorilla, C., & Pasetto, R. (2025). Exploring methods to assess environmental health inequalities in health impact assessments of local interventions: A

systematic review within the JA PreventNCD project. Frontiers in Public Health, 13. https://www.semanticscholar.org/paper/23250506c7c540e715366891fbbe2db3c2826dbc (accessed on 11th June 2025).

40. Prusti, T., de Bruijne, J. H. J., Brown, A. G. A., Vallenari, A., Babusiaux, C., Bailer-Jones, C. A. L., Bastian, U., et al. (2016). The Gaia mission. Astronomy and Astrophysics, 595, A1–A1. https://doi.org/10.1051/0004-6361/201629272.

41. Rachman, R., & Safira, M. (2024). Pembuangan limbah bahan beracun dan berbahaya (B3). Journal Anthologys Hukum. https://www.semanticscholar.org/paper/a95825687615d51498f73c2c11677675dd9c6f67 (accessed on 11th June 2025).

42. Ramji, R., Mangrio, E., Sterner, T., Forss, K. S., Zdravkovic, S., Kottorp, A., Burenby-Yxne, L., et al. (2024). Using a participatory action research approach to explore, understand and evaluate well-being among children living in socially deprived areas in Southern Sweden: A study protocol. BMJ Open, 14. https://www.semanticscholar.org/paper/fbde263901c566832ce60329f111e285f8f385da (accessed on 11th June 2025).

43. Rodríguez-Mireles, S., Lopez-Valcárcel, B. G., Galdos-Arias, P., Perez-Diaz, E., & Serra-Majem, L. (2024). Socioeconomic disparities in diet and physical activity in children: Evidence from well-child visit electronic health records in the Canary Islands, Spain. Journal of Epidemiology and Community Health, 78, 354–359. https://www.semanticscholar.org/paper/97441791b1c958dec6772adf1d1e78295c6422a1 (accessed on 11th June 2025).

44. Satchwell, C. (2013). "Carbon Literacy Practices": Textual Footprints Between School and Home in Children's Construction if Knowledge About Climate Change. https://core.ac.uk/download/9637079.pdf (accessed on 11th June 2025).

45. Schäfer, M., Pacheco, A. R., Künzler, R., Bortfeld-Miller, M., Field, C. M., Vayena, E., Hatzimanikatis, V., et al. (2023). Metabolic interaction models recapitulate leaf microbiota ecology. Science, 381. https://www.semanticscholar.org/paper/76feb99d77f56d8ee07cb9ed55e31fd17fb2b3ae (accessed on 11th June 2025).

46. Sies, H., Berndt, C., & Jones, D. P. (2017). Oxidative stress. *Annual Review of Biochemistry, 86*, 715–748. https://doi.org/10.1146/annurev-biochem-061516-045037.

47. Sonderlund, A. L., Wang, E. A., Williams, N. J., Horowitz, C. R., Schoenthaler, A. M., & Holaday, L. (2025). County incarceration rate and stroke death: A cross-sectional study of the influence of physical environment, health care access, and community mental distress. *Journal of the American Heart Association*. https://www.semanticscholar.org/paper/24fda12b403b6879fba51a9cefffb6ae43c5c7d0 (accessed on 11th June 2025).

48. Stein, K., Miller, R., Bruijnzels, M., Schiff, J., Calamati, S., & Antonelli, R. (2023). Creating a global learning environment to promote integrated care. *International Journal of Integrated Care*. https://www.semanticscholar.org/paper/200cdaacf52072fa80eb99c03908e7d0a1221a82 (accessed on 11th June 2025).

49. Sundqvist, A., Nyman-Kurkiala, P., Ness, O., & Hemberg, J. (2024). The influence of educational transitions on loneliness and mental health from emerging adults' perspectives. *International Journal of Qualitative Studies on Health and Well-Being, 19*. https://www.semanticscholar.org/paper/3a0339aefeb9c37bb0ca5a309677e2dbd5df7ac6 (accessed on 11th June 2025).

50. Tison, G. H., Avram, R., Kuhar, P., Abreau, S., Marcus, G. M., Pletcher, M. J., & Olgin, J. E. (2020). Worldwide effect of COVID-19 on physical activity: A descriptive study. *Annals of Internal*

Medicine, 173, 767–770. https://doi.org/10.7326/m20-2665.

51. Tudi, M., Ruan, H. D., Wang, L., Lyu, J., Sadler, R., Connell, D., Chu, C., et al. (2021). Agriculture development, pesticide application and its impact on the environment. International Journal of Environmental Research and Public Health, 18, 1112–1112. https://doi.org/10.3390/ijerph18031112.
52. Wiederhold, B. K. (2020). Connecting through technology during the Coronavirus Disease 2019 pandemic: Avoiding "Zoom fatigue." *Cyberpsychology Behavior and Social Networking, 23*, 437–438. https://doi.org/10.1089/cyber.2020.29188.bkw.
53. Wong, K., Papachristou, E., Francesconi, M., & Dekkers, T. (2025). Editorial: 'Like a bee and a flower'–The symbiotic relationship between physical environment and children and young people's psychosocial outcomes. *Child and Adolescent Mental Health*. https://www.semanticscholar.org/paper/75bd1835bdf0cb836f77a4907e0f8562564b4744 (accessed on 11th June 2025).
54. Xu, L. D., Xu, E., & Li, L. (2018). Industry 4.0: State of the art and future trends. International Journal of Production Research, 56, 2941–2962. https://doi.org/10.1080/00207543.2018.1444806.

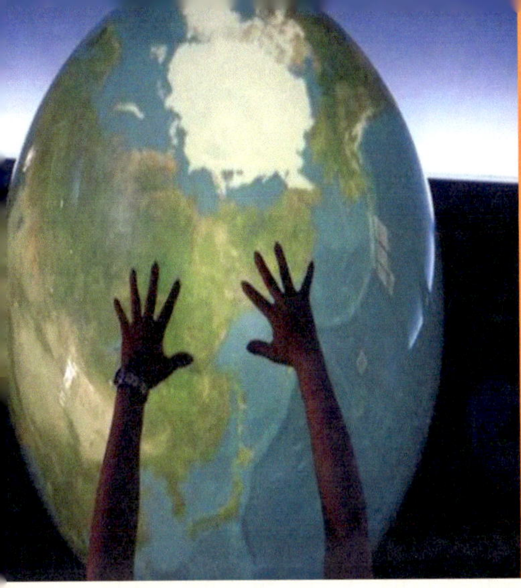

Chapter 2

CLIMATE CHANGE AND IMPLICATIONS ON COMMUNITY HEALTH

Contents

Introduction

Introduction into the topic of climate change and its impact on community health requires an assessment of the multifaceted issues presented by the global phenomenon. Climate change is not just an environmental issue but a significant determinant of health that exacerbates compounded risks in the community. The many implications of climate change, including intense weather, rise in sea levels, and altered ecosystems, pose threats to public health security. Such changes can lead to greater infectious disease levels, air pollution-related respiratory diseases, and climatic-disasters-triggered mental health disorders. The nexus between climate change and community health is significant for comprehending as a means of creating sufficient responses directed towards safeguarding vulnerable individuals, enhancing both their resilience and adaptive competencies in the face of ongoing environmental changes. Moreover, the intersection of climate change and public health reveals a critical intersection that influences the socioeconomic dynamics within communities. As demonstrated in recent studies, the effects of climate change are uneven; rather, they serve to worsen pre-existing inequalities, disproportionately affecting vulnerable populations. For instanceConley et al., 2012 states that climate-driven conflict and migration have the unintended effect of significantly affecting national and local health systems, thereby producing additional insecurity in already volatile regions. Poor communities are particularly at risk because they lack the ability to respond to the twin threats of health emergencies and climate change. This unequal setting demands concerted policy interventions that address environmental sustainability in tandem with social determinants of health, thereby creating an overall strategy that would benefit larger populations and also minimize the consequences of negative climate change impacts. Secondly, the lessons from recent public health emergencies underline the need for integrating climate resilience into health systems. The West African Ebola outbreak underscores the way that environmental degradation is coupled with socio-political forces to create fertile ground for disease emergence and spread. As explicitly outlined in Kay et al. (2016), past context involving colonialism and present-day inequities influences health outcomes across affected nations. This is why there must be a unified response that addresses not just acute health threats, but is working to establish the underlying public health infrastructure. By promoting coordination between local and global organizations, a sustainable infrastructure can be built that prepares communities to meet future health crises heightened by climate change. The introduction thus lays the groundwork for a nuanced examination of these forces, highlighting the value of anticipatory measures in safeguarding public health in a world increasingly marked by climate uncertainty (Figure 2.1).

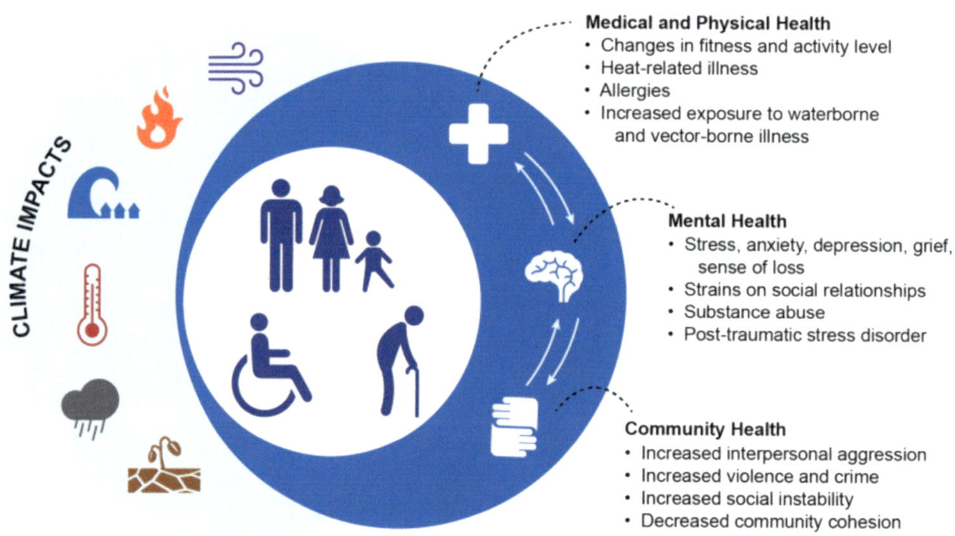

Figure 2.1. Climate change and implications for community health.

Source: https://www.jkgeography.com/uploads/1/0/8/4/108433405/climate-change-and-health_orig.png.

Definition of Climate Change

Climate change refers to the process of the Earth's climate system being radically changed by human activities. The change arises as a result of the emission of greenhouse gases (GHGs) such as carbon dioxide and methane resulting from deforestation, industrial emissions, and agriculture.

The changes have several impacts on weather patterns, oceanic levels, and biological diversity. Climate change manifests as increased mean temperatures, increased frequency of climatic extremes , and shifts in ecological regimes. These alter natural ecosystems and compel populations to adapt or migrate, irreversibly altering community profiles and health status. The need to understand these processes is due to the fact that climate change impacts penetrate deeply into the social, economic, and health fabric of communities. The intérface between environmental health and change demands an interdisciplinary approach to enable the development of proper policy interventions. Further, climate change is heavily rooted in social determinants of health, primarily in vulnerable communities. With ongoing changes in climate, disparities in health outcomes have increased and disproportionately affected vulnerable populations. Such groups are not often endowed with the ability to adapt to changing environments, which is why they are more prone to health emergencies triggered by heatwaves, floods, and food shortages. This intersection of climate disasters and public health poses a significant challenge to local governments and health systems. The implications of climate change are not only immediate environmental effects but also longer-term socio-economic impacts that echo across communities. As highlighted in recent literature, recognizing such relationships is needed to enhance resilience to climate-related health risks, particularly in populations where socio-economic stress may enhance the effects of environmental change, and which indicate a need for targeted policy and interventions in health (Conley et al., 2012). For New Zealand and globally, the population transitions triggered by climate change pose extra challenges to community health. As some areas are becoming uninhabitable due to higher sea levels or more heat, global and internal migration trends will become more accelerated. Past studies point to the fact that such population movements can contribute to severe health outcomes, resulting in higher mortality and exerting further stress on healthcare in receiving communities. For instance, the movement of displaced individuals can overburden the local health system, thus complicating service delivery in times of climate-related events. Besides, the psychological effects of displacement and environmental damage can be reflected in increased levels of mental illness among displaced populations. Hence, preparatory planning and a multidisciplinary public health response to account for these population shifts are necessary to provide assurance that communities are able to adapt to changing climate change-related challenges (Cameron et al., 2013).

Overview of Community Health

Community health is a vital field in the determination of the larger perspective of climate change and public health issues. Examining the determinants influencing health outcomes, community health emphasizes the determinants based on environmental, economic, and social conditions. Vulnerable communities—most commonly low-income groups and marginalized individuals—are subject to greater hazards involved in climate-related events. For example, climate extremes such as floods and droughts can have immediate effects on physical health in the present, but they also amplify underlying social disparities. These conditions cumulatively undermine the resilience of communities, particularly given the shift in the timing and magnitude of climatic patterns. With this framework in mind, policymakers and health professionals can act on these disparities, necessitating interventions that maximize equity and optimize community health gains in the context of climate change. Beyond the direct health consequences of climate change, the long-term impact on community health must not be overlooked. Altered weather trends directly impact significant resources like water supply and agriculture, as noted in the focus given to both built and natural infrastructures that sustain the demands. According to the research findings presented, water quality could be damaged through climate-influenced stresses, leading to significant public health threats. Socioeconomically already disadvantaged groups usually end up at the focal point of such adverse effects, much like flood-risk low-lying communities. Further, the threat of relocation due to environmental degradation can result in erosion of community and loss of identity, thus aggravating health inequities (N/A, 2017). By addressing them, there can be planning of sustainable interventions by community health practitioners for improving the health of affected communities.

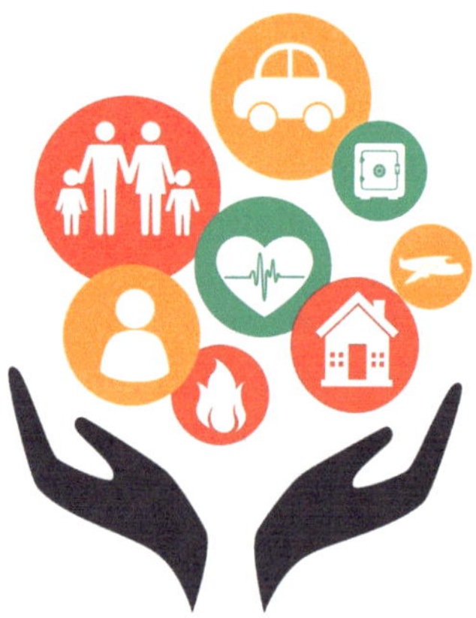

Figure 2.2. Community health.

Source: https://o.quizlet.com/76cxQevpJYrm1i4UvFFmsg_b.jpg.

The potential for adaptation actions for climate change to improve community health is increasingly recognized in the global public health debate. Besides meeting existing health needs, investment in adaptation promotes preparedness to future climate hazards. As it has been discussed, significant funds for climate adaptation actions are being raised, considering a substantial likelihood of closing gaps in health (Kathryn et al., 2012). Nonetheless, making certain that such investments are tailored to community needs entails comprehensive evaluations of prevailing vulnerabilities and social conditions. Through this, it is necessary to have coordination among different stakeholders, such as health organizations, urban planners, and community leaders, in coming up with targeted and effective interventions. By prioritizing research and action on the intersection of climate change and community health, stakeholders can advance equitable health outcomes, thus reinforcing the importance of integrating health considerations into broader climate policies (Figure 2.2).

Importance of Studying the Intersection of Climate Change and Health

The intersection of climate change and health necessitates rigorous examination due to its extensive range of implications for the welfare, or well-being, of populations. Climate change is a critical determinant of health as it exacerbates health inequities and also creates new obstacles. For instance, increased frequency and intensity of natural phenomena such as hurricanes and droughts can lead to direct trauma, deaths, and overwhelmed health systems. Also, climate change influences the disease pattern, resulting in the emergence of pathogens in new areas that were not previously exposed. From the knowledge of these complex interactions, researchers are capable of outlining high-risk groups and designing focused interventions that treat not only the illnesses caused by climate change but also build resilience among populations. This multi-dimensional strategy can finally result in improved public health outcomes in conjunction with more environmentally friendly policy and practice to conserve the environment. The link between health and climate change is a particularly significant one to examine in trying to comprehend the particular problem of marginalized groups. Low-income groups and women in low- and middle-income countries are often disproportionately affected by the health impacts of climate change due to socio-economic inequality. The disproportionate effect on women, for example, requires mainstreaming gender imperatives in climate resilience interventions, considering that women are disproportionately exposed to health risks exacerbated by climate pressures. Initiatives to promote women's digital health literacy, access to essential healthcare services, and voice empowerment in decision forums can enhance community health resilience. By addressing these intersections, stakeholders are able to make policies that not only protect public health but also empower people to adapt to a shifting climate environment. The understanding of the intersection between climate change and health guides the creation of effective sensitization and education programs. Education programs aimed at signaling environmental health effects can mobilize people to demand climate action and use collective obligation towards sustainable practices. There is evidence that education on climate change can lead to increased knowledge, competence, and adaptive capability in individuals, particularly youth, to engage in productive climate discourse and action. Furthermore, integrating community-based practice is beneficial in pursuing collaborative work among various actors and enhancing a holistic view of the effect of climate on health. Thus, such educative programs must emphasize the importance of adaptability and resilience in a climate change scenario , ultimately leading to improved individual health as well as community health as a whole. As such, a good education system has a critical role to play in getting communities ready to respond effectively to the interconnected climate change and health challenges.

2.1. The Science of Climate Change

Climate change science is an integrated study of atmospheric, environmental, and social processes triggered by rising global temperatures. In essence, climate change is primarily triggered by the high concentration of greenhouse gases, such as carbon dioxide and methane, that lead to trapping heat in the Earth's atmosphere. This results in alterations in weather patterns, sea-level rise, and heightened instances of extreme weather events. Knowledge of these scientific principles is the bedrock of comprehending the effect of climate change on public health. As scientists compile and analyze data on climatic system changes, it becomes evident that links between environmental changes and consequential health effects are apparent, prompting coordinated research and policy response that considers not only short-term but also long-term effects on community well-being. Societies faced with the adverse effects of climate change are subjected to a gamut of health-related challenges due to environmental degradation. Temperature rise contributes to the spread of vector-borne diseases, worsening air quality exacerbates respiratory illnesses, and disasters associated with climate might precipitate mental health crises. Moreover, vulnerable populations like the aged and those with underlying health issues are disproportionately affected by these changes. It is important to note that climate change not only threatens the environment; it also poses a great risk to the health of people, particularly in disadvantaged communities. It is through a synergistic response of acknowledging the direct and indirect health consequences associated with climate change and building resilience among communities through evidence-based adaptations and interventions that such challenges can be addressed. The adaptation landscape concerning climate change has evolved dramatically over the past two decades, transitioning from a theoretical concept to a recognized mandate aimed at reducing societal vulnerability. This shift in focus underscores the need for diverse strategies to address climate impacts across various sectors, including agriculture, resources, and human communities.

For instance, innovation in farming practice to make it more climate resilient has a direct relationship with enhancing food security and health. Additionally, effective policy frameworks must be established to bridge existing gaps in adaptation to ensure community-level resilience. Therefore, community health responses to climate change need to be merged into overall adaptation planning in a way that ensures the resilience of health systems in the face of ongoing environmental change, in keeping with central lessons of the broader literature on climate adaptation, e.g., those outlined in Snover et al. (2013) (Figure 2.3).

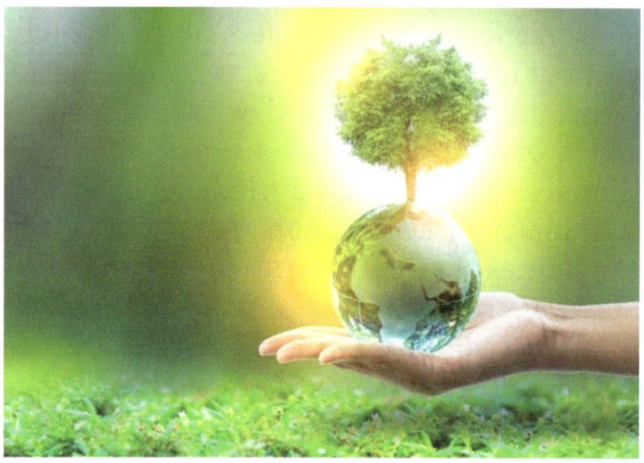

Figure 2.3. Science of climate change for health.

Source: https://www.orfonline.org/public/uploads/posts/image/Climate-Finance-1.jpg.

2.1.1. Greenhouse Gases and Their Effects

Greenhouse gas (GHG) accumulation in the Earth's atmosphere is now a major cause of climate change, with extensive harmful effects on community health. The GHGs, primarily carbon dioxide, methane, and nitrous oxide, are released through human activities including industrial processes, agriculture, and transport. Rising levels of GHGs warm the world by retaining heat, leading to ecological imbalance and weather conditions. Altered climate conditions result in extreme weather events, such as floods and heatwaves, which directly affect public health. Communities, particularly already disadvantaged communities based on socioeconomic status, are placed at greater risk of heat illness, respiratory disease, and vector-borne disease by the changing climate. Knowledge of the impact of GHGs on public health is required to make effective responses and interventions that will be capable of safeguarding community well-being in the midst of these emerging trends. The social and human aspects of climate change also reveal profound meanings for public health. Poor communities and excluded groups are often the worst affected by climate change, exacerbating total health inequities. The intersection of gender, health outcomes, and climate change reveals the necessity for holistic approaches to address such problems. Women, in particular, typically serve as frontline agents to address climate problems and are key stakeholders in establishing community resilience. Initiatives on climate action with strategies that integrate women's visions and leadership can potentially improve not just environmental sustainability but also health. Bringing together these elements emphasizes the need for policies that are equitable in improving both the environment and human wellbeing by addressing inequality as outlined in Deeb et al. (2011). Furthermore, the role that dedicated funds have played in climate resilience initiatives cannot be overstated, especially in pushing for grassroots struggles for gender and climate justice. Increased focus on financing women's climate work supports the important role that grassroots groups play in advancing community wellbeing and strong climate action. As has been witnessed in Davis et al. (2015), financing small- to medium-sized grants can empower women and their communities to initiate localized interventions that counter the effects of climate change. Such projects usually embrace health education, sustainable livelihood, and advocacy, hence community resilience to the consequences of climate change. Emphasizing the complexity of financing in the intersections of climate justice and community health is a central method for creating actual change so that affected populations can evolve and thrive in shifting environmental conditions.

2.1.2. Global Temperature Rise and Its Trends

Rising temperatures globally have been a signature of global warming over the last century, as evidenced by extensive research and observation. Global temperatures have risen by approximately 1.2 degrees Celsius from the pre-industrial era, largely due to human activities such as the combustion of fossil fuels, deforestation, and industrial processes. This temperature increase is not only a figure; it has far-reaching consequences for natural environments and human health. This rise in heat enhances the frequency and intensity of extreme weather conditions, which have been proven to enhance pre-existing inequalities in health among populations. For example, heatwaves can lead to increased death rates, particularly among vulnerable populations, thus highlighting the connection between global warming and community health consequences that are in immediate need of attention and action (Christopher et al., 2012). As global temperatures rise even higher, trends that are observable further reveal the potential impacts on community health. The health-climate change relationship is multifaceted, involving direct effects such as heat illness and indirect effects such as the transmission of vector-borne diseases. Heat facilitates enhanced transmission of bugs such as mosquitoes, which are vectors of diseases such as malaria and dengue fever. Already disadvantaged populations with low health resources find it even harder to respond to such emergent health threats. The Vermont Climate Assessment underscores the specific vulnerabilities of rural communities and the need for strategic adaptation planning to address these vulnerabilities (Baker et al., 2014). Trends in global temperature increase thus emphasize the need for convergence in health approaches, wedging climate resilience and public health action. With the rising global temperature, its implications extend from acute health effects to impacting the socio-economic structure in communities. Societies must deal with the economic burden of climate-related health issues, such as increased healthcare costs and decreased labor productivity due to climate-related diseases. The farming community is particularly at risk; changing temperature and precipitation regimes have the potential to disrupt food production, exacerbating food insecurity and nutrition issues. Marginalized communities are more affected, thereby increasing existing health disparities. In addition, implications for the increase in temperature complicate local governance structures, calling for concerted effort between environmental planners, public health policymakers, and grassroots leaders to create effective resilience systems. This crisis's intricate nature necessitates comprehension of temperature patterns globally within a broader socio-economic and health context, compelling an urgent interdisciplinary response (Christopher et al., 2012) (Figure 2.4).

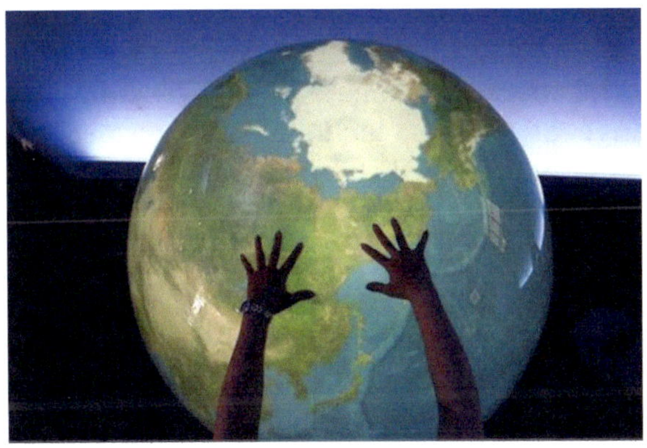

Figure 2.4. Health problems tied to global warming are on the rise.

Source: https://www.financialexpress.com/wp-content/uploads/2021/10/global-warming.jpeg.

2.1.3. Impact of Climate Change on Weather Patterns

The changing climate drastically changes weather patterns, leading to unpredictable and extreme weather conditions with severe repercussions for community well-being. Rising temperatures are responsible for the frequency and severity of heatwaves, leading to increased risks of heat-related ailments as well as aggravation of pre-existing medical conditions, especially among the elderly and those with comorbid conditions. The higher incidence of heavy precipitation and floods also contributes to these challenges, bringing with it an increased potential for waterborne disease outbreaks and contamination of drinking water sources. In addition to these physical health threats, the psychological toll of these events must be determined, as communities grapple with the devastation and disruption of their lifestyle. As stated by Appiah-Brempong et al. (2014), global climate change has a major implication on public health, with a focus on the necessity to implement robust mitigation and adaptation responses at the community level, with a prioritization on health promotion. Moreover, the disturbance of weather patterns also contributes to the transmission of vector-borne diseases. Climate change expands the range of vectors, including mosquitoes and ticks, allowing diseases such as malaria, Zika virus, and Lyme disease to emerge in areas where they would not have previously been present. As temperature increases, the lifespan of these vectors shortens, leading to faster transmission levels. This is concerning in regions that lack adequate public health infrastructure to address emerging disease threats. Findings in a recent survey highlighted in Augustinavicius et al. (2024) show heightened youth anxiety with regard to climate change and resulting health effects, which suggests that the mental health effects are as significant as the physical health effects. Populations must understand these interlinked health risks and be prepared to cope with the wider range of diseases caused by changing weather patterns. In comprehending the relationship between population health and climate change, it is necessary to keep in mind the broader socio-economic implications of these changes. The effects of climate change predominantly fall on vulnerable groups, exacerbating existing health inequities and inequalities. Unavailability of health services and supplies constrains their ability to respond to threats to health posed by changing climatic conditions. Furthermore, local economies' effects due to extreme weather can lead to an increase in poverty levels, thereby affecting community resilience and health levels. It requires addressing these connected problems through the coming together of public health professionals, policymakers, and activists from communities. As discussed in Appiah-Brempong et al. (2014), engaging local communities in climate action projects may encourage resilience and empower them to diminish the adverse effects of climate change on their well-being and health.

2.2. Direct Health Impacts of Climate Change

The direct health impacts of climate change happen primarily through the effects of extreme weather and alteration of environmental conditions. As more intensification of climate change arises, the frequency and severity of heatwaves, floods, and storms rise, having the potential to directly threaten existence and well-being. Along with physical damage, these events also add to the already present levels of stress and anxiety in the affected people. For instance, respiratory illnesses such as asthma are becoming more common due to poor air quality, which is a consequence of warming and pollution. Other than that, infectious diseases are transmitted through climate change, where warming temperatures can expand the range of disease carriers, such as mosquitoes, making it more difficult for public health interventions. Counteracting these direct health impacts necessitates a comprehensive appreciation of the interlinkages of climate change with an array of health impacts (Fortunato et al., 2015). Also, the mental health impacts of climate change cannot be disregarded because they significantly affect people. The direct effects that emanate as a result of climate-related hazards have the potential to bring about psychological trauma, articulated in terms of anxiety and depression among victims. Marginalized groups are disproportionately affected, with higher challenges in accessing mental health care following a disaster. Climate change's emotional toll, including helplessness and trauma from weather extremes, also highlights the imperative for mainstreaming mental health issues into climate response planning. The patterns through which these direct health effects restructure community dynamics are critical to developing the interventions needed. Investment in climate-focused mental health services can offer a forward-thinking approach to counteract these adverse effects on public health (Blashki et al., 2008).

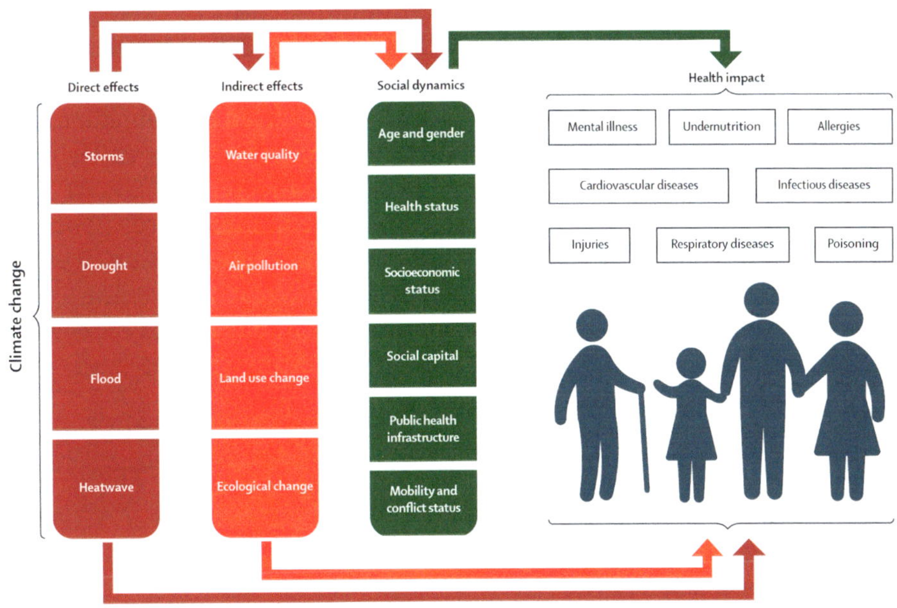

Figure 2.5. The direct and indirect effects of climate change on health.

Source: https://www.researchgate.net/profile/Maria-Nilsson-20/publication/279060470/figure/fig1/AS:998328217108482@1615031403681/The-direct-and-indirect-eff-ects-of-climate-change-on-health-and-wellbeing-There-are.png.

Furthermore, climate change extends into important determinants of health, such as nutrition and economic stability. Changes in agricultural yields due to unpredictable weather patterns undermine food security, leading to malnutrition and related diseases in vulnerable groups. In addition, as regional economies are economically affected by climate disturbances, the follow-on impact on the availability of healthcare worsens inherent health disparities. The potential to combine philanthropic efforts into effective action against climate change offers a window of opportunity to enhance the health of communities. By prioritizing funding efforts to fortify infrastructure, improve agricultural resilience, and support mental health, we can slow the direct health impacts of climate change today and tomorrow. This integrated strategy not only addresses proximal threats to health but also lays the groundwork for sustained improvement in health for populations (Fortunato et al., 2015) (Figure 2.5).

2.2.1. Heat-Related Illnesses and Mortality

The increased incidence of heat-related illnesses is a severe health concern amidst the widespread problem of climate change. With rising global temperatures, heatwave rates have skyrocketed, leading to heightened cases of heat exhaustion, heat stroke, and other related illnesses. Such high temperatures disproportionately affect susceptible populations like the elderly, individuals with existing medical conditions, and low-income groups. It indicates the urgent necessity to connect the influence of climate change on extreme heat to the overall socio-economic disparities typically encountered in the most-at-risk groups, or the Climate Gap (Sadd et al., 2009). There is a need to rectify these disparities in an effort to mitigate the adverse impacts of climate change, particularly on health outcomes as a result of heat exposure. Furthermore, public health impacts of heat illness do not consist only of acute health crises but also generate long-term issues of resilience in communities and the health infrastructure. The Centers for Disease Control and Prevention (CDC) emphasizes that the adverse effect of climate change on health is bound to expand while global emissions aggravate, stressing the importance of comprehensive approaches to offsetting these challenges (Aytur et al., 2014). Through frameworks like the Building Resilience Against Climate Effects (BRACE), people are able to develop resilient policies that increase capacity to manage heat-related morbidity. These have to consider urban planning, resource management, and community involvement in developing environments where populations can thrive, irrespective of rising temperatures. In order to manage heat-related mortality properly, it is important to step up public awareness and adaptation strategies. Educational campaigns that alert citizens to the dangers of heat exposure and hydration needs are necessary to eradicate instances of heat-related sickness. Additionally, communities must make it a priority to create cooling shelters and green areas, which can provide relief during a heat wave and promote health. Inter-segment collaboration, as highlighted in the visionary State Health Improvement Plan, can ensure interventions are not only focused on immediate health outcomes but also respond to the underlying determinants of health affected by climate change. Through building community resilience through multi-dimensional intervention, we can mitigate the impacts of heat illness and eventually lead to improved public health outcomes in a changing climate setting (Figure 2.6).

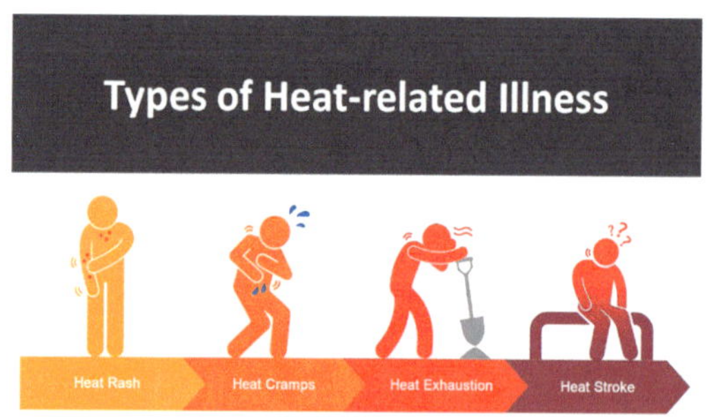

Figure 2.6. Heat-related illnesses.

Source: https://pbs.twimg.com/media/FwL3yvdXsAYDgmy.jpg.

2.2.2. Respiratory Issues from Air Quality Deterioration

Air quality deterioration, in addition to climate change, is a significant contributor to the weakening respiratory health of populations worldwide. Elevated levels of pollutants like sulfur dioxide (SO_2) and ozone (O_3) have been linked very firmly with elevated rates of respiratory conditions such as asthma and bronchitis. The facts indicate that pollutants like nitrogen oxides (NO) and carbon monoxide (CO) are most detrimental as they result in long-term diseases and continue to aggravate other disorders. Because urban residents are more likely to be exposed to pollution, the consequences for public health are serious, adding to the urgency of integrating stricter air quality standards into policies against climate change to mitigate the risks. Decreasing emissions and raising awareness of air quality among the public can both be huge measures in safeguarding respiratory health in risk groups.

In addition, the intersection of air quality deterioration and climate change has important implications for vulnerable groups like the elderly and children. Such groups are likely to be more susceptible to respiratory illnesses resulting from polluted air. Maintaining the public's health in such a case, therefore, requires effective measures that can target the socio-economic determinants of the exposure disparities. Interventions aimed at lowering pollutant levels in communities residing in their homes, especially for lower-income communities, are crucial to promoting health equity. Community education campaigns also have the power to inform communities and enable them to require cleaner air policies and become environmental guardians. A combination approach considering both the outcomes on health and the environmental policies can lead to a substantial decrease in community health outcomes, including hospitalizations and overall health costs due to respiratory issues. The challenge to address the issue of air quality deterioration calls for collaborative action by government agencies, public health organizations, and community participants. It is crucial to tap authoritative information on air quality markers and respiratory disease markers to inform specific policy interventions. There is evidence that measures in environmental management and policymaking can significantly reduce the health risks associated with air pollution. Particularly, assessing the air quality situation and how it directly affects public health results imposes urgency in acting on solutions. Experiences of the transition economies of Eastern Europe and Central Asia introduce the consequences of environmentally poor management and the imperative to act with urgency in addressing climate change. With concerted action and more stringent compliance with air quality regulations, communities can move towards healthier environments that lighten the burden of respiratory illnesses, ultimately enhancing public health resilience in the context of climate change (Akaike et al., 2010; Markandya et al., 2025) (Figure 2.7).

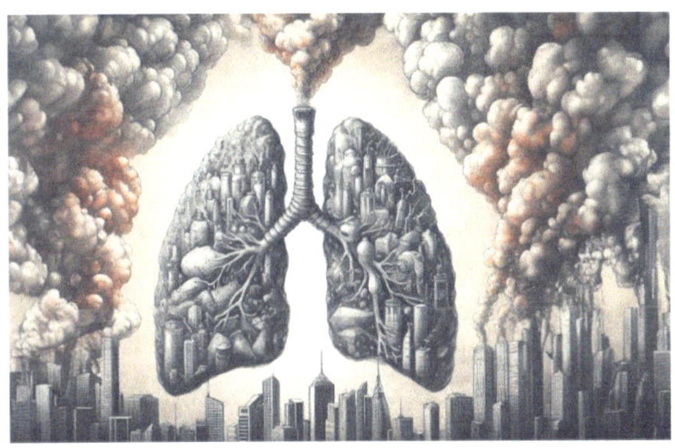

Figure 2.7. Respiratory issues from air quality deterioration.

Source: https://akm-img-a-in.tosshub.com/indiatoday/images/story/202311/during-diwali--the-air-quality-in-many-parts-of-india-deteriorates-dramatically-due-to-the-widesprea-085623834-16x9_0.jpg?VersionId=2uBArmB65as1M.P8Buecd4Wi_E0lvyVs.

2.2.3. Vector-Borne Diseases and Their Spread

The rising rates of vector-borne diseases are a leading effect of climate change that has a major influence on the health of communities. While the world is warming up, the distribution of vectors—like mosquitoes and ticks—has increased geographically, enabling these disease-carrying agents to move into new areas. Climatic conditions brought about by warming favor the growth of vectors, with evidence showing an association between temperature rise and the spread of diseases like dengue fever and malaria. So far, untouched populations are now witnessing outbreaks, overwhelming local health facilities, and increasing morbidity and mortality levels. This shift demands the urgency of implementing public health strategies to monitor and respond proactively to vector populations and their consequent disease in the midst of a changing climate (N/A, 2009). Climate change not only allows the transmission of existing vector-borne diseases but also causes new infectious diseases to emerge. Changes in precipitation and humidity levels might create favorable breeding sites for the vectors, resulting in alterations in transmission patterns. Flooding, for instance, can induce standing water conducive to the breeding of mosquitoes transmitting West Nile virus and Zika virus outbreaks. Furthermore, the increased frequency of extreme weather events such as hurricanes and heatwaves disrupts the established ecosystem balance, providing space for more complex interactions between vectors, hosts, and pathogens. This introduces potential threats for zoonotic transmissions and public health issues as communities adapt to new diseases and control them (Abouzaid et al., 2009). Strategies to mitigate the impacts of vector-borne diseases in the face of climate change need an integrative approach involving public health policy, community education, and collaborative research. Local health authorities must place an emphasis on data collection and surveillance to identify vulnerable populations and maintain accurate estimates of vector populations. Furthermore, community action programs, including education on preventive measures such as the use of insect repellents and window screens, play a fundamental role in enabling individuals to protect themselves. Since healthcare providers are increasingly faced with the consequences of climate change, it is necessary that they embrace their roles not only in the curative of disease but also in agitating and championing for systemic change at the community, state, and federal levels (N/A, 2009).

2.3. Indirect Health Impacts of Climate Change

The secondary or indirect health impacts of climate change are progressively recognized as a higher priority, affecting various dimensions of population health. They are not merely the byproduct of immediate environmental changes but are caused by complex interactions between socio-economic factors, mental health dimensions, and community resilience. For instance, as weather-related catastrophes such as hurricanes and wildfires increase in severity, populations are subject to heightened levels of trauma and stress related to loss and displacement. Research emphasizes the importance of studying cumulative trauma burdens, demonstrating how prolonged impacts of climate exposure create a multiplying factor for existing vulnerabilities in a population. These issues emphasize the importance of intervention that targets the psychological and emotional cost to the communities, leading eventually to a framework for understanding climate-related health issues and resilience efforts (O'Donnell et al., 2024). Moreover, indirect health effects of climate change are most perilous among vulnerable populations in economically developing nations. Where societies are experiencing extreme changes in the environment—such as increased temperature, floods, and droughts—issues of climate change, food security, sanitation, and clean water become salient.

The relationship between environmental issues and health is extensive; for instance, contaminated water may bring an increase in water-borne disease. But concern about climate change may potentially not be synchronized with the urgency of the local health crisis. It is henceforth necessary to bridge the gap between the overall climate change narrative and the emergency public health concerns within communities. Processes that can bridge consciousness about climate change with local health heterogeneity have the potential to maximize responses and enhance communities' resilience (Nash et al., 2019). In mental health emphasis, the indirect effects of climate change manifest in terms of greater anxiety, depression, and other mental disorders as a result of environmental disruptions, as well as associated socio-economic stressors. With further advancing impacts of climate, communities can experience a common trauma that will interfere with their mental health and social cohesion. For example, the loss of familiar environments and social structures can lead to helplessness and hopelessness, particularly among those who perceive their worlds as ever under threat. These psychological consequences can compound physical health issues, hence becoming a compounded public health issue. Therefore, it is crucial to recognize the interdependence of physical and psychological consequences of climate change for the purposes of developing integrated public health interventions. Recognizing these secondary health impacts, policymakers can better prepare communities to deal with the challenges of the impending volatile climate (O'Donnell et al., 2024).

2.3.1. Food Security and Nutrition Challenges

With global ecosystems being transformed due to climate change, the threat to food security becomes increasingly urgent. Altered weather patterns disrupt agricultural cycles, and yields of staple foods essential for human nutrition diminish. In most regions of the world, heightened frequency of extreme weather events like floods and droughts destabilize food systems. This precarious situation is exacerbated by socio-economic factors such as poverty and inequalities, which further limit access to nutritional foods and increase vulnerability for previously disadvantaged groups. Addressing the impact on public health is serious, particularly among children and malnourished groups who are vulnerable to food-related health issues. Therefore, tackling these interconnected food insecurity and nutrition problems becomes a priority to establish community resilience to the adverse effects of climate change and ensure a secure food supply for all individuals (Hassan et al., 2024). Besides crop productivity challenges, climate change affects the availability and safety of food resources as well. Variations in climatic conditions can enhance foodborne illnesses due to decreased food safety and poor water supply, which are necessary for effective preparation and processing of food. The rising temperatures and unpredictable patterns of rainfall further increase the activity of pests and diseases, further degrading the quality and safety of crops. Communities, therefore, are left to contend not just with the risk of starvation but also with the possibility of adverse health effects from consumption of spoiled food. These crossroads of climate, agriculture, and public health call for collaborative responses among agricultural, public health, and environmental actors. Unless strategies that consider both nutrition and food security are brought together, communities will be contributing to the prevalent health inequities that undermine their overall health (Committee UNSS on Nutrition, 2020). Climate change is also contributing to the maldistribution of resources and exacerbating food and water inequities, and it is bringing about human rights abuses in terms of access to nutrition. The most recent data indicate an alarming trend with growing incidences of undernourishment and higher levels of overweight and obesity due to inadequate diets. The two issues highlight the importance of an exhaustive understanding of the interlinkages between public health and food systems. In order to enhance the battle against these issues, enhanced collaboration between the United Nations programs focused on nutrition and water sustainability is inevitable. An integrated process allows for optimization of efforts addressing SDG 2 (zero hunger) and SDG 6 (clean water and sanitation) together, ultimately resulting in a resilient, health-oriented approach capable of enduring the stresses presented by climate change (Committee UNSS on Nutrition, 2020) (Figure 2.8).

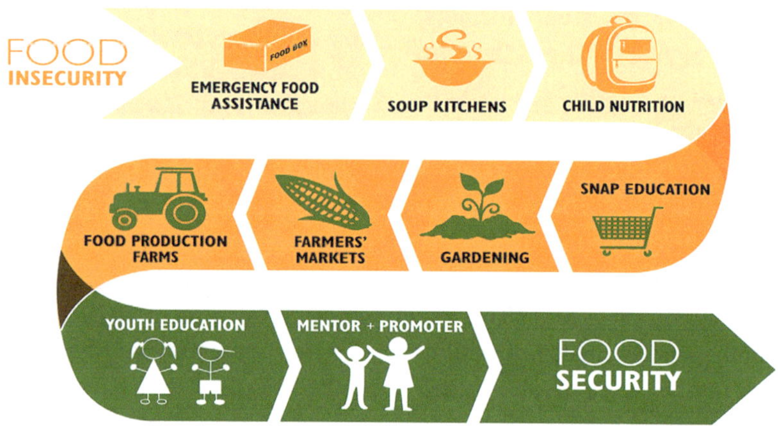

Figure 2.8. Food-and-nutrition-security.

Source: https://www.iasexpress.net/wp-content/uploads/2019/10/Food-and-nutrition-security-in-India-upsc-ias-notes-essay-mindmap-state-psc-cds-1.jpg.

2.3.2. Water Scarcity and Sanitation Issues

Shortages of water and sanitation issues have become significant public health concerns, particularly in the context of climate change. Decreasing supplies of freshwater are aggravated by rising temperatures, changed precipitation patterns, and dangerous weather conditions, which cumulatively destabilize clean and safe drinking water accessibility. Already marginalized groups suffer most, as most of them lack access to basic sanitation facilities. The World Health Organization has established a clear link between water scarcity and the spread of waterborne disease, and there is a straightforward health consequence in the community. This vulnerable condition necessitates prompt interventions that alleviate short- and long-term needs for sustainability in the face of continued climate change effects. In the case of Bangladesh specifically, there was a manual that was specifically developed to assist governmental and non-government institutions in capacity development to deliver safe water and sanitation in the face of climate pressures. The handbook presents operational solutions for upgrading water supply infrastructure and hygiene practices, which are tailored to the rural setting where the impacts of climate change are most vulnerable. By equipping local practitioners with the necessary information and resources, the handbook aims at mitigating the adverse effects of water scarcity and sanitation problems, thereby enhancing community resilience. The project indicates the importance of disaster risk management in integration with water supply and sanitation programs, and how preventive intervention could significantly enhance community health outcomes. At an overall level, the business houses' contribution to water resource management cannot be stressed enough. Increasingly, companies these days are coming to recognize the operational and reputational risks stemming from bad water management, and this is underlining the need for sustainable means of working. A recent paper outlines a number of strategies through which businesses may mitigate such risks and emphasizes that sectoral cooperation is the key to addressing the global water crisis. Case studies illustrate the way multinational firms are taking proactive measures to improve their water management processes, not only boosting their operations' sustainability but also contributing to community health. Leaning on corporate capacity and skills, businesses can play a leading role in addressing water scarcity and sanitation issues, eventually enriching healthier communities in the face of climate change challenges.

2.3.3. Mental Health Effects Due to Climate Anxiety

The psychological effects of climate change, notably climate anxiety, are now a significant topic in the broader discussion of community health. Climate anxiety is defined as the feelings of fear, helplessness, and worry experienced by individuals when reacting to perceived danger due to climate change. This anxiety has the potential to manifest as an overall sense of fear for the future, leading to stress-induced illness, depression, and even PTSD in extreme cases. The psychological effect of climate anxiety falls unevenly on different groups and has a largely negative impact on vulnerable populations who may already be facing socioeconomic disadvantage. These psychological impacts highlight the need to increase awareness and education concerning the psychological dimension of climate change, encompassing both community and individual levels of knowledge, to address the issue of mental health within the context of environmental stress to effectively combat the challenge. It is essential to understand the multi-level impacts of climate change on mental health to develop effective intervention programs. Research has shown that the mental health outcomes are determined by a variety of factors encompassing personal experiences, social networks, and broader societal environments. For instance, workers' psychological well-being may be shaped by the work environment and extrinsic stressors induced by climate change, which represents the interplay among several levels of analysis (Arnetz et al., 2014). Thus, climate anxiety solutions require an integrated approach that considers both the psychosocial work environment and community resilience. Through the integration of individual worries with community measures, efforts can be made to stem climate anxiety while simultaneously fostering conditions conducive to sustaining mental health and resilience in the face of ongoing climate change. Besides, training and supervision of mental health practitioners play a vital role in equipping them with responses to the unique challenges that define climate anxiety. It is found that the experiences and backgrounds of the practitioners significantly influence how they understand clients' psychological distress about climate issues (Ayers et al., 2018). As there is growing awareness among mental health professionals of the impact of climate change on mental health, they will be in a position to develop effective coping strategies and therapeutic interventions. Developing an environment where clinicians learn about the nuances of climate anxiety will not just make them better professionals but will also contribute to larger community health initiatives. In this regard, strengthening training programs to respond to climate-associated mental health problems is an important step towards the development of psychological resilience and enhancing community health outcomes as nations confront the intricacies of climate change (Figure 2.9).

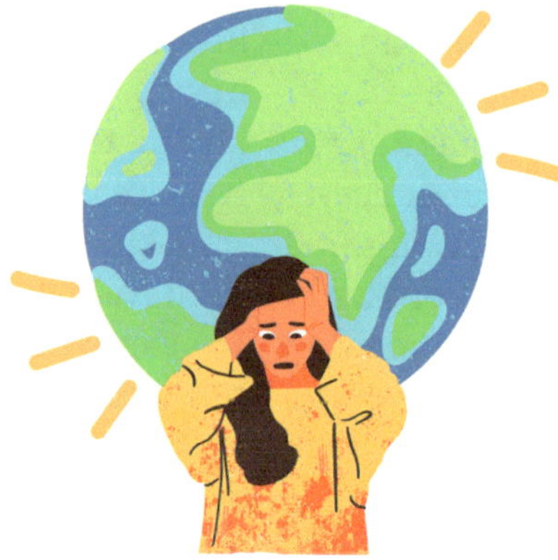

Figure 2.9. Mental health effects due to climate anxiety.

Source: https://external-content.duckduckgo.com/iu/?u=https%3A%2F%2Fmiro.medium.com%2Fv2%2Fresize%3Afit%3A750%2F1*gxEA4IqCxgpWgYZKXD7vuw.png&f=1&nofb=1&ipt=5463d7dfc10dbf8e2f078b62cf1db6df63bca4b3c09e2df4e266fc0373a6cd96.

2.4. Vulnerable Populations

Climate change is threatening to increase complex threats that disproportionately affect vulnerable populations, mostly those in lower socioeconomic groups. These populations are likely to face underlying health disparities and limited access to healthcare centers, further enhancing their susceptibility to the impacts of climate change on health. For instance, poor people are less likely to possess the economic means to act on the impacts of climate change, for instance, purchase air conditioning during heat waves or relocate from flood-prone areas. Centers for Disease Control and Prevention (CDC) is at the forefront of addressing such disparities through initiatives that aim at the identification and empowerment of populations most vulnerable to climate change effects. Targeted interventions against the same populations, the CDC aims to create specially formulated strategies that build resilience and health equity as the climate grows increasingly uncertain (N/A). Moreover, geographic and demographic factors have a crucial role to play in subjecting certain groups to climate change. Rural areas, for example, could face challenges of remoteness from critical services such as transport and health centers, hence rendering the population more challenged when it comes to preparing and recovering from extreme weather patterns. Consequently, societies with underlying health issues or disabilities are further burdened by climate impacts, which have a propensity to worsen current problems. According to reports from the CDC, these location-specific vulnerabilities must be measured so as to create tailored adaptation strategies that prove effective in mitigating risks in diverse regional environments. These integrated assessments support public health professionals and community leaders in implementing operational plans that place priority on ensuring the safety and well-being of vulnerable populations (N/A). With the extensive implications of climate change for community health, it is essential to engage vulnerable groups in developing adaptation strategies that address particular needs. Building the capacity of vulnerable populations to participate in decision-making enhances resilience and agency. Local stakeholders can apply their knowledge of the particular impacts of climate change in their environment to inform effective interventions. The CDC Climate and Health Program directly involves community members in such dialog and empowers them with resources and tools that enable them to articulate their own health needs and priorities. This participatory approach not only generates more effective public health interventions but also fosters ownership and empowerment among vulnerable populations when addressing the complex dimensions of climate-impacted health risk (N/A) (Figure 2.10).

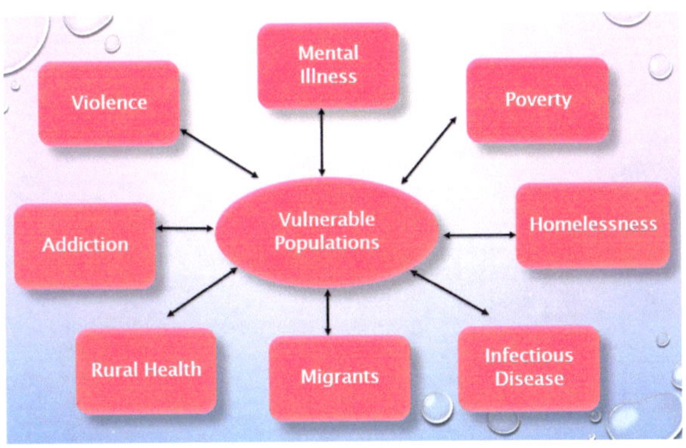

Figure 2.10. Vulnerable populations.

Source: https://external-content.duckduckgo.com/iu/?u=https%3A%2F%2Fi.ytimg.com%2Fvi%2FTps0eqdAYQA%2Fmaxresdefault.jpg&f=1&nofb=1&ipt=5dfc2406b7ed5e1adff0ea8455c028b7340e95c713dd8f91303b7db9f19293f3.

2.4.1. Low-Income Communities and Their Risks

The intersection of public health and climate change presents severe threats, particularly for poor communities. Those at risk are typically residing in areas that are disproportionately affected by the changes in the environment, so they are more exposed to weather events. For instance, the increasing number of extreme heat events poses a critical issue. Lower-income communities are less apt to have adequate cooling equipment or health care access, and therefore, during heat waves, they experience more severe health impacts. Research indicates that severe heat impacts all populations disproportionately; lower-income communities and marginalized groups, including communities of color, are the most impacted by these changes. With climate models projecting a significant rise in summer temperatures, the need for targeted intervention and protection for these groups becomes increasingly urgent (Bond et al., 2023). In addition to heat extremes, variability in water availability itself is an important contributor to public health risks among low-income communities. The lingering effects of climate change reorganize precipitation regimes, leading to droughts and heavy rainfall. These alterations exert stress on essential water infrastructure, threatening access to clean and reliable water sources. Additionally, already disadvantaged groups lack the infrastructure to adjust to these alterations, thereby leading to reduced water quality and an increased risk of waterborne infections. This synergistic action further reinforces health inequities since poor communities are potentially exposed to long-term conditions linked with dirty water and unsanitary conditions. Thus, management of such systemic vulnerabilities calls for holistic measures focusing on the establishment of resilience and fair resource distribution within urban planning (N/A, 2017). Climate change is a spotlight for the already existing socioeconomic disparities, particularly in low-income communities. The combined impacts of environmental deterioration can lead to forced displacement and economic insecurity, further entrapping individuals in poverty chains. These families are most likely to be found in flood-vulnerable, low-lying areas, further increasing the risk of loss of property and displacement. In addition, the lack of funds limits the capacity to adjust, either by investing in flood defense or migrating to higher ground. Unless certain interventions addressed to the specific issues facing low-income groups are made, the cycle of vulnerability under the influence of climate change will persist. Therefore, facilitating community health improvement by equity-based policies and practices is not only necessary for reducing risks but also essential for constructing durable community resilience to climate-related threats (Bond et al., 2023; N/A, 2017).

2.4.2. Elderly Populations and Health Vulnerabilities

The older population is at greatest risk of adverse health impacts of climate change, and it highlights the intersection of environmental and public health concerns. As the global temperature rises, older individuals are placed under greater risks as a result of heatwaves that cause heat illness and exacerbation of pre-existing illnesses. This risk is compounded with physiological alterations in aging, such as compromised thermoregulation and comorbidities. Furthermore, the increased severity and frequency of intense weather phenomena, including hurricanes and flooding, disproportionately impact the elderly, who may be immobile or reside in facilities lacking in emergency preparedness. All these highlight the need for a proper assessment of interventions aimed at enhancing the resilience of aging populations against climate-related dangers (Culp et al., 2015). Aside from the physical health outcomes, climate change has an impact on the mental well-being of elderly individuals as well.

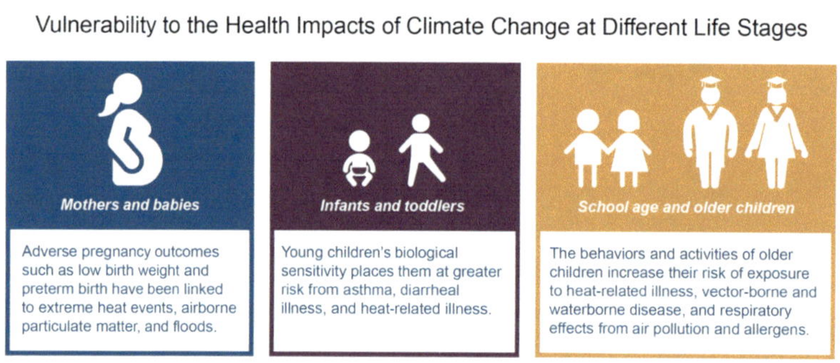
Vulnerability to the Health Impacts of Climate Change at Different Life Stages
Mothers and babies
Adverse pregnancy outcomes such as low birth weight and preterm birth have been linked to extreme heat events, airborne particulate matter, and floods.
Infants and toddlers
Young children's biological sensitivity places them at greater risk from asthma, diarrheal illness, and heat-related illness.
School age and older children
The behaviors and activities of older children increase their risk of exposure to heat-related illness, vector-borne and waterborne disease, and respiratory effects from air pollution and allergens.

Figure 2.11. Elderly populations and health vulnerabilities.

Source: https://health2016.globalchange.gov/sites/default/files/styles/large_figure/public/figure/f3-cropped_19.png.

Stress and anxiety resulting from natural disasters, migration, and uncertainty regarding the effects of climate change can exacerbate or initiate existing mental health disorders or create new ones. Isolation further exacerbates the effect since elderly individuals may not have access to social support groups or resources when experiencing climate change. This isolation can decrease their resilience, diminishing their ability to recover from trauma and manage health challenges effectively. Public health interventions must therefore prioritize mental health resources to support elderly populations facing climate-induced stressors. Understanding the social determinants that influence the vulnerability of this demographic is essential for addressing their unique needs during climate crises (Aytur et al., 2014). Finally, the development of resilience among the elderly must be a multi-faceted effort based on readiness, investment in resources, and education. A multisectoral collaborative partnership with public health organizations, community associations, and local governments is needed to establish a general climate adaptation plan. This plan should involve the production of assistive physical environments, e.g., accessible shelter facilities during weather disasters, and education among communities that empower older adults to take anticipatory action. It is equally important to integrate healthcare systems that meet both physical and mental healthcare needs and provide such care for older groups during and following climatic events. Through prioritizing these collaborative, resilience-enhancing measures, we can reduce the impacts of climate change on older groups and secure their health and well-being amid rising environmental stressors (Culp et al., 2015) (Figure 2.11).

2.4.3. Children and Their Susceptibility to Climate Impacts

Exposure of children to climate impacts is an urgent matter since children are exposed to special health vulnerabilities that will have lasting effects. The increasing climate change is causing more adverse effects of environmental degradation, with increased levels of food insecurity, respiratory illness, and exposure to severe weather conditions, which affect the developing minds and bodies of children more. An infant born today, says Lancet Countdown, could experience severe threats to health if the climate crisis is not addressed properly, including increased risks of undernutrition and increased morbidity of infectious diseases and air pollution.

This evidence calls for the children to be put at the forefront of climate action efforts since their health outcomes directly relate to the changed ecosystem of the planet and therefore, stakeholders need to take a comprehensive adaptation and mitigation approach that protects this vulnerable group. Additionally, the psychological impacts of climate change on children cannot be ignored. Evidence indicates that children experience fear and anxiety about the deteriorating state of the planet, commonly known as eco-anxiety. In a survey conducted in March 2020, it was revealed that 73% of children aged between 8 and 16 years were worried about the future of the world, with a significant majority claiming to have nightmares about climate-related issues. Such psychological distress is a growing mental health crisis, driven by the continued media coverage and occurrence of climate disasters, including fires and hurricanes. Such mental stress places additional pressures on children's welfare and well-being and therefore requires parents, teachers, and policymakers to address these matters in caring conversation and active civic engagement and promote resilience and empowerment among young people amid adversity (Cohen, 2021). To address these challenges with their multi-dimensional layers, communities must adopt a health equity approach that emphasizes the centrality of supportive systems. Disparities in access to mental health care, driven by social inequities, can further contribute to the vulnerabilities of children who have been exposed to climate change. Findings suggest that fewer privileged and marginalized youth are likely to experience unwanted negative effects of ecological anxiety and grief, and thus, there is a vital necessity to ensure that mental health services and interventions are culturally responsive and accessible. By creating cross-sector collaborations among health workers, teachers, and community organizations, it is possible to achieve inclusive frameworks that promote the emotional and physical well-being of children within the climate change context. Such a collective endeavor not only addresses existing inequalities but also draws on mutual resilience to ensure that children are equipped to deal with a more complex world and to foster sustainable responses (Cohen, 2021).

2.5. Community Resilience and Adaptation Strategies

The community resilience concept encompasses the capacity of a community to prepare for, respond to, and recover from adverse situations, particularly those exacerbated by climate change. Effective resilience relies on the capacity of a community to adapt its strategy in relation to local needs and circumstances, especially for environmental degradation. Public spaces are the essentials in which to quantify this flexibility, and they indicate a community's health and capacity for resilience. Function and design of the same tend to enhance interaction between the community, be inclusive, and support multi-form activities, leading to emotional and social well-being. Research has demonstrated that engaging communities in the process of planning and undertaking the adaptive measures is vital in initiating a feeling of possession as well as guaranteeing strategies directly address local exposures (Van et al., 2014:374). The participation is further emphasized through schemes in developing available public space for enhancing resilience towards the impacts of climate change. Adaptation initiatives must be cognizant of the unique socio-economic contexts of communities, particularly those that are vulnerable within systems. Those communities with extreme poverty and marginalization will display less ability in putting in place effective adaptations. This was the case in a study conducted in Dhaka, Bangladesh, which displayed how poor households suffering from chronic poverty cannot adapt to climate change, highlighting the imperative for nuanced adaptation initiatives that can be tailored to their specific condition (Hossain et al., 2014). If they have inadequate access to resources such as savings, credit, and insurance, these households might feel compelled to resort to destructive coping mechanisms that compromise their long-term health. Creating social policies and enhancing protective mechanisms for these populations could therefore be one of the most important things in developing resilience. This will give the vulnerable populations an opportunity to accumulate the assets that enhance their adaptive capacity, ultimately translating their vulnerability into resilience to present and future climatic stresses. Effective adaptation within a community also relies on collective actions at multiple scales, including micro (household), meso (community), and macro (institutional).

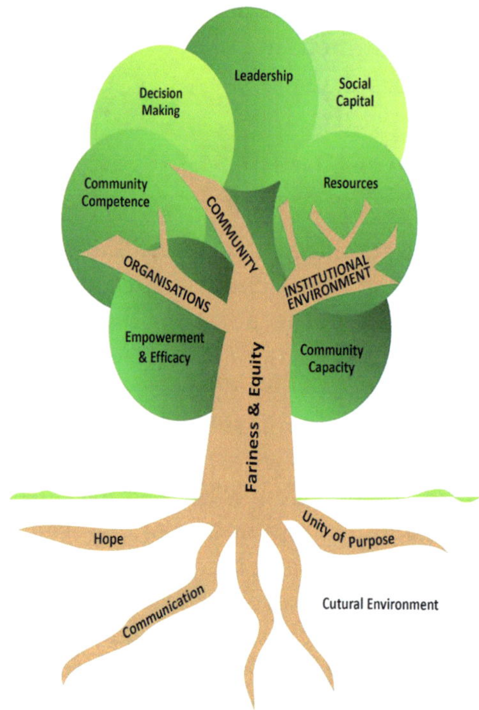

Figure 2.12. Community resiliency.

Source: https://image1.slideserve.com/2631870/slide3-l.jpg.

This multi-level approach recognizes that resilience must be based not just on individual or local interventions but also on general policies and institutional mechanisms reinforcing communities (Hossain et al., 2014). Through planning inclusive systems where marginalized groups may participate and influence decision-making, communities are able to most effectively cope with exposure to climate impacts. In addition, matching community-based action with targeted public policies may facilitate the development of required infrastructure to mitigate climate danger. Communities will need to develop robust social networks and collective organizations in order to cope with climate change, but these will play a central role in overcoming entrenched social inequalities. Such an integrated strategy illustrates how a common strategy towards resilience can yield long-term sustainable health and well-being benefits under climate change (Figure 2.12).

2.5.1. Importance of Community Engagement in Health Initiatives

Community participation is a bedrock in health programs that respond to the complex issues presented by climate change. When communities take part in health intervention planning, their experiences and perceptions become part of the agenda. These programs must mirror the true needs and concerns of the population being served. For instance, health programs that incorporate community perceptions are likely to establish strong trust and foster cooperation among the populace. With the understanding of local customs and interpersonal dynamics, healthcare professionals are able to maximize their outreach and, hence, have greater sustainable health effects. This community-based approach not only makes communities stronger but also translates into greater public health resilience, particularly against climate-linked health threats such as heatwaves and vector-borne diseases, which are set to increase under the new climate realities. Community engagement also becomes critical for its role in supporting local ownership and accountability for health interventions. Active communities can more effectively monitor and evaluate the effects of health interventions, providing feedback that can instigate desired modifications en route. These alliances can produce a more adaptive public health response, one tailored to the evolving climate and its associated health implications. For example, plans to mitigate the adverse effects of flooding would be greatly assisted by local understanding of historical occurrences of flooding and the socio-economic drivers behind vulnerability. Strategies that draw on residents' context-specific knowledge are likely to succeed in building resilience against climate change health impacts. Accordingly, the integration of community participation into the program structure of the health initiative makes the program more relevant, in addition to enhancing the collective capacity to address arising health problems related to climate change. In addition, community participation has the ability to mobilize beneficial social capital that can empower individuals and groups to act collectively in the pursuit of improved health. When individuals come together, they can combine resources, intelligence, and expertise that sum to an integrative response to climate change as well as health effects. Initiatives that foster collaboration among different actors, such as public health experts, local governments, and non-state actors, can lead to the development of pioneering solutions to health challenges exacerbated by climatic conditions. The CGIAR Research Program is a relevant example, demonstrating how community-led research can center on local demands for health and promote sustainable behavior patterns (Andrew et al., 2013). Similarly, the local concentration of resources within flood-concentrated environments can make a place more resilient by leveraging local and external support (Amaratunga et al., 2013). Through developing a sense of cooperation, community engagement supports not only health at the individual level but also strengthens the resilience of the community to adapt to the threats posed by climate change.

2.5.2. Infrastructure Improvements for Climate Resilience

The interface between public health and climate change demands a robust response through large-scale climate resilience infrastructure upgrades. Those communities that have been affected by extreme weather events need carefully planned strategies with the aim of recovery as well as long-term preparation for the future. Here, the Sandy Regional Assembly is a good example of this bottom-up strategy in planning resilience. The Recovery Agendas of the assembly address the necessity to integrate local priorities of resiliency into regional rebuilding to support vulnerable populations while opposing public health threats. The recognition of hardest-hit communities requiring unique solutions underscores the critical imperative for systemic infrastructure upgrades that serve climate resilience and access to healthcare directly, ultimately in pursuit of long-term well-being for citizens (N/A, 2013). The infrastructure landscape in most cities, especially older ones, is increasingly being undermined by climate change, with very serious public health implications. New Jersey is a prime case where extensive use of combined sewer systems presents an enormous challenge. Older systems are vulnerable to combined sewer overflows (CSOs) during storm events, discharging raw sewage directly into water bodies and presenting a tremendous public health risk. Societies that are faced with CSOs are not merely coping with the implications of the decreased quality of water but are also fighting the issue of aging water infrastructure that is insufficient to deal with the increased frequency and severity of precipitation due to climate change. This reality highlights the necessity for strategic investments in infrastructure, which addresses these vulnerabilities and creates community welfare (N/A, 2014). Enhancing urban infrastructure for climatic resilience is a complex process that requires the coordination of different stakeholders like government departments, community organizations, and the private sector. The need for one strategy is also seen in initiatives such as the Agenda for Change in New Jersey, which attempts to address the problems of urban water infrastructure through collective action . By bringing together representation from a wide range of sectors, this initiative aims to offer guiding principles for the modernization and upgrading of city infrastructures. The emphasis on partnership guarantees that any resultant improvements are not merely effective but also equitable, bridging the needs of the most disadvantaged sections of society. As communities adopt these new strategies, they are better placed to mitigate the health impacts of climate change while creating cities that are sustainable to future challenges (N/A, 2014) (Figure 2.13).

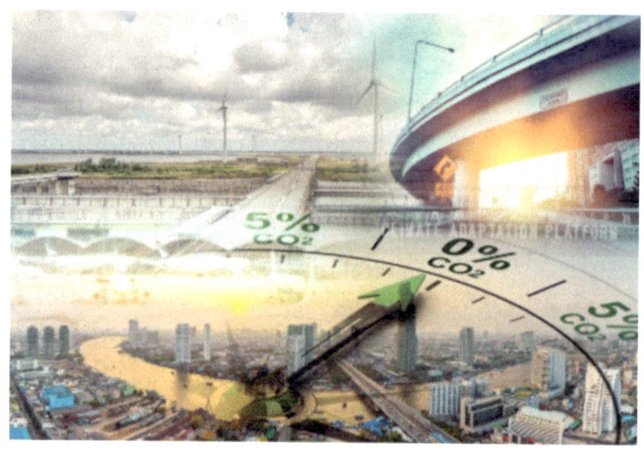

Figure 2.13. Massive infrastructure investment is needed for climate resilience.

Source: https://external-content.duckduckgo.com/iu/?u=https%3A%2F%2Fclimateadaptationplatform.com%2Fwp-content%2 Fuploads%2 F2022%2F01%2 Fclimate-adaptation-net-z ero-resilient-infrastructure.jpg&f=1&nofb =1&ipt= 943432704 68fc0dd 81ff2a0c3f1dff14b2e44b06f3d a973f2f231abac1e8f455.

2.5.3. Public Health Policies Addressing Climate Change

In comprehending the highly interconnected relations between climate change and public health, it is critical to develop focused public health policies that address these challenges. Where populations are fighting against the adverse effects of climate change, policymakers are faced with integrating health outcomes into climate adaptation and resilience efforts. These policies must focus on populations at risk that are disproportionately affected by climate-related health risk factors. For instance, the health equity context of climate response can expose the unique issues of women and vulnerable groups, who are most impacted by climate injustice. If health programs can develop principles that help the above groups become integral to decision-making, then they can effectively combat the disparities brought about by climate change and enhance general resilience in communities against environmental stressors. Also, public health policy must highly prioritize the collection and analysis of complete data to inform climate response actions. Where data are not disaggregated along gender and other intersecting dimensions of vulnerability, the unique needs of specific groups may be overlooked in the midst of climate-change-compounded health crises. There are certain regulations to enhance health equity through the guarantee that data captures various demographic determinants, thus facilitating interventions that are responsive to various individuals in communities. Eliminating loopholes in existing data enables policies to react to crucial environmental and social health determinants, enabling practitioners and policymakers to come up with more suitable responses to health concerns triggered by climate change. More analysis of data also provides a mechanism to predict future health trends driven by climate change, ultimately allowing for more anticipatory public health policy. Lastly, successful public health policy to address climate change needs to encourage coordination across many stakeholders, from the government to communities and non-governmental organizations. Having multiple actors at the table in climate and health negotiations can build an integrated awareness of, and reaction to, climate-related health impacts. Secondly, incorporating people's input can have the effect of having the policy reflect the experience of the people most directly impacted by climate change. For example, efforts towards equity of access to healthcare, mental health care, and disaster preparedness can be essential in mitigating the effects of climate change. Lacking a democratic, equity-fostering political agenda, much of the desired health benefit through climate adaptation would be inaccessible to the most marginalized populations (Perkins et al., 2019; Birnbaum et al., 2011). Through being proactive and advancing equity-focused public health policy, communities are empowered to build resilience and defend the health of their populations against long-term climatic stress (Figure 2.14).

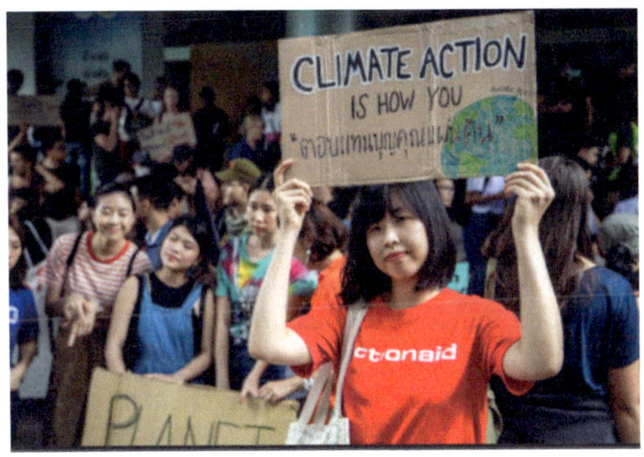

Figure 2.14. Public health policies addressing climate change.

Source: https://external-content.duckduckgo.com/iu/?u= https%3A%2F%2Fdynaimage.cdn.cnn.com%2Fcnn% 2Fdigital-images%2Forg%2Fe88 87564-efd3-468b-811d-8128a5d18e1c.jpeg&f=1&nofb=1&ipt=d419fd8d1b685ce01821e35266e876ab7535e7ce9b71d74b5a9f6ed30c430a96.

2.6. Role of Government and Policy

It is through government and policy that the solution to the intricacies presented by climate change can be achieved, particularly community health. Government regulation can guarantee the transition to green practice while, at the same time, protecting the public from the adverse health effects of environmental depletion. For Ontario, the mining industry, as much as it is ready to propel green energy technology, poses a threat to the environment and the health of communities as well. The subtleties of state priorities illustrate the need for finding a balance between health advocacy and economic development, and for public health to be an even more paramount guiding principle in policy for extractive industries. In taking a leadership role in health when crafting climate policies, policymakers can avoid unintended health consequences and promote healthy practices for the mining sector, ultimately promoting local communities and ecosystems (Hutchuk et al., 2023). Moreover, the effectiveness of climate initiatives is contingent upon identifying the impediments that discourage the active participation of public health at policy levels. Stakeholder participation, according to recent research, exhibits negligible inter-sectoral coordination amongst industries, health units, and government ministries in Ontario, presenting inconsistencies and an incapacity to respond to people's needs. These constraints present critical challenges to public health advocates who seek to incorporate health considerations into climate action policy. For this reason, it is crucial to spot and overcome these barriers so as to construct an enabling environment where public health can openly be applied to guide the mining industry towards safer and more sustainable practices. By addressing such concerns, government authorities can more effectively advance health results among individuals most intimately impacted by extractive activities and climate change (Hutchuk et al., 2023). To effectively close the gap between public health outcomes and government policy, strong assessments such as Scotland's current annual reviews of various policy areas might be a good model to follow. These assessments also engage experts and stakeholders, as well as produce an organized method of understanding the impacts of diverse policies on public health. Based on evidence-based recommendations from various domains, governments are able to create effective climate policies prioritizing local community health in combination with economic, social, and environmental factors. This combined method guarantees fulfillment of requirements for local nearby communities as well as enhances resilience against the impacts of climate change. Since communities are now more and more dealing with the impacts of climate change, government and policy intervention become forefront in addressing public health and advocating for activities that can bring about positive changes in the environment and society (Figure 2.15).

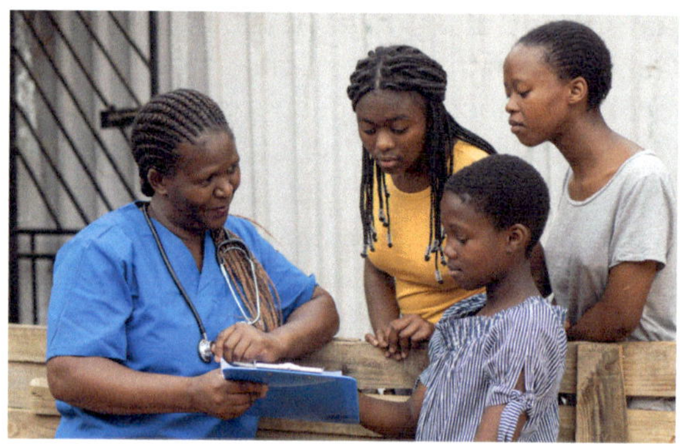

Figure 2.15. Economic case for community health workers.

Source: https://www.newyorkfed.org/medialibrary/media/newsevents/events/regional_outreach/2023/062323/community-health-workers-06232023event-eventpage.

2.6.1. National and International Climate Agreements

Success in international and national climate agreements is crucial to limiting climate change and its effects on community health. Agreements such as the Paris Accord and the Kyoto Protocol are milestones in the global crusade against reducing greenhouse gas emissions, and they underscore the necessity of a unified effort from nations. These frameworks not just set emission reduction targets but also call for transparency and accountability in achieving them. The targets under these agreements directly influence the policies of countries, which can enhance public health by reducing air pollution and, consequently, lessening the cases of respiratory diseases. The alignment of health goals and climate action highlights the synergistic relationship between environmental activity and health outcomes at a community level, since improved environmental policies can also lead to healthier populations. In addition to enhancing health outcomes, international climate agreements facilitate technological and economic support to developing nations so that they can shift towards more environmentally friendly practices without compromising their economic development. Mechanisms such as the Green Climate Fund aim at channeling resources to such countries that are victimized by the extensive effects of climate change. Not only do these investments strengthen sustainable development policies, but they also improve local health infrastructures. Outfitting such countries with such vital resources as clean technologies and access to clean energy, climate agreements can significantly cut back on the risks of climate change-related health. Such collaboration highlights the interconnectedness of climate policy and global health and has it say that addressing the health impacts of climate change is an international issue that requires a unified international response. The proliferation of global environmental agreements since the early 1970s has provided the backdrop for a heightened global response to combat climate change. Ninety international legal documents now deal with environmental concerns, illustrating the increased priority placed on climate legislation (Weiss et al., 1993). This expansion signifies comprehension that climate change is a transnational concern and one that presents serious health hazards to populations globally. Through the formulation of strong law structures, states are able to collaborate to promote science-based strategies and respond to regional health concerns. These arrangements, however, must be in constant evaluation and revision to be effective. With the progress of climate science, national and global policies need to be extremely flexible and reactive towards new evidence, such that the health of people remains at the forefront of climate action plans without the undesirable effects of climate change (Duyck et al., 2013).

2.6.2. Local Government Initiatives for Health and Climate

Local government action is critical in addressing the converging challenges of climate change and public health at the community level. Local governments are uniquely situated to develop regionally specific strategies that improve community climate adaptation and enhance public health achievements. For instance, municipalities can engage in urban green initiatives that not only enhance biodiversity but also mitigate heat exposure, thereby protecting vulnerable populations such as the elderly and those with pre-existing medical conditions. The local governments can also launch emergency response programs, considering the specific needs of marginalized groups, who are usually more vulnerable to risks in the event of natural disasters. These efforts emphasize the necessity of the incorporation of health considerations in climate policy so that the benefits of climate action are shared equitably and so that the health of communities is suitably safeguarded. The involvement of marginalized peoples in decision-making is a central feature of good local climate and health governance. Valuing knowledge in such populations due to their experiences can enhance the impact of climate and health programs. Involving a diverse range of voices, local authorities can get to know the unique requirements of vulnerable populations, including those who have been affected by housing instability and diminished access to healthcare. This inclusive approach can help develop more robust interventions that specifically address the environmental injustices that cause health inequalities. Resilience support programs can be modified by local governments to incorporate fundamentals such as clean water and sanitation, which play a critical role in the mitigation of climate change effects. These approaches with marginalized communities facilitate increased equity and enable policies to be informed, fair, and inclusive at all levels. Finally, local governments can enhance public health systems by multi-sectoral involvement aimed at the reduction of climate change effects on health. Collaboration among agencies such as health, housing, and environmental services can result in innovative solutions that are more holistic. For example, initiatives promoting active transport options such as cycling and public transport use not only curtail greenhouse gas emissions but also influence active lifestyles that can combat health deficiencies. These combined initiatives can produce strategies that address the sources of health disparities driven by climate change. Local government initiatives, when framed around health equity, are able to spur systemic change, ultimately creating strong communities prepared to meet the challenges that a changing climate presents.

2.6.3. Funding and Resources for Climate Health Research

Concentration of resources and finance on climate health research is central to understanding and limiting the impact of climate change on the health of communities. As climate-induced health issues intensify, funding for research projects becomes an emergency. Effective mechanisms of funding can trigger innovative responses and stimulate cross-disciplinary alliances towards understanding local vulnerabilities. In particular, projects involving paradigms with a focus on gender equality and social inclusion, like in Sub-Saharan Africa AI-driven agricultural innovations, identify the way targeted funding can address specific issues within communities while fostering sustainable activities (Ozor et al., 2025). By engaging diverse stakeholders and leveraging technological advancements, funding can speed up research and application of health interventions directly addressing climate change's implications. There are huge gaps in Sub-Saharan climate health research because of insufficient funding. A recent review indicated that there have been very few relevant studies conducted among the many countries in the region, with some nations being unrepresented in climate health debates (Kilungo et al., 2024). This under-financing, along with repressing research, also represses the development of adaptive capacities to safeguard public health from climate dangers. The way forward in these failings is a commitment to the development of dynamic funding systems that will address place-specific requirements, something that can encourage researchers to study under-studied spheres of climate health, such as air and natural disasters. This approach not only facilitates the expansion of knowledge but also permits communities to create tailored climate adaptation plans that reflect their unique contexts. Moreover, planning infrastructure for long-term funding of climate health programs is essential to facilitating resilience in communities. Alternative modes of funding, including through public-private partnerships and collaborative grants, can facilitate knowledge sharing and the convening of resources across sectors. These collaborations can optimize the production of research and enhance a culture of cooperative responsibility in the context of climate change issues. Furthermore, long-term investment in training and capacity building, especially among scientists in underrepresented regions, will ensure societies are able to properly implement evidence-based policy. By building this support system strongly, stakeholders can develop a solid framework that not only meets short-term health goals but also creates long-term solutions for future climate challenges (Kilungo et al., 2024) (Figure 2.16).

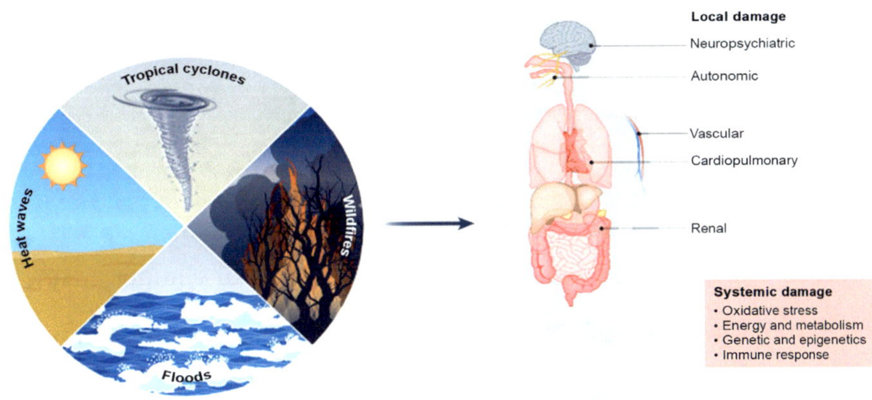

Figure 2.16. Climate change and health.

Source: https://media.springernature.com/m685/springer-static/image/art%3A10.1038%2Fs41591-024-02925-8/MediaObjects/41591_2024_2925_Fig1_HTML.png.

CLOSER LOOK

FUTURE OUTLOOK ON CLIMATE CHANGE AND COMMUNITY HEALTH

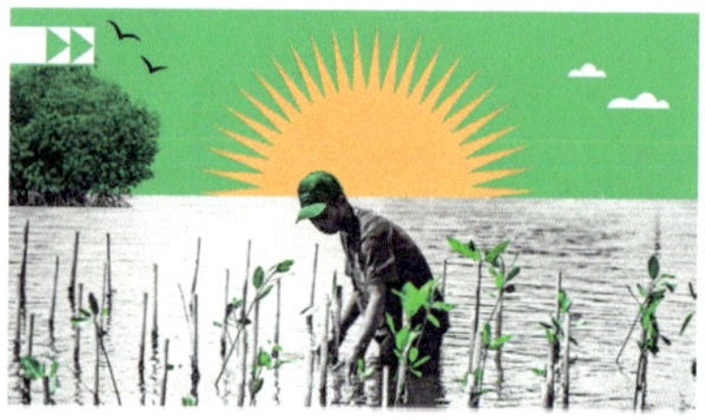

Figure 2.17. A person engaged in mangrove restoration as part of climate adaptation efforts.

Source: https://www.un.org/sites/un2.un.org/files/adaption-narrow-page-header.jpg.

The future projection of climate change presents formidable challenges for community health in various locations, particularly where extreme weather patterns are prevalent. For instance, the increasing occurrence and magnitude of heatwaves that have been witnessed in Western Australia are anticipated to result in adverse effects on public health outcomes. With a record high temperature and a 50% increase in heatwave days since 1950, the danger of heat illness, including heat stroke and exacerbated chronic disease, becomes a pressing concern. If carbon emissions are not drastically reduced, the long-term trend is that populations will be confronted with increasing numbers of heat-related fatalities, which could double from approximately 20 to 40 annually in some regions. This trend raises the imperative need for strategic public health interventions to mitigate the impacts of climate change among vulnerable groups. Besides heatwaves, the risk of extreme bushfire weather is another extreme danger to the health and well-being of populations. The forecast is for a near-doubling of extreme fire danger days in south-western Western Australia by 2090 if emissions are not significantly cut back. With bushfires burning increasingly for longer and across larger areas, long-term air quality and respiratory health consequences are severe. As their smoke pollution encircles populations, the underlying disease is aggravated, and healthcare systems become strained. Moreover, as land becomes uninhabitable due to growing fire risk, there is potential for the displacement of populations with associated social and health-related exposures as communities are left grappling with the consequences of climate change-induced migration. Finally, it is essential to address the community's attitudes towards water resources in the light of climate change to preserve public health and ensure the availability of resources. As the driest populated continent, Australia possesses unique water management challenges in which consumer attitude knowledge can influence policy and action. The Australian Water Consumer Outlook emphasizes the importance of consumer engagement in conversations about water supply and usage, underscoring the need for shared governance. Prioritizing water policy driven by community considerations can help stakeholders better prepare to meet future scarcity, creating resilience against climate fluctuation. Additionally, with the intensification of global warming, the intersection of water management measures with regard to health will be important in promoting community well-being and safeguarding future resources. Thus, an informed public will allow communities to become actively involved in creating effective climate adaptation measures.

SUMMARY

The intersection of climate change and community health underscores a central tenet of public health that requires immediate attention and action. As many areas, particularly those inhabited by Indigenous communities, have single exposures to environmental change, the health consequences are immense. Detection of the specific challenges these groups are experiencing is critical, as demonstrated through attempts to create participatory frameworks for assessing the impact of climate change. These frameworks facilitate action by the community members, researchers, and policymakers together to enhance local capacity to act in response to the health effects of climate change. Ultimately, in the absence of a collective and inclusive response, the health detriments of the climatic changes will only further exacerbate existing disparities and erode good public health responses. In addition, the collected evidence through working with the community in regions like Nunatsiavut captures detailed information on climate-sensitive health priorities. The participatory research methods applied, such as PhotoVoice workshops, reveal the intricate interaction between environmental change and social determinants of health in Indigenous societies. Research findings indicate that important areas like food and water security, mental well-being, and protection are influenced directly by climate change. Health researchers and policy-makers have the ability to design targeted interventions to tackle these areas with the utmost priority. This approach not only makes communities resilient but also makes climatic adaptations informed by the realities they face when it comes to climate change, leading to better health outcomes. In the long term, dealing with the implications of climate change on community health is required through a multi-faceted and integrated approach. Stakeholder coordination—going from local community members to governments—is critical in formulating plans that can withstand the test of time. Data from projects undertaking climate vulnerability highlights that participatory methods need to be used in guiding health research and adaptation planning. With a comprehensive and EcoHealth framework, communities can develop resilience and capacities tailored to their unique requirements and thus more effectively handle the complexities of a shifting climate. In the future, it is necessary to maintain the voices and experiences of the most impacted, to create a more just and health-based approach to the dilemmas of climate change.

As climate change escalates, its impact on community health becomes a top priority. The alteration of climatic systems brings about unequal exposure to extreme weather events such as flooding and violent storms that disproportionately affect the vulnerable group, particularly from low- and middle-income countries. The loss of essential infrastructure, like sources of clean water and sanitation facilities, exacerbates public health crises in communities. For example, in the Fuveme-Keta District of Ghana, there has been recurrent flooding that destroyed Water, Sanitation, and Hygiene (WASH) facilities, thereby increasing population vulnerability to health risks and the occurrence of water-borne diseases. The interplay of environmental hazards and community health emphasizes the urgent need for adaptive processes that can aid in strengthening resilience against increasing climatic risks, highlighting the fact that successful interventions would have to address not only physical health but psychological health as well within affected communities (Dzokoto et al., 2025). Further, community perceptions and climate change beliefs also play an important role in shaping wellbeing. Research indicates that people's own assessments of climate change threats depend on numerous factors, including political beliefs, socioeconomic status, and immediate experience. In Australia, it was decided in one study that clusters were established on the basis of what they believed about climate change and public health policy. These are indicators of a nuanced awareness of how cultural and political conditions affect people's and society's reactions to climatic adversities. Of special note, willingness for climate action would have been highly associated with more inclusive worldviews, and that indicates interventions must consider these complex systems of belief. Through communities' management of the impacts of climate change, increasing public awareness, and fostering group participation can enhance adaptive capacities and maximize health benefits (Lee et al., 2025). Lastly, the urgency of an integrative, multidimensional approach to community health, here, climate change, cannot be overemphasized. This involves integrating climate-resilient infrastructure with specialized mental health intervention and alternative livelihood promotion among vulnerable sections. In the Fuveme-Keta District, for instance, strong, coherent community networks have managed to significantly mitigate the psychosocial impact of climatic disaster, though the lack of alternative livelihood opportunities has been shown to constrain adaptability. It is vital to instate and implement targeted policies that foster mental health and resilience at the community level and intervene against socio-economic determinants of health. Prioritizing climate-resilient WASH systems and mental health services, communities will be well-positioned to survive the danger posed by climate change, thereby translating into improved health outcomes and greater resilience against threats in the future (Dzokoto et al., 2025).

REFERENCES

1. Abouzaid, S., & Sarfaty, M. (2009). *The Physician's Response to Climate Change*. https://core.ac.uk/download/46966943.pdf (accessed on 11th June 2025).
2. Akaike, A., Anderson, B., Bell, M., Box, G., Braat, L., Braga, A., Brunekreef, B., et al. (2010). *Effects of Air Pollution and Meteorological Parameters on Human Health in The City of Athens, Greece*.
3. Amaratunga, D., & Ingirige, B. (2013). *Minimizing Flood Risk Accumulation Through Effective Private and Public Sector Engagement*. https://core.ac.uk/download/30733249.pdf (accessed on 11th June 2025).
4. Andrew, N., Govan, H., Harohau, D., et al. (2013). *Solomon Islands: Malaita Hub Scoping Report*. https://core.ac.uk/download/16384844.pdf (accessed on 11th June 2025).
5. Appiah-Brempong, E., Okyere, P., & Tsiboe, M. (2014). *Should 'Climate Change' Change Health Promoters? Lessons For the Developing World*. https://core.ac.uk/download/234681849.pdf (accessed on 11th June 2025).
6. Arnetz, B., Bacharach, S., Bamberger, P., Biron, M., Biron, M., Biron, M., Biron, M., et al. (2014). *The Psychosocial Work Environment, Employee Mental Health and Organizational Interventions: Improving Research and Practice by Taking a Multilevel Approach*. https://core.ac.uk/download/30650323.pdf (accessed on 11th June 2025).
7. Augustinavicius, J., Carpenter, C., Clayton, S. D., et al. (2024). *Climate Emotions, Thoughts, And Plans Among Us Adolescents and Young Adults: A Cross-Sectional Descriptive Survey and Analysis by Political Party Identification and Self-Reported Exposure to Severe Weather Events*. https://core.ac.uk/download/620955153.pdf (accessed on 11th June 2025).
8. Ayers, S., Hinze, K. A., et al. (2018). *Adult-Child Sexual Contact: Examining Mental Health Trainees' Perception of The Impact on Adult Psychological-Emotional Status*. https://core.ac.uk/download/215491234.pdf (accessed on 11th June 2025).
9. Aytur, S., Bucci, J., & Wake, C. P. (2014). *An Assessment of The Impact of Climate Change on Human Health in New Hampshire*. https://core.ac.uk/download/84123597.pdf (accessed on 11th June 2025).
10. Aziz, M., & Anjum, G. (2024). Transformative strategies for enhancing women's resilience to climate change: A policy perspective for low- and middle-income countries. Women's Health, 20. https://www.semanticscholar.org/paper/041bdd4308423b3e4c177a82b45870293abefb63 (accessed on 11th June 2025).
11. Baker, D. V., Carlson, S., Ford, S., et al. (2014). *Considering Vermont's Future in a Changing Climate: The First Vermont Climate Assessment*. https://core.ac.uk/download/215155341.pdf (accessed on 11th June 2025).
12. Birnbaum, N., Masterson, E., & Schoomaker, H. (2011). *State of Health Equity Movement, 2011 Update Part C: Compendium of Recommendations DRA Project Report No. 11-03*. https://core.ac.uk/download/pdf/18491812.pdf (accessed on 11th June 2025).
13. Blashki, G. A., Burke, S., Fritze, J. G., et al. (2008). *Hope, Despair and Transformation: Climate Change and The Promotion of Mental Health and Wellbeing*. https://core.ac.uk/download/pdf/8195783.pdf (accessed on 11th June 2025).

14. Bond, N., Bumbaco, K., Cunningham, R., et al. (2023). *In the Hot Seat: Saving Lives from Extreme Heat in Washington State.* https://core.ac.uk/download/640913801.pdf (accessed on 11th June 2025).
15. Bowen, K. J., & Friel, S. (2012). Climate Change Adaptation: Where Does Global Health Fit into The Agenda? https://core.ac.uk/download/pdf/30678285.pdf (accessed on 11th June 2025).
16. Weiss Brown, E. (1993). *International Environmental Law: Contemporary Issues and The Emergence of a New World Order.* https://core.ac.uk/download/70375508.pdf (accessed on 11th June 2025).
17. Cameron, M. P. (2013). *The Demographic Implications of Climate Change for Aotearoa New Zealand: A Review.* https://core.ac.uk/download/29201665.pdf (accessed on 11th June 2025).
18. Cohen, M. H. (2021). The sum of us: What racism costs everyone and how we can prosper together. Harvard Educational Review, 91, 540–543. https://doi.org/10.17763/1943-5045-91.4.540.
19. Conley, L., & Werz, M. (2012). Climate Change, Migration, And Conflict: Addressing Complex Crisis Scenarios in the 21st Century. https://core.ac.uk/download/71356959.pdf (accessed on 11th June 2025).
20. Cook, A., Cunsolo Willox, A., Cunsolo Willox, A., Cunsolo Willox, A., Deckert, A., Downing, A., Durkalec, A., et al. (2015). *Climate-Sensitive Health Priorities in Nunatsiavut, Canada.* https://core.ac.uk/download/157728423.pdf (accessed on 11th June 2025).
21. Culp, D., Ebi, K. L., Petkova, E. P., et al. (2015). *Climate Change and Health on the U.S. Gulf Coast: Public Health Adaptation is Needed to Address Future Risks.* https://core.ac.uk/download/161451343.pdf (accessed on 11th June 2025).
22. Cunsolo, A., Harper, S. L., Minor, K., Hayes, K., Williams, K. G., & Howard, C. (2020). Ecological grief and anxiety: The start of a healthy response to climate change? *The Lancet Planetary Health, 4*, e261–e263. https://doi.org/10.1016/s2542-5196(20)30144-3.
23. Davis, A., Roper, L., & Miniszewski, U. (2015). *Climate Justice and Women's Rights: A Guide to Supporting Grassroots Women's Action.* https://core.ac.uk/download/75780604.pdf (accessed on 11th June 2025).
24. Deeb, A., French, A., Heiss, J., et al. (2011). *Responding to Climate Change: The Economy and Economics–Part of the Problem and Solution.* https://core.ac.uk/download/19441204.pdf (accessed on 11th June 2025).
25. Duyck, S., Heinämäki, L., Koivurova, T., et al. (2013). *Addressing Climate Vulnerability: Promoting The Participatory Rights of Indigenous Peoples and Women Through Finnish Foreign Policy.* https://core.ac.uk/download/29574458.pdf (accessed on 11th June 2025).
26. Dzokoto, R., Paintsil, M., Peprah, E. K., Ahiabor, S., & Norvivor, F. A. (2025). Climate change and flooding nexus: Water, sanitation, and hygiene (WASH) and mental health implications in Fuveme, Ghana. BioSocial Health Journal. https://www.semanticscholar.org/paper/a5959ff6c524d513555a8068fd9d3bfa5fb32dda (accessed on 11th June 2025).
27. Field, C. B., Dokken, D. J., Plattner, G. K., Mach, K. J., Ebi, K. L., Tignor, M., Mastrandrea, M. D., et al. (2012). *Managing the Risks of Extreme Events and Disasters to Advance Climate Change Adaptation: Special Report of the Intergovernmental Panel on Climate Change.* https://core.ac.uk/download/75777469.pdf (accessed on 11th June 2025).

28. Fortunato, K., & Sessions, K. (2015). Achieving a Climate for Health: Philanthropy to Promote Health and Justice Through the Challenges of Climate Change. https://core.ac.uk/download/480182799.pdf (accessed on 11th June 2025).

29. Gannon, G., Gearheard, S. F., Gerlach, S. C., et al. (2017). *Staying in Place During Times of Change in Arctic Alaska: The Implications of Attachment, Alternatives, and Buffering*. https://core.ac.uk/download/215529076.pdf (accessed on 11th June 2025).

30. Hassan, N. A., Ibrahim, F., Ismail, R., Mohd Tohit, M., et al. (2024). Symposium 3: Unmasking the Climate Change Challenge: Insight from Malaysia. https://core.ac.uk/download/639867581.pdf (accessed on 11th June 2025).

31. Hossain, M. Z. (2014). Pro-Poor Urban Adaptation to Climate Change in Bangladesh: A Study of Urban Extreme Poverty, Vulnerability and Asset Adaption. https://core.ac.uk/download/77035708.pdf (accessed on 11th June 2025).

32. Hutchuk, N. (2023). Exploring the Role of Public Health in Climate Change Initiatives and The Mining Industry in Ontario, Canada. https://core.ac.uk/download/581135735.pdf (accessed on 11th June 2025).

33. Kay, A., Mabin, A., Petherick, A., Saéz, A. M., Poteete, A. R., Price-Smith, A. T., Israel, B. A., et al. (2016). *The Social and Political Dimensions of The Ebola Response: Global Inequality, Climate Change, And Infectious Disease*. https://core.ac.uk/download/287659558.pdf (accessed on 11th June 2025).

34. Kilungo, A., Chukwuonye, G. N., Okpanachi, V. P., & Hussein, M. (2024). *Assessing Sub-Saharan Africa's Readiness to Address the Impact of Climate Change and Health: A Scoping Review*. https://www.semanticscholar.org/paper/9c1665868e829e66e1fd8e743561e365bf84123d (accessed on 11th June 2025).

35. Lee, A., Sheppard, M., Naughtin, C. K., Rebuli, M. A., & Brindal, E. (2025). Key predictors that characterize different stances on significant global scientific challenges: Comparing vaccine and climate change beliefs. *SAGE Open, 15*. https://www.semanticscholar.org/paper/a63209c12727bd93a7a48434f4dc5f78fba9e904 (accessed on 11th June 2025).

36. Luthfia, S. (2025). Learning approach to climate change education as a framework for sustainability education: A systematic review of literature. IJCER (International Journal of Chemistry Education Research). https://www.semanticscholar.org/paper/08d1a70cfa86760e2b516332f7080fa07578b85f (accessed on 11th June 2025).

37. Markandya, A., & Chou, W. J. (2025). *Eastern Europe and the Former Soviet Union Since the Fall of the Berlin Wall: Review of the Changes in the Environment and Natural Resources*. https://core.ac.uk/download/pdf/6291888.pdf (accessed on 11th June 2025).

38. Nash, N., Capstick, S., Whitmarsh, L., Chaudhary, I., & Manandhar, R. (2019). Perceptions of local environmental issues and the relevance of climate change in Nepal's Terai: Perspectives from two communities. Frontiers in Sociology, 4. https://www.semanticscholar.org/paper/238eb676870291baf0782968f77d5434f1e7471e (accessed on 11th June 2025).

39. O'Donnell, M., & Palinkas, L. A. (2024). Taking a trauma and adversity perspective to climate change mental health. European Journal of Psych traumatology, 15. https://www.semanticscholar.org/paper/a6018256c37940822f7ad10275bcf34d6757e050 (accessed on 11th June 2025).

40. Ozor, N., Nwakaire, J., Nyambane, A., Muhatiah, W., & Nwobodo, C. (2025). Enhancing Africa's agriculture and food systems through responsible and gender inclusive AI innovation: Insights from AI4AFS network. Frontiers in Artificial Intelligence, 7. https://www.semanticscholar.org/paper/4473fdee40c851a8edd67a07e949ec15d3089859 (accessed on 11th June 2025).

41. Pearce, A., Hughes, L., & Steffen, W. (2025). *The Heat Is On: Climate Change, Extreme Heat and Bushfires in WA.* https://core.ac.uk/download/pdf/30672522.pdf (accessed on 11th June 2025).

42. Perkins, P. E. (Ellie). (2017). University-Community Collaboration for Climate Justice Education and Organizing: Partnerships in Canada, Brazil, and Africa. https://core.ac.uk/download/287659513.pdf (accessed on 11th June 2025).

43. Sadd, J., Pastor, M., Morello-Frosch, R., & Shonkoff, S. B. (2009). The Climate Gap: Inequalities In How Climate Change Hurts Americans & How to Close the Gap. https://core.ac.uk/download/71342763.pdf (accessed on 11th June 2025).

44. Schorr, L. B., & Marchand, V. (2007). Pathway to Successful Young Adulthood. https://core.ac.uk/download/75786157.pdf (accessed on 11th June 2025).

45. Snover, A., Hansen, L. J., Jackson, L., Gregg, R. M., Ellworth, S., & Arroyo, V. (2013). *The State of Adaptation in the United States: An Overview*. https://core.ac.uk/download/71361521.pdf (accessed on 11th June 2025).

46. Sustainable Development Commission Scotland. (2012). Sustainable Development: Fourth Annual Assessment of Progress by the Scottish Government. https://core.ac.uk/download/1586739.pdf (accessed on 11th June 2025).

47. United Nations System Standing Committee on Nutrition. (2020). Water and Nutrition: Harmonizing Actions for the United Nations Decade of Action on Nutrition and the United Nations Water Action Decade. https://core.ac.uk/download/288633623.pdf (accessed on 11th June 2025).

48. White, A., Curcio, A., Lambert, D., McCredie, F., McGill, G., & Reinhardt, W. (2025). *Australian Water Consumer Outlook 2015.* https://core.ac.uk/download/pdf/30670969.pdf (accessed on 11th June 2025).

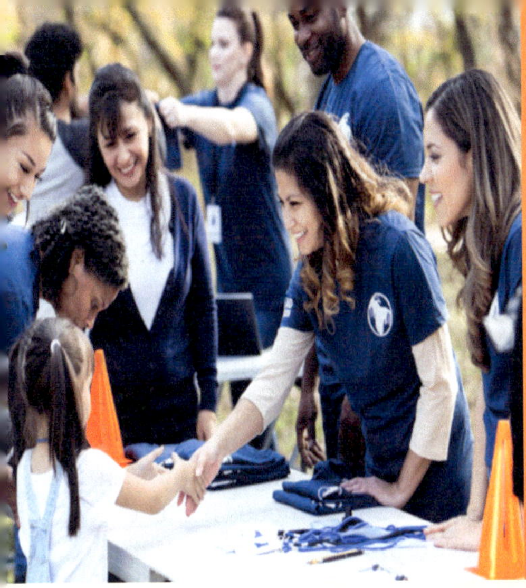

Chapter 3

SOCIAL DETERMINANTS OF HEALTH

Contents

Introduction

The social determinants of health are a group of interconnected factors that play a central role in influencing the health and well-being of people and communities. The determinants include economic stability, education, access to healthcare, and the built environment, among others. Understanding the engagement of these social determinants matters since they have a tendency to create inequalities in health, particularly among vulnerable populations. For instance, individuals with intellectual or developmental disabilities (IDD) face distinctive challenges that are magnified by social determinants, resulting in strong health disparities. The study showcased in Williams et al. (2024) illustrates the manner in which racial and ethnic minorities with IDD have aggregated obstacles to healthcare access and quality, which necessitates a more sophisticated answer to solving health inequities from an integrative viewpoint. On this aspect, the shift towards integrated models of care, as outlined in Rintjema et al. (2022), also lays emphasis on health and social care systems effectively collaborating to deal with social determinants of health. Through awareness of broader structural and institutional determinants of health results, integrated care strives to provide comprehensive solutions that extend beyond traditional models of healthcare. The move towards a population health management model is evidence of a growing recognition that health is more than mere absence of disease but is significantly influenced by social and economic determinants. Implementation of such models requires open governance structures, robust streams of funding, and the establishment of communication channels between stakeholders to ensure effective delivery of services and patient-centered care. Lastly, interventions that address social determinants of health need a multi-faceted approach, with policy reforms, enhanced participation by the community, and targeted health interventions. The findings by Williams et al. (2024) and Rintjema et al. (2022) necessitate the identification of specific obstacles to vulnerable populations and the development of differentiated interventions that ensure the fair provision of health. Placing these determinants center stage of health discussions and policymaking, the stakeholders can build a fairer and more equitable health setting. When efforts towards furthering an understanding of these social determinants are put into action, they will be a central impetus for furthering the realization of improved health benefits for all, particularly for those who have historically been underrepresented and disadvantaged in the healthcare system (Figure 3.1).

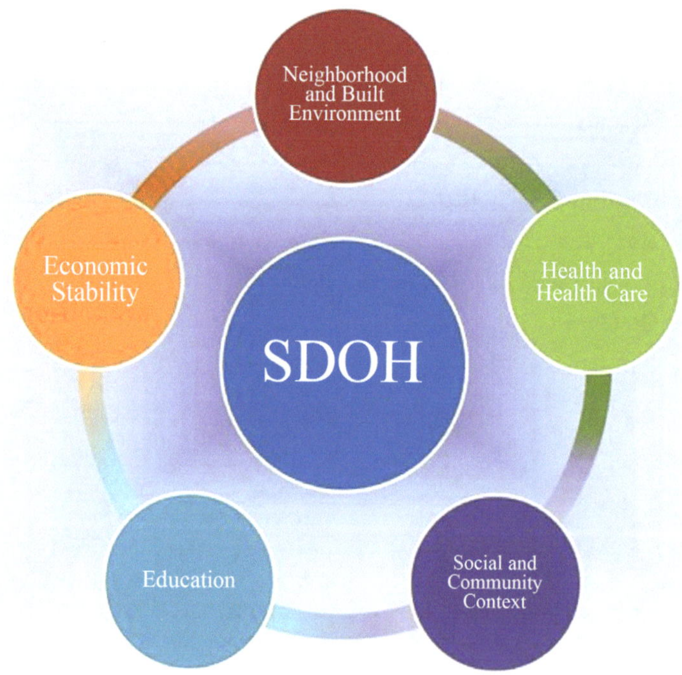

Figure 3.1. Common social determinants of health.

Source: https://bunny-wp-pullzone-3xue3q6yzy.b-cdn.net/resources/wp-content/uploads/2019/07/Social-Determinants-of-Health.jpg.

Definition of Social Determinants of Health

The concept of social determinants of health (SDOH) entails the various conditions where individuals are born, develop, live, work, and age, and they have a tremendous influence on their health.

Such determinants encompass a wide array of components such as socioeconomic status, education, physical setting and neighborhood, work, social support networks, and access to care. Awareness of such determinants is important, as the outcome of health is not directly determined by individual behaviors or by biological factors but is heavily affected by the social context within which people reside. For instance, children who grow up in socioeconomically deprived residential areas tend to do poorly in terms of their health, and this necessitates looking into the regional disparities in health status within different groups (Bryant et al., 2005). Recognition of these social determinants allows for a comprehensive response to public health policy for equity and improving the overall health of communities. Furthermore, some groups, such as the homeless, demonstrate the profound impact that social determinants have on health. Homeless individuals generally have multiple barriers that they must contend with, including limited availability of healthy food, inferior healthcare coverage, and housing instability, which all enhance their health risks. Evidence indicates that organizations serving this population increasingly include SDOH in intake assessments, and this indicates a growing recognition of such issues in determining health outcomes (Williams et al., 2024). Such organizations, leveraging their connections with community partners, are able to bridge resource gaps, although inconsistencies in the measurement of associated SDOH needs persist. Grasping and intervening upon these inequities is critical to enhancing health interventions and to guaranteeing that the most vulnerable groups are treated with the holistic support they need. The relation between SDOH and health equity is pertinent because variation in social conditions can strongly influence the creation of inequities in outcomes of health. For instance, geographic location is a key driver in the health of individuals, with regions in the southern United States consistently reporting poorer health indicators. This regional disparity is used to highlight the need to place health interventions within the relevant social and economic contexts (Bryant et al., 2005). Policymakers are going to have to consider the varied effects of SDOH when designing to address health disparities. Increased insight into such determinants among healthcare workers and the population can help in more effective health advocacy for policy change to address the root causes of health inequities, thereby leading to improved health and well-being for all groups.

Importance of Understanding Social Determinants

Social determinants are essential to be known to mitigate health inequities and promote health equity between various groups of individuals. Social determinants are heterogeneous factors like socioeconomic status, education, availability of medical care, and the built environment that all affect individual and community health outcomes. Knowing the determinants provides a framework for knowing the determinants of health inequities so that policymakers and health professionals may develop interventions to address them. Through the comprehension of the intricate interaction between these variables, stakeholders can direct action towards improving the conditions that lead to enhanced health outcomes, eventually building a more equitable society. The acknowledgment that health is influenced by determinants other than clinical care recognizes the value of intersectoral approaches integrating social determinants with health policy and practice, thereby transforming the broader context of public health interventions (Toaiamoandani et al., 2022). Exaggeration cannot be laid on the need for community engagement and collaboration in valuing social determinants. It has been witnessed through evidence that individuals' health behavior and status have powerful determinants within their immediate surroundings as well as within adjacent social networks. The engagement of the community within prioritization and determination of social determinants provides them with the authority to claim ownership of their health and voice changes needed. Moreover, encouraging cooperation among healthcare professionals, government, and civil society organizations can lead to innovative solutions to the multifaceted issues posed by social determinants. The partnerships can facilitate knowledge, data, and resource sharing and hence encourage public health programs' effectiveness. Hence, it is crucial to embrace community engagement as a means of creating sustainable interventions that respond to the individualized needs of disparate populations in a manner that promotes health equity and overall health outcomes (N/A, 2025).

The incorporation of social determinants in policy for health is not an exercise of the mind; it has profound practical utility. A review of urban health policy defines that such knowledge can inform the creation of more effective health interventions. A scoping review of the terminology used in urban health policy identified 83 determinants of health, a broad set of themes that included physical activity, safety, and access to basic services. This systematic approach helps to reduce the interdependence of the different determinants and their collective effect on health outcomes. Putting such issues at the forefront of policy agendas will allow decision-makers to implement evidence-based interventions tackling the root causes of health inequities. The resulting conceptual models are applicable in practice as well as in research, and they enable stakeholders to question the complex linkages between social determinants and health and ultimately affecting changes in population health (Toaiamoandani et al., 2022) (Figure 3.2).

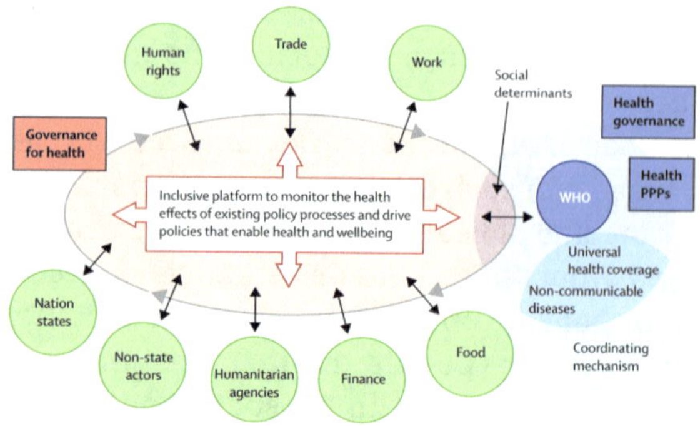

Figure 3.2. The political origins of health inequity.

Source: https://www.thelancet.com/cms/10.1016/S0140-6736(13)62407-1/asset/ded3ce15-ad8d-4cdf-97ee-f7ca7132f84e/main.assets/gr1_lrg.jpg.

3.1. Economic Stability

Economic stability is a foundation of the overall welfare of populations and plays an important role in establishing the social determinants of health. Economic stability provides access to essential determinants of good food, secure housing, and quality health care that are crucial for maintaining and improving health outcomes. Economic determinants shape resilience at the individual and collective level, defining their ability to respond to health adversity and adopt healthier lifestyles. The existence of secure employment opportunities not only provides economic security but also social integration and support systems, which reduce exposure to health risks through stress. It is therefore critical that policymakers recognize the determinants of economic stability in order to be able to minimize health inequalities and bring about equitable health outcomes in diverse populations. The relationship between economic stability and health outcomes is once more confirmed through the relationship between life expectancy and income inequality. Economic regions with high inequality have poor health among their population due to the fact that wealth concentration means restricted access to healthcare services and goods. Longitudinal data available here shows that areas with more income equity tend to enjoy improved longevity and improved general health status because individuals have greater access to education, stable employment, and social mobility. Further, the interaction between economic determinants such as health expenditures, nutrition, and food availability has a direct influence on life expectancy, which implies that economic stability is an important determinant of health in various contexts. This brings a focus on the intricate interactions between economic policy and its impacts on public health. Overcoming the challenges posed by economic insecurity requires cohesive policies to achieve economic growth as well as social justice. Policies such as investment in education, health, and infrastructure can have a positive impact on a stronger workforce, which ultimately leads to improved health outcomes. The adverse effects of unemployment and poverty on health can be mitigated with preventive measures such as policies aimed at employment and family support programs. Further, the implementation of social safety nets can provide a crucial input to vulnerable populations, thereby contributing to stability in their socioeconomic status. By recognizing economic stability as a part of the broader social determinants of health, stakeholders are able to develop targeted interventions that promote not only improved health outcomes but also sustainable long-term economic growth and social justice (Figure 3.3).

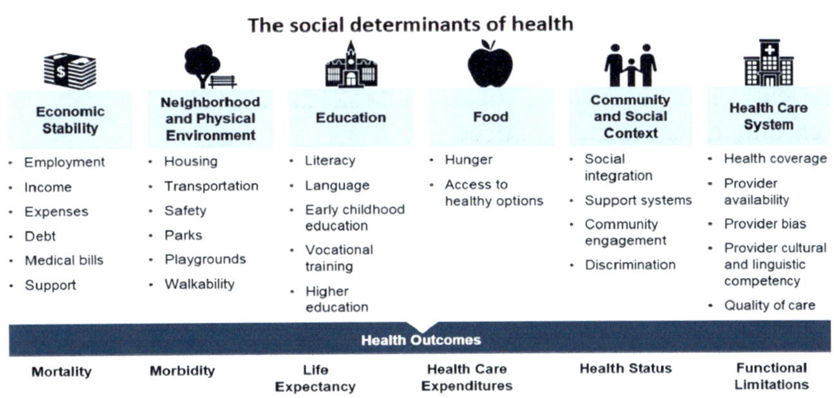

Figure 3.3. Economic stability for social determinants of health.

Source: https://www.center4healthandsdc.org/uploads/7/1/1/4/71142589/published/sdoh-graphic.png?1528489655.

3.1.1. Impact of Income on Health Outcomes

Income levels are a key factor in influencing health outcomes as an important social determinant of health. Individuals with higher income are more likely to have access to better health care facilities, good food, and a better environment, which results in good overall health outcomes. Individuals with lower incomes are more likely to face barriers that keep them from being able to access good health care and follow a healthy life. Such inequality transcends a matter of individual choice and is one of the structural disparities that produce health consequences from economic conditions. While health inequalities persist along socio-economic gradients, understanding the role of income provides valuable lessons into the complicated dynamic between economic status and health. In order to counter these disparities, a comprehensive approach with policy interventions toward improving healthcare and other resource availability among economically disadvantaged populations is essential (Toaiamoandani et al., 2022). Besides, the impact of income on health status extends beyond individual choice to encompass broader environmental and social determinants. Economically disadvantaged neighborhoods generally experience substandard housing conditions, limited access to play spaces, and excessive exposure to environmental risk factors such as pollution. These drivers, in aggregate, contribute to poor health outcomes such as respiratory disease, obesity, and mental illness. Zoning policy all too frequently exacerbates these issues, generating environmental injustices that disproportionately fall on low-income urban minorities. Low income is also associated with poor health outcomes via stress induced by financial instability that potentially fuels elevated rates of chronic diseases and reduced overall health. The environmental determinants of income bring to light the quintessential need for convergent solutions to economic as well as health inequalities (Rodriquez et al., 2020). To understand comprehensively the implications of income on health outcomes, it is critical to look into the intersectionality of certain social determinants. The convergence of income, education, and access to healthcare yields a complex platform where each affects the others. For instance, improved income usually goes hand in hand with better opportunities for education, which further enable one to make healthy choices and access quality health care services. Conversely, restricted income can restrict chances for education and spread a cycle of health inequity that is difficult to break. With the intricate interactions between these determinants, policy interventions that target income alone without targeting education or access to healthcare may not translate to creating substantial improvements in health outcomes. A multifaceted approach, therefore, which acknowledges and accepts various social determinants of health, is necessary in enhancing health equity and outcomes in populations with varying backgrounds (Toaiamoandani et al., 2022) (Figure 3.4).

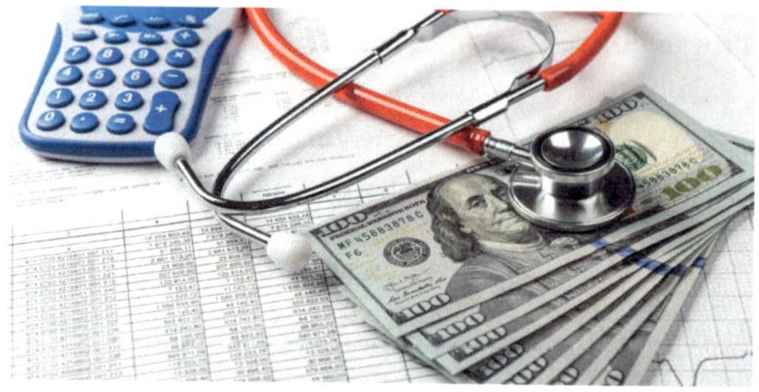

Figure 3.4. Income and health.

Source: https://external-content.duckduckgo.com/iu/?u=https%3A%2F%2Fcdn.magloft.com%2Fpdf-import%2F850%2Fimages%2Fimg_22-1.jpg&f=1&nofb=1&ipt=01b98608b21efe381e2270e32dfce07e5709a286bc2a515ba444a24df14a66a2.

3.1.2. Employment Status and Access to Healthcare

Employment status plays an important role in determining the availability of healthcare to individuals, not just in the availability of health insurance but also in the quality of care received. Employees typically have health insurance provided by their employers, and this helps significantly in reducing the expense of healthcare as well as in overall access to necessary medical treatment. Conversely, the unemployed and the under-employed are often without health insurance, creating heightened economic barriers to medical care. The gap is even greater in times of economic downturn, as higher rates of unemployment are joined by higher unmet medical care needs. For instance, studies discover that work status and income are good predictors of unmet health needs, particularly within austerity settings, as is the case in Greece during its recent economic crisis (Kyriopoulos et al., 2016). Such findings fit the dramatic influence of employment on access to health care, highlighting a key point of the social determinants of health. The COVID-19 pandemic has also complicated the relationship between healthcare access and employment status, particularly with the increased use of work-from-home policies. As employees transitioned from working to working from home, their employment status changed in a way that affected access to health insurance coverage and healthcare. Research revealed that telecommuting workers suffered from productivity and psychological challenges that are interwoven in their work environments (Graham et al., 2024). Lack of in-person interactions and minimal social support often left individuals feeling isolated, which might have adverse consequences for their willingness to seek care when needed. This case indicates that there should be robust employer support systems in place that are able to campaign for mental health units and uphold access to healthcare services. The problems are vital in the context of improving the well-being of workers within the context of shifting employment circumstances. Lastly, the relationship between employment status and the accessibility of healthcare is a key area for policy intervention. Legislative action toward ensuring employment security and comprehensive coverage of all healthcare for all individuals, regardless of employment status, is the solution to reducing health disparities. All evidence demonstrates that expanding income and employment is directly related to improved healthcare access, as also noted by research that studied economic factors affecting healthcare needs (Kyriopoulos et al., 2016). Moreover, designing an employee-friendly work environment can overcome remote work issues and promote overall mental well-being (Graham et al., 2024). Hence, integrating employment programs with health policy initiatives will be pivotal in containing the broader social determinants of health, aiming to create a fairer health care system for multisectoral populations.

3.1.3. Housing Stability and Its Effects on Well-Being

The stability of housing is currently considered one of the fundamental determinants of health outcomes, with particular implications for individuals' physical and mental health. The lack of housing stability can potentially lead to chronic stress, anxiety, and other negative health-related consequences. In circumstances where individuals are subject to housing instability, they may incur disruptions in their capacity to receive essential services like healthcare, education, and employment opportunities. As signaled in the social determinants of health framework, stable housing serves as a foundation for healthier lifestyle promotion and health disparity reduction. This is particularly relevant for vulnerable populations, who frequently experience a layered set of socioeconomic forces that amplify their threat of eviction and homelessness and further reinforce poverty and poor health cycles (Hernandez et al., 2023). The New Beginning Educational Workshop illustrates the critical intersection of housing stability and empowerment. The workshop focuses on educating tenants whose lives have been harmed by eviction histories and highlights the importance of education to temper barriers to stable housing. By providing tenants with mechanisms to expunge eviction records, the workshop addresses embedded inequities blocking access to secure and affordable housing. This initiative is a heightened recognition of how structural factors lead to housing instability and its corresponding health impacts. In bringing education and advocacy together, these initiatives aim to dismantle barriers to stable housing, leading to improved health outcomes and allowing individuals in communities to reclaim their narratives (Hernandez et al., 2023). Moreover, research underscores the connection between the characteristics of neighborhoods and overall well-being, with a focus on the contribution of place-based concerns to the discussion of housing stability. Research identifies that people who live in traditionally disadvantaged neighborhoods with poor housing conditions and fewer resources have higher levels of health disparities and chronic disease. The relationship between area disadvantage and housing instability demonstrates how the underlying disparities are reflected in community well-being as well as health at the individual level. Recent research emphasizes that minimizing these disparities with targeted policies has the potential to create stable living situations that enhance community health. Investments in housing infrastructure and neighborhood development are essential in crafting balanced living conditions that foster overall well-being and health equity (Rao et al., 2024) (Figure 3.5).

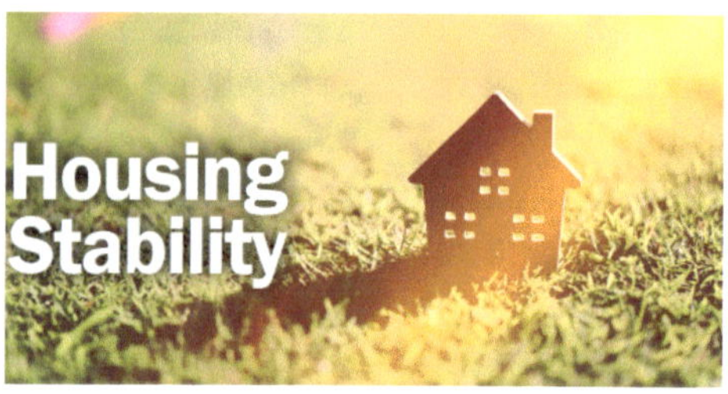

Figure 3.5. Housing stability and its effects on well-being.

Source: https://humanservices.vermont.gov/sites/ahsnew/files/styles/500_/public/2023-08/HousingstabilityWIDE1920%20890%20FS48.png?itok=YGBFvz_f.

3.2. Education

Education is a social determinant of health that has a profound impact on individual and community well-being. Further education is linked to improved health, with those who attain increased levels of education tending to have increased levels of health literacy and being better able to access and use healthcare services. It is not simply a matter of personal responsibility but also one of the societal environment that determines how much education one can gain. For instance, disparities in education access perpetuate poverty and poor health outcomes, demonstrating how education levels become imbricated with socioeconomic conditions. A health equity framework should identify such disparate opportunities in education, particularly among vulnerable groups, to address the root causes of health inequalities (Calender et al., 2016). In addition, educational institutions have an important role to promote better health. Schools are not only places for learning but also environments where children acquire health education and health services, in an attempt to highlight the importance of healthy living choices. An implementation of school health education programs can equip students with knowledge about nutrition, physical activity, and mental well-being, eventually leading them to transform habits of long-term health. Nonetheless, challenges that cross-cut encompass underfunding and scarce resources, disproportionately affecting schools in poor communities. Addressing such obstacles is central to creating learning environments that foster scholastic and health successes among students (Saeed et al., 2023). Other than physical schooling experiences, community support systems play an essential role in forming educational accomplishments and, consequently, health outcomes. Having access to ancillary materials, such as tutoring, mentorship programs, and after-school activities, can enhance students' performance and engagement at school. These types of resources are particularly important to low-income students who may face many barriers to success. Furthermore, community involvement in education can lead to a culture of health that transcends the school day by creating collaborative activities between schools, families, and community organizations to improve overall health outcomes. Whenever schools and communities collaborate to support learning as well as health-related projects, the chances of contributing positively to public health in the long term are significantly heightened (Calender et al., 2016).

3.2.1. Role of Education in Health Literacy

The crossroads of health education play a critical role in addressing social determinants of health. Education equips individuals with the skills for understanding and navigating complex health information, critical to making effective decisions about health. For instance, well-educated individuals are likely to be well-placed to read health-related information, adhere to medical advice, and engage in preventive health practices. Such basic information not only forms individual health but also promotes community awareness and overall health outcomes. As noted by Doosti et al. (2018), interventions that are health literacy-oriented and directed towards enhancing the same have proven to increase health-promoting behaviors substantially, suggesting that customized educational programs can empower individuals to take control of their health. Second, education is also important beyond individual advantage in that it has a bearing on public health equity. Health literacy is firmly grounded in the social determinants model that emphasizes contextual determinants of health outcomes. School and community-based educational interventions can potentially decrease health disparities through improved equitable access to health information and resources. Professional practice in education, as explained in Cummings et al. (2023), promotes the implementation of measures that facilitate health literacy within communities through the application of methods that guarantee social justice. Through this type of education, empowering vulnerable communities is a possibility in a way that enables them to move against barriers to well-being and health that come with the unjust social organization. Finally, the connection between education and health literacy is mutual, with either providing a catalyst that facilitates progress in the other. Education systems that are health literacy-minded assist in building well-educated citizens who engage actively within society. Active engagement is necessary for fixing systemic health issues and promoting policy reforms leading to better health outcomes. Curricula that include health education as part of their programs serve not only as a medium of information but also as a location for the building of critical thinking and self-efficacy among future generations. Last but not least, an integrated program of health education fosters resilience and empowerment with a foundation for lifelong health-promoting behavior, according to studies in Doosti et al. (2018); Cummings et al. (2023) (Figure 3.6).

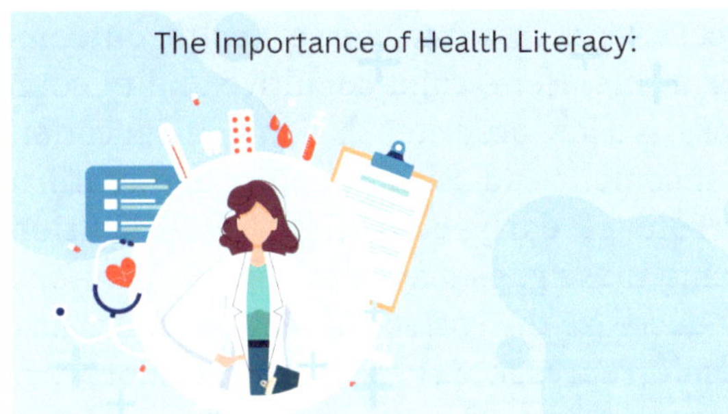

Figure 3.6. The importance of health literacy.

Source: https://www.cspmsolutions.com/wp-content/uploads/2023/05/hghg.png.

3.2.2. Correlation Between Educational Attainment and Health

The relationship between educational attainment and health is a central element of the assessment of social determinants of health. Educational attainment is associated with better health, such as lower chronic disease rates and better mental health. This relationship can partly be attributed to persons having more education having more desirable occupations, which typically provide not only greater earnings but also such things as health insurance. As a result, more well-educated individuals are likely to embrace healthy living and be more aware of health issues. In contrast, less well-educated individuals may be subject to a range of types of deprivation, which can result in poor health and compound cycles of ill health and poverty. Thus, education effectively functions as a modulator between general health and socioeconomic status and is extremely valuable in providing equitable access to quality education. Most importantly, the interaction between education and health is further influenced by the broader social and economic determinants. Studies have shown that early influences such as cognitive function and social environment profoundly affect educational attainment, and, in turn, this affects the health status in adulthood. For instance, disadvantaged children typically face many obstacles that can discourage academic success, and in turn, worse health outcomes later in life. Here, child cognitive ability comes across as a key predictor that shapes educational advancement and social mobility and reaffirms the role of early educational interventions. Closing these gaps may entail systemic reforms that decrease the socioeconomic obstacles faced by underrepresented groups. Furthermore, what occurs to people during their early years might prove to be the key to unlocking means through which education can facilitate or contribute to health throughout life and general community health. There has been evidence linking a mixed and even contradictory relationship between education levels and obesity, which yet again adds another layer of complexity to the controversy regarding education and health outcomes. While some studies indicate a weak negative correlation between obesity and education, consideration must be given to the variables that may confound this relationship, e.g., socioeconomic status and mental well-being. The impact of obesity on education may be because of many issues, e.g., mental illness, stigmatization, and exclusion. (Caird et al., 2011) points out that students who perform poorly academically tend to be obese due to lifestyle choices influenced by their residential areas. Conversely, poorer academic performance in obese children may be caused by reduced participation in physical activities and social interactions. These intricate relationships need to be determined in order to design comprehensive public health interventions in addressing academic inequalities and health disparities, ultimately towards a healthier population.

3.2.3. Access to Quality Education and Community Health

Availability of good education is an important column in the broader picture of community health and influences various social determinants of health. Good education equips one with information and capabilities that allow them to make appropriate health decisions, leading to healthier living and preventive health practices. Besides, educational levels are positively related to socioeconomic status; more educated persons are more likely to get employment in good companies, leading to greater economic stability. This relationship is revealed when consideration is given to the gaps that are suffered by the disadvantaged groups, which in turn usually suffer from barriers to accessing good-quality education, leading to a cycle of poor health. The interaction between health and education elucidates that enhancing educational opportunities is not something that can be addressed in isolation, but is an essential component of enhancing general community well-being. At the community level, the availability of quality education directly impacts the social environment that influences well-being and health. Schools are significant providers of health education, providing learners with education regarding nutrition, physical activity, and mental health, which may constitute long-term healthy habits. Schools in areas with access to resources also have a tendency to offer adolescents extensive health services ranging from mental guidance to physical examination. Educational inequities can mirror and consolidate health inequities, as poorly funded schools might not possess the programs to fight health issues with optimal efficacy. Thus, the community investment in education plays a vital role in eradicating health disparities as well as enhancing population resilience through more even access to healthcare services and improved health outcomes. In addition, the interconnect between education, economic stability, and health emphasizes the multifaceted nature of social determinants. As stated, individuals with lower levels of education often experience a chain reaction of disadvantages in the form of poor employment opportunities and inadequate health insurance coverage that significantly erode health outcomes. Their interconnectedness is, nevertheless, also further stressed by research detailing how obstacles to education, such as food insecurity and harmful neighborhoods, contribute to increased risks of mental disorders like anxiety and depression. Interventions into problems of access to and quality of education are therefore offered to potentially lead to improved mental health and well-being, stressing the need to intervene into these social determinants. Where communities seek more health improvements, an ambitious approach addressing educational inequalities can be instrumental in designing healthier, more equitable societies (Liu et al., 2025; LaManna et al., 2024) (Figure 3.7).

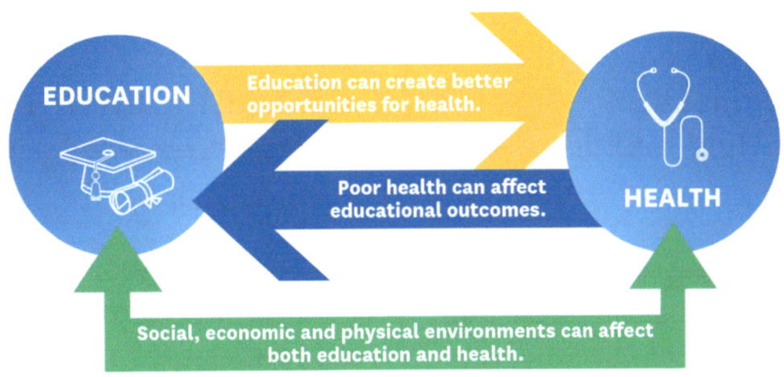
EDUCATION
Education can create better opportunities for health.
Poor health can affect educational outcomes.
HEALTH
Social, economic and physical environments can affect both education and health.

Figure 3.7. Access to quality education and community health.

Source: https://external-content.duckduckgo.com/iu/?u=http%3A%2F%2Fcohealthinitiative.org%2Fwp-content%2Fuploads%2F2019%2F10%2FEducation-Health-1024x512.png&f=1&nofb=1&ipt=cd51f9b173e5e60bc12f9f011403ef68cb4ac3f6596e31f020132a68d1ec2a5d.

3.3. Social and Community Context

The social and community context is one of the central frameworks in the broader universe of social determinants of health, encompassing the numerous ways that an individual's social environment influences their health outcome. The context includes the networks of family, friends, and neighbors, and the cultural and societal norms existing within a community. For example, behavioral health issues have a tendency to occur not solely from individual decision-making but are determined substantially by social conditions of living. The interconnectedness of the social factors creates environments that support and detract from health. Health improvement mechanisms must then account for the varying social dynamics at play, with the acknowledgment that health itself is not an individual problem but one of community concern and collaboration in the promotion of healthier environments and lifestyles (Storie et al., 2017). Beyond this, an awareness of the context of the community permits effective mitigation of specific health concerns in differing populations. Socio-economically disadvantaged groups or those with trauma histories can be prone to disparity in health outcomes. Experiences of Aboriginal and Torres Strait Islander peoples, for instance, are indicative of the urgency to address the socio-historic determinants that are integrated into health. Social and emotional well-being is a model that extends beyond traditional measures of health to encompass cultural identity, relationship to place, and family as core elements of health and health-seeking behavior. By comprehending the unique social dynamics that influence certain populations, stakeholders can create more effective, culturally sensitive health interventions. This holistic method is important in being capable of empowering communities with a degree of agency over health outcomes, enabling resilience and social determinants that fundamentally redefine improved decisions regarding health (Brodie et al., 2023).

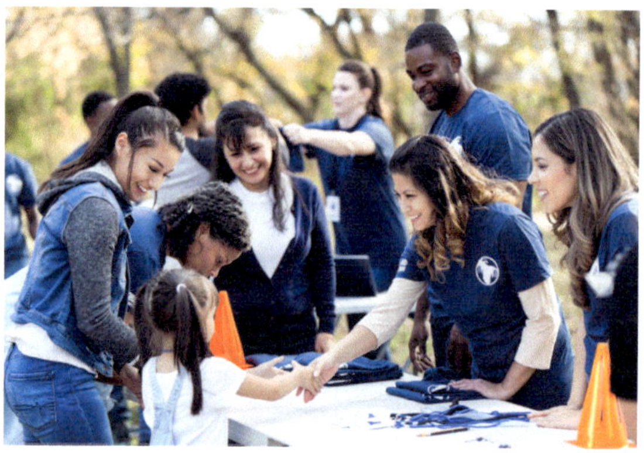

Figure 3.8. Social and community context.

Source: https://cwig-prod-prod-drupal-s3fs-us-east-1.s3.amazonaws. com/public/images/94- community.jpg? VersionId= TdX793mkLKUoneln23 XGEEyDuVmH0JKY.

Finally, by effectively mitigating the impacts of detrimental social determinants, partnership at the community level must be prioritized. This requires building partnerships among community agencies, government agencies, and residents to create health-promoting settings. Cross-sector initiatives can address not only individual behavior but also the structural determinants that sustain health disparities. For example, holistic programs in housing, education, and employment sectors can offer a sustained support system that encourages marginalized communities. Systemic change can only be realized through the exploration of existing data and evidence to act upon set priorities. By embracing an integrative strategy that considers various perspectives and comments, health programs can be better aligned with the unique needs of communities and ultimately lead to long-term gains in health outcomes for all (Storie et al., 2017) (Figure 3.8).

3.3.1. Influence of Social Networks on Health Behaviors

Influence on health behavior of social networks is a most important but underemphasized component of social determinants of health. Social connections, such as family, peer, and community relationships, play a significant role in the individual's health habits and attitudes. Studies have shown that people are more likely to develop healthy habits when they have strong social networks in favor of these habits. For instance, the ones with health-conscious friends eat healthier and exercise more. Poor or negative social connections lead to increased stress, unhealthy eating, and prolonged periods of sitting.

The social network and health behavior connection confirms the importance of health-supporting community relationships and demonstrates that being healthy involves much more than an individual process but is well-rooted in social environments. In addition, the intersection of mental health and social networks provides additional detail on the potency of social determinants. Healthy social relationships have the ability to lower depression and loneliness, which are central components of the overall picture of health. Gerontology studies highlight that older persons with dense social networks perform better in mental health and the control of chronic illness. Moreover, shared social experiences within social groups can yield a consensus perception of health-related concerns, facilitating talk about coping and lifestyle interventions. This is particularly relevant for marginalized social groups, where social support might be less accessible but is paramount in the promotion of mental health resilience in the face of adversities. Such a symbiotic relationship between social networks and health behavior, therefore, necessitates an integrated model of health promotion that is sensitive to the strength of social ties. Secondly, the impact of social determinants also extends to the function that social networks have in bridging health inequities. Socioeconomic status, for instance, significantly factors into both the formation and quality of social relationships with implications for resources that beget health. Adolescent women, during pregnancy, face particular stresses that can challenge social relationships, testing maladaptive coping responses like tension-driven, poorly nourished diets. Awareness of the stressors inherent in specific social contexts is essential to developing effective interventions for health. Strengthening efforts in communities can stimulate healthy behavior and thus have a lasting influence on health. As highlighted in the symposium, the inclusion of social and cultural determinants other than race only is important in determining health behavior among various groups (Baker et al., 2020; Bucciarelli et al., 2024). Understanding these intricate forces allows public health interventions to be better designed to foster facilitating environments to enhance health outcomes through increased social networks.

3.3.2. Effects of Discrimination and Social Cohesion

Discrimination is a powerful social determinant with wide-ranging impacts on health outcomes, particularly for oppressed groups. The effects of discrimination can be both acute and chronic and lead to various conditions of psychological distress. Studies, for example, that of migrants in Sweden, indicate that various forms of discrimination increase the risk of mental illness, particularly when combined with other social determinants like socioeconomic status and social cohesion. The findings indicated that differences in native and migrant psychological distress were significantly mitigated when the aforementioned social determinants were accounted for, illustrating the central role that acceptance and integration play in shaping health experiences. Specifically, analysis suggested that efforts to enhance social cohesion would be able to mitigate more effectively the detrimental effects of discrimination, thus resulting in improved overall health among affected groups (Honkaniemi et al., 2020). Social cohesion, or social relation quality consistency, and sense of belonging to a community, is one of the main determinants that promote health and well-being. In such settings characterized by strong social relations, individuals are in a position to utilize available resources, adopt health-protective behaviors, and continue being supportive of one another during an emergency. The relationship between social cohesion and health behavior, particularly among heterogeneous Latino communities in America, reflects this importance. Evidence has indicated that higher neighborhood cohesion is related to less prevalent smoking and more prevalent quitting, particularly in some Latino groups. This suggests that communities supporting high connectivity may buffer individuals against health-damaging behaviors linked with discrimination and stress. Social cohesion is thus central to the creation of supportive environments that can lead to improved health outcomes across different populations (Delva et al., 2012). The dynamic of discrimination and social cohesion illustrates the necessity of intervention and policy towards systemic concerns in marginalized groups. With high priorities assigned to interventions that minimize discrimination and maximize social cohesion, public health interventions can directly intervene on health disparities. Some potential interventions include community development initiatives that build inclusive environments, expanding mental health access, and promoting civic engagement of marginalized groups. These efforts can help to significantly mitigate the psychological burdens carried by those who are discriminated against and create a healthier social fabric conducive to overall well-being. As findings indicate, addressing these interrelated problems may not only promote individual health but also create healthier communities that can thrive in spite of societal challenges (Honkaniemi et al., 2020; Delva et al., 2012) (Figure 3.9).

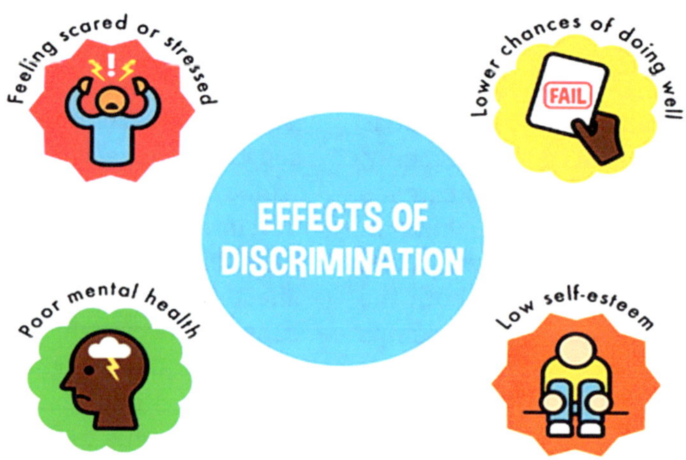
Feeling scared or stressed
Lower chances of doing well
FAIL
EFFECTS OF DISCRIMINATION
Poor mental health
Low self-esteem

Figure 3.9. Effects of discrimination.

Source: https://external-content.duckduckgo.com/iu/?u=https%3A%2F%2Fichef.bbci.co.uk%2Fimages%2Fic%2F480xn%2Fp0gsqdbd.png&f=1&nofb=1&ipt=bcb16fefa20c7028da28cc9a6e73b1f019873c01f10d020aafd681e7973d1809.

3.3.3. Community Engagement and Health Outcomes

The complexities of health outcomes are likely to reverberate in the framework of community engagement, which is a pivotal factor in addressing most of the social determinants of health. Community engagement is about the active involvement of individuals within a community in making decisions that affect their health and lives. It is not merely the dissemination of information but also the facilitation of an environment where the people are empowered and fully informed. Such empowerment is particularly crucial when dealing with health disparities because vulnerable groups tend to face obstacles that limit their access to quality health care. By means of an acknowledgment of the impact of social determinants such as economic stability and access to healthcare, community-based interventions can be strategically implemented in a bid to counteract these disparities, hence improving overall health outcomes in heterogeneous groups. Research has further illuminated the importance of social determinants in shaping health-seeking behavior, especially during times of public health crises. The Rapid Acceleration of Diagnostics-Underserved Populations (RADx-UP) initiative, for instance, shows how community engagement helps illuminate pathways between social determinants and health outcomes, specifically with respect to COVID-19 testing accessibility. Guided participation, via participatory approaches, allowed researchers to identify salient variables that influenced testing behaviors, such as health literacy and resource access. These results demonstrate that the reaction to the social determinants of health through proactive community action not only increases access to core services but also creates an informed and healthy community. In demonstrating such correlations, stakeholders are able to better plan interventions, closing gaps in health care access and generating equitable health outcomes, underscoring the value of integrating community voices into public health policy.

In addition, the widespread discussion of aging populations further emphasizes the massive impact of social determinants on health outcomes. As increasing numbers of elderly cancer survivors have complicated care needs, being aware of their social determinants works to enhance survivorship outcomes. Evidence reveals that neighborhoods, social networks, and access to healthcare significantly affect these individuals' health trajectories. Through the inclusion of community engagement in cancer care models, healthcare professionals are more likely to target the social determinants. Initiatives that align with access to high-quality care and the development of supportive community networks advance survivorship outcomes but also general well-being. Thus, developing a participatory environment that recognizes the complex nature of social determinants provides the potential for innovative interventions that can improve health outcomes for older adults and other vulnerable populations, which reiterates the critical importance of public health community engagement.

3.4. Health and Healthcare

Social determinants of health are inherent in affecting health outcomes, particularly in vulnerable populations that experience many challenges. Economic stability, being a component of these determinants, plays a great role in individuals' health-related quality of life (HRQoL). As an instance, one recent study found that higher family income correlates with improved HRQoL outcomes for cancer survivors, indicating that economic resources not only facilitate access to healthcare but also enhance overall well-being. Participants from more affluent backgrounds boasted better physical and mental health, underscoring the importance of addressing economic disparities as a component of health policy. By developing comprehensive interventions that account for economic differences, the health system can improve health equity and improve the well-being of individuals moving through transformative health states, such as cancer survivorship (Peitz et al., 2024). Apart from economic concerns, education is also a determinant of health outcomes. Quality education access is influential, as it equips people with the skills and knowledge required for informed health decision-making, thereby influencing their engagement with healthcare systems. A strong correlation of healthcare access with socioeconomic status (SES) was observed in a study of glioblastoma patients, with the result indicating that patients in lower SES quartiles had longer hospital stays and poorer outcomes. The disparities still prevailed, indicating that education and awareness regarding healthcare are needed to promote the well-being of underprivileged communities. Closing educational disparities enables healthcare interventions to achieve an educated patient population, which in turn leads to healthier behaviors and better health outcomes (Zerubabbel et al., 2024). Access to health also remains a fundamental component of the social determinants of health. Patients from lower ethnic and racial groups generally experience challenges in accessing good healthcare services, resulting in enormous health disparities. The data for glioblastoma patients revealed the disproportionate number of non-White individuals as part of the lowest SES, which had a direct impact on the outcomes of treatment. Insurance status—higher outcomes for privately insured patients—is only one of the indicators revealing how access to care can overcome the pernicious effects of adverse social determinants. Enhancing health care access via policy reform aimed at minimizing disparity can significantly boost health outcomes and quality of life for all, particularly those under systemic barriers (Zerubabbel et al., 2024) (Figure 3.10).

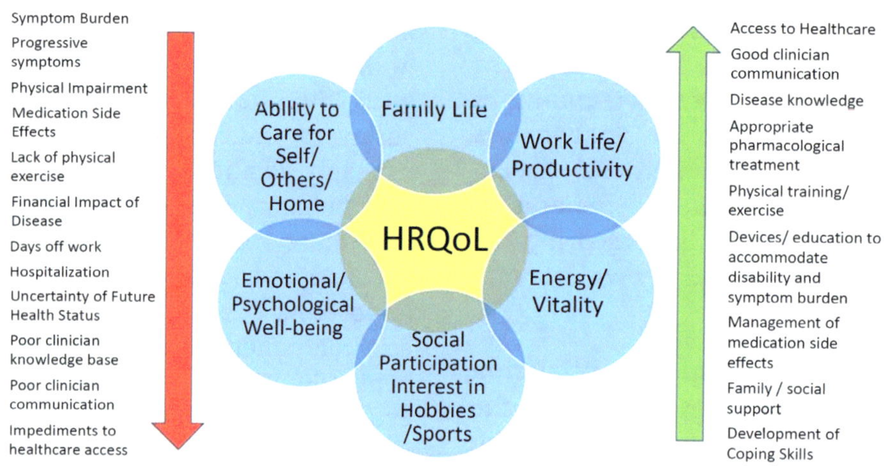

Figure 3.10. Health-related quality of life (HRQoL).

Source: https://www.mdpi.com/diagnostics/diagnostics-11-01089/article_deploy/html/images/diagnostics-11-01089-g002.png.

3.4.1. Access to Healthcare Services

Healthcare access is a critical component in social determinants of health research, as various obstructions can be present to prevent people from getting suitable medical attention. Socioeconomic status, location, and availability of healthcare services are accessibility factors. Individuals of lower socioeconomic status often experience more than one barrier, including a lack of transport and a lack of finances to pay for services or insurance. This non-uniform access is also sustained by structural determinants such as policies that fail to accommodate the needs of the most disadvantaged populations. Additionally, variation in healthcare access can enhance health disparities, necessitating interventions of inclusive practice by healthcare systems to confront these inequities and enable all individuals, regardless of their socioeconomic status, to access the healthcare services they require. Cultural background is also just as vital in shaping individuals' healthcare experience, particularly for multicultural ethnic groups. Research indicates that cultural practices and beliefs significantly influence how communities talk about health, obtain care, and comprehend health information. For instance, caregiving practices within the Asian American communities may vary from those common among Caucasian communities, affecting their sexual and reproductive health service access. A sense of these differences is required by health care providers who want to deliver good quality patient care. Findings from a study that included female college students from diverse cultures underscore the importance of culturally competent health communication strategies that not only acknowledge but respect such differences. Tailoring health care to take into account cultural variations can encourage a more inclusive environment, ultimately enhancing access to necessary services for all (Ly et al., 2024). Besides cultural factors, experiences of immigrant populations demonstrate the intricacy of accessing health care. Evidence indicates that Hispanic Latino immigrants typically experience strong barriers due to their unique sociocultural situations. Health barriers like language, fear of discrimination, and economic instability can compromise their ability to access healthcare. Political and historical background further contribute to this complexity and shape the healthcare environment for these groups. Understanding the perceived facilitators and barriers to healthcare access can guide the planning of culturally tailored and effective interventions. Further, surmounting these obstacles necessitates acquaintance with the broader social frameworks that sustain health disparities in access, such as race, ethnicity, and the legacies of colonial histories in the Americas. Through a critical examination of these factors, healthcare systems can strive to eliminate disparities and promote a more equitable health landscape for all individuals (Edward et al., 2013).

3.4.2. Quality of Healthcare and Its Implications

Health care quality is a critical determinant of general health outcomes and has a significant influence on the impact of health disparities across various populations. Quality health care access can reverse the negative impacts of socioeconomic disadvantage and eventually lead to improved health status and quality of life. In regions with higher unemployment and poverty levels, such as in the case of Italy, individuals also have poorer health since the living standards and the healthcare system are substandard (Franzini et al., 2025). Regional measures directed at quality access to healthcare and addressing general social determinants can then address inequalities and enhance the health of vulnerable groups. The interconnected nature of healthcare, social, and economic determinants underscores the importance of an integrated approach to quality improvement in healthcare that would form the basis for reducing health disparities. Moreover, the impact of healthcare quality is not only on individual health but also reaches workforce participation and economic production. For instance, adults with serious mental illness (SMI) have poorer health outcomes and higher healthcare costs compared to the general population, and these can further perpetuate unemployment among this group (O'Neill et al., 2018). The liaison between physical well-being and employment among SMI individuals highlights the requirement for integrated healthcare policies that address not only mental illnesses but also physical health conditions. By considering the dynamic interplay between employment status, healthcare quality, and health-related quality of life, policymakers can devise specific interventions that stimulate both health and economic participation of marginalized populations. In this manner, healthcare quality emerges as an important propellant of broader social and economic processes. Finally, healthcare quality has implications for community health since differences in access to consistent and effective healthcare services create systemic health inequities. Socioeconomic and geographic factors significantly impact the quality and amount of healthcare services delivered to different populations. For the majority of cases, the marginalized groups are faced with barriers such as transportation limitations, insurance policies, and services not being accessible, rendering the services hard to access (Franzini et al., 2025). These need to be overcome through consistent and coordinated strategies that extend beyond the improvement of healthcare delivery but also encompass supportive actions to modify living circumstances and health behavior within the groups. By achieving this, we can create environments favoring health equity and empower individuals to improve their health outcomes, thus defining the long-term implications of healthcare quality as a social determinant of health (Figure 3.11).

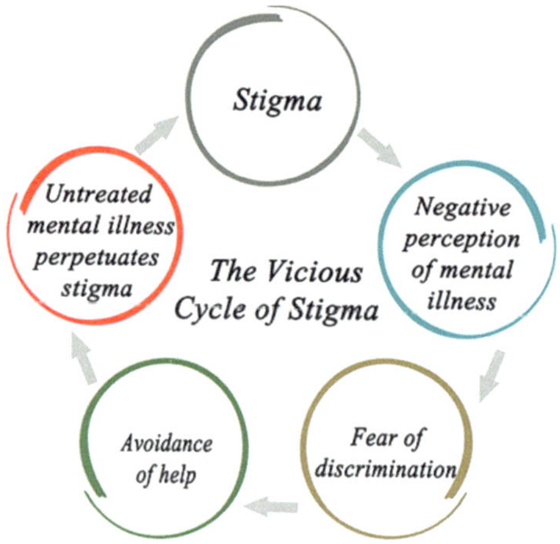
Stigma
Negative perception of mental illness
Fear of discrimination
Avoidance of help
Untreated mental illness perpetuates stigma
The Vicious Cycle of Stigma

Figure 3.11. Serious mental illness.

Source: https://external-content.duckduckgo.com/iu/?u=https%3A%2F%2Fwww.cvhnc.org%2Fwp-content%2Fuploads%2F2023%2F08%2FThe-Impact-of-SMI-on-Families-and-Society.jpg&f=1&nofb=1&ipt=ede138ba957ab603523f5bfb2435adc99a22db84b8bac9d36b046804f6d20548.

3.4.3. Health Insurance Coverage and Disparities

The interconnection of health insurance coverage and health disparities represents a critical axis in determining social determinants of health. Despite significant reforms, such as the Affordable Care Act (ACA), that aimed to increase healthcare access for all Americans, structural disparities continue to be widespread across racially marginalized populations. The COVID-19 pandemic revealed these existing gaps and their impact on specific demographic groups experiencing disproportionately poor health outcomes. For instance, research indicates that such populations with deep-seated inequities in access to healthcare and public health infrastructure were at higher risk of contracting severe illness and death due to the virus.

Even researchers have begun questioning whether insurance reform alone is sufficient to overcome such deep-seated inequities, and if the structural barriers built up by systemic racism can realistically dislodge the effectiveness of healthcare policies targeting equity to a determining degree (Johnson et al., 2025). In addition to the structural racism effects, health insurance differences significantly cut across most social determinants of health, including economic stability, education, and access to medical care services. For LGBTQ individuals, narrowing such disparities entails not just numerical changes in insurance status but also qualitative improvements to healthcare experience. Attempts at boosting the cultural competence of health providers are instrumental in ensuring that LGBTQ populations receive equal treatment at all healthcare institutions. This involves staff training to understand the unique challenges faced by these groups, thereby establishing an environment where patients feel free and accommodated while seeking healthcare. These advances are pivotal to bridging the gap in stigma reduction and overall health outcomes among these groups, very much tied to an enlarged vision of health equity (Maulbeck et al., 2015). The challenge for collaborative policy platforms extends beyond minimum insurance coverage and into the structural underpinnings that frame health outcomes. Policymakers must undertake a poly-pronged approach in order to dismantle the deeply entrenched health inequities facing marginalized groups. This entails not just expanding insurance coverage but also enhancing social determinants of health, such as access to quality education and economic empowerment. Health interventions mustn't be designed in isolation; rather, they should be viewed as part of a connected system that aims to tackle broader social inequalities. Effective advocacy and investment in public health infrastructure are also key in developing a solid response to the issue of vulnerable populations. Only through such system-level interventions is substantial progress made in achieving goals of health equity and disparities based on the social determinants of health (Johnson et al., 2025) (Figure 3.12).

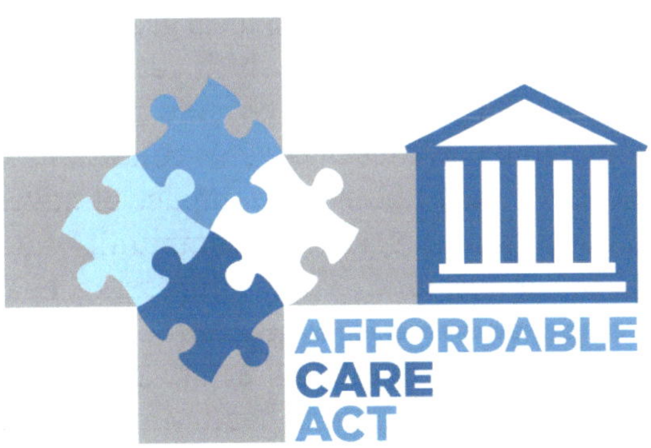

Figure 3.12. Affordable Care Act (ACA).

Source: https://coherecommunity.com/wp-content/uploads/2013/10/ACA-Logo.jpg.

3.5. Neighborhood and Built Environment

Residential environment and built community are inherently involved in the social determinants of health, influencing every aspect of day-to-day living. They refer to the physical neighborhoods where one lives, works, and socializes with others, having a direct impact on the accessibility of resources such as nutritious foods, recreational facilities, and health care. Poorly planned neighborhoods can potentially increase sedentary activity by discouraging walking or cycling, and their impact on public health can be significant. More and more evidence indicates that incorporating active lifestyles into city design is essential, stimulating mobility and social contact. By creating livable, prosperous public places, populations have the ability to counteract adverse health effects attributed to a stationary lifestyle, thereby emphasizing the necessity of incorporating health factors into urban planning strategies (Alves et al., 2019). In addition, as the population of cities grows, it is increasingly important to understand the intricate dynamic between neighborhood health and conditions. Urban environments, through sheer scale, density, diversity, and complexity, shape health outcomes by controlling living conditions that systematically reflect system-wide socioeconomic disparities. For instance, lower-income neighborhoods typically lack adequate space for green areas and safe play areas, directly impacting decreased physical activity rates among the residents. This disparity needs an integrated response that takes into consideration local and national policy influence on the health of the urban population. Intervening on the determinants of these intricacies, public health interventions can positively address the determinants of health inequalities of urban life, thus enhancing general well-being and community health (Freudenberg et al., 2005). Lastly, the interactive relationship between neighborhood environments and health outcomes emphasizes the importance of synergistic intervention to improve such environments. Stakeholders, including urban planners, public health professionals, and residents, must interact to develop innovative solutions that tackle health within the environment of community development. Such intervention results in environments that not only promote physical health but also social cohesion and mental well-being. Healthier communities guarantee more equitable resource distribution, thus reducing cases of chronic diseases caused by sedentary lifestyles. With further urban development, the need for sustainable and health-enhancing design strategies will be key in shaping futures that enable all individuals to achieve their full capabilities, further reinforcing the public health debate on the pivotal role played by the built environment (Alves et al., 2019) (Figure 3.13).

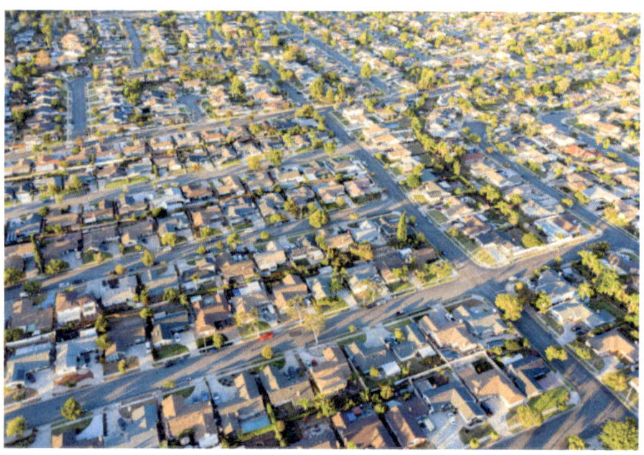

Figure 3.13. Neighborhood and built environment.

Source: https://www.networkforphl.org/wp-content/uploads/2020/06/iStock-1182778603-1238x0-c-default-q40.jpg.

3.5.1. Impact of Neighborhood Safety on Health

The effect of neighborhood safety on health consequences is a critical field of study when using the social determinants of health. Safety in the environment entails not only the absence of crime but also a general feeling of safety with which residents feel secure on a daily basis. When individuals perceive that their neighborhoods are unsafe, they will limit outdoor activities, thereby lessening opportunities for exercise and social communication. This restriction can lead to higher rates of obesity and associated illnesses like heart disease, in effect lowering the overall health of communities. Moreover, violent neighborhoods can induce chronic stress, which has been linked to numerous physical and mental illnesses, including anxiety, depression, and cardiovascular diseases. Last, enhancing neighborhood safety is more of an issue of public safety rather than law enforcement, but a consequential health concern that demands multi-disciplinary responses mirroring the determinants of insecurity. Lastly, the interface between neighborhood safety and health outcomes overflows into areas of access to resources and health equity. In safer communities, there is improved access to recreational facilities, healthcare facilities, and healthy food establishments—all of which are vital in ensuring a healthy life. In contrast, risky communities do not have such resources, thereby reinforcing health disparities among vulnerable communities. For instance, individuals who live in communities with more crime may struggle to get to local grocery stores that have healthy foods, which leads to poor diets and a higher risk of chronic diseases. As highlighted by studies of chronic conditions like congestive heart failure, the impact of adverse social determinants, such as community safety, must be understood when addressing health outcomes and constructing effective public health policy (Pierre-Louis et al., 2022). Such understanding can inform health interventions aimed at improving community well-being. Besides, neighborhood safety promotion by policy and community participation can bring about a healthy culture that offsets the adverse effects of environmental stress. This is achievable through initiatives to enhance community policing, the creation of secure public spaces, and fostering local social networks. Health equity movements recognize that policymakers should consider social settings like crime levels and community cohesion (Birnbaum et al., 2011). As environmental safety is enhanced within the community, residents may become more actively involved in health-enabling behaviors, which lead to enhanced quality of life. Ultimately, the relationship between determinants of health outcomes and environmental safety underscores the significance of resolving the broader social determinants of health, including not just physical safety but psychological security and social cohesion.

3.5.2. Availability of Healthy Food Options

Availability of healthy food options is central to the identification of the social determinants of health since it has a direct influence on food consumption and overall well-being. The population with low exposure to fresh produce and nutritious food has high rates of diet-related diseases, such as obesity and diabetes. Food deserts, characterized by residents having no easy access to healthy, affordable food, create these health disparities. It is established in research that factors such as the food store location, prices of healthy food, and product variety have a significant effect on food choice and diet. Enhancing the supply of healthy food requires undertaking activities to increase options for local food availability, which can assist in filling the food security gap and subsequently improve health, particularly for vulnerable individuals (Bureau of Statistics et al., 2017). Besides, the availability of food carries a sense beyond access; it entails aspects such as quality, cost, and location of food retailers. When taking college environments into consideration, for example, studies identify price, meal quality, and accessibility as significant influences on healthy food options among students. The link between these determinants and diet reflects that even if healthy food is present, it needs to be accessible and affordable too in order to work. It is shown through research that women are most sensitive to healthy food availability, reflecting the subtle processes whereby gender influences food access (Brandão et al., 2021). Hence, merely increasing the number of healthy food outlets is not sufficient; policymakers must also ensure that they are offered competitively and at convenient locations in order to induce healthier dietary habits. Finally, the extension of raising healthy food option availability is a public health promotion intervention. Conquering the barriers to healthy eating, time constraints, and shortages of cooking skills can also increase food utilization. Interventions aimed at food literacy, quick and nutritious meal preparation skills, and budgeting behaviors can help empower people to make health-protective choices. Through learning by doing and community support systems, these interventions can endow individuals with the capacity to access and effectively utilize their food places. Last but not least, establishing a culture in which healthy foods are readily accessible can result in long-term change with an effect on food patterns and improving the health of those with social determinants (Bureau of Statistics et al., 2017) (Figure 3.14).

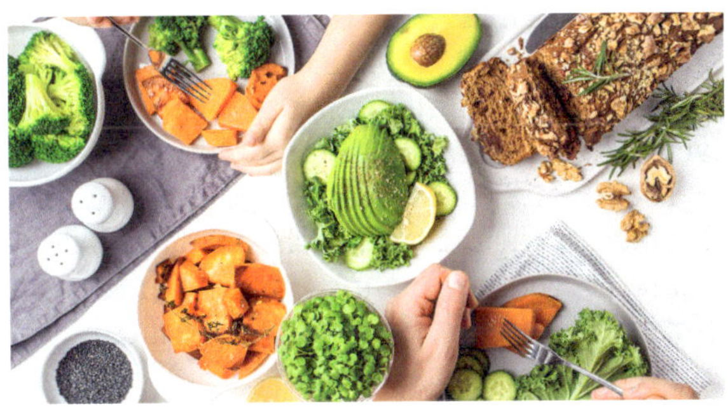

Figure 3.14. Healthy-food-choices.

Source: https://mytunbridgewells.com/wp-content/uploads/2021/05/Healthy-Food-Choices.png.

3.5.3. Access to Recreational Spaces and Physical Activity

Recreational space access plays a crucial role in the facilitation of physical activity, playing an important role in determining public health outcomes. The built environment has a direct impact on residents' ability to engage in physical activity, with parks, pedestrian paths, and sporting facilities being contributory attributes to general well-being. An appropriately designed urban environment with accessible recreational facilities can encourage individuals to become part of active lives. This is particularly crucial in impoverished communities where such facilities may be in short supply, leading to disparities in health gains among socioeconomic groups. By developing equitable access to recreational spaces, cities can develop an environment to facilitate physical activity, ultimately reducing the risk of chronic diseases and enhancing the well-being of residents, as the meta-analysis of the evidence-based literature concluded on the basis of the relationship between the built environment and the health status of subgroups (Claudia, 2007). In addition to health benefits associated with physical activity, access to leisure space can facilitate improved mental health outcomes. Municipalities that emphasize green spaces and recreational facilities allow citizens to engage in activities that serve not only to improve physical fitness but also function as stress reduction mechanisms. For instance, local parks provide critical venues for social interactions, encouraging positive relations among citizens. Such social interaction is able to combat feelings of loneliness and depression, which have been associated with poorer academic performance and general health among adolescents. Research indicates that positive relationships in various contexts, including schools and communities, can buffer the effect of depressive symptoms on academic achievement (Delva et al., 2013). Therefore, recreation facilities are not only places for physical exercise but also central to the strengthening of community cohesion and mental resilience. Moreover, the problem of access to recreational facilities is further compounded with concerns of social equity, as marginalized groups are typically faced with obstacles to physical activity that are different from those for their more advantaged counterparts. Poor infrastructure, inadequate transportation, and safety concerns can discourage users from visiting existing recreation facilities. Remedying these imbalances involves more than improving access to present facilities, but allocating funds to new facilities in low-service areas. By ensuring all groups have access to safe, clean, and welcoming recreation spaces, policymakers can help ensure a more equitable distribution of physical activity-related health benefits. As such, recreational area access is a cornerstone piece in working to address broader social determinants of health and assist in leading to a more equitable society where physical and mental health outcomes may be optimized for all individuals, regardless of socioeconomic status or geography.

3.6. Policy and Governance

Policy and governance influence on social determinants of health is highly significant, particularly in the education field. Schooling program structure and organization are essential determinants that influence children's health outcomes. For example, sound policies are capable of offering access to quality educational facilities and guaranteeing learning environments that are secure. Moreover, the interpersonal relationships established in school environments are accountable for social and emotional development, which are antecedents of well-being. Rectifying the determinants of structure, such as differences between gender, race, and social class, becomes essential for achieving fair health outcomes. The review points towards the necessity of policymakers prioritizing the development of child-friendly education policies that are aware of and respond to such social structures and, in so doing, maximize the potential of education as an instrument for health gain among children (Fillol et al., 2024). Governance systems significantly influence resource distribution and prioritization of public health programs, especially among marginalized communities. The success of health interventions typically relies on the interlinkage of various systems of governance, public policy, and the needs of the community. For example, where health education and preventive programs take priority with governments, especially in health disparity-ridden areas, the impact can be significantly increased at the community level. But for this to occur, robust governance systems must exist, with stakeholder consultations and evidence-based practice that are also apt to local health requirements. Moreover, as changing health conditions arise, governance frameworks must be elastic and adaptable so that interventions such as vaccination programs are performed safely and effectively. Policymakers have to weigh hoped-for benefits from health programs against risks and realities in communities (Hasan et al., 2011). Ultimately, good synthesis of policy and governance must come together to counteract broader social determinants of health. As reflected in the evidence, the fact that such determinants are multifaceted calls for a multidisciplinary program that connects health, education, and socioeconomic factors. For example, healthcare policies for increased healthcare access, coupled with effective educational reforms, can be employed to move the overall health status in communities forward. This not only calls for the commitment of state institutions but also for the engagement of community entities and health professionals. Furthermore, constant evaluation and update of such policies are critical, so stakeholders can gain insights from outcomes and refine strategies that address persistent disparities. Subsequently, a policy and governance emphasis is critical in formulating inclusive public health policies that can effectively counteract health disparities among diverse populations (Fillol et al., 2024).

3.6.1. Role of Government Policies in Shaping Health Outcomes

Health outcomes are influenced by government policies, and these are further influenced by affecting many of the social determinants of health, including healthcare access, quality of environmental conditions, and socio-economic stability. State, local, and federal policies can influence the construction of systems that facilitate or discourage providing basic health care. Local government, above all, has a critical leadership role to play in developing public health systems that focus on the upstream determinants of health for the community. Through the enactment of policies that are specially responsive to the needs of the population, e.g., improved sanitation, safe shelter, and availability of healthy food, governments are able to construct environments conducive to physical and mental health. Therefore, effective governance is central to ensuring that social structures support healthy living, and therefore, is an integral part of public health policy (Gamsu et al., 2014). Moreover, urban living creates its own unique challenges and opportunities, which have significant effects on public health outcomes. With much of the world's population still moving to city environments, government policies need to shift to respond to the health requirements of varied populations in these environments. Urbanization usually coincides with complicated health dynamics that are linked to socioeconomic status, environmental quality, and availability of services. Policymakers must deal with the means through which urbanization influences health, especially considering that large parts of the densely populated areas are typically plagued by increased levels of pollution, fewer options for nutritious foods, and weaker healthcare infrastructure. Through an understanding of the interconnected nature of these determinants, governments can create specialized policies that reduce health disparities and ensure equitable access to resources vital to citizens in improving the overall quality of life of city inhabitants (Freudenberg et al., 2005). In addition to local and city-level strategies, national policies must be created to directly address structural health inequities. These policies must extend beyond health access exploration to a greater integration of education, labor, and transport infrastructure, which are all determinants for health outcomes. For instance, housing policy that enables housing affordability and increased public transit has a significant effect on one's ability to access health care, hence overall health status. Strategies to reduce socioeconomic disparities using tax incentives, the law on minimum wage, and education policy changes can also be used to ensure vulnerable population segments receive the support they need for healthier living. The integration of these various components of public policy allows governments to craft an integrated strategy for health that understands the interconnectedness of social determinants and promotes a healthier population (Gamsu et al., 2014) (Figure 3.15).

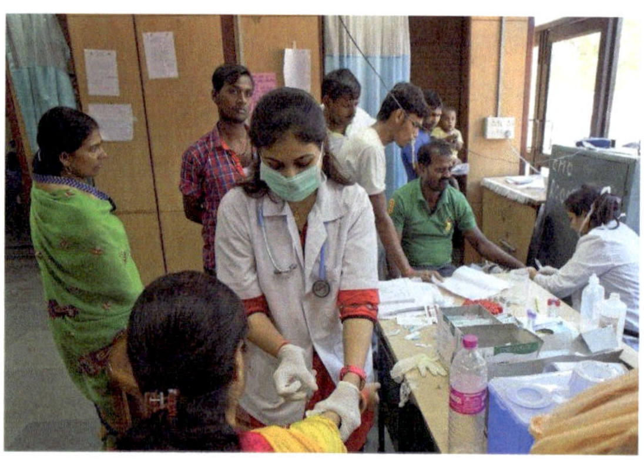

Figure 3.15. Public health care system.

Source: https://resize.indiatvnews.com/en/resize/newbucket/1200_-/2016/09/PTI9_15_2016_000267B.jpg.

3.6.2. Importance of Public Health Initiatives

Public health measures are important in resolving the social determinants of health, which include the different economic and social circumstances that affect people's and populations' health. Through a focus on these determinants, public health measures can address the causes of health inequities and not merely their consequences. Examples of measures that advance improved health outcomes include efforts toward increasing access to quality education and jobs. There is evidence to show that when populations are given better resources and support systems, their health improves, further consolidating the worth of healthcare programs based on a better understanding of social determinants. Therefore, prevention of these underlying causes by intentional public health action becomes paramount in making communities healthier and bridging health gaps that have persisted among different groups of populations. Successful public health programs are implemented through an intersectoral strategy that involves government agencies, health providers, and community organizations working in coordination. This intersectoral approach is necessary to tackle the multiple layers of social determinants, including income inequality, housing stability, and access to healthcare services. For instance, programs that improve housing quality among disadvantaged populations not only facilitate improved physical health outcomes but also improve mental well-being. These concerted actions have been shown to be in concord with effective actions that are advantageous to health, hence advancing the value of addressing social determinants comprehensively. As more debate in recent health reform discussions, a focus on the interconnection between social determinants and health can ultimately lead to revolutionary improvements in population health outcomes, making public health interventions essential in pursuing health equity (Philip, 2005). Moreover, the worth of public health programs is best exemplified in high-risk groups, such as Indigenous communities, where social determinants play a considerable role in determining health disparities. Successful programs aimed at addressing the particular hardships these groups experience demonstrate the prospect of greater health outcomes through targeted efforts. For example, by incorporating aspects such as community participation and culturally adapted education, public health interventions may be efficiently employed to address the disparities experienced by Indigenous people. As noted in comprehensive reviews of evidence, such comprehensive and goal-specific programs are required in terms of being part of initiatives aimed at bridging the gap in health between Indigenous and non-Indigenous peoples. Thus, the identification and reaction to the significance of social determinants through robust public health action is of critical significance in realizing long-term health equity and encouraging all communities to thrive in a healthier and equitable society (Baum et al., 2013).

3.6.3. Advocacy for Health Equity and Social Justice

Social justice and health equity advocacy are central to addressing the social determinants of health (SDOH). Determinants encompass various factors such as education, socioeconomic status, community, and systemic inequality impacting total health outcomes. In this, advocates seek to identify and eliminate structural barriers to health disparities in marginalized groups. The Multicultural and Social Justice Counseling Competencies highlight the importance of responding to issues of equity through advocacy that promotes social justice in healthcare environments (Goktan et al., 2024). Advocacy in this manner not only creates awareness but also allows communities to participate actively in attempts that seek to rectify injustices in health. Through inclusive debate and building platforms for marginalized voices, campaigners can facilitate improved access to resources necessary for optimal health, ultimately resulting in equitable health outcomes for everyone. One of the critical frameworks used to conceptualize health equity is the health justice framework, which points to how legal and social systems create health inequities. By recognizing that unmet legal needs are formidable obstacles to the attainment of health equity, advocates can effectively bridge the connection between legal rights and health. Laws regulating housing, employment, and education exert a significant influence on the health of individuals and communities. Robust examination of these intersections illustrates how low-income individuals and individuals of color suffer from cumulative health problems fueled by structural racism (Cannon et al., 2022). Thus, advocacy should not only work towards transcending acute injustices but also rectify the legal frameworks perpetuating inequality. The two-pronged approach facilitates a better understanding of health justice that encompasses specific cases as well as the overall systemic issues that hinder equitable access to health. In addition, the necessity of legal representation in health issues cannot be overstated. Access to representation is especially important for individuals with legal issues that disrupt their health and well-being. The health justice model illustrates how representation can reverse the adverse effects of unmet legal needs, ultimately improving the health of marginalized communities. While it is essential to encourage individual legal aid, however, it must be complemented by efforts towards structural change. This involves sticking to policymakers, activists, and legal professionals' alignment to seek a multitiered strategy that includes addressing current problems in addition to addressing structural injustices (Cannon et al., 2022). In concerted advocacy efforts, which integrate legal representation into broader public health agendas, stakeholders are able to actively promote health equity and social justice where everyone, regardless of socio-economic status, can achieve ideal well-being (Figure 3.16).

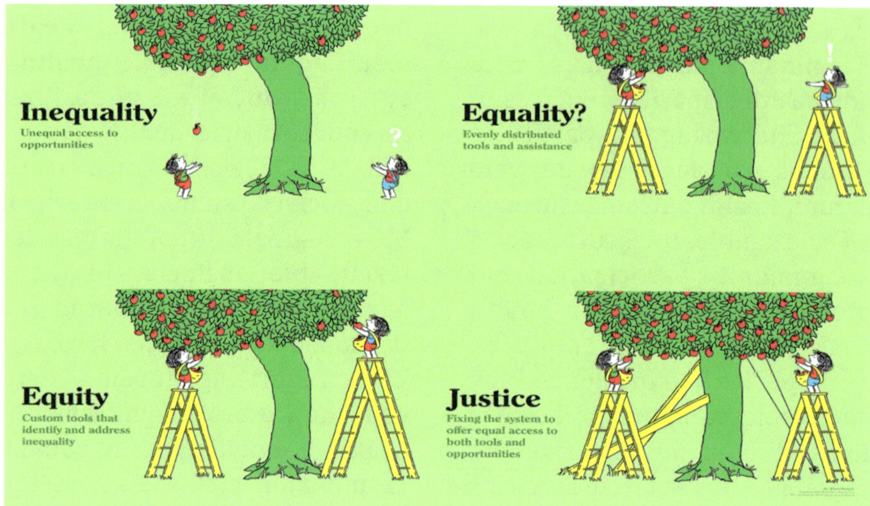
Inequality
Unequal access to opportunities
Equality?
Evenly distributed tools and assistance
Equity
Custom tools that identify and address inequality
Justice
Fixing the system to offer equal access to both tools and opportunities

Figure 3.16. Advocacy for health equity and social justice.

Source: https://www.rwjbh.org/images/health-equity/justice-infographic.gif.

CLOSER LOOK

SOCIAL DETERMINANTS AND MINORITY HEALTH

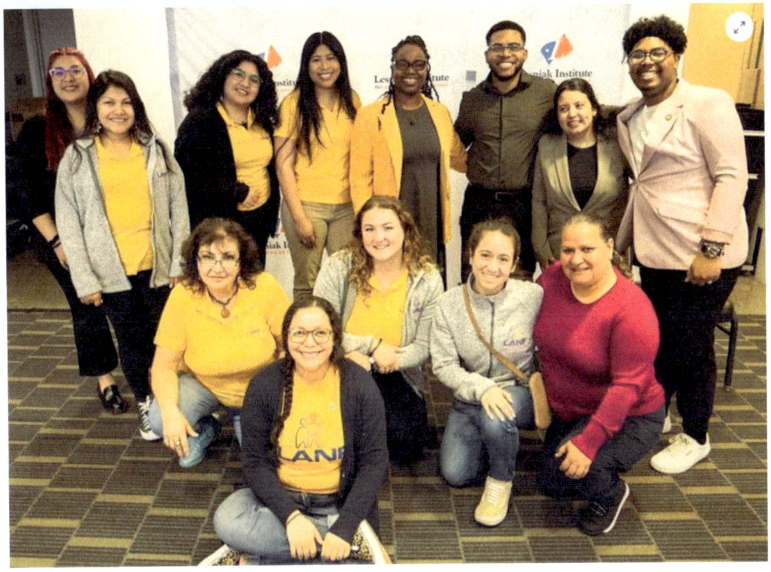

Figure 3.17. Community health advocates gathered to address health disparities and promote equity through social determinants of health.

Source: https://www.lanfoundation.org/post/addressing-health-disparities-a-closer-look-at-social-determinants-and-minority-health.

Social determinants of health are the places where people are born, grow up, work, and age, and significantly impact an individual's overall well-being. These include education, income, occupation, housing, access to healthcare, and social support. Minority populations disproportionately face disadvantage in all these aspects and thus end up with poorer health than the general population. For example, racial and ethnic minorities may live in deprived neighborhoods with limited quality healthcare access, healthy foods, and safe living. Educational and employment opportunities are also likely to be limited, which affects income levels and access to health insurance coverage. Systemic racism and discrimination also contribute to chronic stress and limit paths of upward mobility, creating a cycle of disadvantage. Thus, minority groups are more likely to have higher levels of chronic diseases, such as diabetes, hypertension, and heart disease, and receive poorer-quality care. Closing these gaps will have to be the goal of targeted actions to improve the conditions that affect health, such as investment in education, assuring access to health care services on a more even basis, expanding available and affordable housing, and building economic opportunity. Public health interventions must be culturally appropriate and community-based and involve minority participation in planning and programming. In addition, policies that eliminate systemic barriers and provide social justice will be necessary if health equity is to be achieved. By focusing on the social determinants of health and minority-specific issues, we can work toward ending health disparities and giving all individuals an opportunity to live a healthy and productive life.

SUMMARY

Emphasis on social determinants of health is important in achieving equitable health results among diverse groups. Economic, social, and environmental determinants cross and greatly affect the health and well-being of individuals. Targeting and identification of these determinants assist in achieving equity in significantly better health outcomes, particularly among vulnerable groups. For instance, Indigenous health evidence synthesis has found a number of areas in which interventions have the potential to close the life expectancy gap between non-Indigenous and Indigenous Australians. These actions, while not necessarily only for direct health gain, demonstrate that focusing on areas such as education and housing can have dramatic long-term payoffs in the way of health gains, as suggested in conceptual models in relevant studies (Baum et al., 2013). This requires an approach that attends to the immediate need but also fosters an environment conducive to improved health. Furthermore, no element of advancing public health initiatives is as crucial as the role of local government. Local governments are the best fit to undertake interventions in the determinants of health at a larger scale through community action. Such leadership entails building health systems with the ability to handle local-specific issues, thereby making interventions locally effective and suitable. As identified in many studies, local government initiatives have been proven to show promise in developing comprehensive public health systems to address these social determinants (Gamsu et al., 2014). By applying local resources and providing programs suitable to communities, local governments have a great influence on health outcomes, hence the significance of these institutions' involvement in health promotion and policy formulation processes. Lastly, it is crucial to know that better health in the long run requires an entire effort through the collaboration of numerous partners. Residents, health care providers, community organizations, and policy makers must work together to address the social determinants that affect health outcomes. Through partnership and cross-disciplinary collaboration, communities can establish holistic strategies aimed at reducing health inequities. Strong programs will not just enhance existing health conditions but also bring about enduring social change, thereby enabling a healthier society. Within this holistic context of determinants of health, it is emphasized that successful public health initiatives need to be fair and address the root causes of health disparities, advocating for a more just and fair health environment for all.

A profound appreciation of social determinants of health recognizes that health outcomes are to a significant degree shaped by the social environments in which individuals live. Socioeconomic status, schooling, neighborhood environments, and social connections make up the fabric of health disparities. For instance, people belonging to lower socioeconomic strata are likely to suffer from poor access to healthcare services, which tends to exacerbate health statuses. This cross-cutting strategy emphasizes policies directed towards addressing such determinants in a comprehensive way, and not merely through interventions focused on individual health behaviors. Secondly, the recognition of social determinants as an integral component of health is in line with a process of consensus-building among health professionals and policymakers advocating systemic change in order to minimize health inequities. Cross-sector collaboration is an effective tool for lessening health inequities, in addition to the premise that social determinants of health can be confronted solely through action by various stakeholders in concert. Methods such as cross-sector collaboration are increasing, particularly between governments and communities. The Federal Interagency Health Equity Team (FIHET) demonstrated this in September 2015 with a Roundtable forum that explored collaborative approaches. Key suggestions from this discussion referenced mission and goal alignment, investment in local infrastructure, and stakeholder harmonization in one language. Through emphasis on cooperation and coordination of resources, these methods can enable an integrated public health response to the determinants of health disparities, as noted in social determinants discussions (Nweke et al., 2017). The leadership role of local governments plays a central part in developing public health systems that address wider determinants of health efficiently. Local government is able to mobilize resources and formulate policies that directly affect social determinants, leading to healthier results within communities. Research points out the importance of local governance in tailoring health interventions to meet particular community needs, as it is found that one-size-fits-all approaches are typically insufficient. Funding local health outcomes through the integration of health considerations in local planning can greatly increase the ability of communities to develop healthier environments. Therefore, empowering local authorities to initiate such efforts is important in promoting sustainable improvement in the community's health outcomes, according to studies on the roles of local governments in public health systems (Gamsu et al., 2014).

REFERENCES

1. Alqahtani, A. S. S., Alanazi, A. M., Asiri, H. M. S., Alruwaili, J. M., Alqahtani, M. S. F., Asiri, M. H. A., Asiri, M. M. M., et al. (2023). *Social and Economic Factors That Influence Health Outcomes in Family Medicine*. https://core.ac.uk/download/603897538.pdf (accessed on 11th June 2025).
2. Alves, S., Bento, T., Cid, L., et al. (2019). *Ejercicio Físico Y Estilo De Vida Sedentario: Consecuencias Para La Salud*. https://core.ac.uk/download/286590210.pdf (accessed on 11th June 2025).
3. Asfaw, Z. K., Hernandez-Marquez, G. C., Naik, A., Vega Perez, R., Bickell, N., & Germano, I. M. (2024). 100 The impact of race and social determinants of health on clinical outcome of glioblastoma multiforme patients over a decade. *Journal of Clinical and Translational Science, 8*, 28–28. https://www.semanticscholar.org/paper/a1c310f7bb628669dee12b25c7e74a7faf2ec63a (accessed on 11th June 2025).
4. Australian Bureau of Statistics, Australian Institute of Health and Welfare, Beaulac, J., Blisard, N., et al. (2017). *What Are the Determinants of Food Security Among Regional and Remote Western Australian Children?* https://core.ac.uk/download/84887935.pdf (accessed on 11th June 2025).
5. Baker, T. A., & Minahan, J. (2020). *Interest Group Session—Mental Health Practice and Aging: Integration of Social Determinants of Health in Defining Health Behaviors and Outcomes Among Diverse Older Adults*. https://core.ac.uk/download/344443750.pdf (accessed on 11th June 2025).
6. Bartley, M., Baum, F., Bentler, S., Blane, D., Blane, D., Blau, P., Bourdieu, P., et al. (2005). *Intergenerational Social Mobility and Mid-Life Status Attainment: Influences of Childhood Intelligence, Childhood Social Factors, And Education*. https://core.ac.uk/download/1393703.pdf (accessed on 11th June 2025).
7. Baum, F., Osborne, K., & Brown, L. (2013). *What Works? A Review of Actions Addressing the Social and Economic Determinants of Indigenous Health*. https://core.ac.uk/download/pdf/30675270.pdf (accessed on 11th June 2025).
8. Birnbaum, N., Masterson, E., & Schoomaker, H. (2011). *State of Health Equity Movement, 2011 Update Part C: Compendium of Recommendations DRA Project Report No. 11-03*. https://core.ac.uk/download/pdf/18491812.pdf (accessed on 11th June 2025).
9. Brandão, T. R. S., Costa, S. A., Lima, J. P. M., et al. (2021). *Food Consumption Determinants and Barriers for Healthy Eating at The Workplace: A University Setting*. https://core.ac.uk/download/421872552.pdf (accessed on 11th June 2025).
10. Brodie, T. (2023). *Knowledge to Action: Addressing the Social Determinants of Health to Promote Aboriginal and Torres Strait Islander Social and Emotional Wellbeing*. https://core.ac.uk/download/590280309.pdf (accessed on 11th June 2025).
11. Bryant, T., Dailey, A. B., Goldhagen, J., et al. (2005). *The Health Status of Southern Children: A Neglected Regional Disparity*. https://cupola.gettysburg.edu/cgi/viewcontent.cgi?article=1019&context=healthfac (accessed on 11th June 2025).
12. Bucciarelli, V., Coppi, F., Gallina, S., Mattioli, A. V., Nasi, M., Nodari, S., Pinti, M., et al. (2024). *The Impact of Stress and Social Determinants on Diet in Cardiovascular Prevention in Young Women*. https://core.ac.uk/download/614162600.pdf (accessed on 11th June 2025).

13. Caird, J., Kavanagh, J., O'Mara, A., et al. (2011). *Childhood Obesity and Educational Attainment: A Systematic Review*. https://core.ac.uk/download/pdf/14349752.pdf (accessed on 11th June 2025).

14. Calender, C., & Barker, R. (2016). *Health Equity Series: Food Insecurity December 2015*. https://core.ac.uk/download/75783718.pdf (accessed on 11th June 2025).

15. Cannon, Y. (2022). *Unmet Legal Needs as Health Injustice*. https://core.ac.uk/download/543557545.pdf (accessed on 11th June 2025).

16. Cummings, C. A., & Reilly-Chammat, R. (2023). *Perspective Chapter: Strengthening and Empowering Professional Health Educators' Capacity and Practice*. https://core.ac.uk/download/553310024.pdf (accessed on 11th June 2025).

17. Damayanti, E., Rohani, S. T., Rosyid, A., et al. (2025). *The Contribution of Education, Health, And Unemployment on HDI in East Java, Indonesia*. https://core.ac.uk/download/639972034.pdf (accessed on 11th June 2025).

18. Delva, J., Granillo, M. T., Grogan-Kaylor, A., et al. (2013). *The Role of Social Relationships in The Association Between Adolescents' Depressive Symptoms and Academic Achievement*. https://open.bu.edu/bitstream/2144/31341/1/nihms482635.pdf (accessed on 11th June 2025).

19. Delva, J., Horner, P., & Li, S. (2012). *Social capital And Cigarette Smoking Among Latinos in the United States*. https://core.ac.uk/download/215934561.pdf (accessed on 11th June 2025).

20. Doosti, H., Jahani Eftekhari, M., & Peyman, N. (2018). *The Effect of Educational Intervention Based on The Self-Efficacy and Health Literacy Theory on Health Promoting Lifestyles Among Female Health Volunteers of Neyshabur, Iran*. https://core.ac.uk/download/159123293.pdf (accessed on 11th June 2025).

21. Edward, J. S. (2013). *Understanding Social Determinants of Healthcare Access from The Perspective of Hispanic Latino immigrants in Louisville, Ky*. https://core.ac.uk/download/143832184.pdf (accessed on 11th June 2025).

22. Fillol, A., Rivadeneyra-Sicilia, A., Ferron, C., Brandler-Weinreb, J., Cambon, L., Wallerich, L., Larose, M. P., et al. (2024). *The Influence of Educational Determinants on Children's Health: A Scoping Review of Reviews*. https://core.ac.uk/download/615443471.pdf (accessed on 11th June 2025).

23. Franzini, L., & Giannoni, M. (2025). *Determinants of Health Disparities in Italian Regions*. https://core.ac.uk/download/pdf/6309596.pdf (accessed on 11th June 2025).

24. Frerichs, L., Akiwumi, A. M., Kaz, L., Kim, D., Florick, L., Lucas, V., Layer, M., et al. (2025). A systems perspective of how community-engaged public health addresses social determinants of health: A case study of a population-based COVID-19 testing program. *Journal of Public Health Management & Practice, 31*, E169–E178. https://www.semanticscholar.org/paper/38fac830074e4694d5037de596fc1d17adcf8639 (accessed on 11th June 2025).

25. Freudenberg, N., Galea, S., & Vlahov, D. (2005). *Cities and Population Health*. https://core.ac.uk/download/323072008.pdf (accessed on 11th June 2025).

26. Gamsu, M., Hunter, D. J., & South, J. (2014). *Need to Know Review Number Two: What Local Government Needs to Know About Public Health*. https://core.ac.uk/download/29018952.pdf (accessed on 11th June 2025).

27. Goktan, A. J., & Henry, M. C. (2024). *The Social Determinants of Sexual and Reproductive Health in Integrative Sex and Couples Counseling: A Structural Competence Perspective.* https://core.ac.uk/download/624082332.pdf (accessed on 11th June 2025).

28. Graham, J. (2024). *Employees working From Home During COVID-19 and Potential Mental Health Challenges.* https://core.ac.uk/download/639356118.pdf (accessed on 11th June 2025).

29. Guerron-Gomez, G., Rojas-Fierro, M., Parra-Medina, R., Mosquera, A., & Gomez Suarez, M. (2025). A reflective analysis on the inequities in cancer diagnosis and treatment in Latin America: A call to action for public health. *International Journal for Equity in Health, 24.* https://www.semanticscholar.org/paper/a07ca87203d0c6f8a416416a3da536192b318db7 (accessed on 11th June 2025).

30. Halicioglu, F. (2025). *Modelling Life Expectancy in Turkey.* https://core.ac.uk/download/pdf/6621027.pdf (accessed on 11th June 2025).

31. Hasan, H., Neogi, S. B., Sheikh, K., Zodpey, et al. (2011). *Scope for Rotavirus Vaccination in India: Revisiting the Scientific Evidence.*

32. Hernandez, E. (2023). *New Beginnings: Educational Workshop.* https://core.ac.uk/download/568006821.pdf (accessed on 11th June 2025).

33. Honkaniemi, H., Juárez, S. P., Katikireddi, S. V., Rostila, et al. (2020). *Psychological Distress by Age at Migration and Duration of Residence in Sweden.* https://core.ac.uk/download/287595383.pdf (accessed on 11th June 2025).

34. Johnson, N. (2025). *Reformed But Not Repaired.* https://core.ac.uk/download/645536979.pdf (accessed on 11th June 2025).

35. Kyriopoulos, I. I., Kyriopoulos, J., Zavras, A. I., Zavras, et al. (2016). *Economic Crisis, Austerity and Unmet Healthcare Needs: The Case of Greece.* https://core.ac.uk/download/59740019.pdf (accessed on 11th June 2025).

36. Labonté, R., & Schrecker, T. (2007). *Globalization and Social Determinants of Health: Promoting Health Equity in Global Governance (Part 3 of 3).* https://core.ac.uk/download/578117069.pdf (accessed on 11th June 2025).

37. LaManna, S., Hatfield, B., & McCann, E. (2024). Considering the influence of social determinants of health on parent feeding practices. *Advances in Neonatal Care, 24*, 110–118. https://www.semanticscholar.org/paper/5da6e0c5bc1d0b6dcbb56581068815cc7aa6df39 (accessed on 11th June 2025).

38. Liu, J., Tanarsuwongkul, S., Spaulding, M., Perea-Schmittle, K., Lohman, M., & Wang, Q. (2025). Associations between social determinants of health and mental health disorders among U.S. population: A cross-sectional study. *Epidemiology and Psychiatric Sciences, 34.* https://www.semanticscholar.org/paper/5a155fb31337e7e6ba24607cda3bcdf8425df7f0 (accessed on 11th June 2025).

39. Ly, E. (2024). *Exploring the Cultural Influences on Sexual and Reproductive Health Behaviors: A Cross-Cultural Study of Asian American and Caucasian Female College Students.* https://core.ac.uk/download/618164680.pdf (accessed on 11th June 2025).

40. Maulbeck, B. F., & Avrett, S. (2015). *Vital Funding: Grantmaking Strategies for Improving LGBTQ Health, Part Two.* https://core.ac.uk/download/87085567.pdf (accessed on 11th June 2025).

41. McGhan, S., Gustafson, K., Scott, L. A., Hokanson, T., Patterson, S., McDougall, L., & Lacombe, C. (2023). Community and healthcare team partnership addressing financial worries as a barrier to health. *International Journal of Integrated Care*. https://www.semanticscholar.org/paper/ff5c51b1de5cd3e9f36c5b68ae0fa52fe7777717 (accessed on 11th June 2025).

42. N/A. (2025). Options for meeting longitudinal information needs: A preliminary investigation. https://core.ac.uk/download/pdf/30674776.pdf (accessed on 11th June 2025).

43. Nweke, O. (2017). A roundtable on cross-sector collaboration and resource alignment for health equity: Meeting summary. https://digitalscholarship.unlv.edu/cgi/viewcontent.cgi?article=1681&context=jhdrp (accessed on 11th June 2025).

44. O'Hara, P. (2005). Creating social and health equity: Adopting an Alberta social determinants of health framework. https://core.ac.uk/download/71343870.pdf (accessed on 11th June 2025).

45. O'Neill, E. A. (2018). Health and employment for adults with serious mental illness: An examination of physical health conditions, healthcare utilization, health-related quality of life, and employment. https://core.ac.uk/download/213426840.pdf (accessed on 11th June 2025).

46. Peitz, J., Zhong, M., Adebamowo, C. A., & Adebamowo, S. (2024). Impact of social determinants of health on health-related quality of life among cancer survivors in the United States. *Research Square*. https://www.semanticscholar.org/paper/a0b9c5f9cdd61b3d6e46cb41a444b079de13fdde (accessed on 11th June 2025).

47. Pierre-Louis, S. (2022). Identifying gaps in social determinants of health among patients 65 years and older with congestive heart failure: A secondary data analysis. https://digitalscholarship.unlv.edu/cgi/viewcontent.cgi?article=5457&context=thesesdissertations (accessed on 11th June 2025).

48. Rao, N. (2024). The place-based impacts of social determinants of health: An examination of social and structural influences. https://core.ac.uk/download/614713283.pdf (accessed on 11th June 2025).

49. Rintjema, J. (2022). Integrated primary care and social care services. https://core.ac.uk/download/639178678.pdf (accessed on 11th June 2025).

50. Rodriquez, T. J. (2020). Environmental injustice's impact on asthma disparities in NYC. https://core.ac.uk/download/345953598.pdf (accessed on 11th June 2025).

51. Seraphim, A. P., Niu, H., Morgado, P., Miranda, B., & Silva, E. A. (2025). Mapping urban health policies: a scoping review of environmental, behavioral and socioeconomic determinants of health. https://core.ac.uk/download/635798188.pdf (accessed on 11th June 2025)

52. Siegel, Z., Smith-Nuñez, A., & Lewis, M. W. (2025). Social determinants of health and health outcomes in older cancer survivors. *Current Opinion in Supportive and Palliative Care, 19*, 19–24. https://www.semanticscholar.org/paper/9db72a03af7999f8a9dee53c71f9fb91b1786afe (accessed on 11th June 2025).

53. Storie, H. (2017). Community behavioral health integration initiative program plan. https://core.ac.uk/download/210607269.pdf (accessed on 11th June 2025).

54. Toaiamoandani, P. (2022). Exploring the interplay of social determinants and health outcomes towards equitable well-being. https://core.ac.uk/download/578907552.pdf (accessed on 11th June 2025).

55. Williams, C. H. (2007). *The Built Environment and Physical Activity: What Is the Relationship?* https://core.ac.uk/download/71346268.pdf (accessed on 11th June 2025).

56. Williams, D. (2024). A comparative analysis of oral health disparities among Caucasians and African Americans with intellectual disabilities. https://core.ac.uk/download/599632121.pdf (accessed on 11th June 2025).

57. Williams, M. (2024). Promoting health in the unhoused community: Assessing the screening process for social determinants of health for the houseless. https://core.ac.uk/download/619687926.docx (accessed on 11th June 2025).

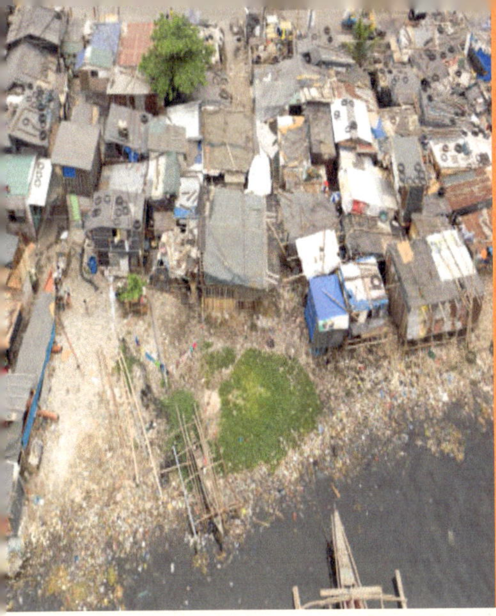

Chapter 4

SOURCES OF COMMUNITY/ PUBLIC HEALTH PROBLEMS IN RURAL AND URBAN AREAS OF LESS DEVELOPED COUNTRIES

Contents

Introduction

The variations of public and community health issues between urban and rural areas in less developed countries are complex and substantial. They are also compounded by numerous socio-economic factors, lack of infrastructure, and varying access to health facilities. Rural settings are likely to experience limited access to health facilities, which corresponds to less access to fundamental medical care. For instance, medical staff can be drastically restricted from their presence, and this aids in enhanced mortality of preventable illness. Urban areas, as much as they typically possess a greater number of healthcare facilities, have congestion, air pollution, and disparity in levels of quality healthcare. The difference in accessibility and quality of care clearly illustrates the pressing need for targeted interventions that consider the differential characteristics of rural and urban areas of less developed countries. Moreover, the position of socio-economic conditions in influencing the health indicators in these regions must not be minimized. The poverty level is often higher in rural areas, and this has a direct correlation with the deterioration of health statistics, such as malnutrition, infant mortality, and others. Urban regions may have other problems, such as high rates of unemployment and informal employment, which equate to unstable living standards. The COVID-19 pandemic has similarly revealed these inequities, affecting levels of physical activity and overall health differently in these settings. It has been found that adherence to social distancing measures in urban areas was often structured by socioeconomic status and individual behaviors, leading to an overall decrease in physical activity and corresponding health outcomes (Geoffrey et al., 2020). Thus, it is important that addressing community and public health issues be addressed with a profound understanding of the unique determinants that affect each community. In addition to socio-economic determinants, environmental as well as cultural determinants also play significant roles in health issues. Rural cultural practices and beliefs can also influence health behavior, such as eating habits or healthcare access, and this could translate to resistance in implementing contemporary health programs. Urban dwellers, however, are burdened by noise pollution and a physically inactive lifestyle that erodes overall well-being. The convergence of many diseases—ranging from communicable diseases to chronic conditions—calls for an integrated approach strategy that harmonizes public health interventions between urban and rural areas. Involvement of people and stakeholder collaboration are essential as these initiatives may lead to sustainable health benefits along with literacy in health. By embracing the results from accessible health data and diversity in intervention methods, communities can address the complex web of health determinants (Zhu et al., 2017) (Figure 4.1).

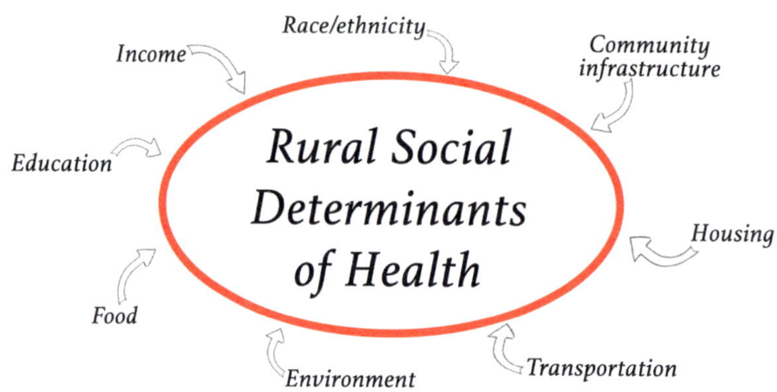

Figure 4.1. Rural social determinants of health.

Source: https://www.ruralhealthinfo.org/assets/526-1475/rural-social-determinants-of-health.jpg.

Definition of Community/Public Health Problems

An in-depth appreciation of community and public health concerns necessitates a review of the many factors that affect health outcomes among populations. Public health essentially resides as endeavors made to foster and increase the health of communities by informing, researching, and disseminating healthy living. This categorization spans a range of health conditions like infectious diseases, long-term conditions, and environmental causes, each varying quite significantly by rural and urban settings in low-income countries. All can be accounted for by differential access to healthcare facilities, social class, and the health infrastructure. This discussion unbundles the multifaceted essence of community health issues and the necessity of interventions tailored to the unique conditions of populations. The increasing openness of mental health issues in the public eye represents a new front in the issues of community health that should be tackled immediately. Recent studies, such as the National Mental Health Survey, made known the incidence and burden of mental illness, citing that cities are more likely to be afflicted with these problems, particularly in poor communities (Murthy, 2017). This is compounded by stigma and inadequate provision of services, which complete the circle of neglect and aggravate mental health conditions. Conceptualization of mental health as part of public health, therefore, necessitates a holistic approach that incorporates various social determinants like poverty, education, and social support systems into the design and provision of programs and health implementation. Healthcare disparities also contribute to the conceptualization of community/public health problems. In developing countries, particularly in rural areas, geographic remoteness, poverty, and limited resources are common causes of a high treatment gap for both physical and mental illnesses (Zhu et al., 2017). For instance, the majority of the patients are not willing to seek care due to insufficient finances or available healthcare providers, which leaves them with a significant burden both on themselves and on the health facilities. The closure of such gaps requires innovative strategies for enhanced healthcare delivery, including mobile health interventions and community health worker programs, which can significantly bridge the gap between health providers and disadvantaged groups. Ensuring accessibility and equity, public health interventions can effectively contribute to the mitigation of the health disparities that define community health concerns in contemporary times (Figure 4.2).

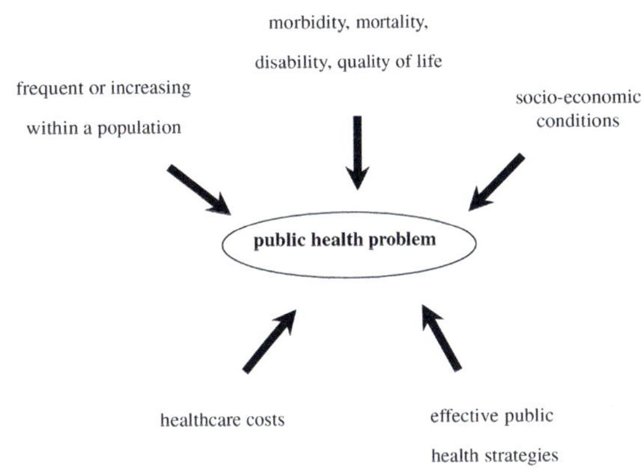

Figure 4.2. Community/public health problems.

Source: https://www.researchgate.net/profile/Kamyar-Kalantar-Zadeh/publication/236090540/figure/fig3/AS:667090390355970@1536058151097/Characteristics-of-a-public-health-problem.png.

Importance of Addressing Health Issues in Less-Developed Countries

Health issues in less developed countries are significant for numerous reasons, including the betterment of general quality of life and financial stability. Malnutrition, infection, and the unavailability of clean water greatly hamper development and productivity. Often, these health issues create a cycle of poverty that is difficult to escape from. Public health interventions can be a force for change, as evidenced by effective vaccine programs and strengthened maternity healthcare systems. These not only reduce morbidity and mortality rates but also free up economic resources from being wasted on them for more productive purposes in education and economic growth. Besides, by giving priority to health, these countries are able to align themselves with global health targets, forging alliances that are quintessential for sustainable development. Last but not least, addressing health issues results in social stability and security within such societies. Epidemics and endemic health emergencies can potentially trigger civil unrest, emigration, and strained social services. By fixing these health-related issues, governments and institutions are able to boost public trust and facilitate citizen engagement. Better health systems, which are capable of managing both communicable and non-communicable diseases, make the social system more robust. Investments into health infrastructure not only improve the immediate care enjoyed by communities but also make them better placed to manage future health demands. With the threats of climate change and new infections occurring, healthcare prevention will result in a safer and more secure tomorrow for every citizen in less developed countries (Intergovernmental Panel on Climate Change, 2023). Education is crucial in health problem-solving by empowering citizens and communities to make proactive moves in health management. By providing health education in schools and through community programs, developing nations can build a culture of well-being oriented towards prevention instead of treatment. Sanitation, nutritional, and disease prevention education can significantly lower the incidence of diseases. Public health interventions, through awareness campaigns on vaccination, access to clean water, and nutrition, can lead to healthier generations. In addition, the development of health education programs can be made specific to address the local culture, making it more effective in delivering important information. Lastly, health problem-solving in developing countries should be addressed in a multi-faceted approach and give prominence to education as the key to long-term health improvement in communities and serve as the foundation for societal advances (Zhu et al., 2017).

Overview of Rural and Urban Health Disparities

A clear picture of rural-urban health disparities is crucial for the response to community and public health issues in developing countries. Health care provision in rural areas tends to be limited due to geographical remoteness, inadequate transportation networks, and a shortage of health workers. These issues result in poorer health indicators, compounded by inadequate provision of education and poor preventive care. Urban areas, however, possess their own inequalities, commonly characterized by congestion, pollution, and blended access to health services, particularly on the part of marginal groups. These inequities call for dedicated interventions for both extremes of the continuum because health inequities experienced by populations are rooted in socio-economic and system-related causes, and therefore, an integrated strategy in addressing health care reform is called for (Chino et al., 2010). Determinants of health disparities analysis reveal a complex nexus of social determinants, including income, education, and work. In the rural regions, poverty is particularly acute, which limits access to health food and housing safety, thereby influencing health outcomes. For urban populations, the problems of inequality of affluence and insecure labor conditions prevail, leading to differential exposure to health resources. This means that not only are the urban and rural populations vulnerable, but that the imbalances themselves are rooted in broader socio-economic patterns that perpetuate inequality. Addressing these determinants is important in crafting effective healthcare plans, particularly to each community's requirements and thereby improving health equity. Ongoing surveillance of the impact of socio-economic interventions is essential to establish effective means of eradicating health disparities (Birnbaum et al., 2011). Lastly, the recognition of health disparities as health inequities reinforces the need for policy interventions aimed at social justice. Health inequities, rather than differences in health outcomes, are due to socially constructed and inequitable processes that must be addressed systematically. This necessitates a paradigm shift from addressing causes of health inequities to understanding causes of health inequities, where provision of healthcare resources alone, without addressing such systemic issues, is insufficient. As in global health debates, community participation in deciding what they want and perhaps how it should be addressed is the key to sustainable health interventions. An overall plan addressing policy reform, community engagement, and comprehensive health education must bridge health disparities between the urban and rural poor in developing nations (Chino et al., 2010). This plan not only improves health outcomes but also creates a more equitable health system overall (Figure 4.3).

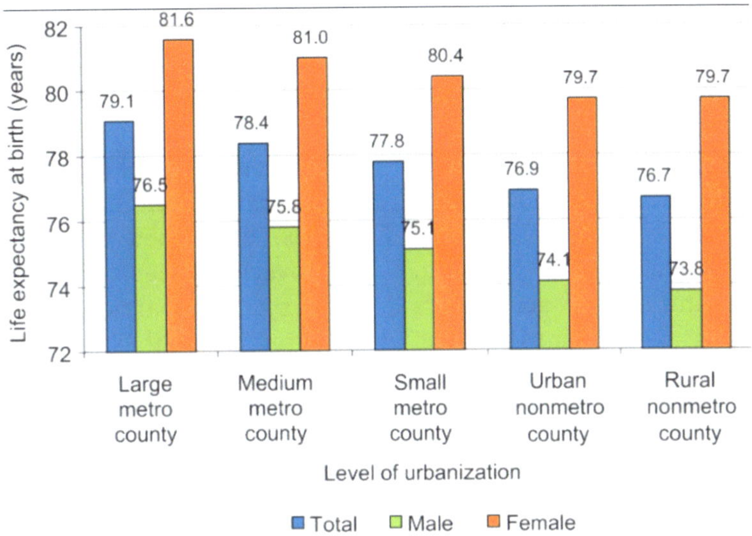

Figure 4.3. Rural and urban health disparities.

Source: https://els-jbs-prod-cdn.jbs.elsevierhealth.com/cms/attachment/b7d7cf26-37bb-4059-812d-d3c08782733b/gr1_lrg.jpg.

4.1. Socioeconomic Factors

Socioeconomic status is at the forefront in determining public health problems in the urban and rural areas of less developed countries. With nations moving along with the waves of globalization, differences in incomes, levels of education, and healthcare access are highlighted, particularly among vulnerable populations. Economic and social transition without the capabilities for some groups to adapt can lead to pathological consequences, particularly if it is brought about without adequate mechanisms for adaptation by specific population groups. For instance, the less educated masses may struggle with understanding health messages, and that impacts their ability to implement preventative action towards health and take advantage of timely medical services. This point is important in highlighting why interventions aimed at addressing socioeconomic disparities should be adopted as a means of mitigating issues of community health amidst periods of change, as established in existing studies correlating intense change with health-related outcomes (Vogli et al., 2004). Aside from that, socioeconomic status-linked environmental and behavioral determinants significantly add to community health issues. A study in Malawi uncovered the increased prevalence of cryptosporidiosis in under-fives, where certain risk factors had a link with increased infection rates. The risk factors involved unhygienic practices, i.e., taking baths from polluted water sources and not having formal education within the household (Grimason et al., 2008). The consequences of the research extend beyond individual health, reflecting community public hygiene practice and educational deficiency. Socioeconomic status and health determinants are relevant; neighborhoods with poor sanitation and availability of clean drinking water are at higher risk of infectious disease, illustrating how socioeconomic factors foster a cycle of causes of health challenges that are difficult to escape. Besides, the influence of socioeconomic conditions trickles down to mental well-being in these populations. Imbalances of financial stability, employment, and shelter are factors that lead to anxiety and mental illness, riding on top of the already existing physical health complications brought about by poor healthcare access.

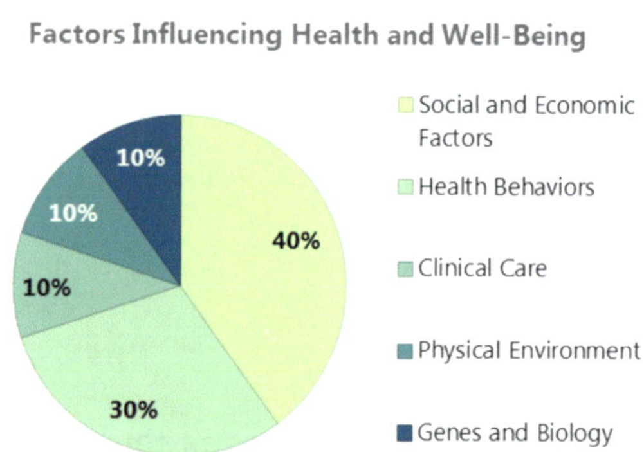

Figure 4.4. Socioeconomic factors, health, and well-being.

Source: https://www.health.state.mn.us/communities/practice/resources/chsadmin/images/_factors_rev.png.

With globalization and high-speed change affecting regional economies, workers are bound to be unemployed, leading to a rise in anxiety, depression, and other mental illnesses. This situation can be self-perpetuating, with deteriorating mental health further worsening an individual's ability to seek out and adhere to medical treatment. Eradication of socioeconomic conditions is thus not only essential to the improvement of physical well-being but also to the advancement of mental health in rural and urban areas of developing countries, ultimately resulting in healthier populations (Figure 4.4).

4.1.1. Poverty and Its Impact on Health Access

The intersection of poverty and health access is a profound dilemma in rural and urban areas of less developed countries. Individuals from impoverished backgrounds are generally faced with systemic barriers that restrict their access to primary health care, further exacerbating the gap in prevailing health inequalities. Economic limitations can lead to a poor standard of living, an inappropriate diet, and increased vulnerability to disease. Additionally, limited resources for funding discourage low-income groups from accessing medical care in a timely manner, leading to increased rates of morbidity and mortality. Peri-urban regions are characterized by infrastructure shortages and high levels of poverty, whose interactions contribute to health access hindrances, thereby fostering a cycle of poor health among the poor population (Allen et al., 1999). This inequality of structure points to the necessity of targeted intervention to improve access to health among poor individuals, which would go a significant distance towards their health and quality of life overall. In the context of global health targets, Sustainable Development Goals (SDGs) also emphasize the necessity to counter poverty as a determinant of health access. The SDGs are explicitly aiming to eliminate poverty and shared prosperity, indicating the interrelation between health and socioeconomic status (Kullman et al., 2017). Effective delivery of healthcare to poor populations is required in order to reduce disparities and establish healthier environments. Systematic approaches considering social, economic, and environmental factors are most crucial when addressing multifaceted issues facing poor groups. By evidentiary reforms that act on imbalances in service delivery, including water, sanitation, and hygiene, we can make a profound impact on the health outcomes of the poor. These reforms must be backed by end-to-end data to inform resource distribution and to make strategic health investments among the most vulnerable. Finally, to solve the issue of poverty and its impact on access to health, there needs to be a comprehensive response that addresses both the immediate health needs as well as the underlying socioeconomic determinants. Enhancing access to health care services among poor populations can be supported through innovative funding sources, private-public partnerships, and community-level interventions. With the mobilization of resources and stakeholders coming together in collaboration, efficient strategies can be developed to bridge the gap in health service delivery. When we encounter the public health challenges that are prevalent among the rural and urban areas of less developed countries, we must commit ourselves to strategies that diminish poverty and ensure equal access to health for every citizen, irrespective of their socioeconomic status. Then alone shall we be able to develop a healthier and more just society.

4.1.2. Education Levels and Health Literacy

One of the most significant determinants of both public and community health in the rural and urban regions of less developed countries is the educational level, which is directly connected with health literacy. Health literacy enhances the capacity to understand and make efficient use of health information, thus greatly impacting health outcomes. Tertiary levels of education are generally found to have improved health literacy, enabling them to access and navigate health systems as well as make health-related decisions themselves. This is particularly evident in developing regions, where false or misleading information around health issues leads to adverse health behaviors and outcomes. Effective health literacy is a foundation for disease prevention and disease control, and also for controlling health conditions since it provides individuals with the capacity to access preventive care and adhere to treatment protocols. Thus, as there is growing sophistication in health issues within these settings, an increase in levels of education becomes critical to the maintenance of an educated and health-literate population (Margaret et al., 2018). Further, differences in levels of education across groups also expand health inequities among populations. Disadvantaged areas usually have more limited opportunities for education and hence more avoidable disease and poorer health. Such a lack of education is merely a symptom of more widespread disadvantage within society, as excluded groups—feminine, rural dwellers, and poorer families—are often denied any access to good-quality education.

Therefore, such populations are disproportionately represented in experiencing health issues, as they not only lack higher health literacy but also fewer means to acquire and receive necessary health information and care. For instance, findings in the National Mental Health Survey present proof of the connection between reduced levels of education and increased prevalence rates of mental illness, as well as limited access to care, to imply that enhancing education channels can lead to enhanced mental well-being among such individuals (Murthy, 2017). Coordination between stakeholders—governments, NGOs, and healthcare providers—is key to addressing both the issues of education and literacy on health. The resources need to be focused on implementing education programs that integrate health information into curricula, particularly where the greatest disparities in health exist. Community health programs can also play a critical role in enhancing health literacy by contributing through place-based education that is respectful of cultural context and leverages community strengths. Such an integrated approach can help to demystify information related to health and facilitate more effective public health interventions. Lastly, increasing education levels is not merely an educational goal; it is a key public health intervention that will help to raise the well-being of populations and reduce the prevalence of conditions in rural and urban areas of less developed countries (Margaret et al., 2018).

4.1.3. Employment Opportunities and Health Outcomes

In addressing the intricate nexus between employment opportunities and health outcomes of less developed countries, it is becoming increasingly important to recognize the multi-dimensional interlinkages that characterize this nexus. Employment has a determining effect not just on the economic well-being of individuals but also on the health of communities. When individuals are in a position to gain employment, they become capable of accessing means that better position them to purchase care, buy nutritious food, and enjoy secure housing circumstances.

These problems have a significant contribution to improved health outcomes. Unemployment at high levels, however, contributes to a health spiral downwards as individuals lack the means of buying essential services, resulting in the depletion of both physical and mental health. This vicious circle further affirms the need for specialized employment programs that address the unique issues found within rural and urban settings of less developed countries. Moreover, the quality of employment being offered has a significant impact on overall health. Work conditions, including job security, safety, and working hours, influence not only incomes but also psychosocial health. Informal sectors tend to dominate labor markets of less developed countries with poor work conditions and minimal or no health benefits. Workers in such cases will tend to feel more anxiety and stress about job insecurity, which is likely to have a detrimental effect on mental health and overall well-being. Furthermore, inadequate protection may also result in an increased risk of accidents and chronic health issues, particularly in physically demanding work. Good-quality labor policies are required not only to spearhead economic growth but also to build healthier communities, particularly among the most vulnerable groups that are typically disproportionately affected by poor working conditions. Increasing the status of social determinants of health within employment policy can bring about long-term health gains in developing nations. Jobs-training programs that combine job creation with vocational education and health instruction can double both economic and health prospects for populations. For instance, skills training programs can increase employability with the addition of health literacy components to promote enhanced health-seeking behaviors. Subsequently, as an educated and economically empowered labor force takes shape, communities can see declining health disparities and overall better public health. Therefore, for meaningful progress in health outcomes to be achieved, employment strategies must be integrated into health and social policies that consider the major contribution made by economic factors, as was highlighted in recent conceptualization around quality in health systems (Margaret et al., 2018). Through focusing on employment opportunities alongside related health decision-making factors, there is a holistic approach made, and at last, it improves the lives of citizens in rural and urban life in less developed countries (N/A, 2016) (Figure 4.5).

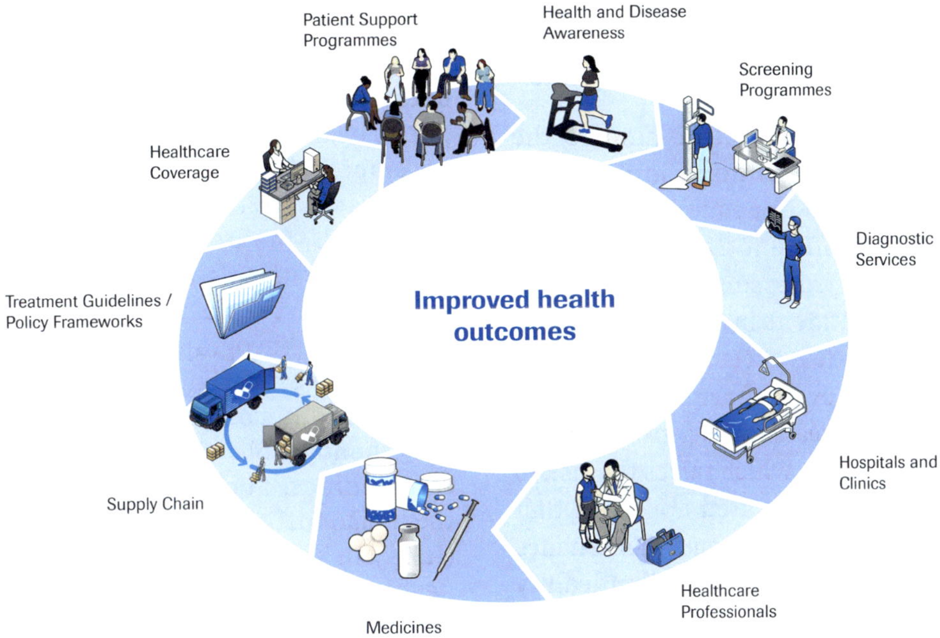

Figure 4.5. Employment opportunities and health outcomes.

Source: https://i.pinimg.com/originals/58/3d/67/583d67f8c1a080aac9767ed58cad1c02.jpg.

4.2. Infrastructure and Resources

The relationship between infrastructure and resources plays a crucial role in the health outcomes of both urban and rural regions in less developed countries. In most cases, non-existent or substandard infrastructure is a major contributor to the public health challenges, in which the lack of roads, sanitation, and healthcare facilities makes disease transmission difficult. Within peri-urban contexts where there is the convergence of rural and urban conditions, a lack of inclusive infrastructure is not only responsible for environmental sustainability issues but also for poverty cycles, overburdening local public health means and systems. This results in a large gap in access to health care among vulnerable populations, with priorities for interventions in order to bolster key infrastructure delivering public health (Allen et al., 1999). No less important is strategic resource allocation, notably in the context of SDGs. As a system of goals established with the aim of eliminating all types of poverty, the SDGs require an integrated strategy encompassing social, economic, and environmental aspects. This vision of integration is critical in closing gaps in service delivery, especially for sectors like water supply, sanitation, and hygiene (WASH). Such management not only enhances improved health outcomes but also strengthens communities through equitable access to basic services. Prior investment in WASH infrastructure, alongside sound data-driven approaches, is essential for human capital promotion and prevention of existing inequalities that disproportionately accrue to marginalized groups (Kullman et al., 2017). The interaction of infrastructure and public health is of particular significance in less developed countries, as infrastructure shortfalls are often correlated with high morbidity as well as mortality rates.

Moreover, bad infrastructure hinders the impact of health interventions intended to mitigate communicable endemic diseases. For instance, the lack of efficient transport systems means that medical professionals are not able to offer medical treatment in a timely manner, while patients cannot access the required treatments. This is even more important in urban slums, which already have a crowded and unhygienic environment, which raises the risk to health. Therefore, an integrated approach that makes sure there is investment and maintenance of infrastructure can contribute significantly to an increase in public health impacts and community resilience at a wider level to ensure long-term health equity (Allen et al., 1999) (Figure 4.6).

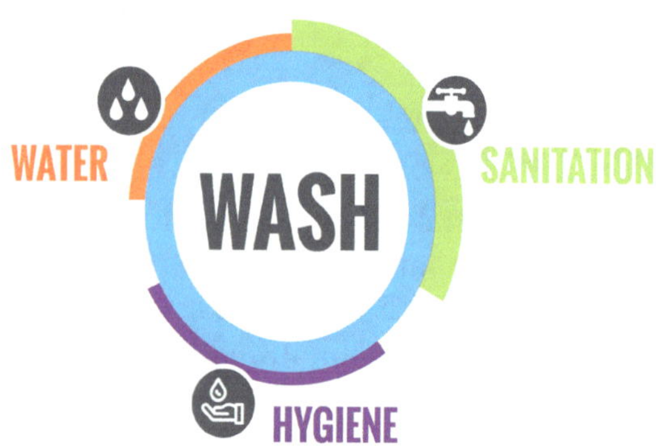

Figure 4.6. The WASH foundation.

Source: https://external-content.duckduckgo.com/iu/?u=https%3A%2F%2Fthewashfoundation.org%2Fwp-content%2Fuploads%2F2018%2F04%2Fctwf-major-components-of-proper-handwashing.png&f=1&nofb=1&ipt=6401a4406b0811de9198c88e763b55ead5a337c0de9b4d18bb350c5b2933df00.

4.2.1. Availability of Healthcare Facilities

Availability of medical facilities is an important determinant that influences the outcomes of public health in general and particularly in less developed countries, where access to health services is typically poor or fragmented. In rural areas, the reality that few hospitals and clinics exist means that the gaps in access to health services are wide compared to urban areas. These geographical and infrastructural issues can exacerbate health issues, making interventions come too late for preventable and manageable disease burdens' affected communities. Such inequalities are noted by the Indian Institute of Management, Ahmedabad (IIMA), in its demand for managerial concerns in healthcare delivery and ensuring robust health policy systems that are able to respond to the unique needs of different communities (Malek et al., 2025). The limitations of healthcare facilities contribute to already prevalent public health problems, furthering morbidity and mortality among rural communities. In urban communities, despite a greater concentration of healthcare facilities, accessibility is also an issue due to socioeconomic considerations. The standard of accessible healthcare tends to be reliant on economic status, leaving the urban poor to end up in a healthcare system that not only has an overspill but cannot meet their needs. These are clearly more severe in informal settlements, where public health systems tend to collapse because they are underfunded and lack infrastructure. In addition, the relationship between urbanization and healthcare access commonly leads to overcrowded facilities and few healthcare workers, hence making it cumbersome to deliver quality care and, in turn, exacerbating the community health issues. These interactions cast a light on the need for targeted interventions toward ensuring the equitable delivery and quality of healthcare services, particularly in overcrowded urban areas (Malek et al., 2025). The consequences of insufficient availability of health facilities extend to public health crises, such as epidemics of infectious diseases, which are disproportionately worse in vulnerable populations. For example, a study conducted in Malawi reported stunning connections between poor access to healthcare and higher risks of disease such as cryptosporidiosis in rural children. Interventions like poor sanitation, inadequate education, and reliance on contaminated water sources were seen to greatly enhance infection prevalence and thus health gaps. The findings highlight the need for comprehensive intervention measures that not only enhance care accessibility but also encompass education and community participation in public health interventions. Addressing these issues in an integrated fashion is the way to reduce the disease burden and promote health equity in both rural and urban areas of less developed countries.

4.2.2. Transportation Challenges in Accessing Care

Health care access remains a prevailing issue in rural and urban areas of less developed countries, primarily because of mobility hindrances. Individuals needing medical attention are then confronted with public transportation that is rare and limited, extended travel distances, and the cost of private transport. The hindrances tend to affect more vulnerable populations, where the lack of transport can lead to delayed or missed medical intervention. Furthermore, apart from this, the issue is also exacerbated by the inappropriate timing of transport services, which fail to match healthcare appointment times, further making accessibility an issue. In the majority of instances, those who are able to access healthcare facilities feel frustrated and powerless due to the inefficiencies of transport systems, thereby impacting their health outcome and quality of life, and therefore, a serious public health issue.

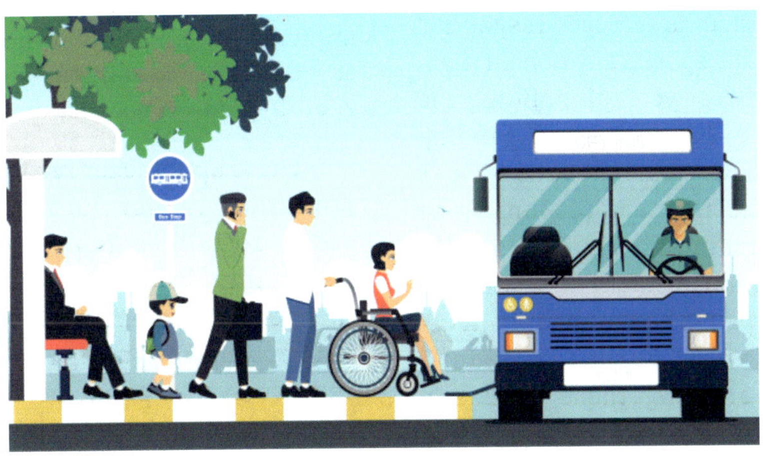

Figure 4.7. Transportation barriers limit opportunities in accessing care.

Source: https://external-content.duckduckgo.com/iu/?u=https%3A%2F%2Fbloustein.rutgers.edu%2Fwp-content%2Fuploads%2F2020%2F02%2 Ftransportation-autism-lubin.jpg&f=1&nofb=1&ipt= 95375b9d4802 abaaf4ad5d2952a4 5d3d95b814941a8b0b9448 a6a6546c1c42b6.

The significance of transport problems transcends logistics; it intersects with socio-economic reasons that determine health-seeking behavior. In another study of maternal health in India, economic accessibility and perceived care quality were the main determinants for where to seek medical treatment. Women are likely to opt for private health centers, which they see as offering quality services, even if at a price, while public centers are marked by inequalities such as disrespect and bribery. In such settings, it becomes necessary to learn about transportation systems because it is usually the case that better-provided individuals manage to get access to improved health care services. Hence, addressing transportation deficiencies must entail boosting the image of healthcare quality and reducing associated costs in order to ensure equal access to all members of a community (Barge et al., 2016).

In rural populations, such as the Homer Area of Alaska, transportation challenges pose unique barriers to access to healthcare, on top of already existing issues related to overall healthcare provision. As reported in research directly focusing on this region, travel expenses, specialist shortages, and suspicion of medical practitioners exacerbate the transport issue. A high proportion of residents surveyed responded that transport problems specifically denied them access to health care last year, pinpointing the multifaceted nature of the problem. Expanding health access necessitates innovative ways of providing services that are responsive to the specific geographic and cultural setting of rural dwellers. Improvement in transport infrastructure, as well as establishing trust between patients and health providers, is paramount for bridging these gaps and enhancing healthcare access in remote areas (Zatz et al., 2016) (Figure 4.7).

4.2.3. Water and Sanitation Issues

Clean water and proper sanitation facilities are still a fundamental problem in rural and urban areas of less developed countries. The lack of steady sources of water and proper sanitation facilities worsens the problem for public health, leading to increased cases of waterborne diseases such as cholera and dysentery. For instance, according to the World Health Organization, a significant majority of such diseases can be traced directly back to unsatisfactory water and sanitation facilities, which disproportionately affect the most vulnerable parts of the population. Secondly, the processes of attaining water quality and sanitation access are also frustrated by insufficient infrastructure and funding, which limit the proper application of public health interventions. Addressing such issues requires an intersectoral solution that not only improves access to safe water but also integrates education on hygiene behavior to build better communities (Evans et al., 2010). Proper application of sanitation and hygiene behavior change interventions is key to preventing waterborne diseases. Recent systematic reviews have outlined a variety of methods that can be used to bring drastic improvements in sanitation programming and induce behavioral change within communities. These approaches encompass community outreach initiatives that engage local stakeholders in the planning and implementation of sanitation projects, as well as education campaigns intended to enforce good hygiene practices.

These approaches recognize that improving sanitation is not just a technical matter but a socially complex problem involving community buy-in and sustained behavior change. Implementation of these strategies can potentially mitigate health risks and improve overall public health results, having a measurable impact towards disease reduction in rural and urban settings (Evans et al., 2010). The Sustainable Development Goals prioritize the targeting of inequalities in Water Supply, Sanitation, and Hygiene (WASH) as a method of combating poverty and promoting health. SDGs shift the focus from merely increasing access to WASH services to ensuring that the services are for the benefit of the most disadvantaged. The WASH Poverty Diagnostic

Initiative indicates how targeted investment can reduce such disparities and improve the provision of services. Through focusing on resource allocation and promoting cooperative institutional arrangements, this initiative will strengthen human capital in marginalized communities, thus enhancing health benefits and overall social stability. In this respect, effective water and sanitation resource management and allocation continue to be essential in meeting both the SDGs and the wider public health goals in less developed nations.

4.3. Environmental Factors

Environmental factors are most important in deciding public health experience in rural and urban areas of less developed countries. The physical environment's state, for example, the availability of clean water, sanitation, and the level of pollution, has a direct impact on the health of populations. In cities, population growth is rapid, and it most often leads to overpopulated living conditions where facilities are behind demand.

This environment is likely to enhance the transmission of infectious diseases and aggravate long-term health issues by exposing people to higher concentrations of contaminants and scarce healthcare resources. Moreover, the effect of urbanization is complex and multifaceted, with determinants varying greatly based on context and location. The dynamic interactions of scale, intensity, and heterogeneity of urban settings may create unique health risks worthy of close analysis (Freudenberg et al., 2005). In rural areas, the environmental landscape contains special health concerns that are often overlooked. Limited access to healthcare may lead to delayed treatment and unwanted health outcomes. Natural systems, critical in offering resources such as clean water and food, are increasingly compromised by climate change and unsustainable exploitation. As rural societies are heavily dependent on their local environments to support livelihood, any loss in environmental quality can pose health risks, including malnutrition and disease outbreaks. Interventions to such problems require innovative solutions that consider both the ecological balance and socio-economic vulnerability of such populations. Without a complete understanding of such environmental conditions, interventions to enhance public health impacts among rural communities may fall short (Long et al., 2013).

The inclusion of environmental factors in public health policy is paramount when creating sustainable solutions for cities and rural areas. Public health practitioners and policymakers must adopt an all-encompassing approach that acknowledges the interconnectedness of environment, health, and socio-economic status. Urban design, in the urban environment, must prioritize green spaces, promote environmentally sustainable transport, and provide access to basic services to offset health risks. Concurrently, rural development programs need to target restoring ecosystems, improving agricultural methods, and upgrading infrastructure so that health can be better accessed.

By helping vulnerable groups become resilient and adaptable, these kinds of efforts can actually minimize the negative health impacts caused by environmental factors. Lastly, commitment to these approaches will enhance health equity and offer a broad improvement in the health of populations in less developed countries (Freudenberg et al., 2005; Long et al., 2013) (Figure 4.8).

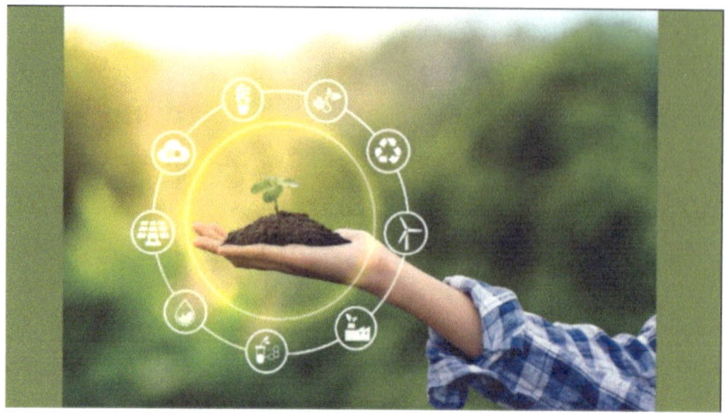

Figure 4.8. Environmental factors affecting human health.

Source: https://external-content.duckduckgo.com/iu/?u=https%3A%2F%2Fwww.verdantixsummit-ehs.com%2Fwp-content%2Fuploads%2F2023%2F02%2F8-Environmental-Factors-Affecting-Human-Health-1.jpg&f=1&nofb=1&ipt=c64094af3126ff00e9138db2c211fc203c8e849cf3ed4c501cdc465d662bcb49.

4.3.1. Pollution and Its Health Effects

Less developed countries are facing the issue of pollution, particularly in urban areas where populations grow at a rapid rate, promoting unsustainable practices. Urbanization, characterized by high population concentration, results in a perfect storm of pollution-related public health issues. Air pollution, generated from transport, industry, and biomass combustion, gives rise to a spectrum of ailments ranging from respiratory diseases, cardiovascular ailments, and even premature mortality. The urban pollution levels magnify the impact on weaker sections, i.e., children and the elderly, and they are more susceptible to the adverse effects of poor air. This issue requires a multi-faceted solution consisting of regulatory intervention, public awareness campaigns, and public participation to stem emissions at the source and address healthier environments for our cities. At the same time, water pollution is a significant public health concern within the urban and rural contexts of less developed countries. Poor management of waste and industrial effluent leads to pollution of water sources, hence the prevalence of waterborne illnesses such as cholera and dysentery. Excessive deprivation of access to clean drinking water disproportionately affects poor communities most, adding complexity to existing health disparities. Rural areas, where cropland waste has a tendency to seep into the waterways nearby, are most vulnerable. The solutions to the issue should be in the form of investments in infrastructure that promote healthy sanitation and treatment centers for waste. Water pollution is not only an environmental concern; it is one with inherent links to health impacts, economic productivity, and overall well-being for the affected populations within these communities. The combination of urbanization and environmental health puts a priority on targeted interventions. The estimated figure that more and more people will reside in cities than ever before highlights an imminent crisis, particularly in less developed regions. The health effects of overpopulation in urban settings by Songsore et al. (2005) are far-reaching, adding to the prevalence of chronic disease because of pollution. Moreover, with increased population density comes an increased burden of environmental hazards. Historical trends in industry, joined by inadequate city planning, have resulted in environmentally degraded conditions that also affect public health. The consequences of the resultant conditions illustrate the worth of integrated approaches that reconcile both economic development and environmental sustainability, ultimately reaffirming associations between pollution management and improved health outcomes as outlined in Allen et al. (1999).

4.3.2. Housing Conditions and Overcrowding

The relationship between living conditions and public health is most pronounced in poorer countries, where inadequate infrastructure is often the cause of severe community-level health problems. Overcrowding, which is common in rural as well as urban populations, promotes the spread of infectious disease, as close contact among individuals increases the risk of pathogen transmission. In addition, substandard housing usually does not have fundamental utilities such as clean water, sanitation, and good ventilation, further compromising residents' health. It is the most acute vulnerability among children living in conditions like this, whose physical and emotional well-being is strongly connected to their environment. The importance of addressing such issues with multidimensional policy interventions cannot be overstated, as it is through healthy urban living conditions that it is possible to reduce community health concerns and enhance the overall quality of life (N/A, 2012). Cities, despite their promise of economic opportunities, are likely to harbor particular challenges that adversely affect housing standards. Urbanization, driven by rural-to-urban migration in the hope of better livelihoods, leads to extreme overcrowding. Cities get overcrowded, and that results in the growth of slums with poor infrastructure. The conditions not only create cycles of poverty but also introduce a vicious cycle of health hazards, wherein high population density and low-quality housing translate into more cases of infectious diseases and mental illness. The unplanned expansion of cities creates problems in implementing effective policy interventions because local governments can struggle to provide suitable housing options. Therefore, understanding the dynamics of overcrowding in urban areas is essential in planning effective public health interventions that reverse such endemic conditions (Osei-Assibey et al., 2013). Rural areas also have their own set of issues in poor housing conditions that result in public health crises. While not as crowded as in urban areas, rural areas have profound limitations in quality housing due to poverty and limited resources. The majority of communities reside in old houses with poor insulation, toilet facilities, and clean water access, making them susceptible to waterborne illnesses and pneumonia. Moreover, economic reform in countries like Ghana, which has made the shift from agricultural to service economies, has not benefitted the majority of rural communities, leaving them with limited economic prospects. Therefore, remediating rural community living conditions is vital in addressing health inequities and supporting sustainable community development. All in all, interventions that combine housing improvements with health initiatives will be essential to enhancing the health of these communities (N/A, 2012).

4.3.3. Agricultural Practices and Food Security

Agriculture is at the core of food security, particularly in developing countries where rural and urban populations suffer from serious health disorders. Over-reliance on traditional farming methods often leads to poor harvests of crops, which exacerbate hunger and malnutrition among vulnerable populations. The inability to adopt new agricultural technology not only limits food availability but also undermines the nutritional content of foods that are supplied. Empirical data support the fact that increasing agricultural productivity using efficient agricultural practices can raise food security and public health significantly. To this end, it is necessary to understand the connection between public health and agricultural practices because food systems actually have a basic role in affecting health status and nutrition, especially where poverty and resource limitations are the prevailing characteristics (Burlando et al., 2017). Additionally, the use of participatory approaches in agricultural development has been promising in addressing food security concerns. Involvement of local communities in decision-making around agricultural innovations guarantees a sense of belonging and encourages the application of practices suited to specific regional contexts. For instance, the EU-funded H2020 project 'Social Innovation in Marginalized Rural Areas' highlights co-designing models in collaboration with stakeholders, wherein not only agricultural products are considered but also the socio-economic condition of the populace. Such participatory models can significantly contribute to food system resilience as well as enhance public health impact at the same time. With community-based interventions, therefore, such interventions can effectively target the intricate health issues related to food insecurity and poor nutrition, thereby pushing greater health agendas in less developed countries (Burlando et al., 2017). In addition, the interplay between agriculture and public health illustrates the necessity of considering food security comprehensively in less developed countries. If agri-issues are handled in ignorance of their health implications, the outcome may be poor in both areas. For instance, health diseases caused by agriculture, such as foodborne diseases and occupational health, not only threaten health but also likely decrease productivity and enhance food insecurity. Literature establishes the complex interconnections between farm practices and health outcomes, revealing that farm practice improvement decreases health risks while simultaneously enhancing food security. Programs aimed at reducing the occurrence of health problems caused by agriculture should therefore target approaches that connect health and agricultural change, driving towards a more sustainable and equitable food system (Hawkes et al., 2025) (Figure 4.9).

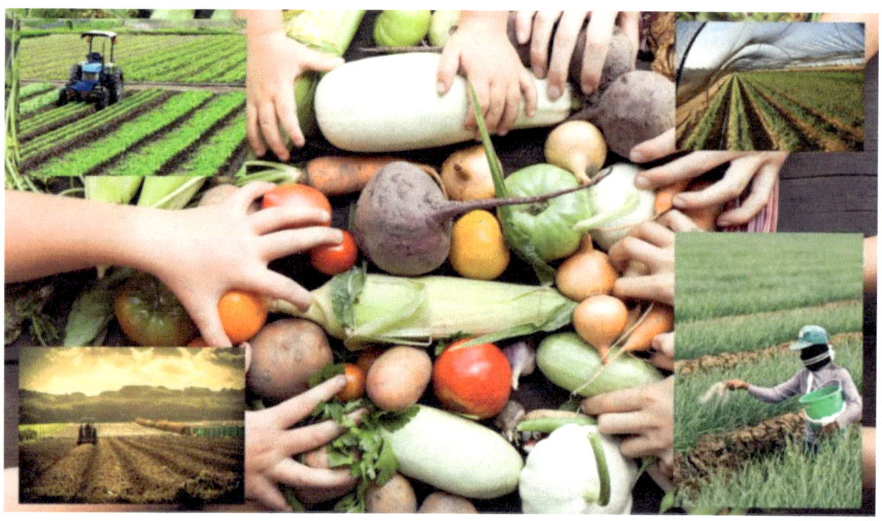

Figure 4.9. Food-security-and-agriculture.

Source: https://just10facts.com/wp-content/uploads/2023/06/Food-Security-and-Agriculture-1.jpg.

4.4. Cultural Beliefs and Practices

Cultural practices and beliefs are paramount in driving public and community health outcomes, particularly in the developing world. Cultural beliefs are likely to dictate the manner in which individuals perceive care in terms of health and the way they respond to health systems. Traditional birth attendants (TBAs), for instance, are central figures in most communities as the first line of care during delivery. While TBAs have a lot of authority, their practice at times conflicts with biomedical recommendations. Such paradoxes result from strongly rooted cultural routines, such as the direct submersion of newborns and the avoidance of colostrum in infant feeding, which can hinder health outcomes for mothers as well as children. Successful public health programs need to be established that respect local norms and promote safer health practices by adequately understanding such complex dynamics (Adamson et al., 2010). Besides, the interaction is such that it leads to a delicate balance that is likely to generate varying public health problems. In the rural areas, widespread reliance on traditional medicine is typically caused by a combination of inaccessibility of healthcare services and lack of confidence in official medical frameworks. Such a reliance can increase public health problems because traditional treatments might not agree with present-day medical data, leading to adverse health outcomes. Improved infant and maternal health, for example, requires a compatibility of contemporary medical education with indigenous practice. Cultural awareness training that instructs residents in the risks of certain cultural practices can empower citizens to make healthy choices consistent with their culture while remaining informed (Vasquez et al., 2014). Public healthscapes in cities are also influenced by the same cultural beliefs. The rapid urbanization rate can bring about massive cultural change, which most often creates conflict between existing norms and modern systems of health. To this change, people may respond with health care inequalities as a means of adjusting to new ones with respect to values and beliefs regarding health care. For instance, as societies in urban cities embrace new lifestyles, they also encounter the old stigma surrounding matters such as menstruation or family planning. Satisfying these cultural sensitivities with specialized health education programs has the potential to advance health outcomes dramatically. Moreover, by engaging community leaders and members in intervention strategy design and implementation, health professionals can ensure that cultural beliefs are respected and important public health concerns are met effectively (Adamson et al., 2010) (Figure 4.10).

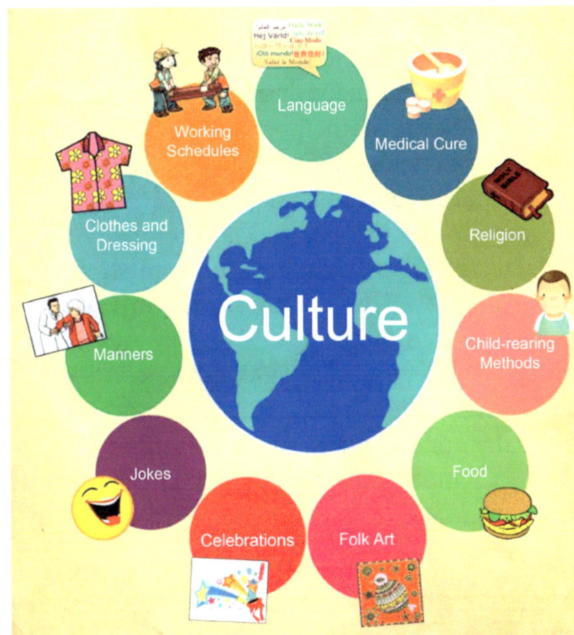

Figure 4.10. Cultural beliefs and practices.

Source: https://i.pinimg.com/originals/d3/85/37/d385374bc7ddc518950eb0287bd3183b.jpg.

4.4.1. Traditional Medicine vs. Modern Healthcare

The debate between traditional medicine and modern healthcare generally reflects society's values and resource availability, especially in developing countries. Traditional medicine is founded on centuries-old practices and relies on indigenous resources and expertise, and is thus more accessible and meaningful culturally. Modern healthcare, however, is founded on high-tech technology and pharmaceutical methods, which are not always available in rural settings. This dualism poses significant implications for public health interventions. With communities facing different obstacles to health, the intersection of these two paradigms of medicine can create tension as well as opportunities that produce varied health outcomes in varying populations. An understanding of this dynamic is necessary for effective policy implementation in regions where resources are limited and indigenous practices persist (Saner et al., 2025). One of the broader dimensions of this debate is the economic one. Where modern healthcare infrastructure does not exist in some areas, traditional medicine is the dominant one for many families. It is not just an effect on health; the sale of medicinal plants in South Africa, for instance, has been calculated to generate between $60 and $100 billion annually, underlining the central role of biodiversity in regional economies. By encouraging sustainable use of these resources, communities can tackle economic development and public health simultaneously. Projects which bring together local economic development and biodiversity conservation, like the Umthathi Africulture Project, illustrate how traditional medicine can be a path to sustainable community health, validating the need for policies that value indigenous medical knowledge equally with modern medicine (Saner et al., 2025). Moreover, modern-day healthcare systems lack social sustainability, an issue increasingly relevant in the present global context. As economies like China gain prominence in biotech, the administration of these systems must address the equitable sharing of benefits from medical advancements. The '3D' approach introduced by The STEPS Centre emphasizes the combination of social, technological, and policy dynamics that can innovate but minimize risks surrounding healthcare inequalities. This, in the context of developing countries, means that although advanced healthcare technologies can potentially facilitate public health, their implementation must be culturally sensitive and include indigenous practices. Through resolving such a complexity, we can develop a more balanced healthcare setting that honors both traditional treatments and modern interventions, thus strengthening community health outcomes across dissimilar settings.

4.4.2. Stigma Surrounding Certain Health Issues

The stigma associated with some health issues is used to significantly exacerbate public health concerns in rural and urban areas of less developed countries. Such stigma typically stems from cultural beliefs, misperception, and ignorance, which lead to the social fear and discrimination of individuals suffering from such disorders. In settings such as Vietnam, in which the HIV epidemic has shown an alarming surge among youth, disease-associated stigma is particularly destructive. The stigma not only impacts the mental well-being of a person but also affects the extent to which they are willing to obtain potentially life-saving medical care or disclose their status, further closing the cycle of infection. The interface of health-seeking behavior and social attitudes demonstrates the utmost necessity for interventions aimed at reducing stigma and creating awareness in communities regarding concerns of health, thereby providing an environment for better health outcomes. Moreover, the impact of stigma is not confined to specific health conditions but permeates across a variety of illnesses, including mental illness and chronic illness. The reluctance to address and treat openly such conditions has a tendency to isolate patients and overburden individuals and communities. In Indonesia, for instance, the mass media play a very crucial role in determining how health issues are perceived, particularly documentaries that have a tendency to give a voice to marginalized groups. But city-dominated stories tend to hide the lives of rural populations, thereby limiting their exposure to health-related stigma. That gap also necessitates representative media that will deconstruct hidden prejudices as well as educate policy and community health programs. Because health issues intersect with socioeconomic determinants, health-related stigma can also be a barrier to relevant services. Marginalized groups, such as migrants or the poor, often face compounded stigma that might push them away from seeking care altogether. From observations of studies focused on Vietnam, the intersection of gender roles and discrimination with post-Doi Moi socio-economic change has increased vulnerabilities related to HIV as well as other health problems. This socio-cultural nexus points to the nature of public health challenges in less developed countries as being intricate, where stigma not only results in health-based discrimination but also in continued wider cycles of poverty and inequality. Untangling this stigma by way of inclusive public health education and community engagement is critical in the dismantling of barriers and provision of access to health services on equitable terms (Figure 4.11).

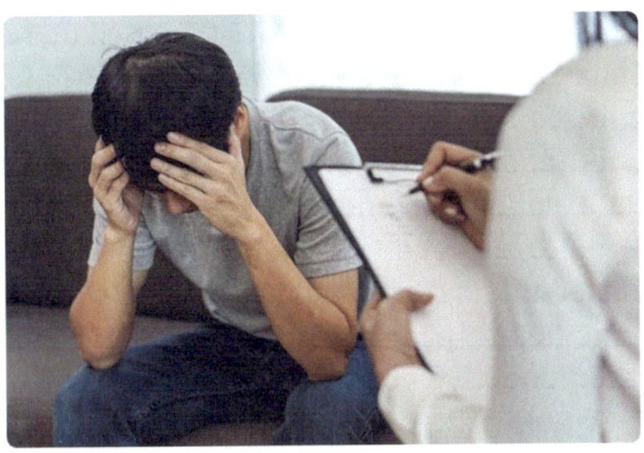

Figure 4.11. Analyzing the stigma surrounding mental health.

Source: https://d2jx2rerrg6sh3.cloudfront.net/image-handler/picture/2021/8/shutterstock_1897694278-1.jpg.

4.4.3. Community Engagement in Health Initiatives

Community participation is critical in health interventions, particularly in rural and urban areas of less developed countries, where health conditions are typically aggravated by structural inequities and scarce resources. Successful health interventions require the active participation of community members, since they are most likely to identify local health issues and help address solutions appropriate to their specific contexts. There is evidence that this community engagement in planning for their own health makes people not just more knowledgeable and confident but also responsible for controlling their own health outcomes. Involvement leads to the blending of modern medicine with the traditional approach and can lead to more effective and appropriate health interventions. Without community engagement, health programs can fail to link, resulting in inappropriate service use and no long-term advantage to public health (Margaret et al., 2018). Moreover, the involvement of local stakeholders in health programs is central to building the capacity of health systems in poor countries. Strong communities can bargain their health needs and affect decisions on policy and resource use. Community involvement also serves to integrate various sectors such as education, agriculture, and housing, which are major determinants of health. Communities are able to construct holistic health plans for both actual medical needs and underlying social determinants of health using local resources and knowledge. These efforts can potentially enhance the capability of health systems to respond to emerging public health threats, like those posed by climate change and environmental degradation, that disproportionately affect the poor sections of society (Whitmee et al., 2015). Furthermore, integrating a community-oriented model in health programs can potentially significantly augment health literacy and preventive care activities. When community members are engaged as active stakeholders, they gain basic knowledge about health behavior, disease prevention, and available health services. Greater awareness allows them to make wise health decisions and encourage healthier behavior change. Furthermore, community involvement fosters solidarity and shared responsibility, leading to improved mental health outcomes and the de-stigmatization of conditions. Because the evidence suggests that the long-term success of health programs is closely linked with the level of engagement that communities have within the planning and implementation process, ultimately leading to healthier outcomes and empowered populations (Margaret et al., 2018) (Figure 4.12).

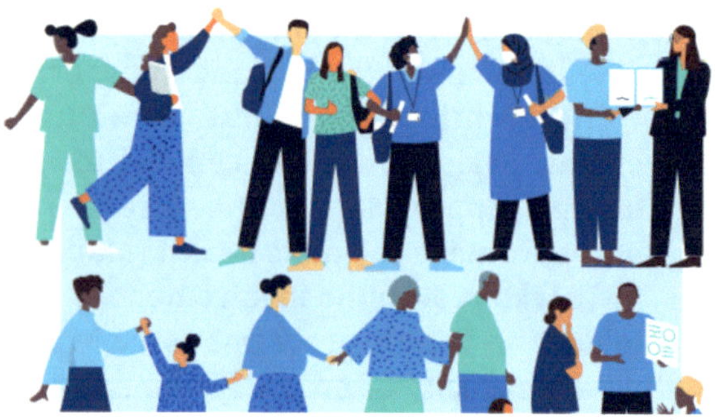

Figure 4.12. Community engagement in health initiatives.

Source: https://global.comminit.com/sites/default/files/cengagewho4.png.

4.5. Government Policies and Health Systems

Good policies of government are crucial in shaping health systems, particularly in the developing world, where disparities in health outcomes between urban and rural areas are greater. Such disparities often emanate from limited funding, inefficient allocation of resources, and poor overall health infrastructure. Governments must commit themselves to policies that respond to the interests of marginalized communities in a way that makes preventive as well as curative care accessible. By constructing health care systems through targeted investments, developing robust health infrastructure, and reinforcing public health programs, governments can mitigate causes that exacerbate public health issues. For instance, overcoming motivational and institutional barriers that deter the large-scale deployment of health services is important in order to gain trust and collaboration from communities (Clancy et al., 2011). Public health issues in developing nations are often a manifestation of broader issues in governance and institutional support. Poorly considered, poorly enforced health policies can lead to badly coordinated health systems that cannot respond to health crises competently. Urban areas with high populations feel the effects of such fragmentation fast, and it means the rapid transmission of infectious diseases, which is a public health threat. Conversely, rural areas may suffer from unavailability and lack of access to health care services, which widens health disparities. The governments must, therefore, ensure that they come up with inclusive policies that include rural and urban health systems and ensure that the distribution of resources and expertise is evenly distributed. Further, the centralized approach of data collection and management of health can reinforce local health care professionals to better understand and react to community-specific health problems (Cramer et al., 2004). Further, effective government policy must take into account the socioeconomic determinants of health, which are most pronounced in less developed environments. Poverty, education, and occupation-related risks have a significant influence on health outcomes, necessitating a comprehensive approach to health governance. Economic growth and education-promoting policies can be the foundation for a healthier public. Investments in training and health education workforces create an educated population that can recognize and neutralize issues of concern to health before they arise. Thus, an integrated policy approach—supported by an understanding of the interconnection between socioeconomic status and health—is capable of facilitating effective improvement in community well-being, thus reducing the prevalence of public health concerns in rural as well as urban populations (Clancy et al., 2011) (Figure 4.13).

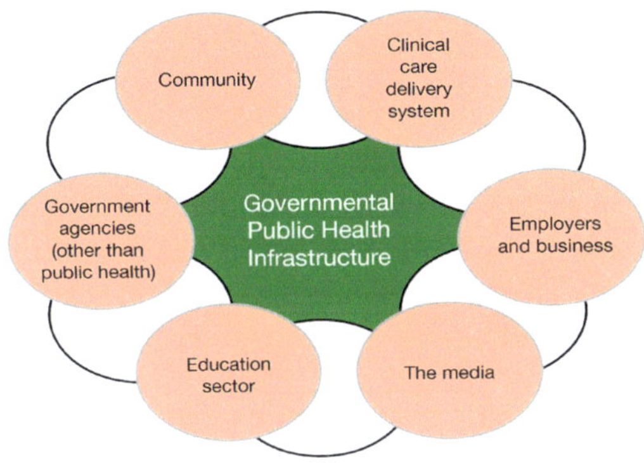

Figure 4.13. Governmental public health infrastructure.

Source: https://nap.nationalacademies.org/openbook/13093/xhtml/images/p17-01.jpg.

4.5.1. Health Policy Frameworks in Less Developed Countries

In developing countries, health policy frameworks are essential in addressing the myriad of public health concerns prevalent in rural and urban areas. The frameworks typically lack the necessary facilities and resources, which compromise the effective delivery of health care services. For instance, in rural settings, hospitals lack proper access to clean water and sanitation, resulting in higher disease transmission and undesirable health outcomes. Implementation of initiatives such as the water, sanitation, and hygiene facility improvement tool (WASH FIT) has been pivotal in enhancing health care services among these populations. According to Ali et al. (2024), prioritization of improving water supply, sanitation, and hygiene behavior can sharply reduce health care-associated infections, hence addressing fundamental health disparities that plague less developed regions. Urban centers within less developed countries also have their own set of health policy concerns that emanate primarily from population explosion and inadequate infrastructure. Overcrowding in healthcare institutions, coupled with inadequate financial management and inefficiencies from the government, exacerbates public health issues in such settings.

Urban-related factors, such as pollution and congestion, exert a major influence on the health outcomes and must be taken into consideration within health policies. Research identifies how even with better-endowed resources, urban healthcare facilities fall under pressure, and the care diminishes as a consequence. Therefore, any health policy system has to address such complex urban processes since both rural and urban healthcare facilities struggle to adapt to global health standards and manage community needs accordingly, as the evidence from rural facilities in Bangladesh reveals (Ali et al., 2024).

The effectiveness of health policy frameworks within poorer countries relies heavily upon a well-refined comprehension of both rural and urban issues. Evidence-based policy formulation is often constrained by factors such as limited resource availability and political necessity, particularly in rural areas. As defined in studies of Australian rural health policy, local experientialism has long, prevailed over scientific inquiry in health policy making, resulting in a possible disconnection between policy and actual community needs. What this implies is an imperative need for policymakers to formulate more evidence-based policy, reacting to contextual factors as well as to unique health issues presented in different settings. By improving the framework of health policy with in-depth situational analysis, poorer nations are in a position to deal with the causative factors of public and community health problems effectively.

4.5.2. Funding and Resource Allocation for Health Services

The face of health services in less developed countries is greatly influenced by funding and resource allocation trends that have a direct impact on public health outcomes. Health service erosion through historical decreases in public spending on health services contributes to existing voids in the sector, further exacerbating the need for efficient mobilization and resource allocation. This evolution has typically been made worse by budget crises that compel governments to seek other ways of raising funds, such as private stakeholders and non-governmental organizations (NGOs) (Kanwal et al., 2025). As a result, there has also been considerable evolution from exclusively public models of health towards hybrid types incorporating private players, but this evolution ends up excluding the economically marginalized. This poses significant challenges to equity of access to health care, particularly in rural areas where government resources are limited and often poorly allocated. More recent frameworks, such as the Sustainable Development Goals (SDGs) have more recently emphasized the importance of targeted interventions to the most vulnerable. By acknowledging the interconnectedness of social determinants and health outcomes, the SDGs encourage integrative means of embedding health in economic and environmental planning (Kullman et al., 2017). The foundations of innovation using this framework have brought about a new paradigm for health service provision, in which data-driven decision-making becomes pivotal to giving equitable resource allocation. For instance, WASH programs illustrate the possibility of putting investment in core services first to achieve remarkable improvements in community health results. Equity reduction-focused models provide useful learnings on how to maximize health financing to serve the interests of disadvantaged populations in the urban and rural settings. For better development of the health services of less developed nations, policymakers are faced with the challenges of how to secure sustainable funding and implement efficient resource allocation policies. The reliance on foreign sources of finance, which is a common observation in various health financing mechanisms, creates volatility and limits governments' ability to create long-term health plans (Kanwal et al., 2025). In addition, the need to establish a social safety net for the vulnerable groups underscores the utmost importance of national governments in setting their health priorities within the budget. The development of local capacity in the governance of health resources and harmonizing the implementation of effective funding models is crucial to enhancing health services. By promoting effective collaboration and drawing on the wisdom of the population, effective resource use actually decreases health disparities immediately, fostering more robust public health systems in rural and urban settings (Figure 4.14).

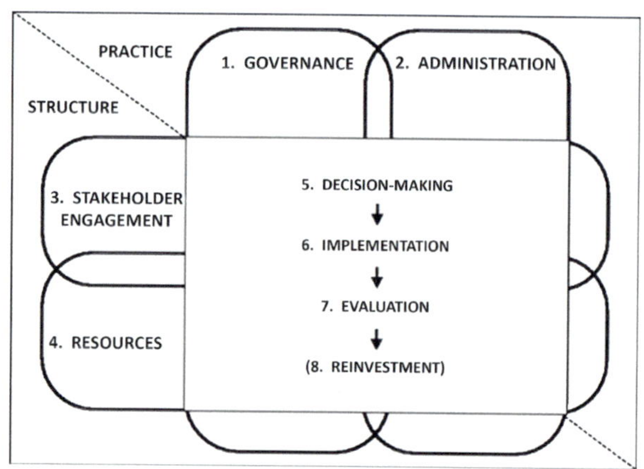

Figure 4.14. Framework for the process of resource allocation in a local health service.

Source: https://www.researchgate.net/publication/316862592/figure/fig3/AS:614063079952420@1523415455779/Framework-for-the-process-of-resource-allocation-in-a-local-health-service.png.

4.5.3. Role of International Aid and NGOs

The roles of foreign aid and non-governmental organizations (NGOs) are key to resolving the public and community health challenges that are prevalent in both urban and rural areas of less developed countries. NGOs share resources, expertise, and strategic interventions that are tailored to dealing with the particular challenges present in these communities. In particular, they specifically address major concerns like child and maternal health, infectious disease control, and access to sanitation and clean water. Through the emphasis on localized health crises and advocacy for systemic reform, international aid and NGOs not only provide short-term assistance but also induce long-term resilience and sustainability within these groups. This dual approach is crucial in environments where government capacity may be limited, thereby managing principal deficits in public health infrastructure and service delivery that are generally founded on socio-economic disparities and poor policy contexts (Schlosberg et al., 2014). Furthermore, the utilization of foreign aid and NGOs allows for the implementation of specialized health programs that are community-focused and culturally sensitive. Such groups tend to involve local stakeholders in the planning and implementation of health interventions in a manner that ensures projects are respectful of local traditions and responsive to local needs. Not only does this participatory strategy improve the impact of health programs, but it also fosters trust and responsibility among communities. Where health issues are likely to be exacerbated by environmental factors and socio-economic restrictions, NGOs can advocate for policy change and resource allocation aligned with the principles of environmental justice. Through enhancing the voice and sovereignty of the community, such organizations can address disproportionate vulnerabilities that constrain health outcomes, thus fostering an improved, fairer, and just public health environment (N/A, 2011). Moreover, the strategic alliance between international organizations and local NGOs has played a critical role in scaling up effective health interventions that test time. NGOs also serve as key facilitators of international aid, ensuring effective and efficient delivery to those who need it most. This partnership work has frequently led to the creation of innovative and novel solutions sensitive to the specific public health matters that least developed countries undergo, for instance, disease outbreaks or maternal health crises. Whether such collaborations are successful is a function of long-term support and commitment from donors and implementing partners alike. It is important to regularly assess the impact of such programs, so that international aid not only acts as a reaction to immediate health needs but also works towards the general goal of sustainable development and improved health systems in the long term (N/A, 2011).

4.6. Disease Burden and Epidemiology

The disease burden in the less developed world, particularly in rural and urban areas, is largely established by many epidemiological conditions. In the less developed countries, infections at very high rates and emerging non-communicable conditions create a complex public health environment. Conditions such as poor nutrition, poor sanitation, and limited access to health services, among others, exacerbate the prevalence of diseases such as HIV/AIDS, malaria, and tuberculosis. Furthermore, the urbanization pattern in such countries accelerates health conditions, leading to heavily crowded houses that facilitate the spread of infection-causing agents. The epidemiology of health in such places calls for certain public health interventions through prevention and early management, emphasizing the need to address the underlying socio-economic determinants of health inequalities that cause health disparities in vulnerable populations. Urbanization, as has been observed in recent studies, has been responsible for both the distribution and burden of disease in developing countries. The transition over historical centuries from agrarian lifestyles to city-based populations has led to cataclysmic changes in health patterns, including the initiation of diseases of lifestyle. By the year 2000, it was estimated that nearly 50% of the global population resided in cities, a figure estimated to reach 5 billion by 2025. Such a rapid transformation has serious health implications because densely populated urban areas lack proper health facilities and infrastructure. Africa particularly illustrates the imperative site of intersection of heightened urbanization, bleak economic development, and the resulting public health challenge, as explicated in newer publications. Not only do such cities entertain physical disease exposures, but they also generate socio-economic exposures that further spread the disease burden among these populations (Songsore et al., 2005). Policies to tackle the multifaceted problems of disease burden and epidemiology in poorer countries need greater emphasis on environmental health and research priority. In nations like Malawi, large gaps exist in examining the environmental health concerns underlying the prevalence of diseases. A systematic evaluation of such gaps can potentially inform directed research toward informing effective strategies for planning action to decrease health risk with regard to environmental concerns. Improved public health policy should encompass not just the built environment but also the overall social determinants of health and their interdependence in the causation of disease. Urban growth will augment the need for interdisciplinary studies that take into consideration epidemiological research in tandem with widely based public health interventions (Lungu et al., 2010). Through the resolution of such complex public health challenges, disease burden may be managed and health improved among populations by communities (Figure 4.15).

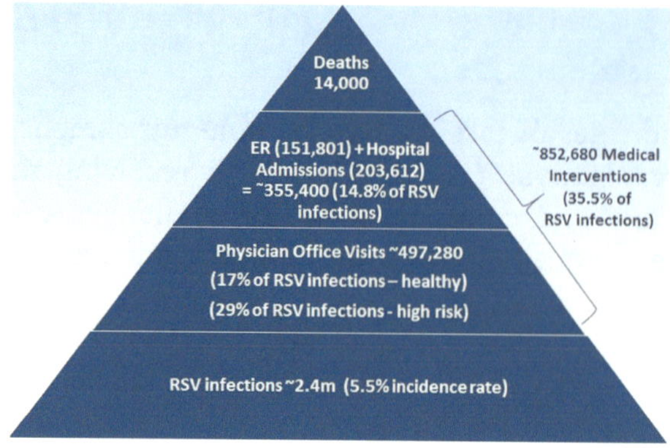

Figure 4.15. RSV F vaccine burden of disease in older adults.

Source: https://www.sec.gov/Archives/edgar/data/1000694/000114420415057166/image_034.jpg.

4.6.1. Prevalence of Communicable Diseases

The prevalence of infectious diseases remains an issue of public health in developing countries, even with the continued urbanization process shaping population dynamics. Urbanization has significantly altered living conditions, and the resulting overpopulation has made efficient living unfeasible, rendering sanitation ineffective in promoting basic health. For instance, the process of urbanization, marked by its potential to culminate in disastrous health consequences, disproportionately impacts the slum dwellers in cities in African and Asian nations. Such densely populated areas lack the ability to absorb the pressing needs brought about by increased population concentration, thus facing increased susceptibility to infectious diseases. Additionally, with the urban settings struggling to cope with infrastructural shortfalls, the linkages between the urban environment and health grow more pronounced and give rise to urgent needs for a robust response in addressing the pressing health problems of vulnerable groups (Songsore et al., 2005). In rural settings, infectious diseases increase their own unique set of problems, adding to them the issues of limited access to healthcare services and decreased levels of awareness of health interventions. In countries like India, there are significant disparities in health outcomes, particularly among rural women. The statistics reveal that illnesses like malaria and tuberculosis are prevalent in these regions, which tend to exacerbate the mortality rates of women in the reproductive age group. Furthermore, the lack of proper healthcare programs tailored to the needs of the populations perpetuates the disease-poverty cycle. Although some relief of mortality has been assured by national health programs, more targeted and localized interventions are needed to act against the complexities of infectious diseases, which overburden rural communities disproportionately (Agnihotram et al., 2004). The intersection of rural and urban disease requires interagency cooperation in addressing communicable diseases in less developed countries. Effective public health interventions must consider the particular characteristics of both environments, realizing that urbanization is both a potential source of opportunities and of issues for disease spread. Multi-sector activities in which local communities are involved in health education and in preventive practice promotion can actually reduce the spread of infectious diseases. Furthermore, dealing with underlying issues such as education and poverty is essential in achieving lasting health outcomes. By integrating community-oriented interventions with holistic policy recommendations, countries can proceed towards reducing the infectious disease burden among rural as well as urban populations (Songsore et al., 2005).

4.6.2. Non-Communicable Diseases and Lifestyle Factors

The expanding disease epidemic of non-communicable diseases (NCDs) across developing countries is a key public health problem, particularly in rural and urban areas. Evidences show that lifestyle determinants are key to the development and occurrence of these diseases, of which diseases like cardiovascular diseases, diabetes, and obesity are top-ranked. Determinants like low diet, physical inactivity, and smoking contribute immensely to the burden of NCDs. In the case of South Africa, healthy lifestyle interventions, including enhanced nutrition and physical activity, are crucial to the reduction of chronic disease incidence. These life changes, along with community health education regarding the importance of health optimization, play a key role in offsetting the impacts of NCDs and maximizing overall population health, as highlighted in recent literature that has concentrated on the potential of lifestyle adjustment towards the prevention of chronic diseases (Parker et al., 2008). Urbanization at high speeds in the urban regions of less developed countries has introduced prospects and issues relating to lifestyle factors affecting health. Urban environments are likely to offer better access to unhealthy diets, inactive lifestyles, and higher pollution levels, thereby driving the increasing rates of NCDs. Nonetheless, there are opportunities for health programs promoting a healthy lifestyle in urbanization, and it is therefore necessary to capitalize on such opportunities. This context is illustrated in rural sub-Saharan Africa, with the beginning of economic transition now beginning to transform healthful traditional ways of life, raising changes in physical activity and nutrition patterns (Lee et al., 2007). These changes necessitate a precise understanding of the impact of urbanization on health behaviors, providing public health interventions set to mitigate the unique problems facing rural dwellers in avoiding or controlling NCDs. Rural villages, however, apparently leading healthier lives, are not spared either from the burgeoning epidemic of non-communicable diseases. The active interaction of social determinants such as education, income, and access to healthcare has a great impact on rural health outcomes. With rising economic levels, lifestyle changes—greater consumption of processed foods and physical inactivity—can become common, leading to higher risks of NCDs. The rural South African context is utilized as a case example, outlining the transition to a phase characterized by high rates of hypertension and obesity, particularly in females (Lee et al., 2007). Interventions through targeted public health measures must address these disparities by increasing awareness of NCD risk factors and promoting healthy lifestyle choices to further improve public health performance in rural contexts. Thus, it is important to comprehend the sociocultural forces influencing health behavior in an attempt to build effective interventions (Figure 4.16).

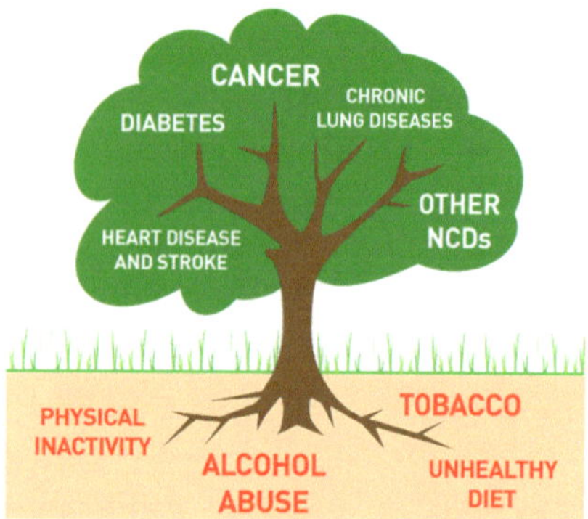

Figure 4.16. Non-communicable diseases (NCDs).

Source: https://www.dianova.ngo/wp-content/uploads/2015/07/Initiatives-citoyennes_non-com-dis-tree-en.png.

4.6.3. Impact of Emerging Health Threats (E.g., Pandemics)

Increased health threats, particularly pandemics, have far-reaching consequences for the public health system in rural and urban areas of less developed countries. The COVID-19 pandemic brutally unveiled the widespread loopholes in the healthcare system, exacerbating vulnerabilities that had gone unnoticed prior to its emergence. In these nations, poor-quality health facilities, a lack of healthcare staff, and inadequate access to essential resources left populations highly exposed to the virus. This was also aggravated by socioeconomic factors because individuals were losing their employment and had no food, limiting their capacity to recover well from the health crisis. According to recent assessments, the dynamics between health, social, and economic systems increase the prevailing disparities, thereby aggravating the effects of pandemics among such groups (Intergovernmental Panel on Climate Change, 2023). The consequences of such health crises extend beyond direct healthcare problems since they impact food security and local economies significantly. The disturbances brought about by the COVID-19 pandemic resulted in serious challenges in local food systems, particularly in low and middle-income countries. Government-imposed lockdowns and mobility restrictions have been said to lead to increased food insecurity among the vulnerable population, particularly the poor (Christophe, 2020). These disruptions are a sign of the fragile nature of local economies and the manner in which public health intersects with food supply chains. As communities lose income, access to an adequate level of nutrition deteriorates, leading to possible long-term health effects that will persist long after the immediate crisis has resolved. To enhance resilience against future health risks, policymakers need to embark on an integrated effort that entails harmonizing health systems with food security initiatives. The COVID-19 pandemic lessons inform us that flexible approaches are important in providing support for the resilience of populations to absorb shocks. A measurement framework for food system resilience can guide the design of interventions intended to enhance local actors, like policymakers, with the ability to address health crises and other shocks (Christophe, 2020). By getting the health and food security sectors to collaborate, lower-income nations can develop more robust systems that not only respond to current health risks but also preventively mitigate the dangers of future pandemics. Such a multidisciplinary approach is required to address the root causes of public health problems and foster overall well-being in the community.

CLOSER LOOK

COMMUNITY HEALTH CARE IN DEVELOPING COUNTRIES

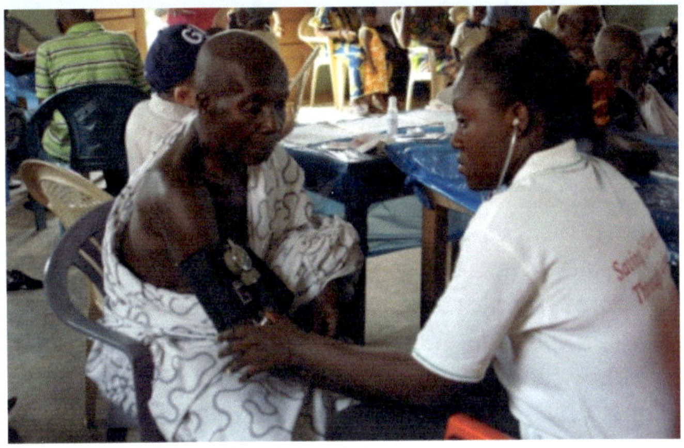

Figure 4.17. Community health outreach providing blood pressure screening for elderly individuals.

Source: https://external-content.duckduckgo.com/iu/?u=https%3A%2F%2Fwww.tms-global.org%2Fdata%2FFileManager%2Fthumbnails%2F_Uploads%2FStories%2FImported%2F2785_16282_404a802656_1435320639_550x350.jpg&f=1&nofb=1&ipt=f21f08f163847731968bba0b3f33ad8802f1084e26bc8bb6a6a9093d844240f2.

Developing world community health care is imperative in the provision of basic health needs, reduction of disease burden, and improvement in quality of life, especially among the poor. Limited availability of resources translates into healthcare provision in the form of a primary health care strategy, with emphasis placed on prevention, education, and community involvement. Community health workers (CHWs) are at the front line, providing essential services like immunization, maternal and child health, nutrition education, and disease prevention at the community level. CHWs fill gaps between formal health systems and rural or disadvantaged communities, with culturally appropriate and affordable care.

Despite challenges of inadequate infrastructure, personnel shortages, and scarce resources, a number of developing countries have managed to succeed through community-based initiatives augmented by government and external assistance. Betterment has been achieved through innovations such as mobile health clinics, telemedicine, and health promotion campaigns, which have enhanced outreach and impacts. Community involvement is crucial—when communities are involved in planning and implementation of health projects, the programs are sustainable and more effective.

However, to ensure even stronger community health care, more investment in training, supervision, supply chains, and health information systems is required. Increased collaboration among public, private, and non-governmental sectors can also enhance service delivery. In general, community health care is a cost-effective, people-centered approach with tremendous scope for improving public health in developing nations if supported by solid policy, infrastructure, and community mobilization.

SUMMARY

Investigating community and public health problems in rural and urban areas of less developed countries, the interplay of social, economic, and environmental forces becomes an important determinant of health outcomes. The SDGs confront interventions that address the sensitivities of poverty and inequality in health, attempting to integrate these dimensions through improved service delivery systems. Appreciation of the nuances of health problems, especially where inequality exists, emphasizes the need for interventions that are targeted for the SDGs. Such a comprehensive approach not only eschews poverty alleviation but also fortifies the robustness of health systems towards further efficiency, which ultimately results in community resilience and overall well-being for marginalized populations (Kullman et al., 2017). Fighting against some of these health problems, such as cryptosporidiosis, is typical of the immediate public health concerns that beset less developed regions. One Malawian study is characteristic of high rates of infection in rural communities, particularly among children under the age of five. The researchers determined significant correlations between the incidence of cryptosporidiosis and some factors, including poor household cleanliness and knowledge. These findings underscore the importance of community-based interventions that not only promote awareness among residents on hygiene practices but also engage local health systems in efforts to deal with these essential issues. This addresses both the short-term health threat and underlying social determinants that perpetuate health disparities (Grimason et al., 2008). The merging of these observations into a credible strategy underscores the urgent need for policymakers and health professionals to meet in developing coordinated solutions. Understanding the deeply ingrained socio-economic vulnerabilities that rural and urban communities in less developed countries suffer is key to developing policies to advance these groups. WASH program investments are paramount in advancing public health outcomes. By providing equal access to these resources, nations can foster healthier communities, reduce the prevalence of infectious diseases, and ultimately build sustainable development. Community involvement and focus on their unique needs will be instrumental in ensuring the successful execution of health policies (Kullman et al., 2017).

In rural and urban regions of poorer countries, a number of different sources create typical health problems, and problems of hygiene and sanitation clearly head the list. Inadequate access to clean water and improper waste disposal radically enhance the risk of infectious diseases. There is a lack of appropriate infrastructure for sanitation, which increases the population's exposure, particularly in high-density urban areas and poor rural villages. Addressing these sanitation challenges involves more than the development of infrastructure; changes in hygiene behavior need to be addressed. A comprehensive review of methodologies and strategies aimed at promoting sanitation and hygiene behavior change underlines the need for developing methodologies in line with community contexts (Evans et al., 2010). Through participation in effective sanitation interventions, communities can effectively remove health risks, resulting in improved overall public health. Still another crucial source of health problems in such populations is associated with environmental circumstances that affect the quality of air and water. Pollution, caused by industrial production in cities or agricultural practices in rural towns, is a long-term public health concern. Poor air quality, exacerbated by weak laws and enforcement measures, leads to respiratory ailments and other associated health complications. In rural areas, excessive reliance on traditional farming and the use of pesticides can lead to water body pollution that affects both human health and biodiversity. Extensive research on environmental health, as in regions of Malawi, uncovers vast knowledge gaps when it comes to these problems and suggests prioritizing applied research to tackle these environmental health risks effectively (Lungu et al., 2010). These targeted interventions are vital in informing policy and practice with the capacity to reduce such health concerns. Socioeconomic status is also vital in exacerbating health problems in rural and urban areas. Poor healthcare services, inadequate education, and poverty create a vicious cycle that enables health problems to flourish. Economic constraints often lead to substandard living conditions, with limited resources to ensure proper nutrition, education, and access to healthcare, perpetuating a cycle of poverty and illness. Social determinants of health, such as housing, education, and income inequality, can markedly undermine efforts at community interventions for health. Understanding these risk factors is essential when developing appropriate public health policies that address the etiology of illness directly. By responding not only to direct health problems but also to root socioeconomic determinants, more durable improvement in community health outcomes can be achieved.

REFERENCES

1. Adamson, P., Armstrong, P., Bajpai, S., et al. (2010). Birthing practices of traditional birth attendants in South Asia in the context of training programmers. https://core.ac.uk/download/10898961.pdf (accessed on 11th June 2025).
2. Agnihotram, V., & Ramanakumar, R. (2004). *Reviewing Disease Burden Among Rural Indian Women*. https://core.ac.uk/download/pdf/86039.pdf (accessed on 11th June 2025).
3. Ali, M., & Shahreen, T. (2024). Implementing WASH FIT in Bangladesh: A study on rural and urban health care facility challenges and opportunities. *International Journal of Science and Research Archive*. https://www.semanticscholar.org/paper/67fe9e24b9af23f01fa95267f803d380b52da436 (accessed on 11th June 2025).
4. Allen, A., Corubolo, E., & da Silva, N. (1999). *Environmental Problems and Opportunities of The Peri Urban Interface and Their Impact Upon the Poor*. https://core.ac.uk/download/1668830.pdf (accessed on 11th June 2025).
5. Alston, L., Nichols, M., & Allender, S. (2019). Policy makers' perceptions of the high burden of heart disease in rural Australia: Implications for the implementation of evidence-based rural health policy. *PLoS ONE, 14*. https://www.semanticscholar.org/paper/f79e3c3f1ed6014a79b72df5232faa7c0a34579b (accessed on 11th June 2025).
6. Barge, S., Beyeler, N., Diamond-Smith, N., et al. (2016). *Decision-Making For Delivery Location and Quality of Care Among Slum-Dwellers: A Qualitative Study in Uttar Pradesh, India*. https://core.ac.uk/download/323077709.pdf (accessed on 11th June 2025).
7. Béné, C. (2020). Resilience of local food systems and links to food security–A review of some important concepts in the context of COVID-19 and other shocks. *Food Security, 12*, 805–822. https://doi.org/10.1007/s12571-020-01076-1 (accessed on 11th June 2025).
8. Birnbaum, N., Masterson, E., & Schoomaker, H. (2011). *State of Health Equity Movement, 2011 Update Part B: Catalog of Activities DRA Project Report No. 11-02*. https://core.ac.uk/download/pdf/18491811.pdf (accessed on 11th June 2025).
9. Burlando, C., Da Re, R., Klovankova, T., et al. (2017). *Co-Constructing A New Framework for Evaluating Social Innovation in Marginalized Rural Areas*. https://core.ac.uk/download/154331243.pdf (accessed on 11th June 2025).
10. Chen, Y., & Ely, A. (2011). *Health Biotechnology Innovation for Social Sustainability: A Perspective from China*. https://core.ac.uk/download/2731317.pdf (accessed on 11th June 2025).
11. Chino, M., Clark, W., Compher, C., et al. (2010). *Indigenous Health–Australia, Canada, New Zealand And the United States: Laying Claim to A Future That Embraces Health for Us All*. https://digitalscholarship.unlv.edu/cgi/viewcontent.cgi?article=1206&context=community_health_sciences_fac_articles (accessed on 11th June 2025).
12. Clancy, J. (2011). *Small-Scale Energy Systems on A Large-Scale in Developing Countries*. https://core.ac.uk/download/pdf/11481471.pdf (accessed on 11th June 2025).
13. Cramer, C., Oya, C., & Sender, J. (2004). *Unequal Prospects: Disparities In the Quantity and Quality of Labor Supply in Sub-Saharan Africa*. https://core.ac.uk/download/2783490.pdf (accessed on 11th June 2025).

14. Vogli De, R. (2004). *Change, Psychosocial Stress and Health in An Era of Globalization.* https://core.ac.uk/download/1670668.pdf (accessed on 11th June 2025).

15. Evans, B. E., Peal, A. J., & van der Voorden, C. (2010). Hygiene and sanitation software: An overview of approaches.

16. Fliessbach, A., & Nicolay, G. L. (2012). Production of innovations within farmer–researcher associations applying transdisciplinary research principles. https://core.ac.uk/download/10932781.pdf (accessed on 11th June 2025).

17. Freudenberg, N., Galea, S., & Vlahov, D. (2005). *Cities and Population Health.* https://core.ac.uk/download/323072008.pdf (accessed on 11th June 2025).

18. Grimason, A., Morse, T., Nicholls, R., et al. (2008). *Epidemiology of Cryptosporidiosis in Rural Malawi.* https://core.ac.uk/download/19610159.pdf (accessed on 11th June 2025).

19. Hawkes, C., & Ruel, M. T. (2025). *Understanding the Links Between Agriculture and Health.* https://core.ac.uk/download/pdf/6288827.pdf (accessed on 11th June 2025).

20. Intergovernmental Panel on Climate Change. (2023). *Climate Change 2022–Impacts, Adaptation and Vulnerability.* https://doi.org/10.1017/9781009325844 (accessed on 11th June 2025).

21. Kanwal, V., & Mondal, S. K. (2025). *Addressing Key Issues in the Light of Structural Adjustment Programmer (Sap) in Health and Family Welfare Sector in India.* https://core.ac.uk/download/pdf/6356578.pdf (accessed on 11th June 2025).

22. Kruk, M. E., Gage, A., Arsenault, C., Jordan, K., Leslie, H. H., Roder-DeWan, S., Adeyi, O., et al. (2018). High-quality health systems in the Sustainable Development Goals era: Time for a revolution. *The Lancet Global Health, 6*, e1196–e1252. https://doi.org/10.1016/s2214-109x(18)30386-3 (accessed on 11th June 2025).

23. Kullman, C., Skoufias, E., Andres, L. A., & Srivastava, V. (2017). *Reducing Inequalities in Water Supply, Sanitation, And Hygiene in The Era of the Sustainable Development Goals.* https://core.ac.uk/download/141922872.pdf (accessed on 11th June 2025).

24. Lee, A., Swai, A. B. M., Bunker, C., Monteiro, C. A., Murray, C. J. L., Reed, D. M., Cappuccio, F., et al. (2007). A cross-sectional study of vascular risk factors in a rural South African population: Data from the Southern African Stroke Prevention Initiative (SASPI). https://core.ac.uk/download/49222.pdf (accessed on 11th June 2025).

25. Long, J., & Vages, N. (2013). *A Critical Scan of Four Key Topics for The Philanthropic Sector: A Study by the Rockefeller Foundation and Accenture Development Partnerships.* https://core.ac.uk/download/71362647.pdf (accessed on 11th June 2025).

26. Lungu, K., Morse, T., & Taulo, S. (2010). Gap analysis of environmental health research in Malawi: Report to the National Commission of Science and Technology. https://core.ac.uk/download/19610167.pdf (accessed on 11th June 2025).

27. Malek, I., Ramani, K. V., & Trivedi, P. (2025). IIMA in healthcare management: Abstract of publications (2000–2010). https://core.ac.uk/download/pdf/6815495.pdf (accessed on 11th June 2025).

28. Murthy, R. S. (2017). National mental health survey of India 2015–2016. *Indian Journal of Psychiatry, 59*, 21–21. https://doi.org/10.4103/psychiatry.indianjpsychiatry_102_17 (accessed on 11th June 2025).

29. Nielsen, M. H. (2009). From peasant society to manufacturing society. https://core.ac.uk/download/11986270.pdf (accessed on 11th June 2025).

30. Osei-Assibey, E., & Grey, S. K. (2013). *2010 Population and Housing Census Report: Millennium Development Goals in Ghana*. https://core.ac.uk/download/75781643.pdf (accessed on 11th June 2025).

31. Parker, W., Puoane, T., Sanders, D., Tsolekile, et al. (2008). Chronic non-communicable diseases. https://core.ac.uk/download/62632955.pdf (accessed on 11th June 2025).

32. Saner, N. (2025). Conservation of biodiversity and African traditional medicine: A market incentives and local economic development approach. https://core.ac.uk/download/pdf/6522489.pdf (accessed on 11th June 2025).

33. Saraswati, A. (Asri). (2012). The urban-rural dichotomy in the Indonesian documentaries Nona Nyonya? and Untuk Apa? https://core.ac.uk/download/639388509.pdf (accessed on 11th June 2025).

34. Schlosberg, D., & Collins, L. B. (2014). From environmental to climate justice: Climate change and the discourse of environmental justice. *Wiley Interdisciplinary Reviews Climate Change, 5*, 359–374. https://doi.org/10.1002/wcc.275 (accessed on 11th June 2025).

35. Songsore, J. (2005). Urbanization and health in Africa: Exploring the interconnections between poverty, inequality and the burden of disease. https://core.ac.uk/download/14504865.pdf (accessed on 11th June 2025).

36. Tison, G. H., Avram, R., Kuhar, P., Abreau, S., Marcus, G. M., Pletcher, M. J., & Olgin, J. E. (2020). Worldwide effect of COVID-19 on physical activity: A descriptive study. *Annals of Internal Medicine, 173*, 767–770. https://doi.org/10.7326/m20-2665 (accessed on 11th June 2025).

37. Vasquez, E., Sommer, M., Sahin, M., Worthington, N., & Dooley, T. (2014). *WASH in Schools Empowers Girls' Education: Proceedings of the Menstrual Hygiene Management in Schools Virtual Conference 2013*. https://core.ac.uk/download/75783637.pdf (accessed on 11th June 2025).

38. Whitmee, S., Haines, A., Beyrer, C., Boltz, F., Capon, A., de Souza Dias, B. F., Ezeh, A., et al. (2015). Safeguarding human health in the Anthropocene epoch: Report of The Rockefeller Foundation–Lancet Commission on planetary health. *The Lancet, 386*, 1973–2028. https://doi.org/10.1016/s0140-6736(15)60901-1 (accessed on 11th June 2025).

39. Zatz, L. M. (2016). Describing barriers to healthcare access in the Homer Area, Alaska. https://core.ac.uk/download/162578813.pdf (accessed on 11th June 2025).

40. Zhu, J. Y., Park, T., Isola, P., & Efros, A. A. (2017). *Unpaired Image-to-Image Translation Using Cycle-Consistent Adversarial Networks*. https://doi.org/10.1109/iccv.2017.244 (accessed on 11th June 2025).

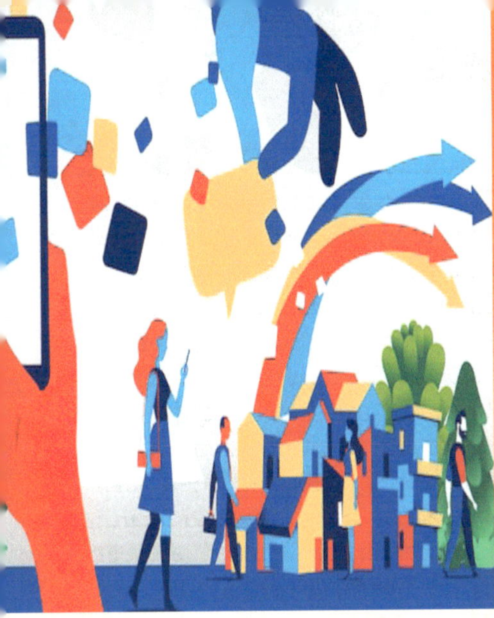

Chapter 5

ENVIRONMENTAL AND OCCUPATIONAL HEALTH

Contents

Introduction

Environmental and occupational health intersect as an important field of research that mirrors our shared experience with environmental policy and public health. With more evidence pointing to the connection between environmental factors and community health indicators, there is a greater need to examine how these fields come together to affect population well-being. This essay examines several risks to both workers and communities, explaining the ways that climate change amplifies already present threats. Environmental health is a broad category of determinants encompassing air and water quality, exposure to toxic substances, and workplace standards of safety. These determinants are crucial in understanding the big picture for public health, particularly for marginalized populations that most frequently bear the brunt of environmental decline. Moreover, the degree to which the dangers outlined can be alleviated by sustainable projects will also be examined, ensuring that the discussion is relevant to contemporary issues relating to health and safety. When faced with the issues of climate change and its relation to occupational and environmental health, mention of poorer communities and heightened exposure to environmental hazards is inevitable. The root connection between health and poverty calls for an integrated approach to investigating the role that socio-economic disparities play in creating health risks and the deficiency of access to protective actions, as described by Green for All. This study indicates that making healthcare accessible is not enough, but that it is a deliberate attempt to address the systematic source of these disparities. By encouraging green job expansion and enhancing community resilience, the Green Jobs Movement is one possible answer to balancing environmental concerns with efforts towards health equity. The blue-green alliances illustrate how various constituencies can work together for the benefit of a common goal: improved health for everyone, particularly in light of mounting climate-related peril. As we navigate the dynamics of occupational safety within the discourse of environmental health, it is essential to forge alliances among labor movements and environmentalists. These blue-green coalitions, in the form of labor-environmental partnerships, prioritize health issues as the core pillars of their platforms. By recognizing the interconnectedness of workplace exposure to toxic substances and broader environmental health concerns, these coalitions construct a politically persuasive argument that emphasizes the need for collective action. By bringing together diverse stakeholders to generate collaborative discussions, it stimulates innovative solutions to reducing exposure to harmful chemicals in community and workplace settings alike. This essay will also examine further how such collaborations result in progressive social transformation and enhanced health outcomes, demonstrating that collaborative efforts are not only desirable but unavoidable in addressing the pressing contemporary environmental and occupational health issues (Figure 5).

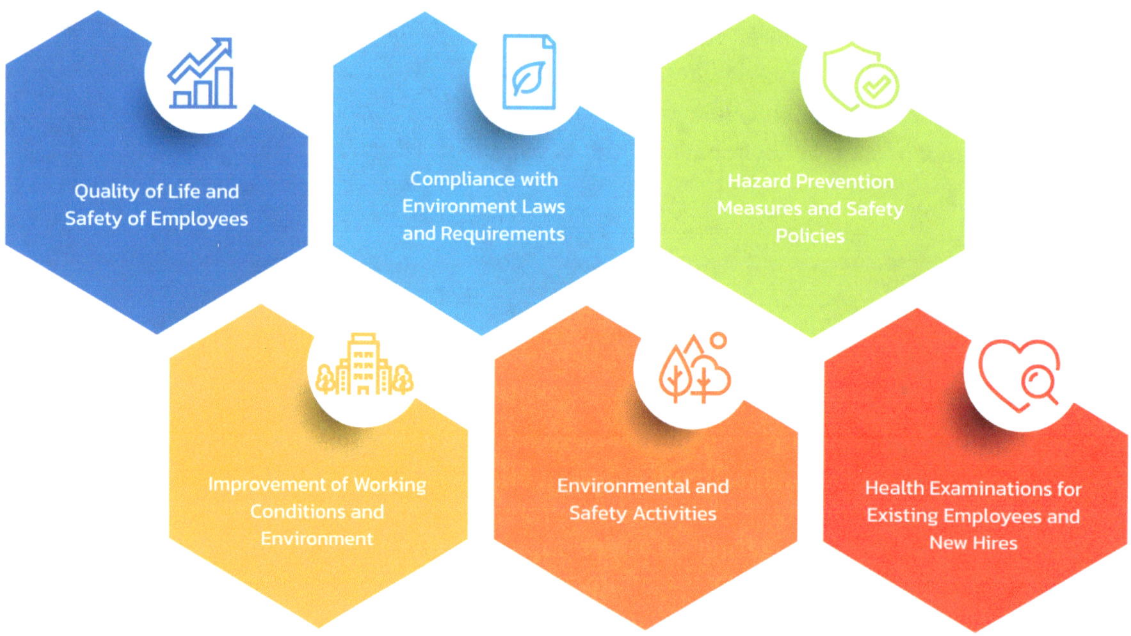
Quality of Life and Safety of Employees
Compliance with Environment Laws and Requirements
Hazard Prevention Measures and Safety Policies
Improvement of Working Conditions and Environment
Environmental and Safety Activities
Health Examinations for Existing Employees and New Hires

Figure 5.1. Environmental and occupational health.

Source: https://www.ckpower.co.th/storage/content/sustainability/management-process/occupational-health-and-safety/sd-2022/en/occupational-health-and-safety-en.png.

Definition of Environmental and Occupational Health

The approach of occupational and environmental health suggests a multidisciplinary approach that examines how exposures in the environment influence the health of workers and populations. The field integrates classical public health with occupational safety and environmental science in an understanding that risks typically intersect across several fields. Practitioners can formulate more holistic solutions for avoiding potential hazards by understanding these interdependencies. For instance, environmental contaminants can penetrate into the workplace and endanger workers' health tremendously. One should thus acknowledge the interaction between occupational and environmental health while designing comprehensive public health interventions. In contemporary discourse, the significance of an integrated approach is more pronounced in the wake of growing labor-environmental allegiances with a common goal of protecting health in the two spheres (Mayer et al., 2009). The impacts of climate change on occupational and environmental health cannot be overstated because it has a myriad of risks that affect workers and communities in general. Climatic pattern fluctuation causes job-related hazards, particularly in climatically sensitive sectors such as construction and agriculture. Higher temperatures, more frequent occurrences of natural disasters, and shifting weather patterns can lead to heightened exposure to hazardous elements and occupational injuries. In light of such problems, the embracement of pro-emergent workplace policies geared toward prioritizing workers' protection while promoting environmental sustainability is crucial. Having forward-looking approaches enables employers to reduce health risks from severe climate events and other climate-related problems, linking job safety with broader ecological aims. Thus, climate change treatment in the occupational health aspect is crucial to develop sustainable community programs (Taylor et al., 2025). Empirical studies and theoretical frameworks also elucidate the interconnection between occupational and environmental health, which can serve as a basis for action-oriented interventions. Several research studies, including the Australian Workplace Barometer project, have contributed to evidence of work environments' effect on workers' health outcomes. This research highlights the importance of psychosocial hazards in occupational settings, with the latter having a connection with overall workforce productivity and well-being. Collecting data from different regions and making these studies a foundation of understanding the complex dynamics that occur within occupational health settings, establishing monitoring and surveillance systems can be conducive to policies countering workplace risks and developing healthier work environments. Such evidence-based approaches are essential to achieving effective, sustainable community health initiatives that link personal well-being with collective environmental stewardship (Taylor et al., 2025).

Importance of the Topic in Contemporary Society

The part played by occupational and environmental health in today's society is underlined by the increasing recognition of the interdependence of workplace conditions and the broader environmental factors. As workplaces gain a greater understanding of the consequences of environmental hazards, a transition from the traditional approach of treatment towards one emphasizing prevention and health-related risk reduction is underway. This shift is especially important because work environment conditions tend to be determined by organizational behaviors like job design, leadership, and general workplace climate. Tackling these factors not only contributes to individual well-being but also fosters a healthier organizational climate. Building on knowledge drawn from public health can generalize intervention strategies aimed at enhancing workplace safety and health considerably. By creating a holistic approach to health incorporating these broader organizational drivers, employers can construct healthier workplaces that, in turn, benefit their employees and their communities (Karanika-Murray et al., 2013). The nexus between occupational health and environmental sustainability is fundamental as society becomes more aware of the consequences of climate change. The recognition that environmental degradation is a direct threat to the well-being of workers and communities has spurred the creation of blue green coalitions that unite the interests of labor and the environment. Such coalitions revolve around health as a focal point in resisting environmental hazards, thus emphasizing cooperative measures to discourage threats from toxic exposures. Through the combination of occupational safety and environmental health, these coalitions heighten the call for an interdisciplinary public health practice that encompasses numerous perspectives. The resultant dialogue enhances prevention measures and environmentally friendly practices with the prospect to influence policy and bring about favorable change on individual and system levels, ultimately contributing to public health improvements on a larger scale (Mayer et al., 2009). Besides, occupational safety and health promotion are important in countering contemporary environmental concerns, particularly because climate change aggravates existing threats to health. With changing climatic patterns, workers across various sectors are faced with emerging hazards, including heat stress, respiratory disease due to increased air pollution, and exposure to toxic chemicals escalated by weather extremes. A focus on sustainable community programs promoting occupational health is essential in preparing work environments to address these challenges. Employers and policymakers must have healthy workplaces with sustainable practices in place in order to protect the health of employees while simultaneously making progress toward broader environmental goals. This policy not only addresses current health concerns but also fosters a culture of health and sustainability that can trigger social change and make workplace safety an axis of public health in contemporary society (Karanika-Murray et al., 2013; Mayer et al., 2009) (Figure 5.2).

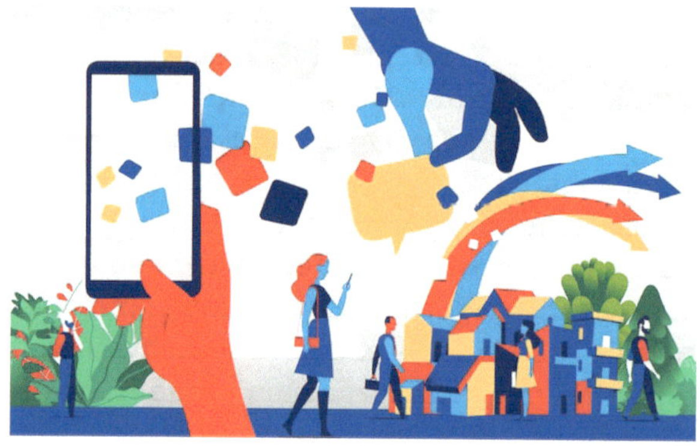

Figure 5.2. Digital technology is shaping modern community interaction and information flow.

Source: https://external-content.duckduckgo.com/iu/?u=https%3A%2F%2Fimage.freepik.com%2Ffree-vector%2Fcontemporary-society_1343-412.jpg&f=1&nofb= 1&ipt=143099f411b7542b1de9b14e3b76b324b8ef0599b2abfd033251e9f201987f10.

5.1. Environmental Hazards

Environmental hazards represent a broad array of hazards coming from natural and human-induced sources, which have direct impacts on the health and safety of the public. Environmental hazards can manifest themselves as chemical pollutants, biological disease-causing agents, or physical threats such as extreme climatic phenomena. Hurricanes and wildland fires are unavoidable events due to weather activities; however, human activities that compromise ecological equilibrium can elevate the scale of their impact. On the other hand, industrial accidents or technological dangers are the outcome of industrial or chemical production processes that are largely preventable by adhering to strict safety conditions and regulations. Legal mechanisms regulating such environmental hazards tend to focus on liability and establish punishment for companies responsible for negligence leading to environmental degradation and community health risks, hence the need for effective labor law and welfare systems to assist concerned groups (Tiraboschi et al., 2015). Climate change has emerged as the top reason for environmental hazards and has initiated a call for re-evaluation of public health strategies. The function of climate change extends beyond weather patterns because a rise in temperature may contribute to more serious and more frequent natural disasters and affect air quality and the availability of water. Occupational Environmental Medicine (OEM) plays a critical role in addressing the intersection of climate change and occupational health, in an effort to prepare health care practitioners to understand and mitigate these risks. Training programs for OEM practitioners increasingly emphasize climate change courses, better equipping them with all the competencies necessary to protect employees and their communities against the impacts of environmental hazards. By integrating climate information into existing models of medical education, OEM aims to create a workforce that can anticipate and counter the dangers a changing environment presents (Ayoub et al., 2025). Sustainable community initiatives form an anticipatory approach to minimizing and adjusting to the hazards of the environment effectively. These initiatives are likely to enhance urban resilience through enhanced infrastructure, promoting green spaces, and the development of grassroots support for caring for the environment. Through the implementation of sustainable practices, communities can reduce their vulnerability to natural and technological hazards as well as improve public health impacts at the same time. For instance, the development of urban green spaces not only enhances biodiversity but also acts as a natural barrier against extreme weather events, ultimately contributing to enhanced community resilience. Moreover, these practices enhance interagency coordination among government departments, non-profit groups, and local residents to encourage a culture of shared responsibility for environmental health. By working together in this way, sustainable community action is able to create safer communities, driving long-term change while it acts on the dynamics between ecological health and public interest (Figure 5.3).

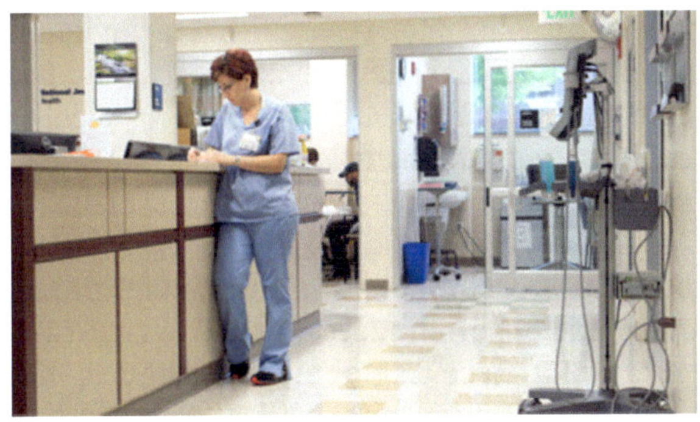

Figure 5.3. The occupational and environmental medicine (OEM).

Source: https://www.nationaljewish.org/getmedia/b19a96ac-c211-420f-bb2b-1ef327807771/Academic-Training-OEM-Residency-Program.jpg?width=428&height=244&ext=.jpg.

5.1.1. Types of Environmental Hazards (Chemical, Biological, Physical)

Classification of environmental risks encompasses three principal types: chemical, biological, and physical risks. Chemical risks are chemicals that are potentially harmful to people and the environment. They are industrial chemicals, pesticides, heavy metals, and volatile organic chemicals. Their exposure can cause acute effects like poisoning or chronic effects like cancer and respiratory diseases. In an occupational environment, chemical hazards are more of a concern in industries like manufacturing and agriculture, where the workers may directly and long-termly be exposed to toxic chemicals. The necessity for stringent regulations and forward-looking safety measures is of utmost importance in curbing these risks and ensuring a safe working environment, particularly against the background of climate change that is capable of altering the availability and concentration of these chemicals in air, land, and water, thereby increasing the intensity of exposure risks (Ayoub et al., 2025). Biological hazards, also referred to as biohazards, are microorganisms like viruses, bacteria, fungi, and parasites that may be harmful to human health. Biological hazards are most typical of healthcare institutions, farming, and laboratories. They are responsible for infectious diseases, allergic reactions, and toxic effects, affecting not only workers but also the neighboring communities of industrial and agricultural operations. Recent global experiences, like the COVID-19 pandemic, have attested to how biological hazards can turn into severe health emergencies and socio-economic effects quickly. Understanding the dynamics and implications of biological hazards in the workplace and in general is a requirement to develop effective preventive measures. In this context, effective training, personal protective equipment (PPE), and efficient health surveillance systems are necessary for minimizing the negative impacts of such hazards on health in the workplace and safeguarding public health (Delclos et al., 2020). Physical hazards are environmental agents that can cause harm but are not necessarily chemical or biological. They include noise, radiation, temperature extremes, and ergonomic hazards like repetitive motion injuries. Physical occupational health hazards present a unique challenge, which in most instances leads to workplace accidents or long-term diseases among the employees. For instance, continuous exposure to loud noise can lead to hearing damage, while inadequate ergonomics can lead to musculoskeletal disorders. Climate change exacerbates physical hazards; increasing temperatures can lead to heat stress among outdoor working individuals, while extreme weather conditions can undermine infrastructure and protective measures.

An effective workplace safety strategy must address physical hazards in an integrated way through risk assessments and mitigation strategies to achieve a safer working environment. It not only protects workers from harm but also promotes their general well-being, which is important to enhance productivity in a changing environment (Ayoub et al., 2025) (Figure 5.4).

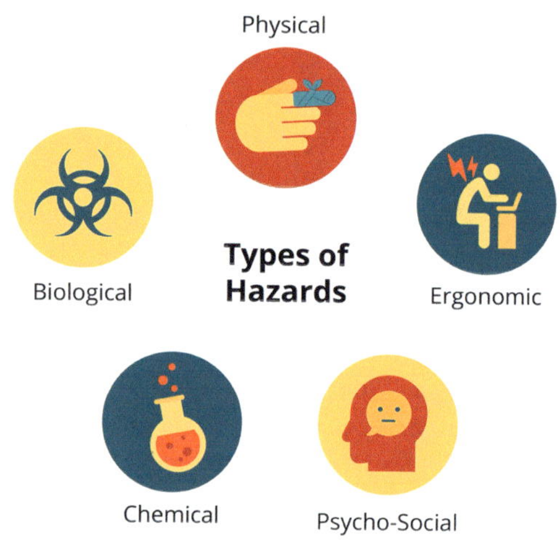

Figure 5.4. Types of environmental hazards.

Source: https://external-content.duckduckgo.com/iu/?u =https%3A%2F%2Fecampusontario.pressbooks.pub%2Fapp%2 Fuploads%2 Fsites%2F2305% 2F2022%2F05 %2FHealthandSafety-Graphic_5-01-1024x576.png&f=1&nofb= 1&ipt= 5da9286be6ef9 f709501 e5b9250374e41e43cc97c6c d9b3fbd958e958510207d.

5.1.2. Impact of Environmental Hazards on Public Health

Environmental risk and public health have a broad-ranging, intricate interaction, perpetuating through numerous mechanisms that affect communities across the globe. Industrial pollution, for instance, introduces dangerous chemicals into air and water systems that yield increased respiratory disease, cardiovascular illness, and cancer in affected populations. Urban populations, typically most burdened by these environmental risks, all too frequently exhibit elevated levels of health disparities.

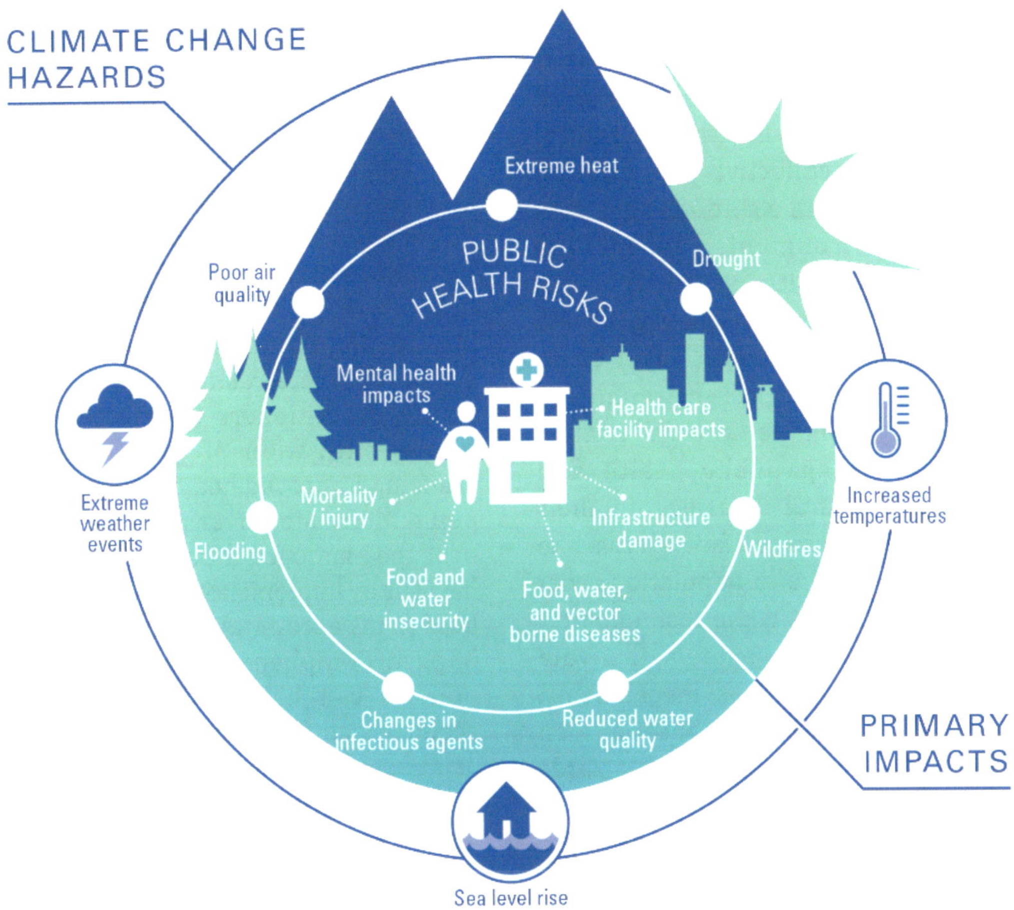

Figure 5.5. Hazards-impacts public health.

Source: https://ecoplan.ca/wp-content/uploads/2017/07/hazards-impacts_public-health.png.

These impacts largely fall on disadvantaged groups, including the poor and minorities, and thus demonstrate the imperative for public health intervention directed towards both environmental justice and health inequity. As components of climate change grow, such as extreme weather conditions and sea level rise, the situation continues to be increasingly vulnerable. It hence demonstrates the imperative to unify environmental and occupational health in order to guarantee public welfare. Besides, the blue-green alliances of labor and environmental movements highlight the synergy between occupational safety and environmental health. Activists in the movement realize that issues related to health link their objectives and advance the agenda for reducing toxic exposures in the workplace and the community as well. These coalitions strive to create comprehensive approaches to solving the root causes of environmental threats to public health, advocating for policy reforms that promote sustainable practices. The framework set by these alliances ensures health as a primary focus, illustrating the potential for collective action to deliver significant improvements in public health indicators. Through encouraging collective coordination and discussion, blue-green coalitions construct more resilient environments, reconciling environmental sustainability with labor rights, thus constructing community resilience in spite of reigning ecological challenges (Mayer et al., 2009). Natural and technological environmental hazards' differences make known critical implications concerning public health and legal frameworks. Natural disasters, in their capricious nature, activate welfare systems to offer immediate assistance to populations that suffer from such disasters, while technological hazards, perceived as preventable, activate accountability through juridical mechanisms. The dualism poses fundamental questions on proactive prevention of environmental hazards and on the part played by industrial relations and labor law in averting potential catastrophes. Studying these nuances can lead to effective measures that not only respond positively to emergencies but also prevent future occurrences by introducing prevention measures across industries. Incorporating workers' perspectives into the debate about environmental hazards not only enhances working environments but also has broad implications on public health within communities, illustrating the interconnectedness of health policy, workers' rights, and environmental justice (Tiraboschi et al., 2015) (Figure 5.5).

5.1.3. Strategies for Mitigating Environmental Hazards

Environmental risk mitigation needs a multifaceted intervention that includes education, policy change, and public engagement. One of the strategies is to enhance educational curricula that provide trainees with information on climate change effects and environmental health. By aligning graduate medical education programs with competency-based skills in climate health, as proposed in recent studies, educators can equip incoming professionals with the competencies necessary to identify and act upon environmental hazards. This convergence not only promotes sensitization but also fosters forward-looking plans for safeguarding worker health and community resilience (Ayoub et al., 2025). Phrasing education in terms of specific climate-related conditions empowers health practitioners to effectively contribute to the mitigation of these risks, ultimately realizing improved health outcomes for affected populations. Moreover, policy interventions also bear the blame for counteracting environmental hazards by implementing regulatory systems that hold firms accountable for their environmental impact. Compliance with tight environmental policies can halt technology and industrial accidents as firms are compelled to adhere to established standards for safety. The standards guarantee that proactive risk assessment and control of possibilities are not only encouraged but mandated as well. The differentiation between natural and technological hazards offers a simplified framework for legal liability and emphasizes environmental regulation compliance as key (Tiraboschi et al., 2015). The regulations have to be regularly evaluated and adjusted to address emerging environmental threats, with the communities remaining safe from both expected and unexpected catastrophes. Community-led initiatives are also a practical approach towards reducing environmental risks through the development of local resilience and empowerment. Involvement of community members in decision-making enhances their awareness of environmental risks and encourages community action. Interventions such as community appraisal and response planning enable residents to personalize plans specific to their environment. Collaboration with local governments and organizations can further aggregate resources and knowledge sharing, amplified by the multiplier effect of mitigation measures. By creating a culture of preparedness and environmental stewardship at the community level, populations become more likely to react to hazards in an effective manner and adapt to climate change more effectively (Ayoub et al., 2025). Community-based movements such as these confirm that sustainable practices and community participation are indeed crucial to sustaining long-term environmental health and safety.

5.2. Occupational Health Hazards

Occupational hazards are crucial in the establishment of a safe and effective workplace as they directly influence the well-being of workers and organizational performance. Occupational hazards are broadly classified into physical, chemical, biological, and ergonomic hazards. These all encompass certain hazards that organizations must overcome in detail. Physical hazards may include noise, radiation, and machine danger, and these may lead to acute injuries or chronic illnesses. Chemical risks, such as exposure to dangerous chemicals, form the nexus of concern for workplace safety. With most workplaces existing at the intersection of a combination of hazard types, an integrated approach towards health and safety management is essential in order to adequately mitigate these risks and have a healthy workforce.

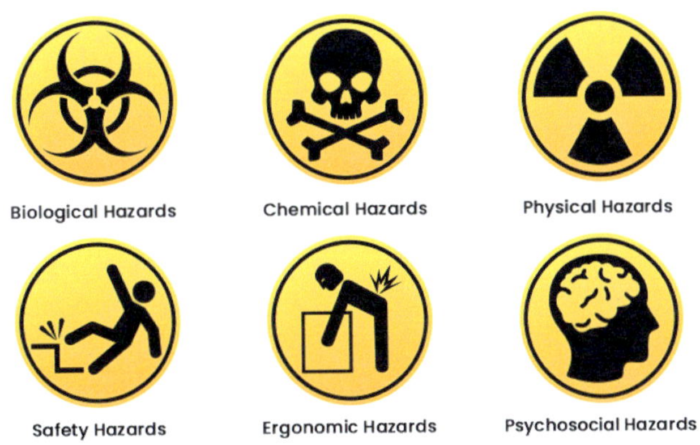

Figure 5.6. Occupational health hazards.

Source: https://external-content.duckduckgo.com/iu/?u=https%3A%2F%2Fmedia.hazwoper-osha.com%2Fwp-content%2Fuploads%2F2022%2F05%2F30122254%2Fblog-banner.png&f=1&nofb=1&ipt=dfd9058fa67732e5721998338254d9d9ffd0ed28db4646685c60225dc2547d6a.

The new emphasis on a whole-system strategy for occupational health puts a great deal of emphasis on the prevention of ill health causes, rather than simply the cure of ill health. Organizations are increasingly being encouraged to adopt frameworks involving job design, management of workload, and leadership style, all of which have a big impact on workers' health and well-being. However, these types of frameworks are hard to implement for most businesses because organizational momentum or enforcement-based methods, as opposed to overall wellness-oriented methods, hinder their effectiveness. Public health principles-based strategies can be particularly valuable because these strategies will generally lean towards a broader concept of health targeted at short-term as opposed to long-term workplace concerns. By expanding their vistas, organizations can create contexts that promote well-being as well as reduce significant occupational hazards (Karanika-Murray et al., 2013). On the issue of environmental and technological hazards, occupational legislation and occupational safety policies are pivotal. As opposed to natural disasters, which call for actions in response, environmental hazards provide opportunistic strategies in management with a prospect for prevention. The difference between these forms of hazards requires an imposition of legal frameworks that mandate organizations to take responsibility for their workplace, such that workers and the surrounding communities are not subject to preventable injuries and sicknesses. Through the establishment of effective regulations and an ethical framework of accountability, economic systems can better foster safety for employees. These actions not only protect individual workers but also guarantee community sustainability, pointing to the interdependence of occupational health and general well-being in society (Tiraboschi et al., 2015) (Figure 5.6).

5.2.1. Common Occupational Health Hazards in Various Industries

Occupational health hazards exist in many different sectors and encompass a range of physical, chemical, and biological hazards. In manufacturing, for instance, workers are commonly exposed to equipment hazards and end up with accidents and musculoskeletal disorders. Exposure to chemicals is also a significant hazard, as workers are exposed to sewage waste without any personal protective equipment (PPE). Similarly, in construction, workers are at risk of hazards such as falls, which may cause severe injury or death. The overlap of physical dangers underscores the need for stringent safety measures and regulations to protect the labor force. Fighting these threats not only promotes a safe workplace but also marks the employer's role in mitigating danger through training and compliance with safety procedures (Tiraboschi et al., 2015). Medical practitioners face a unique set of occupational health threats that arise from interactions with patients and medications. Infectious diseases are the primary fear, as doctors and other staff have to work in areas where pathogens are found everywhere. Moreover, handling cytotoxic drugs, such as chemotherapeutic drugs, in clinical settings necessitates a highly disciplined safety regime to prevent occupational exposure. The healthcare sector is also infested with ergonomic hazards, where repeated motion and heavy lifting lead to chronic musculoskeletal diseases among staff. These risks emphasize the implementation of stringent worker safety measures through training in infection control, PPE, and ergonomic best practices. Through the reduction of such job risks, healthcare facilities can provide enhanced worker safety and quality patient care (Ayoub et al., 2025). Agricultural farmworkers are exposed to various occupational health threats in agricultural environments that are often aggravated by environmental and climate conditions. Pesticide exposure is a significant risk for agricultural farmworkers, and exposure could lead to acute and chronic outcomes like respiratory problems and neurodisability. Moreover, heat stress is also a newly arising problem due to increasing global temperatures, which demands that employees labor in increasingly hazardous environments during peak cultivation seasons. The physical strain of agricultural labor, such as working for extended periods and extensive exposure to heavy machinery, also increases the risk of accidents. Therefore, employers should give utmost priority to promoting the acceptance of security protocols, such as adequate training on using pesticides and managing heat stress. Such initiatives not only protect workers but also promote greenery in the case of evolving environmental issues (Tiraboschi et al., 2015).

5.2.2. Long-Term Health Effects of Exposure to Workplace Hazards

The long-term health effects of worker exposure to occupational hazards include a wide range of physical and psychological disorders that have serious impacts on the health of workers. Workers are most of the time exposed to chemical hazards, ergonomic hazards, and stressful conditions that lead to debilitating diseases such as respiratory diseases, musculoskeletal disorders, and psychological stress. Unless otherwise checked, over time, such effects can escalate to compromised quality of life as well as increased healthcare costs for individuals and systems within society. Furthermore, some occupational groups, such as industrial workers and health workers, are particularly vulnerable to such risks due to the nature of their workplaces. Recognition of these long-term consequences is essential to devising comprehensive safety strategies and risk elimination of occupational exposure, with a view toward healthier workplaces for everybody. The interrelationship between health and work hazards extends beyond individual disease impact to population health and well-being. Prolonged exposure to hazardous conditions has a tendency to exact a high disease burden within specific occupational groups.

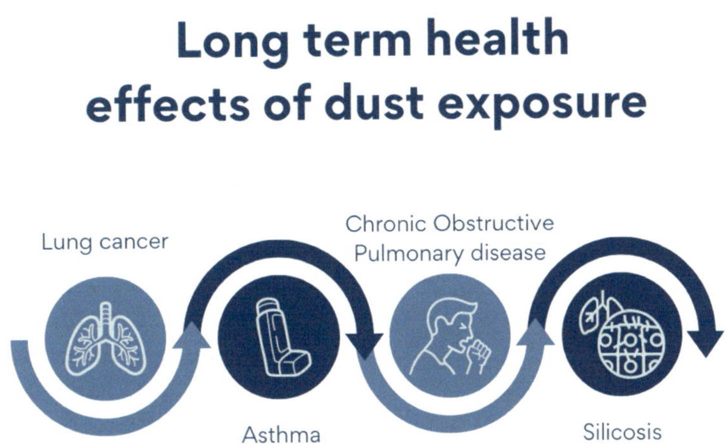
Long term health
effects of dust exposure
Lung cancer
Chronic Obstructive
Pulmonary disease
Asthma
Silicosis

Figure 5.7. Long-term-health-effects-of-dust-exposure.

Source: https://www.wamanagement.co.uk/wp-content/uploads/2023/04/Long-term-health-effects-of-dust-exposure.png.

This is exacerbated by external influences including socioeconomic status and environmental conditions that can further worsen health consequences. For example, low-income communities are often subjected to increased levels of exposure to environmental pollutants, which makes them disproportionately vulnerable to long-term health consequences. The regulatory and legal frameworks that control these workplace hazards must be such that they guarantee accountability, since the response of the legal authorities indicates a basic responsibility to protect worker health. Preventable risk scenarios are a site of intersection where labor law, industrial relations, and health policy meet, under pressure to incorporate preventive stages in dealing with occupational safety, as indicated in Tiraboschi et al. (2015). The evolving environment for occupational safety also points to the value added by education and training in avoiding long-term health effects of exposure to environmental hazards. Existing policy guidelines show that incorporating climate change literacy in occupational and environmental medicine (OEM) training can position healthcare professionals well to respond to emerging environmental issues. Closing existing knowledge gaps regarding health effects from climate change and occupational risks is necessary for workers' health protection and community resilience strengthening. This involves a re-examination of existing educational curricula to include practical skills that equip health caregivers to anticipate and respond suitably to these complex problems, as evident in Ayoub et al. (2025). Foreseeing by modifying training programs not only generates an adequately informed workforce but also contributes to enhancing the overall health outcomes of communities working under toxic conditions (Figure 5.7).

5.2.3. Regulatory Frameworks Governing Occupational Health

Regulatory regimes governing occupational health are essential to ensuring guarantees of employees' well-being and safety across various sectors. These regimes encapsulate a wide scope of legislation and standards meant to eliminate or minimize risks associated with exposure to hazards in the workplace, both physical and chemical in nature. In the United States, regulatory agencies such as the Occupational Safety and Health Administration (OSHA) have a critical role in enforcing regulations in order to prevent workplace illness and injury. By establishing permissible exposure limits and standards for safety training, these regulations play a critical role in establishing a culture of safety in organizations. The complexity of the modern workplace necessitates a robust regulatory context, particularly as technologies are being developed and new hazards emerge, underscoring the need for continuous revisions and harmonization with newly developing scientific understanding of occupational health threats. The intersection of occupational health and climate change merely serves to make the regulation more complicated, calling for a change in perspective as to how the regulations are dealt with. With more dangers from climate change impacting laborers' safety, the regulatory agencies need to adopt a different approach to managing the emerging challenges. For instance, training and education initiatives are being updated to include climate competencies in occupational medicine, as highlighted by new research that reports current curricula have a tendency to overlook such effects. Thus, organizations will be required to make an effort to incorporate training that enhances employees' resilience to climate effects while promoting healthy workplaces. This supports research that stresses the necessity for means not only to address health issues but also to promote well-being through healthier organizational actions, thus overall workplace health and safety. Whereas regulatory mechanisms are typically compliance and sanction-focused, growing recognition is given to the necessity of a more integrated strategy towards workplace health. As in recent practice, the emphasis has changed from the mere symptom management of occupational ill health towards the identification and management of the cause. Integrated models incorporating job design, work-life balance, and organizational culture are increasingly being developed to facilitate sustainable workplace well-being. Through the incorporation of public health knowledge into occupational health interventions, organizations can create more comprehensive approaches to maintaining both physical safety and psychological well-being. These efforts are crucial, especially as corporations start realizing the long-term impact of workplace design and management on the health of workers. This conceptual convergence holds promise in generating stronger regulatory regimes that are sensitive to both current workplace issues and the future of public health.

5.3. Climate Change Effects on Health

Climate change and public health interact increasingly visibly, as temperature increases and extreme weather events contribute to a range of health risks. Respiratory disease exacerbated by air pollution is one of the most visible, tending to worsen in heatwaves. Pre-existing and susceptible groups are most likely to be affected. In addition, climate change promotes the spread of vector-borne diseases, such as mosquito and tick-borne diseases. Notably, climate change effects are not universal, given that poor communities are usually weighed down by cumulative vulnerabilities from socioeconomic causes.

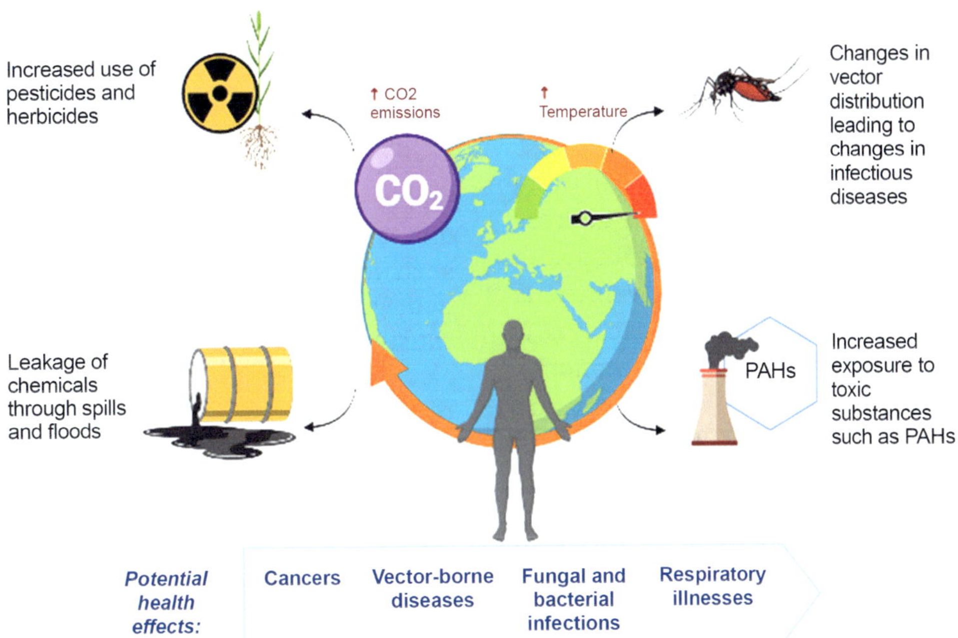

Figure 5.8. Climate change effects on health.

Source: https://www.frontiersin.org/files/Articles/973000/fpubh-10-973000-HTML/image_m/fpubh-10-973000-g001.jpg.

These inequalities require a combined effort to integrate health concerns into climate policy since they are prone to overlap with social determinants explicitly affecting the health implications of poor and minority populations, hence raising inherent disparities (N/A, 2010). Moreover, occupational health and climate change are interconnected and intricate factors. Outdoors and weather-sensitive workers are at higher risk from heat and extreme cold, and a changed pattern of weather. For instance, agricultural workers may get more exposure to heat with longer working hours, leading to heat illness and reduced productivity. In addition, workplaces may be impacted by climate disasters, such as floods and hurricanes, that not only threaten physical safety but also mental well-being through the resultant stress and trauma. In this context, a shift to a more holistic focus on occupational health is imperative. Empowering an understanding of the broader contextual determinants of well being and health has the potential to promote a health-focused and safety-oriented workplace culture that enables an organization to better prepare against challenges posed by climate change while safeguarding the well-being of employees (Karanika-Murray et al., 2013). Finally, sustainable community action helps in averting the health effects of climate change. By promoting green jobs and strengthening community resilience, initiatives can address social and environmental determinants of health simultaneously. The Green Jobs Movement is a classic example of such an approach, as it emphasizes the interconnectedness of economic opportunity, environmental sustainability, and public health. It seeks to lift individuals out of poverty while simultaneously addressing environmental degradation, thus producing a synergistic effect that increases overall well-being. By investing intelligently in community health initiatives through strategic channels, stakeholders can help create healthier environments and move towards health equity. An expanded vision is also reflective of the significance of cross-disciplinary collaboration across sectors, which itself reinforces the understanding that action against climate change is not simply an environmental concern, but a primary public health issue as well (N/A, 2010) (Figure 5.8).

5.3.1. Direct Health Impacts of Climate Change (Heatwaves, Natural Disasters)

The direct impacts of climate change on human health are becoming increasingly urgent, most significantly through increased frequency and intensity of heatwaves. Western Australia has seen a 50% increase in heatwave days since 1950, leading to an overall sharp rise in heat-related illness and mortality. For instance, a study indicates that between 1994 and 2006, the region experienced over 20 heat-related deaths yearly, a figure that would be doubled if the temperature rises by a further 2°C. The extreme heat not only claims lives among the vulnerable populations, such as the elderly, but also strains health systems as they handle a surge of cases of heat stress and heat exhaustion. The threat of increasing temperatures invokes preemptive action in public health policy to mitigate such impacts and protect community health (Pearce et al., 2025). Natural disasters, fueled by climate change, also pose significant direct health risks. Catastrophic occurrences, such as wildfires and floods, are occurring with greater frequency, and they are not only causing immediate injuries and deaths but also long-term health impacts. For example, rescue crews that respond to such accidents are exposed to higher occupational hazards like excessive exposure to heat and toxic smoke. Besides affecting their physical health, this also affects their minds as the psychological toll of violent disasters can lead to conditions like post-traumatic stress disorder (PTSD). Furthermore, the increase in natural disasters can disrupt essential health services and water supplies, leading to outbreaks of disease and exacerbating existing health disparities among populations (Forte et al., 2021). As climate change modifies the number and magnitude of disasters, there is a need for disaster management and public health policy to be aligned so that the issues can be tackled effectively. Additionally, the socio-economic impacts of climatic health effects cannot be overstated. As natural disasters and heatwaves intensify, the cost escalation of healthcare and emergency response imposes unprecedented strain on economies. This trend is most alarming in parts of Western Australia, where economic costs attributed to extreme heat and fire incidence are likely to be monumental. The need for strategic investment in sustainable community initiatives becomes urgent, as these programs not only enhance climate resilience but also public health gains. Sustainable actions, including the promotion of renewable energy and investment in green infrastructure, can both mitigate the effects of climate change and safeguard community health. It is crucial that governments prioritize such efforts to address the pressing challenges brought about by climate change and ensure future generations' well-being (Pearce et al., 2025) (Figure 5.9).

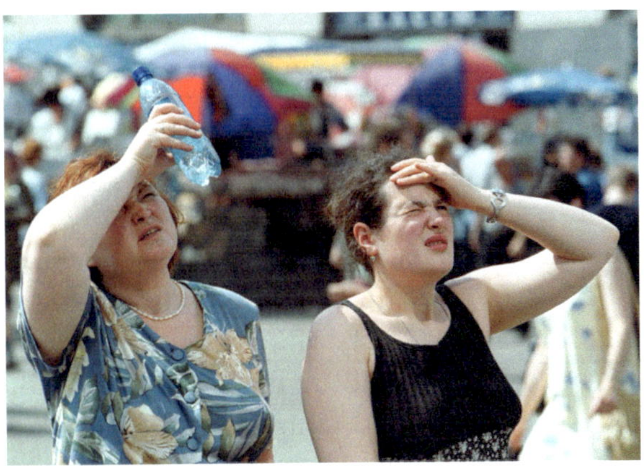

Figure 5.9. Heat waves are replacing drought as the deadliest climate disaster.

Source: https://cdn2.vox-cdn.com/assets/4753970/1603039.jpg.

5.3.2. Indirect Health Impacts (Vector-Borne Diseases, Food Security)

The secondary health implications of global warming, as they pertain to vector-borne disease, are becoming increasingly important and threatening in the environmental and occupational health sphere. Changes in temperature and precipitation patterns create ideal breeding habitats for vectors such as mosquitoes and ticks, which transmit diseases such as malaria and Lyme disease. As climate patterns change, regions that were traditionally thought of as being low-risk are beginning to experience outbreaks. This scenario not only threatens public health but also imposes a burden on healthcare systems.

The need for targeted preventive interventions and research in regions of emerging vector-borne disease risk is of the essence. Following (Lungu et al., 2010), current deficiencies in the research on the environmental health sector lend credibility to placing a high priority on studies that seek to develop successful intervention models. Food insecurity, combined with climate change, is another significant indirect health impact. Erratic weather patterns create fluctuating agricultural output, which may contribute to food shortages and malnutrition. Vulnerable individuals, particularly the poor in developing countries, are disproportionately affected by these disturbances. Restricted availability of multiple and adequate foods aggravates health, resulting in acute as well as chronic conditions.

The interface between food security, agricultural practices, and climatic conditions underscores the need for embracing sustainable community interventions that foster resilience to climatic variability. Implementing measures aimed at enhancing the diversification of food sources and enhancing agricultural efficiency is the top priority in preventing these problems. Research indicates that multi-strategies for food systems can increase food security and health outcomes, and it is in accordance with suggested recommendations by interventions like Nations et al. (2021) for implementing effective policy for health and environmental concerns.

Resolving indirect health impacts caused by climate change needs an interdisciplinary approach that involves collaboration among various sectors. Both vector-borne diseases and food security require collaborative action from environmental scientists, agricultural experts, and public health professionals to design integrated solutions. There has to be a policy formulation that accepts the convergence of environmental health, occupational safety, and community programs. Control measures for vector-borne diseases can be integrated with community programs designed to enhance food security, leading to overall enhanced community health. As mentioned in Nations et al. (2021), WHO and other UN agency directives place strong emphasis on the need for contextualized intervention in respective areas impacted by climate change, again promoting the call for collaborative structures to manage these intersecting health effects effectively.

5.3.3. Vulnerable Populations and Their Increased Risk

Vulnerable groups, historically defined by socioeconomic disadvantage, are at greater risk in both environmental and occupational health settings. These groups routinely inhabit settings with higher exposure to environmental risk factors, such as pollution and toxic waste, with resultant ill health. These environmental exposures are compounded by the denial of appropriate healthcare and provision, limiting their ability to mitigate these risks. The meeting of poverty and health signifies the need for inclusive approaches to remedy the systemic disparities driving these vulnerabilities. As aptly reported by Green For All, such challenges may be resolved through initiatives such as the Green Jobs Movement in order to facilitate the improvement in the health status of low-income communities towards a more equitable occupational and environmental health remedy (N/A, 2010). The impacts of climate change exacerbate the vulnerabilities of specific groups. Rising temperatures, more weather events, and poor air quality disproportionately affect low-income communities, which also have fewer resources with which to adapt to these impacts. These environmental stressors can lead to physical and mental health issues and are causative of a cycle that exacerbates prior disparities.

Moreover, occupational hazards are even more emphasized since individuals from lower socioeconomic groups tend to be more likely to take up work with fewer protective measures. Hence, focus on both environmental interventions and occupational standards for safety is required in order to ensure the reduction of risks and wellness. By broadening the perspective of intervention strategies and combining data from public health, we are in a position to establish specific interventions for the specific problems faced by vulnerable groups (Karanika-Murray et al., 2013). Finally, addressing the needs of vulnerable groups calls for an approach that combines environmental health programs with social justice concepts. Interventions must tackle not just the immediate health risks, but the socioeconomic causes of ill health and poverty that lead to a cyclical repetition of ill health. Providing equitable access to resources, education, and work is essential to empowering such groups to be able to articulate their health needs. Furthermore, collaborative action between environmentalists and health activists, civil rights organizations, and labor unions must be taken to create genuine systemic change. By fighting together against the unequalities embedded in our occupational and societal systems, we are able to develop resilience in vulnerable groups and create healthier communities that are resilient despite environmental and occupational stresses (N/A, 2010) (Figure 5.10).

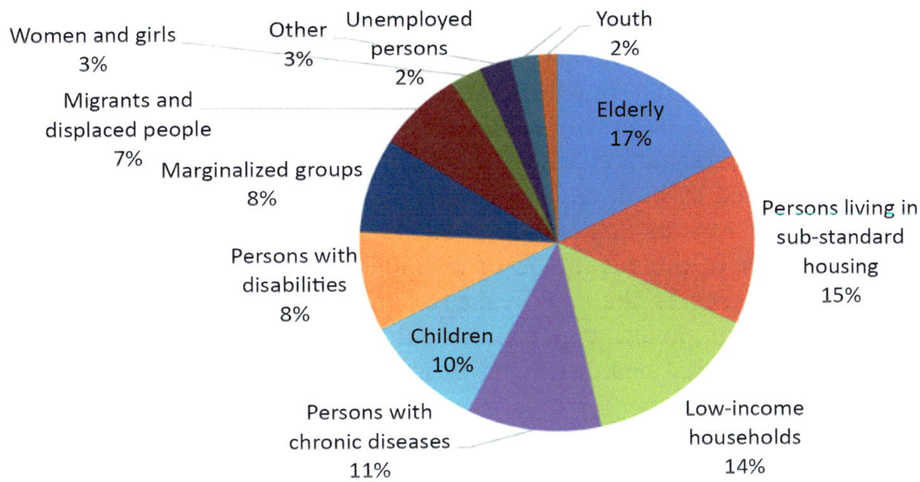

Figure 5.10. Vulnerable population groups.

Source: https://external-content.duckduckgo.com/iu/?u=https%3A%2F%2Fwww.researchgate.net%2Fprofile%2FFabio-Monforti%2Fpublication%2F365353664%2Ffigure%2Ffig28%2FAS%3A11431281096871190%401668356518328%2FMost-reported-vulnerable-population-groups.png&f=1&nofb=1&ipt=6f4b9428506f40023f604c1e847ccd96daeec1ccb56bef33751efdc557d52e8d.

5.4. Workplace Safety Regulations

Workplace safety legislation is profoundly significant in the protection of workers from occupational hazards, thus ensuring physical and mental health across different workplaces. Legal regulations, as established by the Occupational Safety and Health Administration (OSHA), are designed to create standards that minimize chemical, equipment, and environmental hazards. These laws not only require terms of safe work for employers but also grant employees rights for workplace health and safety. A good safety culture can reduce workplace injuries and illnesses, hence resulting in an environment where workers feel valued and safe. Ultimately, the basis of such regulations is an understanding that good workplace safety directly relates to a company's productivity and social responsibility in its operations. The convergence of workplace safety regulations and environmental health becomes increasingly important as climate change adds new risks to the workplace. With weather events becoming more common, the dangers presented in such instances make it necessary to rethink current safety standards. Workers in vulnerable industries, including agriculture and construction, are more vulnerable to climatic threats, and measures need to be made to improve safety standards. With preventive practices, companies are not only adhering to legislative regulations but also doing their share towards the overall objective of protecting the environment. Enhanced security measures that incorporate climatic oscillation can guard against hazards to personnel in attending to the potential long-term impacts of climatic change. This combined approach is paramount to balancing work protection with the pressing appeal of sustainable practices and community resilience in the light of climate adversity. Furthermore, there has been the appearance of blue-green alliances as a coalition among labor and environmentalists based on the foundation of health issues as a bridge between workplace safety and environmental justice. These coalitions highlight the connectedness of occupational health and environmental issues overall, which is of utmost relevance when advocating for more stringent regulations of workplace safety. Discussion and collective action by these coalitions work to reduce exposures to toxic substances that disproportionately affect low-income communities and communities of color, who are disproportionately affected by both environmental degradation and unsafe working practices. By focusing the interests of various stakeholders, such strategies offer windows of opportunity for progressive social change to the advantage of workplaces and the surrounding community at large. This intersection underscores the significant role of inclusive policymaking for maximizing workplace safety and promoting health experience equity, a testament to the fundamental tenets of environmental and occupational health (Mayer et al., 2009; N/A, 2010) (Figure 5.11).

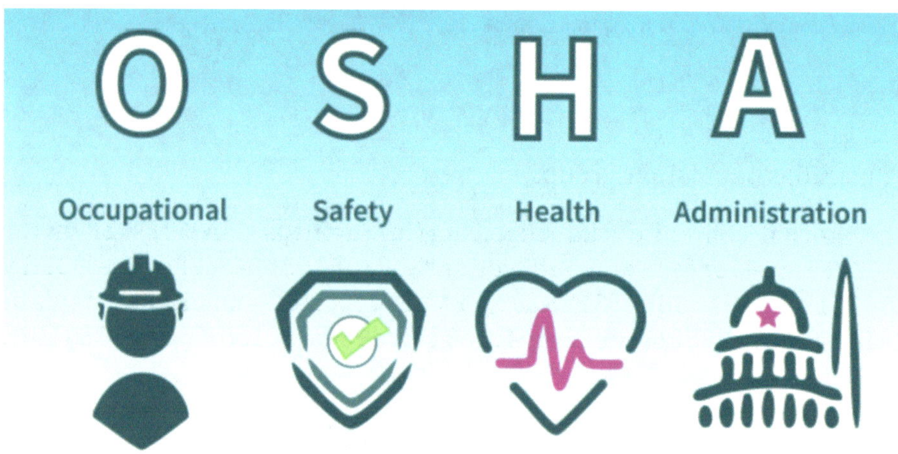

Figure 5.11. Occupational Safety and Health Administration (OSHA).

Source: https://cf-images.us-east-1.prod.boltdns.net/v1/static/777704725001/91141279-35c5-4e85-90ea-39f7120099fc/3366b0ad-64cb-4a19-a339-2c0db454783a/1280x720/match/image.jpg.

5.4.1. Overview of OSHA and Its Role in Workplace Safety

The Occupational Safety and Health Administration, or OSHA, plays a pivotal role in setting safety standards within the workplace in the United States. Established by the Occupational Safety and Health Act of 1970, OSHA's activities revolve around the provision of a safe and healthy working environment for employees. OSHA enforces, sets, and provides training while performing inspections to ensure compliance with safety standards. By offering a solution to potential hazards and promoting best practices, OSHA positively contributes to reducing workplace-related accidents, illnesses, and fatalities. Furthermore, its policies are also directly related to broader concerns of environmental and occupational health, promoting vigilance regarding the impact of hazardous situations in terms of continuous threat possibilities, such as those of industrial pollution and climate change. In its quest for enhancing workplace safety, OSHA is engaged in a broad spectrum of activities dedicated to constant revision of practice and policy. Not only does the agency enforce existing regulations, but it also reacts to new conditions in the workplace and newly evolving hazards, typically with direction from studies and case histories of occupational health hazards. They encompass collaborative efforts that integrate summaries of data from recent reviews, thereby identifying regulatory actions and formulating plans to counter risks of workplace hazards. OSHA's comprehensive strategy highlights the agency's commitment to continuous improvement in workplace safety, presenting a broader view of how environmental conditions and climate change are increasing occupational risks. These programs are critical, as they also fall in line with state and federal recommendations of enhancing the overall safety and health of workers and, at the same time, mitigating environmental-occupational health convergence. Cooperation of OSHA's policy with educational programs ensures enhanced training of the workforce to better sense and manage climate problems. As suggested by the latest studies, the alignment between graduate medical education competencies and climate change impacts becomes more valuable to achieve maximal occupational health strategies. The alignment can potentially trigger recognition of gaps in present education and highlight the importance of transferring skills-related know-how in various occupational health areas. By incorporating climate-related activity into the education of occupational health professionals, there is an urgent plea to safeguard the workers and communities. Notably, this includes an appeal for increased OEM training as a specialty that currently takes the lead in climate-relevant material, affirming the demand for continued education and acclimatization to safeguard against the shifting occupational hazard profile (Kriebel et al., 2011; Ayoub et al., 2025).

5.4.2. Importance of Safety Training and Education for Employees

The importance of safety training and employee education cannot be overstated in the function of creating a sustainable workplace culture. Comprehensive safety training equips employees with the skills and knowledge necessary to recognize and reduce potential hazards, reducing the incidence of occupational injuries and accidents. It has been established from recent studies that inadequate safety measures play a key role in causing workplace accidents and highlight the importance of organizational managers ensuring focus on safety training programs. Through establishing a safety-minded culture and strict safety policies, business organizations are able to foster a healthier workplace environment that not only accumulates benefits for the workers themselves but also for the wider population. As discussed in the findings, adherence to safety training is fundamental in achieving increased safety outcomes, thus overall stability of surrounding communities, which aligns with the grand vision of sustainable community projects (Vaiagae et al., 2020). Moreover, safety training is an integral component of environmental occupational health, particularly in the face of new challenges posed by climate change. As climatic conditions become tougher and as environmental hazards increase, it is essential to keep workers educated on surviving and recovering from the impacts of climate change. Incorporating information on climate into safety training modules is essential in preparing workers to anticipate and adapt to the implications of climate change. For instance, the incorporation of climate change education in organizational development can equip workers with the knowledge to take preventive actions and enable resilient practices in the work environment. Bridging this gap in safety education, organizations not only protect their workforce but also enable them to be contributing forces of change in society (Wainwright et al., 2025). This double focus on proximate safety and general environmental well-being emphasizes the varied benefits of investing in advanced safety training programs. Finally, workplace safety education and training succeed based on their ability to empower employees and engage them. As workers are directly invested in their own safety training, they become more vigilant and sensitive to dangers within their environment. By encouraging participative methods of safety training, organizations are able to enhance employees' hazard recognition and solution recommendation skills in a collaborative framework. This not only creates a more robust safety culture but also stresses empowerment, leading to better morale and job satisfaction. Finally, research suggests that a well-trained workforce can significantly enhance organizational performance through accident cost reduction and enhanced productivity. These findings further augment a healthier more sustainable work culture promoting the goals of local efforts to create safer environments for all to reside. Investments in robust safety training programs therefore become a strategic means of providing not only personal health but also overall society health (Vaiagae et al., 2020) (Figure 5.12).

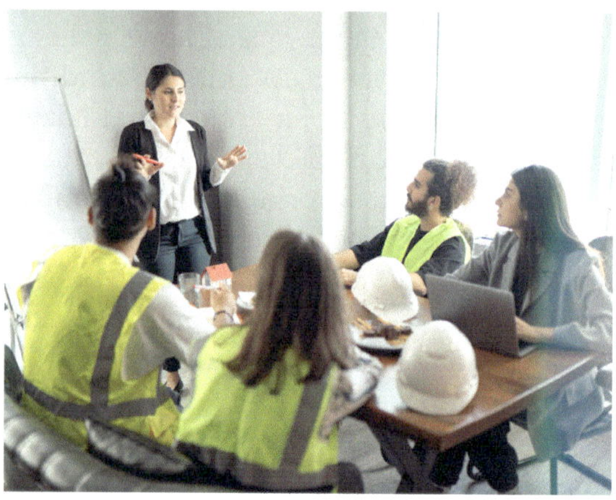

Figure 5.12. Safety training and education.

Source: https://safetyleaderinstitute.com/wp-content/uploads/2023/01/Homebanner2.jpg.

5.4.3. Case Studies of Successful Workplace Safety Programs

Successful workplace safety measures are vital case studies in illustrating the ways in which proactive measures can reduce risk and contribute to well-being in various industries. For instance, a case study of a manufacturing company that implemented an integrated safety management system illustrates the impact of prioritizing safety culture. By adding employee training for equipment operation, emergency response procedure, and routine safety inspections, the company achieved a remarkable reduction in workplace injury by over 40% in one year. Beyond addressing short-term safety concerns, the program instilled a sense of responsibility in workers, leading to increased productivity and employee involvement. These actions are designed to emphasize the essentiality of developing workplace safety programs that are attuned to specific environmental hazards and responsive to the unique requirements of heterogeneous workforce populations. The intersection of workplace safety and environmental health becomes more significant in the wake of climate change and the threats associated with it. A prime example is a building firm that recognized the need to minimize both staff exposure to toxic chemicals and general environmental impact. The company adopted a two-faceted approach: imposing rigorous safety standards and adopting green methodologies, such as utilizing eco-friendly materials and minimizing wastage. By educating workers on potential environmental risk factors and engaging in practical sustainable activities, the organization enhanced both occupational and environmental well-being. This case shows how whole-of-safety programs can also speak to the issue at a wider scale of climate risks, affirming the interdependence of work environments and community health outcomes as highlighted in Bridging the Equity Gap: Driving Community Health Outcomes Through the Green Jobs Movement, Green for all (N/A, 2010). Further, holistic approaches to workplace safety based on public health are effective across various settings. One company transformed its health and safety program by adopting an integrated model that invested in workers' health instead of just treating injuries. The program had its focus on job design, role clarity, and management of workload as being key to a healthy workplace. Unlike traditional methods that addressed injury prevention alone, this framework encouraged intervention that takes into account the psychosocial determinants of the workplace. By identification and control of organizational contextual drivers affecting health, such as leadership style and reward systems, this model addresses the needs of emerging paradigms in occupational health, where an increased integrated understanding of workplace well-being is needed. With its usefulness in responding to contemporary needs for change from the exclusive treatment approach to prevention and promotion of well-being, the utility of this model presents emerging ways of building healthier, safer workplaces (Karanika-Murray et al., 2013).

5.5. Sustainable Community Initiatives

The implementation of sustainable community interventions is a key intersection where social justice and environmental health converge. Prioritizing marginalized communities' interests in such interventions not only promotes ecological sustainability but also addresses historical health disparities driven by environmental hazards. Studies underscore that access to healthcare alone is not enough where underlying societal disparities continue, which means higher risk exposure to health hazards for low-income groups and communities of color. The Green Jobs Movement is an example of how a group of champions from diverse industries can drive overall systems transformation to enhance overall economic, environmental, and health conditions. By integrating job development with the quest for sustainability, such programs will make communities more resilient to climate change impacts while offering self-advocacy for vulnerable communities, ultimately leading to improved health gains and socioeconomic security for such communities (N/A, 2010). Having established sustainable practices within a community framework, workplace health and safety also has much to gain. Recent research suggests an urgent deviation of occupational health towards a whole-systems model aimed at reducing health hazards at their source. Such a model is consistent with the ethos of sustainable community programs, which are also concerned with countering root environmental influences that harm particular groups of individuals. By comprehending and navigating contextual organizational drivers—work design, workload, and leadership style—sustainable community programs can build healthier working environments. Therefore, the possibility lies in translating knowledge from public health into occupational safety, expanding interventions to include variables that enhance individual as well as collective well-being under the strategy of sustainable development (Karanika-Murray et al., 2013). Further, sustainable community programs can become a change agent for policy improvement that enhances environmental as well as occupational health outcomes. By encouraging greener, more equitable public policy, these kinds of initiatives have the capacity to influence legislative frameworks that promote sustainability and community resilience. For example, integrating environmental justice into urban planning can mitigate the health effects of climate change on vulnerable populations. This policy-driven, mutually reinforcing process can help build a culture in which sustainable development is equivalent to just health outcomes. When communities go through such reformative processes, they not only address prevailing environmental hazards but also build the socio-political capital necessary for pursuing public health agendas centered on prioritizing community welfare while addressing climate change concerns. Thus, sustainable community initiatives are tasked with reconstructing the relationship between environmental health, occupational safety, and social justice (N/A, 2010; Karanika-Murray et al., 2013) (Figure 5.13).

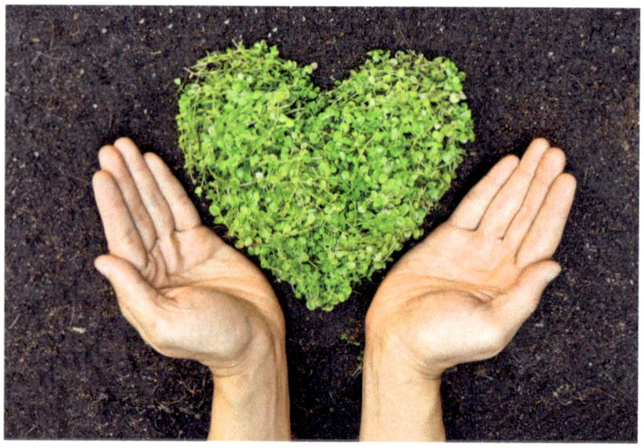

Figure 5.13. Sustainable community initiatives.

Source: https://phswastekit.co.uk/uploads/1/Heart%20shaped%20tree%20-%20eco-friendly%20concept.jpg.

5.5.1. Definition and Examples of Sustainable Community Initiatives

Sustainable community projects illustrate an active approach to solving the environmental and social challenges by enhancing resilience and fairness. Sustainable community projects involve enhancing well-being in communities through enhancing health, economic security, and natural resource stewardship. For instance, community gardens not only provide access to fresh fruits and vegetables but also serve as learning centers, teaching citizens about nutrition and environmentally friendly agriculture. These projects foster community engagement, fight food deserts, and advance mental health. Further, initiatives like community-led renewable energy projects help reduce fossil fuel consumption, aiding environmental well-being and job creation. Through these projects, communities can address neighborhood needs while concurrently promoting universal sustainability goals, literally living up to resilience and equity ideals during climate change and public health emergencies. The interconnection between community sustainability initiatives and public health is increasingly being realized as it relates to climate change and work-site health. Connecting aspects of public health with work-site safety initiatives will enable communities to better protect their citizens from environmental and occupational hazards. Green construction practices, for example, benefit not just energy efficiency but also indoor health. Additionally, these interventions decrease disease prevalence from poor indoor and outdoor air quality and toxic substance exposures. By adopting a holistic health and well-being strategy, as informed by public health models, organizations contribute to a healthier population and work environment. This brings to light the necessity of multi-pronged strategies that address the root causes of health disparities with a view to fostering sustainable models that cater to all stakeholders, especially for disadvantaged communities that have been seriously hit by such issues (Karanika-Murray et al., 2013). The ongoing convergence of social equity and sustainability is seen in various community-oriented programs aimed at disadvantaged groups. While medical access matters, it is not sufficient to address the greater social disparities that contribute to heightened health risks in low-income communities and communities of color by themselves. Sustainable social movements, such as the Green Jobs Movement, strive to counteract these disparities through the unification of environmental action with social justice action. This collaboration promotes the generation of green industry jobs that can improve economic status as well as generate adequate opportunities for vulnerable groups (N/A, 2010). By promoting collaboration between environmental, health, and workers' organizations, these schemes can help produce system changes that support improved health standards in communities, reduce exposure to environmental hazards, and promote climate change resilience. Thus, sustainable community work is excellent for empowering individuals and producing lasting improvement in well-being and health.

5.5.2. Role of Community Engagement in Promoting Sustainability

Community engagement is a key driver for speeding up sustainability initiatives, particularly in occupational and environmental health. It fosters a community sense of ownership of local initiatives and encourages people to take active roles in being advocates for sustainable development. By engaging community members in decision-making, institutions can make their initiatives more sensitive to people's values and needs. This integration not only enhances sustainability programs but also fosters an environmental responsibility culture. As the Healthy Universities Project has implied, organizations can be a major force in this engagement by leveraging resources to connect students, staff, and the wider community. This connection creates a platform of sustainability that goes beyond the classroom and into hands-on engagement in health and wellness through collective action towards environmental stewardship (Doherty et al., 2009). Secondly, maintaining communities through participation in sustainability matters has the potential to address issues at the systems level and particularly at the occupational health level. For business, worker engagement in health and safety matters can lead to more effective interventions that address their respective workplace cultures. Organizations that foster communicative environments will be in a position to obtain constructive feedback on what practices would foster work well-being, which can, in turn, be used to guide necessary policy reforms. By embracing a comprehensive approach to health with involvement from the community, organizations can remove the determinants of occupational damage. The findings show that an open discourse of workplace health can lead to innovative solutions and thus an enhanced working environment conducive to higher sustainability goals (Karanika-Murray et al., 2013).

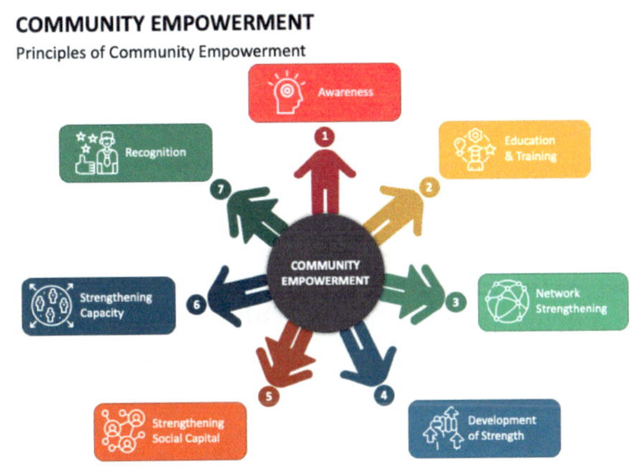
COMMUNITY EMPOWERMENT
Principles of Community Empowerment
COMMUNITY EMPOWERMENT
1 Awareness
2 Education & Training
3 Network Strengthening
4 Development of Strength
5 Strengthening Social Capital
6 Strengthening Capacity
7 Recognition

Figure 5.14. Community engagement.

Source: https://cdn.sketchbubble.com/pub/media/catalog/product/optimized1/c/2/c2cab30db6c57cd885aec91b2012ccd7916030ff275d6450ca735a776edcea1c/community-empowerment-mc-slide1.png.

Finally, the intertwined nature of community involvement and sustainability accounts for the importance of a collective answer to environmental and occupational health issues. Active communities that take part in sustainability initiatives are better able to accommodate climate change and associated health risks. Adaptation depends on local knowledge and shared experience, so that communities can scale up or down solutions to suit their specific circumstances. Through the sudden changes and stresses of climate change, active communities can serve as a cushion against disaster, building resilience in vulnerable groups. As evidenced in many academic and policy discussions, the integration of a community approach into sustainable agendas has profound implications beyond the necessity of mending the environment, hence improving overall public health outcomes and guaranteeing a sustainable future (Doherty et al., 2009) (Figure 5.14).

5.5.3. Benefits of Sustainable Practices for Public Health

Sustainable practice significantly enhances public health by addressing health determinants in the environment that contribute to disease and health inequities. Mitigation of pollution and promotion of clean air and water are among the key pillars of sustainable development. Reductions of air pollutants such as particulate matter and nitrogen oxides play an essential part in the prevention of respiratory diseases as well as cardiovascular disease among communities, most especially in urban communities where they are exacerbated. Besides, access to clean water averts waterborne illnesses that disproportionately affect poor communities. Such risks can be avoided by sustainable infrastructure as they generate healthier environments that are even advantageous to overall well-being, which reflects the need for synergistic solutions addressing environmental and health concerns (N/A, 2010). Social equity, further amplified by integrating sustainable approaches, is therefore necessary in improving public health results. Low-income populations tend to have systematic barriers in accessing healthcare and are subject to environmental hazards, leading them to have an increased disease burden. Green For All, a leading economic and environmental justice organization, states that these disparities can be minimized by sustainable actions and drastically enhance health conditions. Through the creation of green jobs that not only encourage work but also assist with environmental stewardship, communities benefit from increased economic sustainability and a reduction in health hazards brought about by climate change. The interconnectedness here emphasizes the role of integrating social justice within public health intervention and the ability of sustainable measures to enhance levels of community health (N/A, 2010). In addition, sustainable activities support improved mental health through greater community engagement and resilience. Participatory activities, for example, involve the mobilization of local communities to make decisions on their lands—such as urban agriculture, community cleanups, and the development of green spaces in urban areas—are better for social harmony and belongingness. These participatory activities can solve the problems of loneliness and anxiety that are typically related to environmental degradation and poor socioeconomic conditions. Lastly, by encouraging community participation in sustainability, public health programs can help create healthier, more resilient communities and enhanced psychological well-being. By engaging individuals in care for the planet through sustainable practices, not only is there immediate health care, but resilience capacity is built in the long run to ensure that communities will be better able to handle the impacts of climate change, as well as other associated health threats.

5.6. Interconnection of Environmental and Occupational Health

The connection between occupational and environmental health continues to gain prominence as both disciplines influence one another immensely. Environmental shifts, such as climate change, can have a direct impact on the health of workers through enhanced exposure to extreme weather conditions, air pollution, and changing patterns of disease. Farmers are an example of occupational groups that typically face greater vulnerabilities due to climate-related hazards, adding to related occupational risks. As it has been uncovered with the latest studies, an all-encompassing approach allowing the integration of human rights and workers' health can facilitate targeted interventions to protect workers in interactive environments. This takes precedence by emphasizing research and policy reform in order to protect health measures within the interactive risk of climate change, thereby emphasizing occupational health's interactive relationship with environmental responsibility (Landmann et al., 2025). In the anticipation of future work environments, it becomes evident that integration between occupational and environmental health concerns must inform policy practices and structures. Technological innovation and globalization will define future work, offering opportunities and risks. Systematic literature review of this matter reveals that climate change, demographics, and economy are predicted to have a profound effect on the occupation field. Identification of psychosocial risks as prevalent issues within new work settings emphasizes the need for resilience-inducing measures to offset precarious work-induced stressors. Review identifies the need to integrate sustainability and health as strategic concerns within workforce planning, thereby ensuring interventions manage environmental as well as workplace safety comprehensively (Delclos et al., 2020). As community sustainability programs continue to develop, environmental and occupational health become integral to the success of such programs. Successful community outreach aimed at improving worker safety creates a connection with the initiative of establishing a healthier environment. For instance, workplaces that function through green programs are not just protecting their laborers but also working toward public health and ecological goals in general. By working hand in hand with stakeholders like businesses, healthcare providers, and policymakers, communities become capable of implementing integrated health strategies that target occupational exposures as well as environmental concerns. Such interventions show a paradigm shift to think about work environment and ecological environment health impacts, culminating in the end to create a sustainable future towards human and planetary health (Landmann et al., 2025; Delclos et al., 2020) (Figure 5.15).

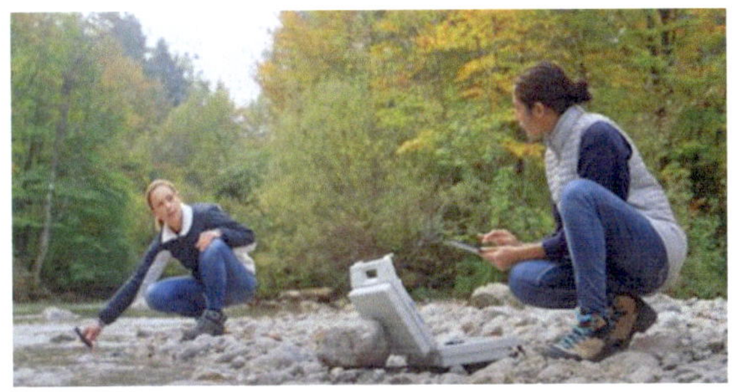

Figure 5.15. Environmental and occupational health.

Source: https://external-content.duckduckgo.com/iu/?u= https%3A%2F%2Ftse3.mm.bing.net%2Fth% 3Fid%3DOIP.zesQfbqciUx9kWNXs6E8NQHaD0%26cb%3Diwp2%26pid%3DApi&f=1&ipt= 776b7d4e275e 2b7d38ed 5cbd6f27 d6032c7ad97bd6 a7c6474a2ecf9449c4aa7a.

5.6.1. How Environmental Factors Influence Occupational Health

Environmental problems have a significant role in affecting occupational health outcomes. They encompass a broad range of aspects that define the physical environment, social relationships, and organizational practices. For instance, organizational environment and job design will have a significant impact on determining the well-being of employees. Poor job design is most likely to lead to high levels of stress and work dissatisfaction, while poor leadership and incentive systems are most likely to encourage unhealthy environments. There needs to be a paradigm shift in occupational health, away from a reactive treatment-oriented focus towards a proactive approach that takes account of underlying environmental causes and promotes well-being (Karanika-Murray et al., 2013). If organizations do not embrace this broader perspective, they may not be able to develop a healthy environment in the workplace and therefore lose productivity and gain absenteeism. Impacts of climate change also complicate the intersection between environmental determinants and occupational health. With more frequent episodes of extreme weather, the risks of outdoor jobs such as construction and agriculture become higher. Jobs are at greater risk of exposure to extreme temperatures, air pollution, and natural catastrophes, all of which are detrimental to their health. Moreover, resource-based industries are particularly vulnerable, and demand adaptive actions to protect the welfare of employees. Consistent practice can mitigate such adverse effects, but investment in training and technology is required to protect workers from harm while adapting to the new environment. Such programs, by doing so, not only protect the safety of the workers but also health outcomes for larger populations (Doyle et al., 2023). Safety culture integration with continuous improvement practices is crucial for developing effective strategies to enhance occupational health against such environmental challenges. An advanced safety culture encourages mutual accountability among employees and management to minimize workplace accidents through employee-management commitment to safety protocols. In small-scale mining, for example, the use of best practice standards for safety protects employees even under conditions of limitations, such as limited resources. Rapid adaptation is achieved through agile management practices that allow for adaptation to quick changes. Environmental change and occupational safety-related intricacies necessitate agile management practices that are meant to allow for rapid adaptation. Through the implementation of an effective safety system and adaptive practices, organizations can significantly enhance occupational health while ensuring sustainable workplace practices. These will benefit workers and the broader community (Doyle et al., 2023).

5.6.2. The Role of Policy in Addressing Both Areas

Good policy is important for bridging the gap between occupational safety and environmental health since both fields are exposed to deteriorating threats of climate change and socioeconomic disparities. Policies that guarantee the integration of health considerations into environmental policies have the ability to significantly contribute to the health conditions of communities, especially vulnerable communities. Low-income communities, for instance, have more exposure to environmental hazards that are worsened by poor access to healthcare and social welfare. These inequalities need to be addressed through a multilateral policy framework that not only provides access to healthcare but also funds for sustainable community investments in order to achieve economic stability and environmental resilience. Investment in these initiatives can empower communities, particularly those who are most suffering from structural injustices, to participate in the creation of healthier living and working conditions. As noted, the Green Jobs Movement can utilize collective action in achieving systemic change in our economic and environmental spheres to eventually foster healthier communities (N/A, 2010). Policy interventions in workplace health should become actively directed towards avoiding workplace illness and towards better overall well-being, as opposed to reactive interventions. Occupational health policy has traditionally been about managing risk once something has occurred; but increasingly, an integrated approach is emerging based on prevention and reducing determinants of ill health. Organizations are better able to manage those systemic influences on worker health, such as job design and organizational climate, by designing environments that care about psychological and physical well-being. There is a significant imperative for policies that reconcile the views of public health because organizational contributors can play a major part in staff well-being. The integration of public health practice into workplace health interventions is a viable path towards constructing healthier workplaces that are attuned to broader public health agendas (Karanika-Murray et al., 2013).

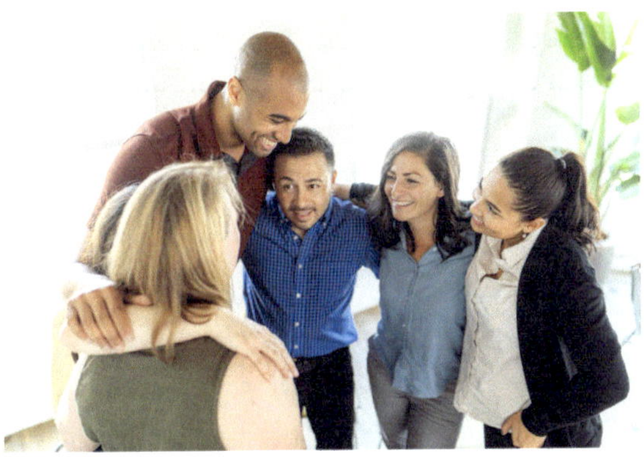

Figure 5.16. Better health outcomes through continuity of care.

Source: https://nurselinecs.co.uk/hahuceq/uploads/2024/06/people-supporting-each-other-2023-11-27-05-28-46-utc-1.jpg.

Last, effective policy must be adaptive, recognizing the interconnectedness of occupational and environmental health and focusing on social justice. Policymakers may require multi-sector alliances that align health and environmental objectives, fostering both community and workplace resilience. Cooperative strategies like these can ensure that health interventions address the determinants of health inequities and environmental risks, particularly among vulnerable populations. To ensure that change is sustainable, policies must address education and advocacy to raise awareness on environmental determinants of health. This entails educating employees on their rights and the impact of climate change on their environment. By creating a framework that is responsive to sustainability as well as results in health, policies are able to create a more just world where occupational and environmental health are addressed together, thereby significantly improving the overall status of health for generations to come (N/A, 2010) (Figure 5.16).

5.6.3. Case Studies Highlighting Successful Integration of Both Fields

Combining occupational and environmental health can involve numerous successful case studies that demonstrate the efficacy of models incorporating both disciplines. An exemplary illustration is a plant that conducted holistic assessments of workplace hazards compared to environmental impacts. By incorporating green strategies such as reducing emissions and recycling waste materials, the plant complied not only with regulations but also improved employees' health outcomes. This proactive approach led to a significant reduction in on-site injuries and illnesses, illustrating the direct correlation of environmental improvement to better occupational health. As well, the implementation of ergonomic designs and safer substitutes for harmful chemicals yielded greater staff morale and productivity, further supporting that sustainable operations can encourage a healthier workforce and fulfill environmental health standards (Kriebel et al., 2011). Still another exemplary case study involves the adoption of Healthy University programs by institutions of higher learning, which is an ideal example of occupational health and environmental sustainability. A close scrutiny of various institutions revealed an increased number of wellness programs that promote healthy living for students and workers. The universities developed better and learning-conducive environments through strategic partnerships and community involvement. The initiative emphasized active living, stress management, and health education, while simultaneously addressing air quality and energy consumption on campus. The research identified that these activities embodied a wellness model of health in which occupational and environmental health interventions are mutually supporting each other. These programs not only enhance psychological and physical health but also facilitate overall aspirations of sustainability in learning settings, highlighting the possibilities of a system-integration approach toward health and environmental standards (Doherty et al., 2009). The role of leadership in maintaining cooperative interaction between occupational and environmental health can be seen in successful cooperation among industries and government organizations. Case studies found that when such organizations came together to address specific health risks, they not only developed compliance with regulatory standards but also came up with innovative options that succeeded in addressing climate change-related risks. Such collaborations exhibited various strategies, such as developing green technology and coming up with workplace safety standards that are environmentally friendly. By integrating occupational health initiatives into sustainability strategies, organizations saw dramatic reductions in health absence and associated costs. Ultimately, the improved stakeholder relations resulted in better comprehension of health's dynamics, thus promoting safety and environmental stewardship culture across industry sectors (Kriebel et al., 2011).

CLOSER LOOK

IMPORTANCE OF A HOLISTIC APPROACH TO HEALTH

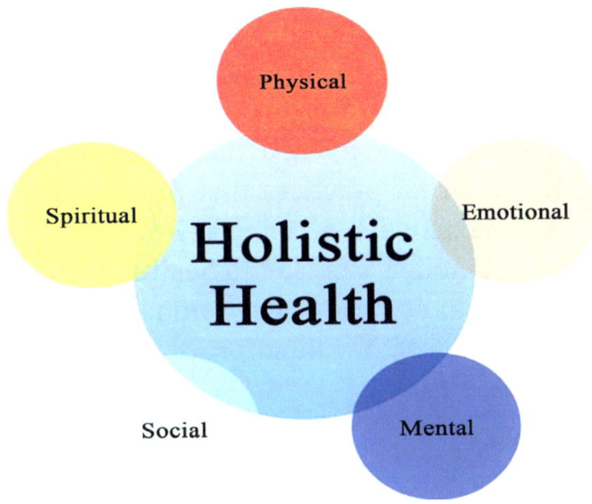

Figure 5.17. Diagram illustrating the five interconnected dimensions of holistic health: physical, emotional, mental, social, and spiritual well-being.

Source: https://media.licdn.com/dms/image/v2/D5612AQFriZMUKyJJPw/article-cover_image-shrink_600_2000/article-cover_image-shrink_600_2000/0/1713777498713?e=2147483647&v=beta&t=yDIqbsJlFAy0WNBHpGrn-vPHuYXecHySPH6dY5ZAB2Q.

Integrative health is essential in addressing environmental and occupational health because it incorporates the interplay of physical, psychological, and social health. In the workplace setting, health cannot be seen solely in terms of physical safety; it must consider psychological factors, work design, and organizational culture, which play a significant role in the well-being of employees. There needs to be a drastic paradigm shift to go from conventional treatment modalities towards preventive interventions, fostering health and well-being at all levels of the organization. This enables acknowledgement that contextual drivers such as workload, leadership style, and job function can both enable or hinder health outcomes. By a comprehensive approach, organizations can construct settings that not only mitigate risks but also enhance a culture of well-being, ultimately resulting in enhanced performance and productivity. Furthermore, the impacts of climate change can be addressed only by a comprehensive health approach that merges environmental factors affecting workplace health and community resilience. Climate-related conditions like natural disasters, impairment of air quality, and heat stress specifically afflict disadvantaged groups, aggravating existing health inequities. By combining environmental health principles with occupational health practices, organizations and policy makers can implement more robust preparation and response mechanisms. This is in accordance with evidence that favors the use of learning from public health approaches to inform workplace health interventions. Environmental sustainability commitment not just makes workplaces healthier but also enables communities to recover and adapt in spite of ongoing climate vulnerabilities. This kind of strategy promotes greater appreciation for how determinants of health interrelate, whether environmental or social, towards the emphasis on the necessity of comprehensive strategies for the promotion of long-term health. Moreover, a holistic strategy is essential in the construction of sustainable community programs promoting public health. Strategies that address environmental issues with respect to health, like air quality and waste, must be paired with occupational safety and health improvement initiatives. This is particularly significant when making comparisons for safety practices across various contexts, e.g., the contrast between Nigeria and Norway's construction industries. A comparison of these two nations allows researchers to identify best practices that highlight the importance of taking into account cultural and regulatory contexts when arriving at health outcomes. Using evidence-based interventions informed by successful models can lead to healthier and more resilient communities. Emphasizing coordination between public health, environmental policy, and occupational safety will ultimately have the ability to spur worthwhile improvement in overall health and well-being, affirming the worth of an integrated strategy.

SUMMARY

Environmental and occupational health research shows a complex nexus of risks, climate change effects, work-site protection, and sustainable community initiatives. As demonstrated in the course of this essay, environmental risks' ubiquity—particularly in vulnerable communities—pose acute public health concerns that need urgent mitigation. Climate change exacerbates the structural injustices that render some groups more vulnerable to health harms from environmental conditions. Therefore, redressing these inequalities must be a component of any overall health strategy. The Green Jobs Movement exhibits a prevention-based approach to alleviating these conditions through creating economic opportunities while simultaneously solving environmental issues, thereby positively influencing community health outcomes in low-income communities (N/A, 2010). In addition to addressing socioeconomic inequalities, it is also essential to incorporate climate change education into occupational health education. With an increase in the frequency of climate events, occupational health practitioners must be equipped with the skills and competencies required to anticipate and deal with these issues. The convergence of ACOEM competencies and the Global Consortium on Climate and Health Education frameworks is a testimony to the developing recognition of the central role that climate literacy plays in occupational health education. This intersection not only prepares future healthcare professionals but also readies them to be advocates for their communities in addressing the multifaceted impacts of climate change (Ayoub et al., 2025). These initiatives can significantly boost climate vulnerability resilience and improve workplace safety standards as companies learn how to adapt to changing environmental factors. Finally, a coherent strategy that brings together environmental health work, occupational education, and community mobilization is the foundation for creating sustainable, healthy environments. By forging alliances between various stakeholders—i.e., health activists, union organizations, and community leaders—strategies can be put in place that not only address short-term health concerns but also create long-term ecological and economic sustainability. In advancing, practitioners and policymakers must prioritize such partnerships, perpetuating the connection between health and environmental sustainability. Without these efforts, health disparities will remain a cycle that will ultimately end up eroding the collective societal desire to produce a secure and healthy future for everyone (N/A, 2010).

As the debate over workplace and environmental health continues, several pertinent points emerge to the forefront, evidence of the multifaceted nature of occupational risk. The contribution of regulatory mechanisms cannot be overstressed; case studies demonstrate that strong regulatory action has often been accompanied by spectacular improvements in working conditions. The convergence of evidence and lessons learned indicates, for instance, that interventions based on redesigning hazardous products have worked to reduce workers' risks to a minimum. Besides, site-specific guidance at the national and state levels also emphasizes continued monitoring and adjustment to safety standards. This ongoing focus on regulation is a foundation for inspiring a culture of safety among businesses, ultimately reducing the risk for workplace accidents and constructing a healthier work culture overall (Kriebel et al., 2011). Impacts of climate change are progressively influencing occupational health, and changes in the environment bring new and compounded hazards in various sectors. Occupational safety standards must evolve to meet these new hazards and guarantee the health of workers. For example, as more severe weather conditions occur, sectors must be prepared for how they affect working conditions and safety measures.

Innovative initiatives promoting resilience and sustainability are essential in preventing potential risks associated with climate variability. This supports the growing realization that companies are not only obligated to meet safety measures but also engage in environmental sustainability measures. Working towards such measures can improve public health benefits, focusing on the integration of workforce protection and environmental responsibility (Doyle et al., 2023). In referring to sustainable community action, the dialogue shifts to action of a multidimensional nature and inter-coordination of stakeholders. Engaging local communities in health and safety activities promotes a shared stake in environmental sustainability and occupational health. Not only do these activities enhance community resilience, but they also enable a means to integrate safety practices into community health initiatives as a whole. Promoting agile management approaches, particularly in small-scale mining operations, demonstrates the flexibility of practice in accelerating best practice adoption in safety and sustainability. By stressing the need for a mature safety culture, organizations can reinforce shared commitments to make actual improvement in occupational health and thereby contribute to the well-being of workers and society as a whole (Doyle et al., 2023).

REFERENCES

1. Akinlade, S. (2024). *How to Improve the Safety Practices in Nigeria Construction Industry in Relation to Europe (Norway)*. https://core.ac.uk/download/646122237.pdf (accessed on 11th June 2025).
2. Ayoub, S., Berenji, M., Chekuri, B., et al. (2025). *The Imperative to Incorporate Climate Change Competencies into Occupational and Environmental Medicine Training to Safeguard Worker Health*. https://core.ac.uk/download/647989308.pdf (accessed on 11th June 2025).
3. Birnbaum, N., Masterson, E., & Schoomaker, H. (2011). *State of Health Equity Movement, 2011 Update Part C: Compendium of Recommendations DRA Project Report No. 11-03*. https://core.ac.uk/download/pdf/18491812.pdf (accessed on 11th June 2025).
4. Delclos, G., Felknor, S. A., Fendinger, S., et al. (2020). *Potential Scenarios and Hazards in The Work of The Future: A Systematic Review of The Peer-Reviewed and Gray Literatures*. https://core.ac.uk/download/604668618.pdf (accessed on 11th June 2025).
5. Doherty, S. H., & Dooris, M. T. (2009). *National Research and Development Project on Healthy Universities: Final Report*. https://core.ac.uk/download/6113091.pdf (accessed on 11th June 2025).
6. Doyle, K. (2023). The safety and sustainability of mining at diverse scales: Placing health and safety at the core of responsibility. https://core.ac.uk/download/591812750.pdf (accessed on 11th June 2025).
7. Forte, S. P. dos S. B. (2021). Extreme weather events, occupational hazards in fire situations and the implications for firefighters' responsiveness: A systematic review. https://core.ac.uk/download/516511564.pdf (accessed on 11th June 2025).
8. Karanika-Murray, M., & Weyman, A. K. (2013). Optimizing workplace interventions for health and wellbeing: A commentary on the limitations of the public health perspective within the workplace health arena [forthcoming]. https://core.ac.uk/download/30633930.pdf (accessed on 11th June 2025).
9. Kriebel, D., Tickner, J., Jacobs, M., & Markkanen, P. (2011). *Lessons Learned: Solutions For Workplace Safety and Health*. https://core.ac.uk/download/71352756.pdf (accessed on 11th June 2025).
10. Landmann, T., Leao, L., & Rodriguez Huerta, E. (2025). Climate change, decent work and workers' health in Brazil: Theoretical considerations. https://core.ac.uk/download/645984772.pdf (accessed on 11th June 2025).
11. Lungu, K., Morse, T., & Taulo, S. (2010). *Gap Analysis of Environmental Health Research in Malawi: Report to the National Commission of Science and Technology*. https://core.ac.uk/download/19610167.pdf (accessed on 11th June 2025).
12. Mayer, B. (2009). *Blue-Green Coalitions: Fighting for Safe Workplaces and Healthy Communities*. https://core.ac.uk/download/5125790.pdf (accessed on 11th June 2025).
13. Pearce, A., Hughes, L., & Steffen, W. (2025). *The Heat Is On: Climate Change, Extreme Heat and Bushfires in WA*. https://core.ac.uk/download/pdf/30672522.pdf (accessed on 11th June 2025).

14. Taylor, A., Dollard, M., Richards, P., McLinton, S., Bond, S., Bailey, T., & McTernan, W. (2025). *The Australian Workplace Barometer: Report on Psychosocial Safety Climate and Worker Health in Australia*. https://core.ac.uk/download/pdf/30670991.pdf (accessed on 11th June 2025).
15. Tiraboschi, M. (2015). *Preventing and Managing Natural and Environmental Disasters: Employment Protection, Welfare and Industrial Relations Systems*. https://core.ac.uk/download/54012384.pdf (accessed on 11th June 2025).
16. United Nations, & World Health Organization. (2021). *Compendium of WHO and Other UN Guidance on Health and Environment*. https://core.ac.uk/download/480451068.pdf (accessed on 11th June 2025).
17. Vaiagae, B. W. (2020). *Workplace Safety Strategies Used by Managers to Reduce Workplace Accidents*. https://core.ac.uk/download/289242708.pdf (accessed on 11th June 2025).
18. van Wyk, D., Cronjé, F., & van Wyk, J. (2009). *Corporate Social Responsibility in The Diamond Mining Industry on the West Coast of South Africa*. https://core.ac.uk/download/75779470.pdf (accessed on 11th June 2025).

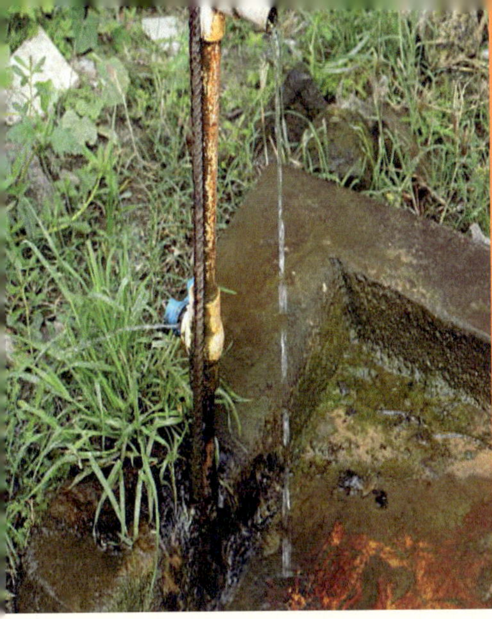

Chapter 6

WATER SUPPLY AND SANITATION

Contents

Introduction

The water supply and sanitation key issues have become a developing concern with increasing urban populations and environmental pressure. The management of the water resource is, most importantly, the determinant of sustainable development and health. Clean water and sanitation are fundamental human rights needs that sustain much of daily life, from hygiene to agriculture. Particularly, surface and groundwater sources form the cornerstone of any effective system for water supply. With an appreciation of diversity in such sources, one is able to better understand water management practices that are suitable in various geographical and climatic conditions, particularly relevant where communities are located under unique challenges, such as Alaskan communities, where traditional systems may face extreme climatic as well as infrastructure challenges (Justice et al., 1977). Water purification and wastewater treatment are crucial to protecting public health and the environment. Treatment processes that convert contaminated water into safe, clean drinking water are complex and involve a range of technologies and methodologies. The purification technologies not only consist of advanced filtration and chemical processes but also natural purification methods that can be applied in rural communities. In addition, effective wastewater management strategies like treatment and disposal are significant in preventing the spread of waterborne disease and preserving ecosystems. It is important to know various wastewater treatment technologies and how they are applied under different environments to enhance sanitation facilities and promote hygiene, particularly in rapidly urbanizing areas in the face of increasing environmental pressures (Figure 6.1).

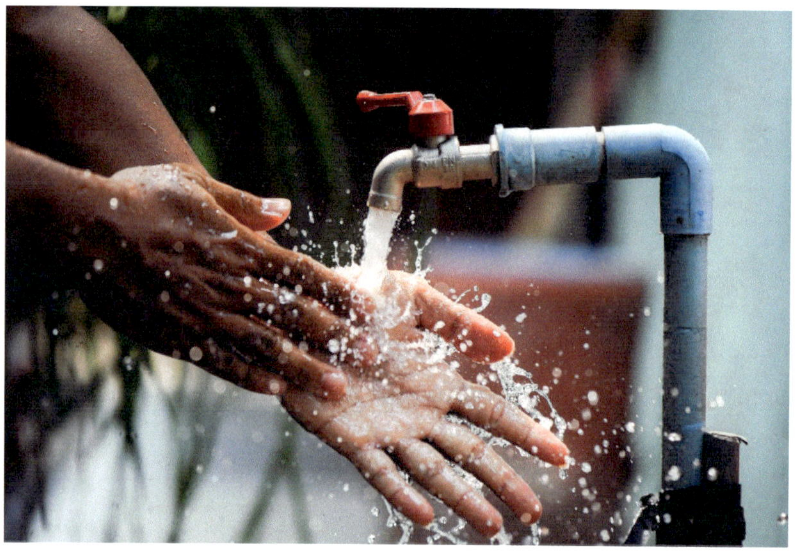

Figure 6.1. Handwashing with clean water as a key practice for hygiene and disease prevention.

Source: https://external-content.duckduckgo.com/iu/?u=https%3A%2F%2Fwww.brookings.edu%2Fwp-content%2Fuploads%2F2022%2F03%2Fshutterstock_1688502520_small.jpg&f=1&nofb=1&ipt=d26bd5a3a4eae2dd2ef774c4b5901771a3f7bec6951f2a6492ab63b8cac60c08.

Importance of Water Supply and Sanitation

The dependency of good water supply and public health cannot be stressed enough because the availability of clean water is a crucial aspect of disease prevention and overall welfare. Groups of people that lack a reliable source of water are likely to experience high levels of waterborne diseases, which cause high morbidity and mortality. The provision of safe drinking water, together with effective sanitation practices, is important in reducing disease occurrences such as cholera, dysentery, and typhoid fever. Furthermore, the need for water, sanitation, and hygiene (WASH) interventions extends beyond the total population to vulnerable groups such as those living with HIV/AIDS. There is evidence available to prove that the enhancement of WASH conditions can greatly improve the health outcome of such individuals, and therefore, healthcare systems should incorporate WASH into their general health agenda (N/A, 2007). Hence, the improvement of water supply and sanitation infrastructure is not only a matter of priority in public health but also a human right. Addressing the water supply and sanitation challenges in developing regions on a recurring basis calls for innovative approaches that are context-specific and demand-responsive. Projects like CuveWaters in Namibia prove the merit of decentralizing water supply and upgrading sanitation through participatory approaches. These interventions recognize the uncertainties of rainfall and the specific socio-cultural dynamics in affected places, allowing stakeholders to adjust solutions that can complement community practices and preferences. Focusing on demand-responsive strategies enables technological measures to support users' everyday practices and mental models of maintenance, thereby advocating long-term sustainable and effective water management (Deffner et al., 2010). Through the application of such locality-based measures, communities are able to enhance resistance to climatic variation while providing enhanced improvements in long-term health through the provision of clean water and sanitation. Moreover, the convergence of sanitation and hygiene behavior is significant to the success of water supply interventions. The enhancement of access to quality sanitation facilities not only protects the contamination of water sources but also empowers the public to change toward improved hygiene behavior, which is significant in reducing the spread of infectious diseases. Mass campaigns to increase public awareness of the necessity of hygiene, i.e., handwashing with soap and safe disposal of human excreta, complement physical water supply and sanitation improvement, and facilitate behavior change. The support of education programs combined with physical water supply and sanitation improvement allows communities to establish a holistic strategy that assists the health benefits achieved with correct WASH practice. The overall upgrading of water supply and sanitation facilities by infrastructural, educational, and participatory interventions ultimately gives rise to healthier and more sustainable communities.

Overview of Global Water Issues

Water crises worldwide are a complex issue that has been brought about by a number of reasons, including population increase, urbanization, and global warming. The rate at which the world population is growing keeps driving the demand for water supply, putting existing infrastructure to its limits and exacerbating the competition for freshwater supplies. The cities, being typically ill-equipped to handle the influx of residents, are especially strained to offer enough water and sanitation facilities. For this reason, effective management methods must be combined with sustainable practices such as urban agriculture and water reuse. Such practices are instrumental in creating societies that can subsist even during times of water scarcity. These practices not only assist in enhancing the existing water supply situation but also provide food security in the long term, showing inter-linkages between water management and broader socio-economic considerations (Bahri et al., 2025). Hygiene and sanitation are core components of public health and are very much reliant upon the availability of clean water. The linkage between water supply and sanitation is evident, whereby unhygienic sanitation facilities have an ensuing negative effect on water quality, with the eventual transference of waterborne disease. Conversely, poorly sanitized communities are more prone to health emergencies, which could clog local health centers, particularly in low-income settings. An excellent case in point is the case of HIV/AIDS and water supply issues, which necessitate intervention from both public health and the WASH community. These issues require a comprehensive solution that entails interagency collaboration to enhance sanitation practices, access to clean water, and consideration of health into broader WASH policy, looking toward imperative research and programmatic emphasis (N/A, 2007). The destiny of water issues globally will be based on advanced technologies that address supply and quality issues simultaneously. Drought, contamination, and inefficient use of water threaten not only individual and group health but also the sustainability of ecosystems. Innovative technologies for water treatment and wastewater treatment can sustain water supply infrastructure, expanding it to withstand external variations. Additionally, engaging communities in participatory management would empower local stakeholders so that water supply and sanitation options are context-specific and culturally appropriate. As the world wrestles with these challenges, emphasis on partnership among sectors, from agriculture production to city planning, will be imperative to developing holistic strategies towards universal access to safe water and sanitation. It is only through collaborative international action that considerable progress toward alleviating the current water crisis can be made.

Importance of Sanitation in Modern Society

Urban growth and successful industries have made it rather self-evident—we need sanitation systems that work. Bad sanitation, especially in lower-income communities, is highly stressful on health services and has a tendency to lead to epidemic levels of disease outbreaks of cholera and dysentery, infecting thousands every year. If water is polluted and waste is not properly disposed of, the whole community suffers. For the most part, investment in quality wastewater management is a sound decision that lifts public health and the environment as a whole. Investment in better sanitation infrastructure isn't just about cleaner water—it's about enhancing the overall quality of life for individuals and communities. For the most part, solid sanitation planning in urban areas can actually reduce the risks of poor hygiene, providing a healthier foundation for all. Techno-strategies for wastewater management are transforming sanitation in much of the world. Smart instruments, especially those associated with IoT, offer novel ways of monitoring and optimizing these systems such that the waste can be dealt with at its optimal level. This might seem technocratic, but these technologies enable farmers to receive safe, treated water for their crops—much like organic farming recycles nutrients naturally. In some cases, using these modern methods not only makes day-to-day life more efficient but also causes less pollution and contributes to a circular economy with the water circulating round and round in useful ways. The marriage of technology and sustainability really offers a solid basis for public health programs and an ecologically cleaner world. It's hard to overstate how deeply sanitation is intertwined with communities' health. Clean and healthy water isn't an extravagance; it's necessary for good well-being, justice, and even economic stability. When sanitation infrastructure fails, the consequences aren't isolated to an individual—it threatens our water supplies and the entire environment. Addressing the challenge involves considering a broad spectrum of solutions, from improved hygiene education to improved management practices. Current digital technologies now aid local communities in gathering meaningful information that, on its part, makes it easier to implement what the communities most truly require. Through the evolving climate and rising populations posing new challenges, it becomes all the more necessary to maintain our sanitation planning sharp and innovative so that everyone gets to benefit from the safe, required resources they deserve (Figure 6.2).

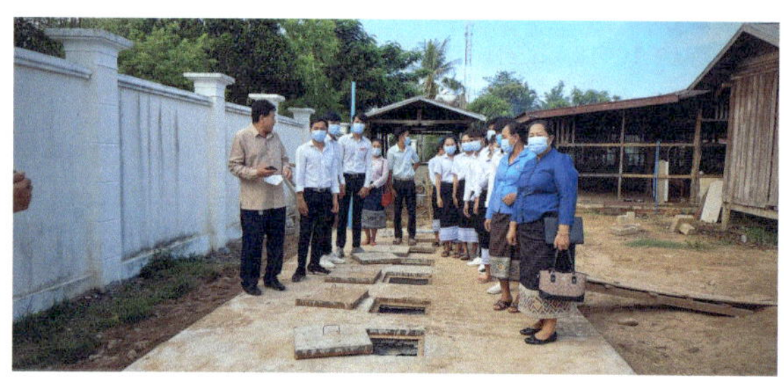

Figure 6.2. Community members and officials inspecting a decentralized wastewater treatment system (DEWATS) facility.

Source: https://siwi.org/wp-content/uploads/2021/05/small-projects_water-and-sanitation-department_dewats.jpg.

6.1. Sources of Water

Water sources form a very crucial component of every comprehensive water supply system, influencing public health and sanitation practice. Water is drawn from different sources, including surface water, groundwater, and rainwater, each possessing specific characteristics and issues. Surface water bodies such as rivers, lakes, and reservoirs are prone to pollution by agricultural runoff, industrial effluent, and municipal wastewaters. Groundwater, obtained through wells, typically suffers contamination from the same sources, and thereby its quality comes to be determined based on surface activities elsewhere. In urban areas, where the density of population increases the demand, the coordination between sourcing and protecting these water sources becomes a priority. The need to understand these sources deeply is essential with regard to water quality monitoring, guiding sanitation activities, and ensuring sustainable water consumption. These problems require joint intervention by water management authorities, public health experts, and civic leaders to implement effective solutions. Rainwater harvesting has emerged as an imperative source of water, particularly in areas facing severe shortages or poor infrastructure. As urbanization continues to grow, traditional water supply sources become overburdened, exacerbating water supply problems. By harvesting rainwater and storing it, communities can effectively augment their water supply, which reduces dependence on conventional sources that are often contaminated or likely to be depleted. Not only does this method enhance access, but it is also an affordable option for ensuring access to clean drinking water. Rainwater harvesting systems can be conveniently integrated into ongoing sanitation facilities and promote hygiene and sanitation behavior among the people in the community, especially among vulnerable groups. The strategic deployment of such systems could present long-term solutions to water shortage, particularly for regions with the impacts of climate change and population growth, underlining the importance of progressive approaches in water resources management (N/A, 2007). Furthermore, the intersection of wastewater treatment and water reuse is a significant area of concentration in the water sources discussion, particularly as cities become increasingly populous.

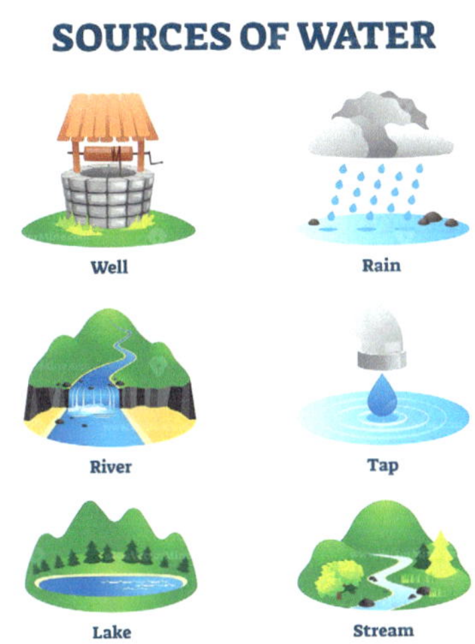

Figure 6.3. Sources of water.

Source: https://vectormine.b-cdn.net/wp-content/uploads/Sources_of_Water.jpg.

Wastewater, which is traditionally considered a menace, can be useful if managed correctly. Practices such as treated wastewater irrigation, apart from recycling water, also support urban agriculture, enhancing food security. As a result of urbanization, the necessity for sustainable water management strategies becomes a necessity; adequate treatment of wastewater makes this possible by rendering water pure to a level that it is fit for reuse. This not only increases the supply of water but also guarantees a holistic reaction to sanitation and hygiene, reduces pollution, and improves public health in populations. The resolution of these issues calls for a clear understanding of the interconnectedness between water resources, sanitation, and community health (N/A, 2007; Bahri et al., 2025) (Figure 6.3).

6.1.1. Surface Water Sources

Surface water sources like rivers, lakes, and streams are an integral component of water supply systems, especially in rural and urban settings. These sources serve as primary providers of drinkable water to support different applications like drinking, sanitation, and irrigation. However, in order to determine the sustainability of these water bodies, it is necessary that these bodies are approached both qualitatively and quantitatively. Pollution, particularly industrial and agricultural effluent runoff, poses a huge threat to the integrity of surface water and needs very tight management controls, taking into account both quality control and good governance. The policies must also address the effects of climate change that enhance water scarcity as well as pollution levels, particularly in vulnerable places. Thus, recognition of such challenges is key in formulating an integrated strategy for surface water resource management in the overall context of water supply and sanitation programs. Treatment and purification of surface water are essential to public health, particularly in urbanized regions with substantial demand for clean water. Advanced treatment processes such as coagulation, filtration, and disinfection are employed to remove impurities that ensure the safety of drinking water abstracted from surface bodies. Surface sources are harder to treat than groundwater due to variability in quality and the presence of organic materials and pathogens associated with surface sources. Furthermore, the effectiveness of these treatment processes must be regularly assessed to adapt to changing environmental conditions and emerging pollutants. Balancing treatment processes with the reality of surface water dynamics not only preserves water quality but also aligns with broader sanitary and hygienic goals intrinsic to community health, particularly within the context of increasing urbanization and population growth (Bahri et al., 2025). Participatory management methods and the involvement of people are necessary for effective utilization of surface water resources. Local citizens, like residents, farmers, and industry, must be involved in decisions that affect water supply and sanitation facilities. Participatory methods promoting local participation not only make water resources sustainable but also enhance transparency and accountability in water governance. Training programs that can introduce more awareness of the importance of surface water conservation can further assist communities, instill sustainable practices, and reduce the risk of contamination. In addition, the inclusion of water reuse practices, e.g., treating wastewater for use in urban farming for irrigation purposes, can relieve pressure on such critical surface water resources, thereby enhancing food security and community resilience overall. In doing so, the interdependence of sanitation and surface water management becomes more evident. It emphasizes integrated approaches in addressing present water challenges (Justice et al., 1977).

6.1.2. Groundwater Sources

Groundwater resources are a significant component of the world's freshwater resources, having significant impacts on water for sanitation and hygiene in societies. Through aquifer access, natural reservoirs, societies can access water naturally filtered by soil layers and typically cleaner than water from the surface. With cities continuing to grow, demand for safe drinking water also increases, putting pressure on these underground systems. Significantly, long-term survival of groundwater as a water source can result in sustainability, albeit at the cost of over-extraction problems and contamination, particularly in areas with inadequate wastewater treatment. Local hydrological conditions and good groundwater management are hence essential to comprehend in order to ensure the sustainability of the resource without compromising public health. The relationship between groundwater sources and sanitation behavior indicates the necessity for integrating water management into community planning processes. Ensuring safe groundwater must include a thorough understanding of technological as well as socio-cultural determinants of local perceptions of water use. Innovative approaches, such as those applied in Namibia's Cuvelai Basin, demonstrate how participatory planning can enable sustainable groundwater sourcing under utilizer conditions. These steps accentuate the need to adapt technological solutions to the circumstances of local environments and societies, for instance, exploiting saline groundwater. By being able to successfully combine scientific knowledge with the socio-empirical circumstances of water consumption, societies can optimize their groundwater availability and further enhance sanitation regulations and hygiene practices, having a beneficial effect on public health ultimately. With increasingly advanced water supply measures, requests for integrated plans incorporating wastewater reuse and groundwater recharge become more critical. Groundwater contribution to crop production, such as urban agriculture, further demonstrates its necessity in crop production in high-density population areas. People, using treated wastewater in irrigation, can reduce the pressure on groundwater sources and enhance sanitation. But that has to be carried out in a careful manner to prevent excessive extraction of groundwater so that there is sustainable utilization. Stakeholder participation in participatory management ensures a democratic process of water resource governance that results in more stable community structures. Emphasizing the role of groundwater not only puts forward its intrinsic value but also underscores the importance of strategic management within the interconnected areas of water supply, sanitation, and public health (Bahri et al., 2025; Deffner et al., 2010) (Figure 6.4).

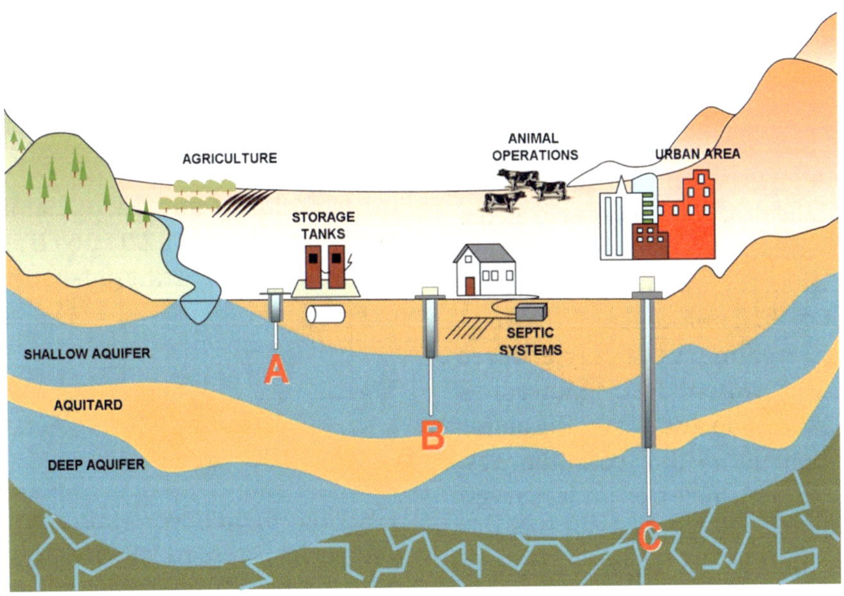

Figure 6.4. Groundwater sources.

https://external-content.duckduckgo.com/iu/?u=https%3A%2F%2Fi.pinimg.com%2Foriginals%2Fce%2F64%2Fbf%2Fce64bf4e43938b8f2b80d1c3030edda3.png&f=1&nofb=1&ipt=a7bfd812cd3d27277a7d5929ed07b8224b680babf38a8a1b2bdc15ebf03990bd.

6.1.3. Rainwater Harvesting

Rainwater harvesting (RWH) has been recognized as a critical strategy to increase water supply and sanitation within communities, particularly in regions experiencing chronic water scarcity. RWH is the collection and storage of rainwater from rooftops and other surfaces, which can be used as an auxiliary source of water for domestic use, irrigation, and sanitation. Implementing RWH systems can reduce reliance on unpredictable municipal supplies, whose levels tend to be irregular. As indicated in some of the research works, schools in Kwa-Zulu Natal greatly depend on rainwater as a significant source of water, citing its importance in accessibility to safe drinking water. However, alongside the constructed infrastructure, aspects such as uncertainty during seasons and the need for constant maintenance of storage tanks are still outstanding factors in the attainment of maximum efficacy in RWH programs (Lindokuhle et al., 2025). Besides, the bacteriological content of collected rainwater can also greatly impact public health and necessitate tight monitoring and treatment regulations. A rural Nigerian study has found that while the physical quality of rainwater usually falls within acceptable limits, sample contamination with *E. coli* indicates a high risk to human health. This underscores the need to integrate treatment processes within communities designed to minimize waterborne disease and antimicrobial resistance (Titilawo et al., 2024). Effective treatment not only ensures the safety of stored rainwater but also underlines the reality that RWH can be a source solution for balancing water demand within communities, particularly those decentralized or underserved by existing infrastructure. Besides, RWH systems will enhance resilience to climate change effects, particularly in poor countries. Through rainwater harvesting and use, communities will be less vulnerable to water shortages and drought. With increasingly variable climate trends, rainwater harvesting is an adaptive and sustainable water supply source. Awareness and community engagement through education are vital in order to promote the utilization of RWH systems so that the inhabitants not only learn about the benefits but are also trained for their management and maintenance. To this end, rainwater harvesting is a key innovation in the overall water supply and sanitation aspect that ensures greater hygiene, health results, and a better water future for communities across the globe (Lindokuhle et al., 2025) (Figure 6.5).

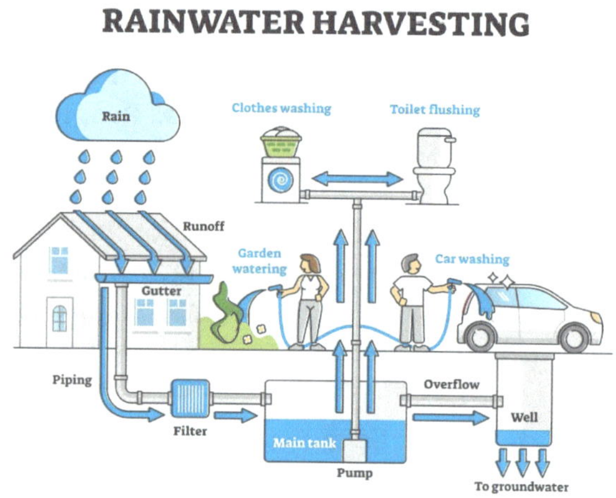

Figure 6.5. Urban-model-of-rainwater-harvesting.

https://cloudfrontgharpediabucket.gharpedia.com/uploads/2020/06/Urban-Model-of-Rainwater-Harvesting-04-0607010001.jpg.

6.2. Water Purification Methods

The value of effective water purification methods cannot be stressed sufficiently, especially as far as global health and environmental sustainability are concerned. Throughout history, human beings have realized the necessity of pure water and established diversified water supply systems and purification methods. These methods have evolved from crude filtering and boiling to sophisticated technologies such as reverse osmosis and ultraviolet treatment. Every process is employed to address specific contaminants with varying degrees of effectiveness, thereby ensuring that water is safe based on quality standards. Ultraviolet treatment, for instance, is most appropriate in eliminating pathogens without the destructive byproducts associated with chemical treatment. The continuous technological innovation in the water purification sector raises the supply of clean water, increasing public health gains and confirming the central position of water purity in raising life expectancy, as analyzed in current studies linking water quality to longevity (Rodr, 2023). In addition, wastewater treatment is also a key component of the water purification context. This process not only cleanses used water of impurities but also recovers valuable resources such as nutrients and energy. The process typically is a multi-step one with the elimination of coarse solids being the first step, followed by biological and chemical treatment to eliminate pollutants and pathogens. Modern-day wastewater treatment facilities apply sophisticated technology to convert waste into bio-methane, which can be used for energy production, thus acting as a resource management strategy in a sustainable manner. As proved by recent studies, effective wastewater treatment significantly decreases the burden on natural water sources by re-circulating and purifying available water (Rodr, 2023). These practices not only conserve freshwater but also enhance overall community sanitation by reducing the risk of waterborne illnesses. Last but not least, the utilization of multiple approaches to purify water emphasizes that there should be an integrated strategy to water management. Those communities that prioritize both water supply and sanitation using new purification technologies can considerably reduce health inequalities. Improved sanitation facilities lead to better hygiene practices, which collectively enhance public health. Studies consistently identify the double connection between improved water quality and increased life expectancy. Improved sanitation and better hygiene practices, fueled by efficient water purifying processes, lead to reduced mortality rates and improved quality of life. As highlighted in recent research, water technology investment is paramount; not only does it address current health concerns but also contributes to medium- and long-term sustainable development goals (Andreas et al., 2021) (Figure 6.6).

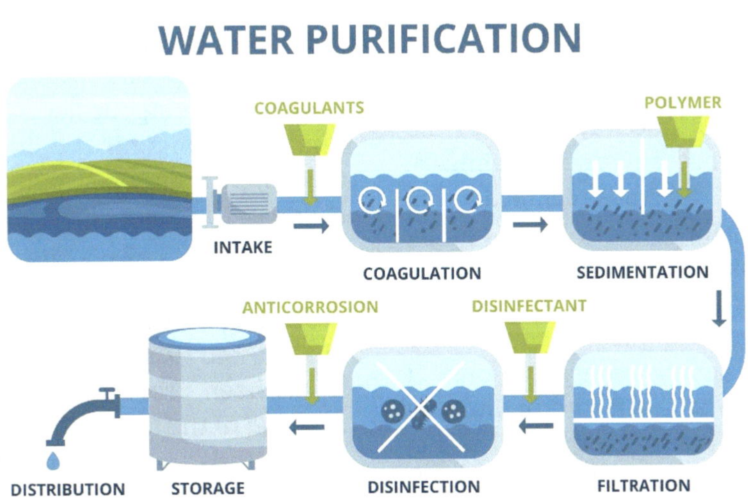

Figure 6.6. Stages-of-purification-process.

https://teslahealthylife.com/assets/images/blog/Stages-of-purification-process.jpg.

6.2.1. Physical Purification Techniques

The role of physical treatment techniques in water supply and sanitation cannot be overemphasized, as they are an important step towards safe drinking water provision. Techniques such as sedimentation, filtration, and disinfection are effective in removing impurities from water sources and thus play a central role in the public health of any community. Sedimentation entails letting particles drop to the bottom of a container; hence, it is simple to evacuate larger pieces of wreckage before additional treatment. Following this, filtration processes—such as membrane and sand filtration—effectively eliminate the remaining impurities, like pathogens. Implementation of such physical filtering techniques reduces the risk of waterborne diseases significantly in developing nations where access to high-level chemical treatments is low. Stable systems utilizing these techniques can reduce the number of waterborne diseases significantly, thus enhancing overall community health and hygiene levels (N/A, 2007). Apart from filtration and sedimentation, there are some physical methods that can be employed to enhance the quality of water in a given geographical environment. For instance, ultraviolet (UV) irradiation is used on a large scale because it has the capability to inactivate most of the microorganisms without any toxic chemicals. While UV disinfection does not technically kill contaminants, it is highly effective in attaining disinfection goals, particularly where chemical agents are unavailable. Physical methods of purification can also be applied to wastewater treatment. Flotation and screening are some of the methods that have been effective in draining solids and oils from effluents, ultimately helping to enhance the quality of water discharged. Where more sophisticated technologies are not available, such approaches offer a less expensive means for communities to effectively treat wastewater, hence protecting environmental health (Justice et al., 1977). Finally, using physical purification techniques in water supply and sanitation offers an important solution to addressing global water quality problems. With the application of these low-cost, simple methods, communities are able to enhance their waterborne disease resilience, and this results in better public health. Sedimentation, filtration, and disinfection are especially valuable in low- and middle-income countries, where waterborne disease is still present. Studies have shown that the application of these physical cleaning methods can significantly reduce health risks associated with contaminated water sources, thereby resulting in healthier populations and better sanitation. As more research continues to evaluate and refine these techniques, their incorporation into integrated water management plans will be instrumental in helping to advance sanitation and hygiene programs across environments (N/A, 2007).

6.2.2. Chemical Purification Processes

The efficiency of chemical processes used for water purification is paramount in enhancing water quality, particularly where resources are strained due to population growth and urbanization. The process typically entails chemicals being utilized to purify water by removing contaminants like pathogens, heavy metals, and organic compounds. Chlorination is one of the most common chemical processes used, which successfully purifies water, rendering it safe for human use. But chemical process operation must be controlled so that it hinders the formation of harmful by-products. It has been proven that defective chlorination can lead to the formation of chlorinated organic compounds, which are toxic to health. The application of chemical purification must thus meet effective disinfection while reducing risk to the general public. In wastewater treatment, chemical purification processes play a crucial role in facilitating the safe return of treated water into the environment or potential reuse. Coagulation and flocculation are two basic chemical techniques that facilitate the union of particulates to facilitate their elimination in the following stages of treatment, thereby making removal easier. In a successful application, the two processes significantly enhance turbidity removal and water clarity in general. Increasing demands of urban agriculture and food security issues demand tertiary treatment of wastewater to reclaim valuable water resources for use in irrigation or other purposes (Justice et al., 1977). Thus, the incorporation of effective chemical purifying processes in wastewater treatment not only addresses sanitation issues but also contributes to sustainable water management in societies. The effectiveness of chemical purification processes depends heavily on the understanding of local impurities and their impact on human health as well as the ecosystem. For example, in regions like Alaska, where the wintry climate presents a unique challenge to water supply and sanitation, local contaminants in water resources need to be understood (Justice et al., 1977). Evidence indicates that water and waste treatment process breakdowns typically result from the lack of knowledge regarding chemical reactions and local conditions. This is indicative of the need for specialized research and specific chemical treatment solutions with sensitivity to the water characteristics of each community. Furthermore, involvement of stakeholders in assessing these processes can enhance transparency and improve the efficiency of community participation in water management policies (Justice et al., 1977).

6.2.3. Biological Purification Methods

Biological treatment processes are a critical component of modern wastewater treatment technologies, which utilize microbial processes for efficient and successful degradation of organic materials and the elimination of contaminants from water. The processes utilize the inherent capability of microorganisms, such as bacteria and fungi, to convert toxic substances into non-toxic products through the utilization of metabolic processes. Through the application of technologies like activated sludge treatment, biofiltration, and constructed wetlands, societies can enhance the quality of their water supply while, in the process, minimizing adverse environmental impacts. Apart from meeting the requirements of wastewater treatment, these systems also serve to promote sustainable sanitation practices towards public health and ecosystem integrity. The efficiency of biological purification is also highlighted through its integration into the circular economy model, where waste products are converted into resources. The Toilet Board Coalition study highlights the potential for upcycling toilet resources as valuable material and presents new business models that align with sustainable development goals. This strategy encourages resource recovery with less pressure on traditional wastewater systems, which tend to depend on chemical treatments that can have adverse impacts on the environment. By focusing on the economic and environmental benefits of biological treatment processes, people can develop a more sustainable water management strategy, which ultimately translates into better sanitation and hygiene standards. Additionally, comparing biological purification processes with other traditional technologies reveals their unique strengths and weaknesses. Traditional systems, such as chemical disinfection and filtration, are able to deal with sudden contamination but are often remiss when it comes to long-term sustainability and resource utilization. Biological methods are able to assist in nutrient recycling, becoming an integral part of wastewater treatment, though. For instance, findings from studies on cold-climate water systems indicate that adapting biological purification to accommodate local conditions can have a considerable impact on system performance and reliability (Justice et al., 1977). Imposing such practices not only increases the public health and sanitation measures but also paves the way for a more sustainable direction in water supply management (Figure 6.7).

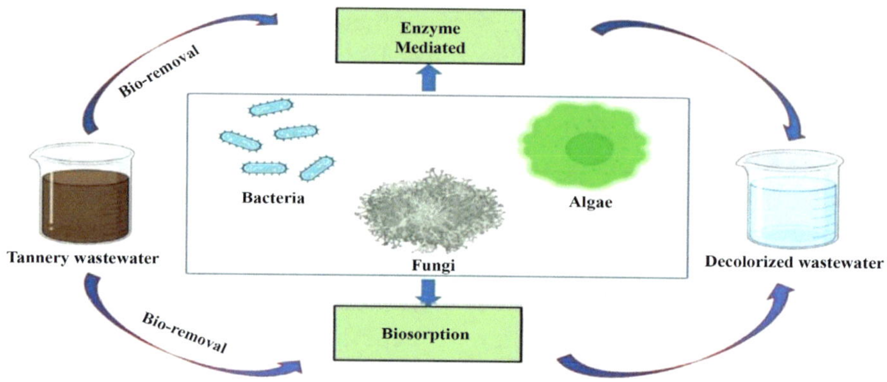

Figure 6.7. Biological treatment methods.

Source: https://external-content.duckduckgo.com/iu/?u=https%3A%2F%2Fwww.researchgate.net%2Fpublication%2F370646001%2Ffigure%2Ffig4%2FAS%3A11431281157194121%401683729602689%2FBiological-treatment-methods.png&f=1&nofb=1&ipt=a992f8f2edd3758409c8a469f623edc4faaed9e8ed94fda91192986fc70bf2ad.

6.3. Public Health and Sanitation

Sanitary hygiene is viewed as being at the heart of healthy communities. If waste is not well managed, a lot of health problems come to the fore, and we see a relationship between inappropriate practice and outbreaks of communicable diseases. There is enough evidence—taken in bulk—to indicate how badly functioning sanitation leads to water pollution and so on. Better sanitation minimizes health hazards, lowers health costs, and even enhances work efficiency, and all of these are good tidings for everyday life. Real change, however, calls upon citizens of all backgrounds to act and create enduring solutions. Breakthroughs in wastewater treatment technology have been a real game-changer for sanitation and public health. New treatment technologies, from fairly straightforward biological processes to some relatively high-tech filtration systems, attempt to kill lethal pathogens before the water ever makes it to the environment. In many cases, communities can even reuse treated water, saving valuable resources in the process. But bringing these innovations to fruition is not trivial—it takes careful planning, good investment, and enough local know-how to keep things running smoothly. Research, for instance, highlights that leveraging previous experience is key to building sanitation programs that address health targets (Gumbo et al., 2012). Politics and finances are clearly major players in how sanitation policies land. Examples throughout the globe show political motivation and how funds are structured tend to shape sanitation initiatives. Take the example of countries such as India and Brazil, where excavating the local political climates led to strategic investments that benefit the most disadvantaged and vulnerable. In most cases, pro-poor policies guarantee adequate access for even the underserved, and this eventually makes a significant difference in health outcomes. All of this serves to serve up the need for collaboration between governments and organizations, if the political waters are occasionally a bit choppy, in order to win long-term health gains for the public (N/A, 2011) (Figure 6.8).

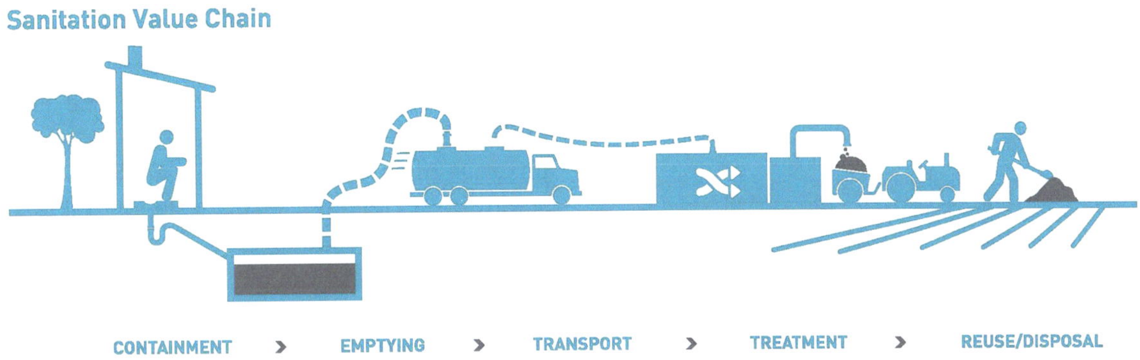

Figure 6.8. The sanitation system: collection, transport, treatment, disposal, or reuse.

Source: https://upload.wikimedia.org/wikipedia/commons/thumb/7/74/Sanitation_Value_Chain.jpg/1920px-Sanitation_Value_Chain.jpg.

6.3.1. Relationship Between Sanitation and Public Health

Cities teeming with people today have a gigantic headache in the shape of sanitation systems that just can't cope. Proper waste management isn't merely a matter of moving garbage—it keeps water sources from being polluted and keeps vulnerable people safe from contracting water-borne diseases. Take Dar es Salaam, Tanzania, for example; its urbanization rate has pulled wastewater management so taut that plants buckle. Under pressure, the plants are regularly letting untreated sewage flow into local creeks, doubling up both health risks and environmental degradation. It's not just a matter of better pipes and plants to correct this problem, but in most cases, it is a matter of reaching out to the community and betting on new flexible technology. Of course, sanitation and public health go together, so sound regulation and stable finance are needed (Azizi et al., 2025). Sanitation issues are more than bricks and mortar; they are mixed up with social and economic factors that determine who gets clean facilities and who doesn't. People in low-income communities bear the brunt of inadequate sanitation, which can lead to nasty episodes of disease like cholera and dysentery. A routine spot check for microbial load in local water can also be a blinding red light that signals just how deep the crisis is. In most developing countries, failure in sanitation lets waterborne diseases run amok, putting additional strain on public health. Predictive modeling now allows officials to pinpoint areas of contamination so interventions may be precisely placed where most needed. With the aid of these innovative tools, stakeholders can enhance balancing acts with resources and also public health interventions, lessening the burden that poor sanitation places on communities (Izah et al., 2025). Emerging technologies in wastewater treatment are upsetting the whole game, confirming yet again the extent to which sanitation depends on overall health. Techniques like Anaerobic Digestion (AD) aren't just treating wastewater more efficiently—they also generate renewable energy as a bonus, ensuring nothing is wasted in the process. These newer systems minimize natural destruction and help eliminate disease transmission that comes with bad sanitation. Community engagement and technology solutions are needed; there is no silver bullet.

If you look at all the facets of sanitation—from collapsing infrastructures to social barriers—it's clear that an inclusive solution needs to be put in place. And by promoting public-private partnerships and investment in robust systems, communities are able to better protect public health and quality of life (Azizi et al., 2025) (Figure 6.9).

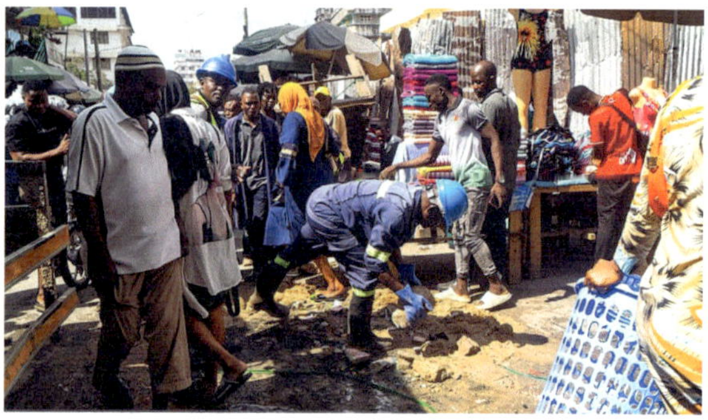

Figure 6.9. In Dar es Salaam, over 90 per cent of residents depend on on-site sanitation systems like septic tanks and pit latrines, many of which are poorly maintained.

Source: https://gumlet.assettype.com/downtoearth%2F2024-10-10%2Fsdnksl6z%2FTanzania?w=768&auto=format%2Ccompress&fit=max.

6.3.2. Key Public Health Issues Related to Poor Sanitation

Sanitation matters—a great deal. Where there are failures of the system, communities are plagued by all manner of waterborne problems that directly originate in dirty sources. In others, unpleasant critters like cholera, dysentery, and typhoid find themselves moving in, which sadly increases sickness and even mortality rates, especially among children and the elderly. People will get absent from work or school when such diseases are on the move, and local healthcare becomes overburdened, too. It's like poor sanitation puts communities in a vicious cycle where good water and proper facilities are a luxury only a handful can afford. In most cases, hitting sanitation head-on is what will turn such trends around (Vosa et al., 2025). Water, sanitation, and quality dance together in a way that determines how healthy a community remains. Without an effective way to treat wastewater, nasty stuff will end up in our water sources—increasing the risk for all. In most African countries, for example, the absence of smart wastewater management has resulted in alarming levels of heavy metals and dangerous pathogens in the water. This kind of contamination, besides playing with human health—sometimes leading to long-term issues like cancer or even neurological disorders—is even dangerous for aquatic organisms. Rural children and women, where medical centers are not always accessible, mostly suffer from it. Overall, improvements in wastewater treatment processes and enforcement by strong rules are needed to minimize such health hazards (Omohwovo, 2024) (Figure 6.10).

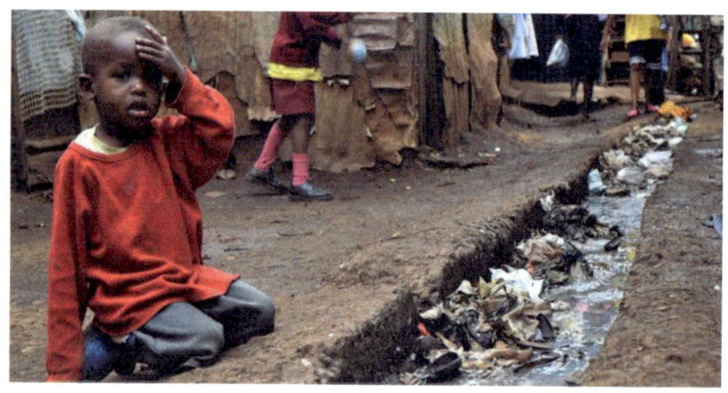

Figure 6.10. Sanitation woes cost Africa 115 lives every hour.

Source: https://media.licdn.com/dms/image/v2/D4D12AQFd3oy6G7gFxQ/article-cover_image-shrink_600_2000/article-cover_image-shrink_600_2000/0/1687001470598?e=2147483647&v=beta&t=_COudCplDjrzk6-_-hUH4qzWQoGjsRnnPLpb4Zqr8pQ.

Sanitation strife isn't just a matter of health—it extends to the manner in which individuals work, study, and live. Children from families that do not have proper sanitation are likely to be absent from school because they are too sick or need to fill in for more tasks at home, which interrupts their learning process. This then ends up trapping families in poverty cycles, with little chance to improve in the long term. Local health systems can become strained also, pushing costs up so that other essential services have to be reduced. A synergy of community mobilization, education applied in hygiene, and investment in water infrastructure will break such cycles. Investing in improved sanitation in all but a few cases lays the foundation for a healthier, more resilient community and even stimulates long-term economic development (Vosa et al., 2025; Omohwovo, 2024) (Figure 6.11).

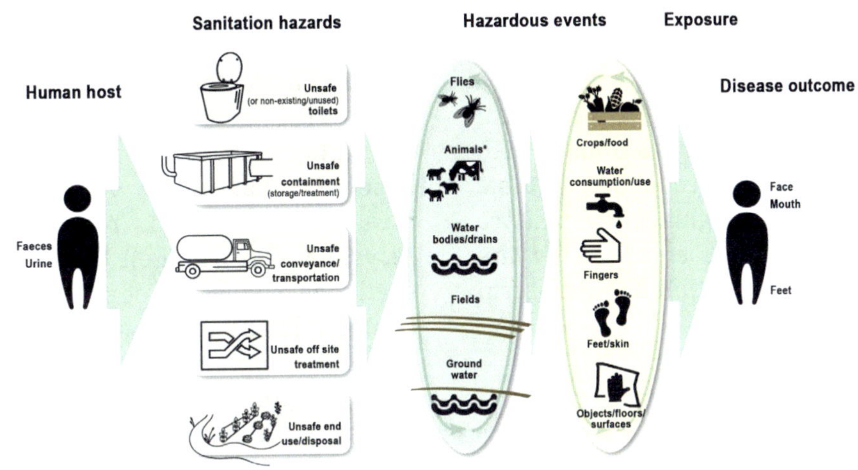

Figure 6.11. The health impacts from unsafe sanitation through various transmission pathways.

Source: https://www.researchgate.net/profile/Richard-Johnston-5/publication/329316603/figure/fig1/AS:703120556441600@1544648412032/The-health-impacts-from-unsafe-sanitation-through-various-transmission-pathways-Figure.jpg.

6.3.3. Role of Sanitation in Disease Prevention

Good sanitation is the best way to keep disease at bay. If neighborhoods do not have effective systems for their waste disposal, it is not just human waste but also a health issue for the general public. Pure water and well-treated wastewater can lower the incidence of outbreaks like cholera, typhoid fever, etc., and studies do seem to substantiate that poor sanitation not only hits individuals hard but also burdens our healthcare systems with a heavy dollar and systemic cost. Installing systems that both treat wastewater and encourage everyday hygiene seems like a smart, sensible step toward the development of communities that can address health concerns—even if the solution arrives on occasion a little disorganized. A growing concern these days is antimicrobial resistance, or AMR, which arises when antibiotics are misused and, all too frequently, when waste management is inadequate. In most cases, having dirty water or poorly treated waste around gives way for resistant bacteria to grow, hence making it extremely hard for clinical therapies to work (Md. Salam et al., 2023). It is discovered that poor sanitation can drive pathogens to adapt in ways that render antimicrobials almost useless. Brushing over hygiene practices and cracking down on poisonous waste may well break this deadly cycle, offering something of an insurance package for communities against these tenacious germs. Innovative ideas in wastewater treatment are shaking up the way we think about sanitation, especially in areas of the world where clean water is not an option. Instead of merely treating sewage, these technologies recycle water and relieve pressure on our declining freshwater resources. In adopting more sustainable modes of working, communities can watch healthier ecosystems emerge naturally. To a large extent, wise policies marrying these innovations with public health interventions are early lines of defense against epidemics – a blessing particularly felt by marginalised groups (Md. Salam et al., 2023). When government agencies, NGOs, and local authorities combine efforts (occasionally with some coordination glitches), providing equitable access to such facilities can significantly enhance community resilience while emphasizing the importance of proper sanitation for long-term health.

6.4. Wastewater Treatment Processes

New technology has literally transformed how we treat wastewater. Today, adding gadgets like membrane bioreactors and oxidation processes isn't just trimming—it decreases contaminants in a manner we never thought possible. Smart tools allow us to monitor systems in real-time, which is essential when things turn ugly with complex setups. Such a digital spin, in general, goes hand in hand with sustainable objectives while serving to save resources and our environment as well. In the meantime, such methods not only enhance water quality but also open up a cycle where beneficial components are salvaged and brought back to life (María et al., 2021). Knowing the process of wastewater cleaning is the most significant part of understanding that it's vital for our health and the planet. Usually, the process starts with letting big particles settle in the primary treatment. Then comes the stage when microorganisms set to work, munching down organics to minimize pollutant levels. Finally, a polishing cycle—in the form of filters or even chemicals—is meant to score high safety marks. Each of these elements, no matter how small they seem to be on their own, contributes to keeping releases minimal as well as making reused water good enough (N/A, 2019). If wastewater is not treated, the effects are too dire. Incompetent treatment will pollute water bodies around and even trigger health crises by spreading waterborne diseases. Nature is not exempt either, with adjacent ecosystems typically impacted and bodies of water spoiled. As our cities grow and more individuals gather, the call for smarter wastewater solutions becomes even more vociferous. Innovative measures like biogas recovery and nutrient recycling offer channels that can help meet the challenge of swelling populations and a shifting climate. These measures, in most cases, can enhance community well-being and keep water clean, aligning with the general principles of environmental stewardship and public health (María et al., 2021) (Figure 6.12).

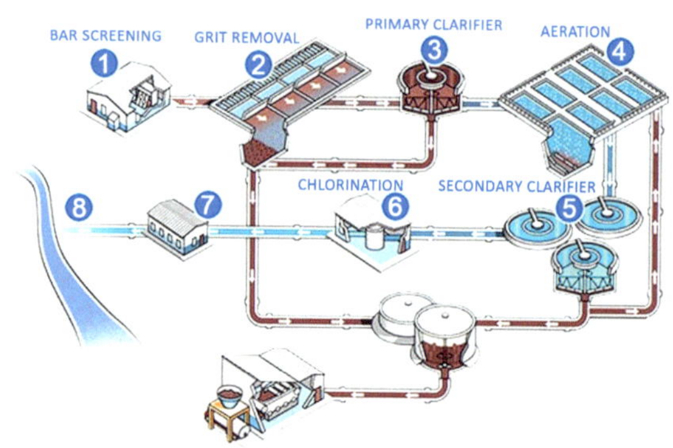

Figure 6.12. The wastewater treatment process.

Source: https://cms-resources.coleparmer.com/a/wastewater-8stage-whole-web.jpg.

6.4.1. Primary Treatment Methods and Their Effectiveness

Effective primary treatment in wastewater management is an important first line of defense against pollution, protecting public health from the get-go. Immediately from the start, sedimentation and flotation treatments serve to extract bulk solid and particle material from water. This rudimentary step lightens the organic load that otherwise might overwhelm ensuing more advanced treatments. In many developing countries where fancy technology is not always on the table, the simple methods end up being the most practical option. Cleaning grime upfront not only preserves regional water security but also aligns with broader initiatives in sanitation and hygiene. The efficiency of those first methods—especially in regions with less advanced infrastructure—irrefutably underscores the importance of tackling high-priority public health concerns (Bahri et al., 2025). Addressing the various problems that accompany poor sanitation actually necessitates an examination of the efficiency with which such rudimentary treatments work. Research indicates that sedimentation tanks are capable of efficiently eliminating solid waste, which in most instances reduces the threats associated with waterborne diseases. Urban settings, where land is limited, often find these primary approaches invaluable as more elaborate solutions simply aren't feasible. Countries that have integrated fundamental wastewater practices in their daily work consistently see tremendous boosts in public health; the linkage of sanitation and communal wellness cannot be overlooked. Promoting broad application of these effective treatments—especially where resources are scarce—not only takes pressure off water systems but also lays groundwork for future, more sophisticated fixes (N/A, 2007). Defying the trend of health concerns, the economic argument adds strength to how starting with quality primary treatment really matters. By removing waste from the water right from the start, cities can take the load off the rest of the process, conserving money and resources at the same time. Clean water can create virtuous loops in healthier populations, and even rattle the cogs of local economies—farming, for instance, benefits when reclaimed water is used. Research in general suggests that investment in primary wastewater management results in immense gains through the reduction of health hazards and enhanced overall production and quality of life. As one of the main elements in the overall scheme of water management, investment in primary treatment not only protects public health but also strengthens the economic foundation required for community growth (Bahri et al., 2025) (Figure 6.13).

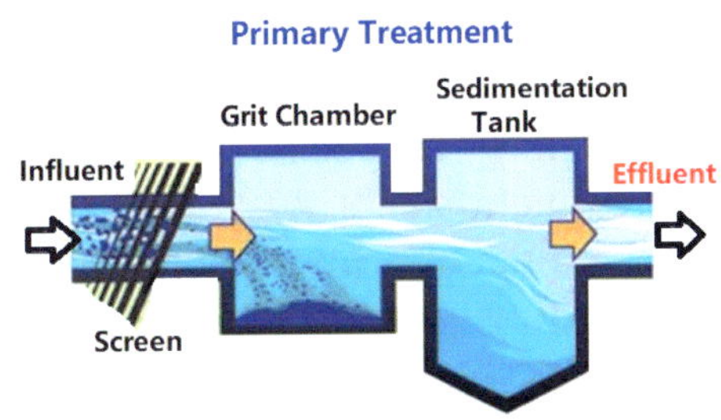

Figure 6.13. Primary treatment of wastewater.

Source: https://www.kelvinindia.in/blog/wp-content/uploads/2023/11/Primary-Treatment-of-Wastewater.png.

6.4.2. Secondary Treatment Processes and Biological Treatment

Effective wastewater management really depends on the efficacy of secondary and biological processes. You've got these processes decomposing organic matter and cutting down excess nutrients so that water that is good enough for nature is in compliance; effluents must be pure. Microorganisms are working overtime here – they basically consume the contaminants, which is much more environmentally friendly than relying on chemicals. Technologies like activated sludge and biofilm reactors were shown to be capable of having a considerable increase in the level of pollutant removed. Furthermore, using locally abundant bio-waste as adsorbents presents an intelligent possibility: wastewater not only may be treated, but this approach may also reduce agricultural waste and decrease its environmental impact. Considering it as a whole, these combined methods remind us that natural materials' utilization can solve the environmental issues while not diminishing treatment efficiency (Nataša et al., 2021). While biological treatment methods seem to be promising, a lot of problems still exist in treating new pollutants when dealing with them, especially in view of the new global health issues. Viruses such as SARS-CoV-2 persist in wastewater – an enormous public health problem – and typical facilities in essence only filter out these risks partially, therefore further disinfection actually becomes imperative. It usually involves an additional check and double-check to verify that pathogens don't get away. Regular screenings of leftover threats might very well lead to management systems explicitly tailored to ensure safe recycling and disposal of water. Generally, the pandemic has shown that secondary treatment cannot only be about organic matter and nutrients; it must also deal with viral invaders in a direct manner (Bogler et al., 2020). Advances in technology for secondary treatment are turning out to be a real game-changer when it comes to sustainable wastewater management. New technologies such as membrane bioreactors and even constructed wetlands jump in to augment the natural ability of biological processes; they harness the energy of specific organisms to break down pollutants, lowering the net environmental effect of treatment plants. As cities grow and the environment gains momentum, merging high-tech solutions with nature's own solution is increasingly a necessity rather than an extravagance. This blend not only helps meet more demanding regulatory standards but also serves a vital role in public health protection through ensuring treated water does not impact surrounding ecosystems (Nataša et al., 2021) (Figure 6.14).

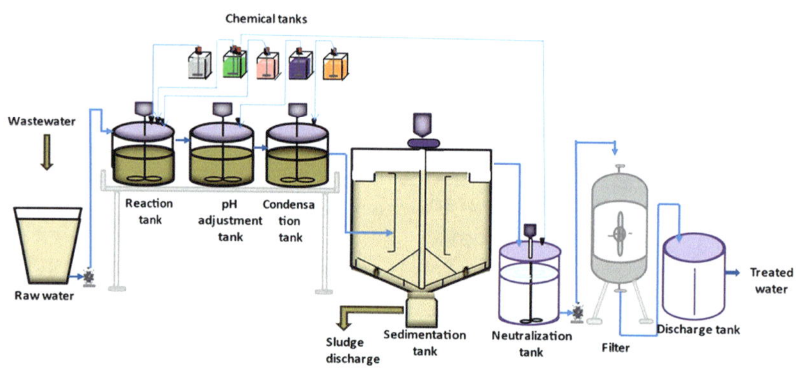

Figure 6.14. Secondary wastewater treatment methods.

Source: https://www.researchgate.net/publication/371970803/figure/fig5/AS:11431281176221609@1690078398310/Secondary-wastewater-treatment-methods.png.

6.4.3. Tertiary Treatment and Advanced Purification Techniques

More wastewater treatment is not an afterthought; it's a game-changer. Tertiary processes extend beyond primary and secondary to deal with the recalcitrant fractions—nutrients, pathogens, and organic contaminants that have made it through. Plants nowadays in most but a minority of situations use techniques like membrane bioreactors and reverse osmosis, which, speaking frankly, are miracles at removing micro-pollutants. Ozonation and advanced oxidation processes (AOPs) come to break down difficult organic molecules that earlier stages may miss. This further degree of cleansing may make treated water acceptable for consumption from irrigation of crops to even (in some cases) drinking water, an important consideration to recall when water is scarce. If sanitation is lacking, the blowback goes on for much farther than local ecosystems. Insufficiently treated wastewater can harbor all types of pathogens, opening doors to waterborne diseases like cholera and dysentery in areas where clean water is not a given. Microbial reduction tertiary treatments have proven in many communities to be the actual solution to such issues. Research overall endorses the application of predictive modeling to locate hotspots of contamination—guiding localized action where the treatment is most needed. In most cases, through the utilization of these directed methods and at times with the use of information that is a bit unconventional, communities can better defend public health against the scourge of waterborne disease. Improved wastewater treatment isn't merely fiddling with what is already in place—it's also about making the most of new, sometimes unconventional natural remedies. Biological nutrient removal systems and wetlands enable nature to handle some of the burden, a strategy that's both resource-and environmentally-savvy; these methods are often coupled with projects that recover valuable by-products like recyclable fertilizers and biogas. For example, research in places like Zambia's Copperbelt Province (Tortajada, 2016) has demonstrated that when mining effluent and sewage effluent combine, such intelligent methods can relieve pressures on regional water bodies. By combining knowledge from multiple disciplines—and yes, sometimes embracing minor idiosyncrasies in data and punctuation—stakeholders are developing wastewater management strategies that balance public health requirements, safeguard ecosystems, and enable sustainable development (Figure 6.15).

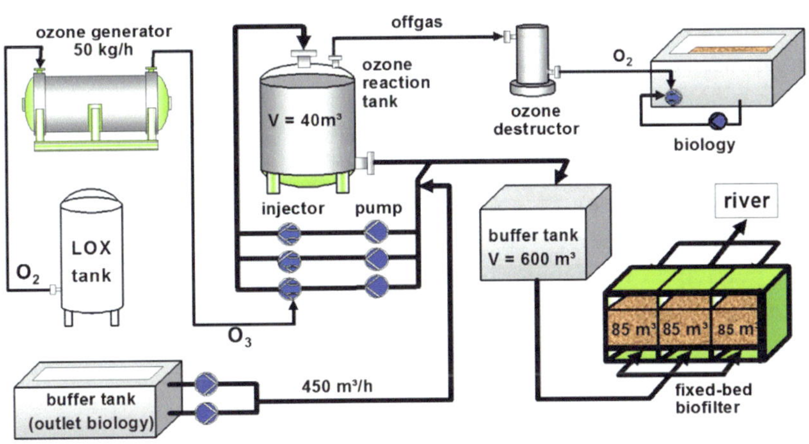

Figure 6.15. Schematic flowchart of the tertiary treatment step.

Source: https://encrypted-tbn2.gstatic.com/images?q=tbn:ANd9GcR_tYgA4KnaLfLvfexbC8bZwSjXNBxtYu4hSX4SrrvjqJJ-Cgpx.

6.5. Wastewater Disposal Techniques

Wastewater management is of great importance in terms of environmental sustainability and public health, especially in regions with less resource access. Disposal methods of wastewater range from conventional systems such as centralized treatment plants to other decentralized alternatives such as septic tanks and constructed wetlands. Centralized systems tend to employ mechanical, biological, and chemical processes in treating wastewater prior to discharge into water bodies or irrigation. On the other hand, decentralized systems present cost-effective and sustainable solutions, especially for rural or underdeveloped areas. They help prevent water pollution and ensure local ecosystems while providing water for irrigation and other non-potable uses. The analysis of cold-climate water and wastewater systems emphasizes the point that understanding problems in the region is essential to designing effective wastewater treatment plants, particularly in remote areas where standard systems tend to malfunction (Justice et al., 1977). New approaches in wastewater management encompass explosive growth in significance as urban populations expand and renewable sources of water become a pressing requirement. One of the key methods is wastewater irrigation, which supports urban agriculture while improving food security concerns in urban areas. It not only reduces the use of freshwater resources but also helps recycle nutrients back into the land. The use of reclaimed water for urban agricultural purposes can significantly improve water disposal management and ensure circularity in the economy. In addition, participatory management with the involvement of stakeholders within the community ensures that their needs and concerns are addressed and accommodated, which results in a responsibility and ownership approach to wastewater management (Bahri et al., 2025). The collaborative process is necessary as it promotes efficient water use while enhancing sanitation and hygiene gains within the community. Technological innovation, ensuring both safety and efficiency of wastewater disposal methods, also enhances the efficacy of wastewater disposal methods. Technologies like membrane bioreactors and advanced oxidation processes are significant innovations in wastewater treatment to a level of quality safe for multiple purposes, such as indirect potable reuse. The technologies are also capable of being modified for application at different scales and capacities, which makes them applicable for use in both rural and urban settings. The policy and regulatory framework addressing water quality and environmental impact will dictate the use of the new technologies. Continuous policy-making and research are imperative to ensure that these technologies remain efficient and sustainable. Confronted with challenges and possibilities for wastewater treatment, not only will this improve water supply and sanitation systems, but also make them resilient to the increasing dangers of climate change and population increase (Justice et al., 1977; Bahri et al., 2025) (Figure 6.16).

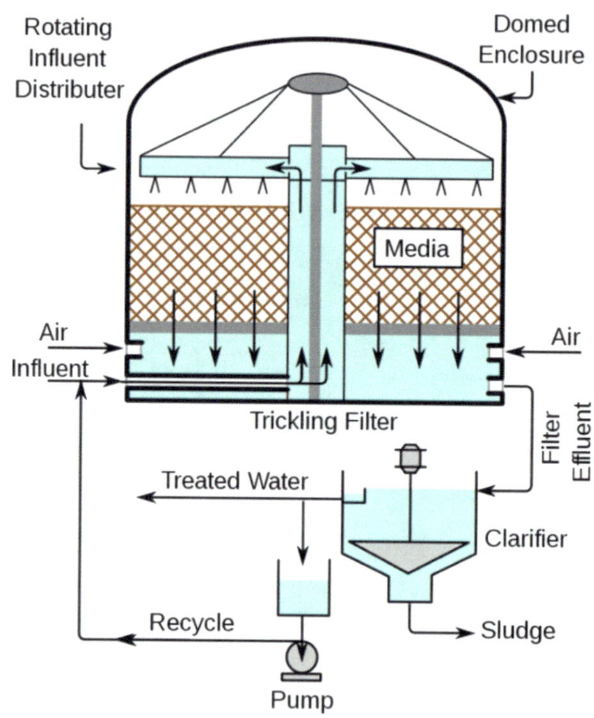

Figure 6.16. Wastewater disposal techniques.

https://media.springernature.com/lw685/springer-static/image/chp%3A10.1007%2F978-3-030-22438-7_90-1/MediaObjects/482133_0_En_90-1_Fig3_HTML.png.

6.5.1. Land Disposal Methods

Land disposal methods play a central role in wastewater handling, particularly in the context of sustainable sanitation systems. Such practices entail numerous strategies for wastewater treatment and disposal through natural ground filtering and absorption. For instance, constructed wetlands use vegetation to filter and uptake nutrients and contaminants from treated wastewater, thus reducing biochemical oxygen demand (BOD) and ammonia levels. This process not only purifies the effluent but also strengthens the surrounding ecosystem, thus representing a feasible substitute for decentralized, small-scale wastewater treatment systems, as evidenced by the usability of domestic systems in aquatic ecosystems management (Magfhira et al., 2021). Through the incorporation of such natural processes in urban planning, cities can promote sustainable water management through adaptation to large-scale environmental goals. Furthermore, land disposal methods are crucial to guaranteeing the safe reuse of treated wastewater, as this emphasizes the practice of appropriate practices in water recycling. The approach is consistent with the Sustainable Development Goals (SDG) principles, particularly SDG 6, which aims to improve water quality through alleviating contamination and enhancing the safe reuse of water resources (Magfhira et al., 2021). In developing countries generally, where traditional wastewater treatment facilities may be lacking, land disposal technologies can circumvent limited-resource limitations. Additionally, they contribute to increased climate change resilience and water scarcity through the provision of a guarantee of treated water availability for irrigation or other purposes, not for drinking. Use of these methods requires meticulous assessments to determine soil condition, environmental impact, and public health, such that at all times, health considerations must be given priority. In situations where proper sanitation amenities are not easily accessible, as is the situation in regions like Kaduna State, Nigeria, land disposal methods offer worthwhile possibilities for upgrading health in the community. A study showed that despite noteworthy complexities, the majority of the population lacked access to advanced water treatment practices and relied extensively on unsafe water sources. Therefore, the integration of land disposal systems along with environmentally focused priority for sanitation and correct management of excreta becomes necessary for reducing waterborne disease-related risks. Promoting educational programs on safe land disposal methods, as well as the provision of affordable sanitary facilities, can be the secret to more effective hygiene and sanitation outcomes. To summarize, the scope for public health benefits and sustainable water handling with land disposal alternatives calls for an engaged cooperation of governments and people.

6.5.2. Ocean Disposal Methods

Ocean disposal is one of the key methods within the broader category of water supply and sanitation management. Ocean disposal methods involve the release of treated wastewater into oceanic habitats, whose currents are believed to rapidly dilute the contaminant. This method comes repeatedly into use in coastal communities where terrestrial-based disposal alternatives may be limited by environmental sensitivity or land availability. However, these measures are cited with valid concerns regarding their impacts on long-term marine environments and water quality. Treatment level prior to disposal is important as untreated or inadequately treated effluents may be toxic to marine life and upset local ecosystems. Once more, the problem of problems caused by growing urbanization highlights the imperative to adopt environmentally friendly methods of disposal that balance human interests against ecoprotection (Justice et al., 1977). While urbanization continues unabated across much of the globe, reliance on ocean disposal methods may be more acute, and thus their efficiency and sustainability need to be examined. Increased population levels mean increased production of wastewater, which causes a strain on the available treatment infrastructure. Coastal populations, being typically low-resource, may find ocean disposal inexpensive. But doing so may overlook the critical role of wastewater management to ensure human health and environmental integrity. To this is added the issue of climate change, which, through rising sea levels and altered ocean current patterns, may exacerbate ocean pollution. The nexus between ocean disposal methods and the grand scale of climate adaptation issues identifies the need for the accommodation of water resource management to the benefit of both sanitation access and environmental sustainability (Justice et al., 1977). Given these challenges, there is increased encouragement of alternative mechanisms to ocean disposal methods like water reuse and reclamation projects.

These actions not only minimize the environmental impacts of ocean disposal but also provide valuable resources for urban agriculture and irrigation, hence enhancing food security in growing populations. Through the transformation of treated wastewater into reusable sources, cities achieve a reduction of pressure on freshwater resources, as well as motivating farmers to sustain agricultural activity. Further, the involvement of the public and stakeholders is important in designing efficient wastewater management systems. Community participation enhances awareness of sanitary and hygiene issues and enables effective implementation of new measures. Ultimately, the elimination of ocean disposal requires an integrated strategy based on public health, environmental conservation, and public involvement in a water supply and sanitation system (Bahri et al., 2025).

6.5.3. Reuse and Recycling of Treated Wastewater

The re-use and recycling of treated wastewater are integral components of modern water supply and sanitation planning, particularly for water-scarce areas. Recycling and treating wastewater allows communities to reuse valuable water resources for non-potable uses such as irrigation, industrial applications, and even for drinking purposes with advanced treatment. Not only does recycling and reusing wastewater avoid the effects of water scarcity, but it also maintains sustainable water management. Societies are increasingly looking at recycling wastewater as a possible economic and environmental prospect since it gives two-fold benefits of reduction in freshwater demand and minimization of wastewater disposal costs. Moreover, such operations follow circular economy principles, which focus on the idea of recycling and reusing resources rather than disposing of them. Efforts to embark on scalable business models for this industry emphasize the potential for economically sustainable opportunities in the management of wastewater (N/A, 2016). Urban agriculture represents a significant field where treated wastewater can be applied, addressing both food security and sustainable management. Because urbanization keeps rising, water resource pressure rises too, and this necessitates innovative solutions. Irrigation of urban agriculture using treated wastewater has the potential to maximize water efficiency and reduce dependency on conventional freshwater sources. The practice has the capability to enhance local food production systems and thus ensure food security in urban areas. Enhanced management of treated wastewater is necessary to ensure public health safety and environmental protection. The integration of participatory management practices that involve local stakeholders is able to bring about community confidence and participation, hence ensuring urban agriculture success fueled by reclaimed wastewater (Bahri et al., 2025).

Additionally, integrating treated wastewater infrastructure into city infrastructure can provide significant socio-economic benefits to communities. By establishing awareness among individuals of the potential utilization of treated wastewater, municipalities are able to encourage public acceptance and participation, which is critical to the long-term sustainability of these programs. Moreover, advancements in treatment processes leading to excellent-quality effluent have the potential for establishing broader acceptance and utilization of recycled water by industries. The findings of current research unveil the opportunities that fall within this sector, as novel business models have the capacity to create additional value from wastewater resources through collaborative relationships. In the future of water supply and sanitation, as societies expect, efficient reuse and recycling of treated wastewater will surely be a major driver in constructing resilience to water scarcity and fostering general community health and well-being (N/A, 2016) (Figure 6.17).

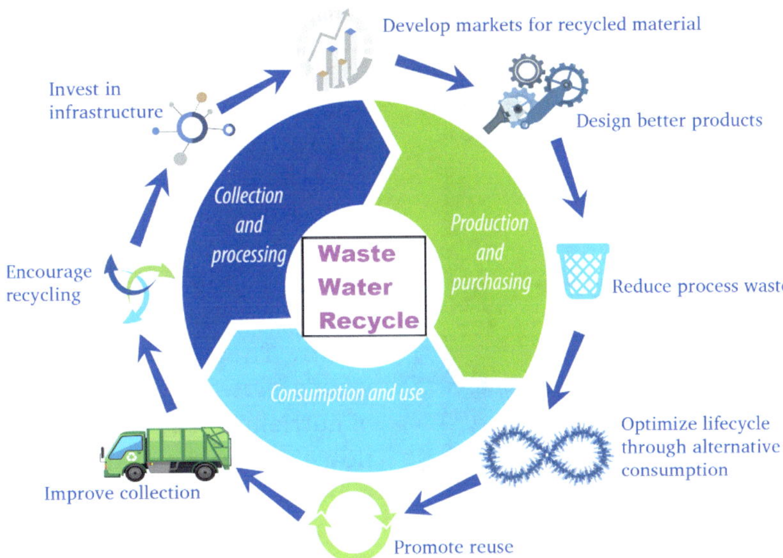
Develop markets for recycled material
Design better products
Reduce process waste
Optimize lifecycle through alternative consumption
Promote reuse
Improve collection
Encourage recycling
Invest in infrastructure
Collection and processing
Production and purchasing
Consumption and use
Waste Water Recycle

Figure 6.17. Reuse and recycling of treated wastewater.

https://www.eawater.com/wp-content/uploads/2022/10/Pic1_Waste-Water-cycle.png.

6.6. The Impact of Poor Sanitation on Water Resources

Poor sanitation actually destroys our water. When wastewater goes into nature untreated, it ends up reaching rivers and lakes—essentially inviting bad germs to the party. You typically see that uncontrolled waste flow acts like a breeding ground for bad microorganisms, and those pesky little guys can seep into our drinking water, making ailments worse. Societies that are suffering from poor sanitation are likely to suffer from heightened waterborne diseases, which not only risk human lives but also overburden regional healthcare as well as impair productivity. Overall, the fact that over 60% of the global population does not have safe sanitation illustrates how dismally water quality and public health can be impacted (Andersson et al., 2018). Getting our water in hand actually starts with a knowledge of how poor sanitation can cause massive problems. Even with the United Nations 2030 Agenda for Sustainable Development efforts toward better water and sanitation control, many areas lack the basic infrastructure needed. The economic, social, and environmental impacts—such as ongoing water quality degradation—demand quick, hands-on intervention. As populations grow and demands for water keep increasing, ignoring sanitation issues only adds to the challenge of providing clean water for everyone. Local practices simply don't align with those global aspirations most of the time, exposing a disparity between grand ideals and real action. It is more than likely that adjusting our focus toward practical, functional policies to deal with water in light of sanitation shortcomings is warranted (Tortajada, 2016).

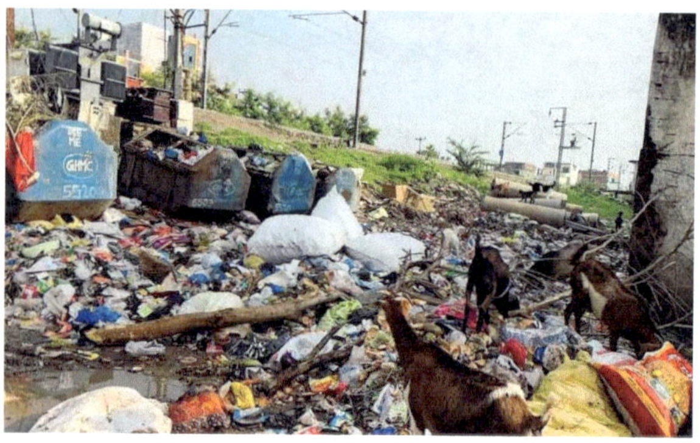

Figure 6.18. Poor sanitation breeds vector-borne diseases.

Source: https://assets.thehansindia.com/h-upload/2022/07/17/1303474-garba.webp.

There is no question that new technologies are needed to minimize the negative impact of insanitary conditions on water supplies. Shifting to a system whereby we reuse water for consumption can actually decrease the amount of wastewater as well as help recover valuable nutrients. New ideas—such as decentralized treatment systems and even low-flush toilets—offer viable options that can greatly improve sanitation results. Such solutions not only expand access to sanitation, but also provide the potential for recycling treated water in practices such as irrigation, etc. Most importantly, an amalgamation of efforts by public agencies, private organizations, and community groups will be required to bring such ideas into practice. In the majority of cases, combining technological innovations with wise policy measures can create an integrated and sustainable system for sanitation and water management that will eventually lead to healthier communities (Andersson et al., 2018) (Figure 6.18).

6.6.1. Effects of Untreated Wastewater on Water Bodies

Untreated wastewater is a significant issue for fish environments as well as for our own health. That waste that's discharged untreated from industry, agriculture, and cities carries a filthy cocktail of chemicals—heavy metals, excess nutrients, and even bacteria—that eventually finds its way into water systems in unregulated forms. These contaminants frequently form what's known as eutrophication, where an excess of nutrients creates surprise algal blooms. These flowers rob the water of oxygen, producing hypoxia and a great deal of aquatic mortality. Suspended bacteria in untreated wastewater can travel considerable distances, occasionally posing a danger to human health while quietly degrading biodiversity. In general, eliminating these environmental hazards is essential if we're to keep our aquatic systems healthy and our communities safe, which means good wastewater management is something of an imperative that we need to address as a priority. The effects of untreated wastewater go far beyond short-term harm to the environment; they also extend to communities on various fronts. Individuals who consume such waters for drinking, bathing, or even some recreation end up with an increased likelihood of waterborne disease. For example, exposure to a mixture of toxins and pathogens suffices to initiate gastrointestinal distress, sometimes even interferes with reproductive health. When water quality fails, local agriculture and aquaculture suffer as well, which could potentially worsen food insecurity and disrupt livelihoods. So the ramifications of neglecting wastewater treatment aren't just about nature out of kilter—it echoes into social injustices and economic stability. For the most part, a well-rounded approach to addressing wastewater has to address both public health and economic concerns if we ever hope to design truly resilient communities. New technologies in wastewater management and sustainable waste management practices have emerged as key solutions to these problems. Technologies today combine biological, chemical, and physical processes to screen out more impurities prior to returning water to nature. The use of bio-based sorbents derived from agricultural waste, for example, is a fascinating example. These sorbents are able to sequester pollutants well, addressing waste disposal and water cleaning at the same time.

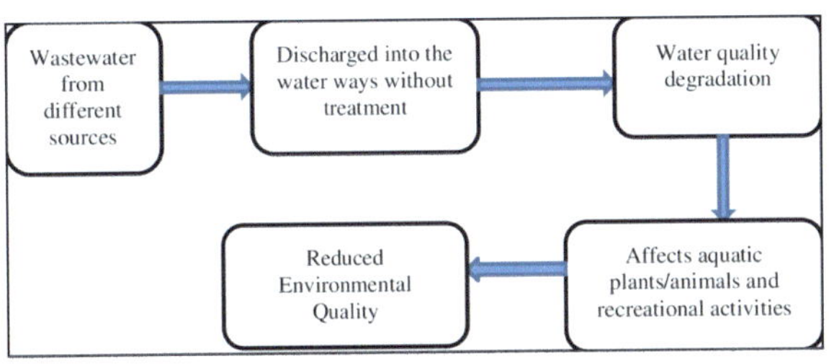

Figure 6.19. Impacts of untreated wastewater on the surface water.

Source: https://www.researchgate.net/profile/Doris-Ogueri/publication/348994672/figure/fig1/AS:987049838530563@161234242882 2/mpacts-of-untreated-wastewater-on-the-surface-water-Developed-by-the-researcher.png.

As some studies indicate (Nataša et al., 2021), adopting local fixes that best utilize available resources can be both eco-friendly and economical. Furthermore, applying measures to manage wastewater discharge on a regular basis and investing in new treatment facilities are key actions toward safeguarding our water. Generally speaking, having access to clean water—to use the words of the Sustainable Development Goals—means embracing an equitable strategy that brings together public health and environmental conservation (Abascal et al., 2021) (Figure 6.19).

6.6.2. Consequences for Aquatic Ecosystems

Hiring out to dump untreated wastewater into our lakes and rivers is not a harmless mistake but has a plethora of unexpected, far-reaching consequences. Typically, when you spill too much of nutrients like nitrogen and phosphorus into these waterbodies, you see an uncontrolled explosion of algae growth, popularly known as algal blooms. These blooms tend, in most cases, to suck oxygen out of the water, strangling aquatic life. And when the algae are dead, the oxygen is depleted even more, and that creates those awful dead zones where life just can't exist. The sensitive organisms disappear first, and that disrupts the whole ecosystem equilibrium. In summary, taking care of wastewater isn't all about cleaner water; it's about protecting the very backbone of aquatic health and resilience (Rodr, 2023). Clean water and sustainable development clearly go hand in hand, and it has been thrown into the global light by the United Nations SDGs—specifically the ones that aim to enhance water quality and healthy ecosystems. If water is not well treated, the danger is not just restricted to fish or aquatic organisms; it spills over to affect communities that rely on such water bodies for consumption, leisure, or even small business ventures. At other instances, pollutants build up—heavy metals and toxins making their way into aquatic life and, ultimately, being transferred to people further up the food chain, thus causing severe health issues. Overall, the whole situation points towards the need for an integrated approach to wastewater management—one that interlaces several SDGs to improve both people's and the environment's health. In a certain way, this integration lays the ground for environmental justice and ecological harmony in the long run (Wang et al., 2022). The cost of uncontrolled wastewater management is far greater than damage to nature—it seeps into our socio-economic existence, too. As water quality worsens, fisheries collapse; they are not only sources of nutrition, but also lifelines for economic equilibrium in the majority of societies. Overfishing combined with polluted water can spark a local fishery collapse, exacerbating poverty and upsetting nutritional levels. Even for recreational use, like swimming and fishing, could be hurt, which in turn could decrease local tourism and other economic opportunities. Investing in new wastewater treatment technologies and sustainable strategies can smooth out these increasing problems, opening the door to healthier waters and thriving local economies. Ultimately, finding an even balance between our daily lives and nature's needs is about adopting smart, effective wastewater and sanitation systems (Rodr, 2023).

6.6.3. Long-Term Implications for Water Quality and Availability

Sanitation and water quality are interlinked in ways that affect our long-term health—big effects that we see in the environment and in health. Sanitation that is not clean, like dirty toilets, typically ends up polluting our clean water, slowly compromising its quality and decreasing its availability. Populations that rely on this dirty water have higher risks of waterborne disease while their health systems are pushed to the limit. (Gumbo et al., 2012) shows some quite clever pairings of water supply solutions with better sanitation practices, which seem to aid people in their recovery. At the end of the day, it's a question of maintaining our water health by treating waste wisely—prioritizing human health and trying to balance nature. Good sanitation infrastructure can also unclog some of the urban pressures on water quality. Urban areas, especially following a significant migration, are overloading their established water systems, as Mosello et al. (2016) state. Additional residents mean that the sanitation equipment is overwhelmed quite often, so waste isn't properly treated, and more runoff ends up in nearby streams or ponds. This slow degradation eventually affects the regional aquatic life as well as the safe water people need to drink, cook, and farm. Most times, simply rethinking how we operate these systems and address city stress proves to be the key to maintaining cleaner water in increasingly dynamic city environments. In the years to come, the problems that inadequate sanitation systems cause will reach beyond short-term health concerns and start playing tricks with the social and economic balance of communities. Clean water, in fact, serves as the keystone of farms, factories, schools—you name it.

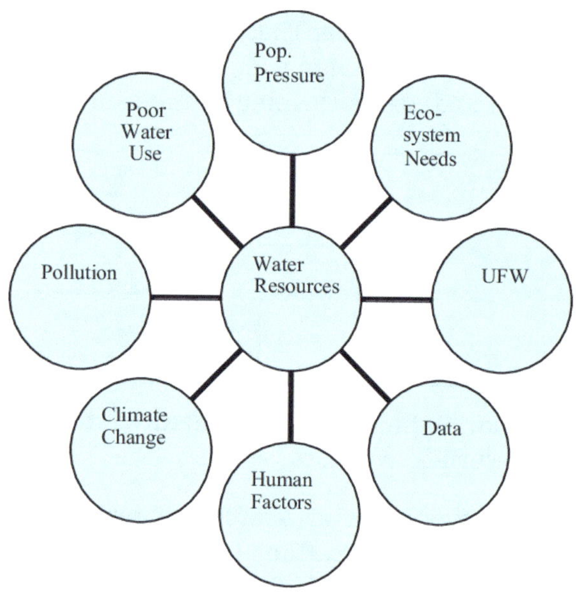

Figure 6.20. Interlinking of factors impacting water quality and availability.

Source: https://www.researchgate.net/profile/Catherine-Zeman/publication/225576583/figure/fig4/AS:872263142350850@1584975147265/nterlinking-of-factors-impacting-water-quality-and-availability.png.

Thus, when water quality declines, its effect percolates to all segments of society, preventing economic progress and, on occasion, actually widening disparities. Gumbo et al. (2012) contend that building knowledge of how to manage water resources is central to building practices to facilitate communities' ability to adapt to these environmental changes more successfully. Generally, investment in better infrastructure and education in sanitation is an investment that can generate a cycle that, in the long run, improves water safety and accessibility for future generations (Figure 6.20).

6.7. Community Health and Sanitation

Sanitation is literally at the heart of keeping communities healthy. Safe waste habits keep people from getting sick by keeping contaminants from reaching sources of drinking water—an especially bad thing to occur in communities lacking adequate infrastructure. Far too often, waterborne illnesses thrive in low-income neighborhoods, where sanitation is subpar and threatens residents. When communities adopt better systems for waste control, rates for these diseases come way down, and overall well-being rises. Effective sanitation, thus, not only promotes health but also improves social and economic conditions with better living conditions. In many cases, the introduction of new technology to save resources efficiently turns sanitation into a true pillar of public health programs (María et al., 2021). Sanitation and wastewater management also walk hand in hand together with the targets for world sustainable development. The United Nations Sustainable Development Goals generally highlight that all human beings—particularly the poor with no adequate services—must be given safe, accessible sanitation. Sanitation innovation and digital technology can step in to simplify data gathering, monitoring, and tracking greatly. For instance, intelligent systems linked to the Internet of Things offer abundant datasets that most frequently, quite naturally, lead to better community health decisions. These innovations not only solve the immediate issues of keeping areas clean but also tackle broader environmental issues, carving a trend of sustainable and equitable health benefits. Such a focus on innovation in sanitation is therefore very critical to enhancing community health worldwide (María et al., 2021). To solve how poor sanitation affects water supplies, one would need to have a blend of policy reform, citizen action, and technology solutions. When water systems become polluted through unsanitary conditions, not only is the health of humans at risk, but the environment of the area is damaged too. Proper wastewater treatment is the key to discouraging environmental degradation and stopping the vicious cycle of disease and poverty. In recent times, treatments like biological treatment and nutrient recovery have been viewed as environmentally sound solutions that can be made feasible. By treating wastewater more creatively, communities can safeguard valuable water sources while gaining benefits for farming, energy, and so much more. Simply put, uniting community well-being with smart sanitation is the foundation for strong environments that ensure the present and future success of individuals around the world (N/A, 2019).

6.7.1. Correlation Between Sanitation and Community Health Outcomes

Good sanitation has a large role in contributing to public health and is identified more today. Sanitation prevents infection and generates healthier everyday surroundings—especially in poorer residential areas, where substandard facilities account for more waterborne diseases like cholera and dysentery. Research generally indicates that investment in better sanitation saves healthcare costs and enhances the standard of living. Interventions in nations like Brazil, India, Indonesia, and Senegal that take sanitation into account both politically and economically tend to show that well-targeted, thought-out interventions can have a certain effect on the most marginalized (N/A, 2011). It's almost as if spending money on sanitation pays off in more than one way. Apart from the obvious health benefits, proper sanitation also overlaps with environmental sustainability and the overall well-being of the community. Not only is human health at risk from unsanitary conditions, but water quality can deteriorate, pollution is augmented, and ecosystems suffer, too. Integrated wastewater management—which means taking into account health benefits as well as environmental impacts—is therefore essential. Evaluations of areas such as Sri Lanka and Ghana indicate, in the majority of cases, that upgraded wastewater treatment is capable of recovering resources as well as meeting sanitation needs simultaneously. When you take these interconnections into account, it is easy to see that integrating sanitation improvement with intelligent environmental approaches is essential to long-term resilience in a community (Merrey et al., 2020).

Sanitation's impact even extends into economic productivity and social justice. Healthy facilities are found in communities that have healthier workers, which means fewer lost workdays and less disease spreading—value factors that can add to overall economic output. At the same time, inadequate sanitation will impact marginalized groups disproportionately, exposing more profound social differences that need to be remedied. In most cases, the gap can be closed by moving towards more equitable sanitation practices, which enable the benefit of health gains as well as economic development to flow more fairly to everyone. Such a large-scale strategy—melding health, economic growth, and social equality—really resonates with the significance of overall sanitation methods in the quest for long-term community health (N/A, 2011) (Figure 6.21).

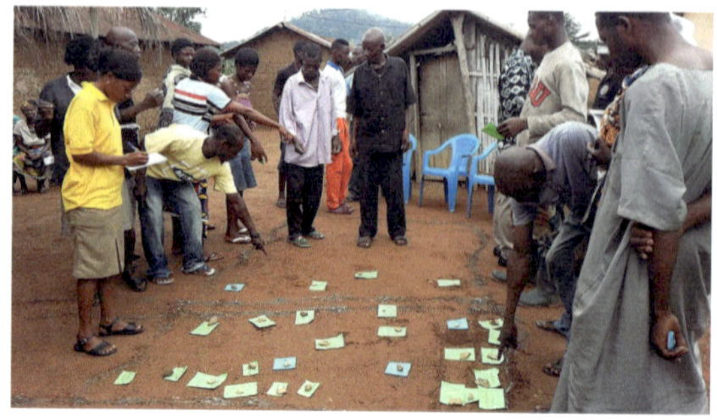

Figure 6.21. Community-led total sanitation (CLTS) triggering process: Community members in Ghana are drawing a map of open defecation for their community.

Source: https://upload.wikimedia.org/wikipedia/commons/thumb/2/22/CLTS_triggering_process_in_the_Volta_Region_of_Ghana.jpg/1024px-CLTS_triggering_process_in_the_Volta_Region_of_Ghana.jpg.

6.7.2. Vulnerable Populations and Sanitation Challenges

Vulnerable populations are left to shoulder the burden when sanitation facilities are not up to par. The majority of the communities in low- and middle-income regions see their basic needs negatively impacted as cities expand, large demand outstrips existing infrastructure. Rapid urban expansion, in most cases, deprives disadvantaged communities of limited exposure to clean, safe sanitation, and that in turn gives rise to aggravated health complications. Poverty, gender, and social status all coalesce to dictate who is being served, women and children most likely to pay the ultimate price. Unpaid care labor and safety issues, for instance, are able to make even something as fundamental as having access to a clean restroom a literal nightmare. The cycle even achieves mental hardship, trauma, and chronic stress coming in during the fight for basic needs (Batra et al., 2025). Apparently, leaders have to base choices on fresh, representative thoughts if they have any hope of plugging gaps. Take Dar es Salaam, for example—its growing population, set to hit 8.5 million by

2025, has pushed wastewater infrastructure far beyond its limits. Its growing population has, in effect, overwhelmed treatment plants and, in the majority of cases, permitted raw sewage to enter nearby waterways. This filthy image is not just one of technological failure; it is symptomatic of an even more intrinsic link between environmental collapse and disastrous health crises that overwhelmingly devastate the most vulnerable populations. Research generally recommends a total reformation of the way wastewater is dealt with. New technologies like Anaerobic Digestion (AD) might improve treatment efficacy, but only if these technology solutions are coupled with active community involvement and regular, stable financing (Azizi et al., 2025). Skip these bigger steps, and the cycle of suffering continues for the most vulnerable. Poor sanitation does more than harm the health of individuals—it can undermine social bonds and local economies, too. Most frequently, the individuals who need decent facilities are those left in facilities that have less than minimum infrastructure, and that is, disaster writing under the guise of waterborne illness. When health is compromised, productivity in communities drops because scarce resources go towards healthcare instead of other things on the list. This problem shows, quite emphatically, that one solution will not cut it; instead, a blend of tech innovation and socio-economic solutions must be used. Entering with some mental health support in sanitation policies may make it easier to recover from setbacks and lower the cost of poor infrastructure on a daily basis (Batra et al., 2025). In the end, solving all of these problems on every front isn't a nice-to-have—it's necessary to promote equity in sanitation access and protect the public health for all, especially the most vulnerable.

6.7.3. Case Studies of Communities Affected by Poor Sanitation

Bad sanitation actually leaves its imprint on communities in ways both seen and unseen. A number of case studies illustrate the numerous layers of effect on public health. In rural Vietnam, for example, sanitation suppliers and water operators face daunting infrastructure hurdles and high operating costs that leave them financially at risk. That typically triggers the necessity for donor-supported projects assisting low-income residents – a necessity difficult to ignore. Conversations during survey interviews and focus group interviews with fifteen public–private partnership suppliers reveal how complex it is to manage sanitation services. Volatile material prices, coupled with tight household budgets, tend to create a cycle of poor access. Overall, intentional financial and policy interventions seem to be of vital importance here, as they can enhance service availability without ruining market mechanisms. Generally, these findings underscore that secure sanitation facilities are a top priority for public health protection and fair access to water (Pham, 2025). Climate change as a lens makes things more complicated. Under warmer temperatures, populations already beset by inadequate sanitation tend to see their systems burdened, with a surge in waterborne diseases. Environmental degradation, compounded by poor sanitation infrastructure, exacerbates the situation. There is a desperate need for new, innovative engineering solutions to urban planning. A range of solid studies, for example, have found that when health programs and engineering methods come together, populations are generally well prepared to overcome climate challenges. Globally, successful interventions encourage us to remember that public health principles married with smart engineering can minimize the dangers from both failed sanitation infrastructure and climate change. As a rule, collaboration between disciplines is most needed in fighting overall public health in areas most impacted by poor sanitation (Irene, 2025). Some examples are especially reminiscent of the larger, systemic problems at play when sanitation fails. Imagine that there exists a city community in a poor country where cholera is too common, and that is mostly because of the failure to treat wastewater effectively. The effects do not stop with immediate health consequences—it also goes out into economic insecurity and even disruption of communal bonds. Many families are often faced with huge medical expenses, and lost workdays due to illness only make matters worse. And to boot, that lingering stigma of poor sanitation can reduce social mobility and inclusion. These instances clearly prove that the solution is not just a matter of upgrading sewer infrastructure; it's about addressing the deep connection between sanitation, community health, and resilience. If we can direct efforts towards more capable, more effective wastewater management solutions, we might be establishing the preconditions for healthier communities and mitigating some of the public health issues we face in comparable settings (Pham, 2025) (Figure 6.22).

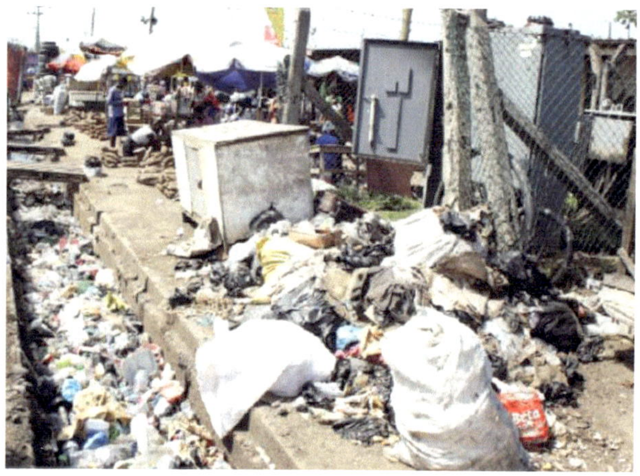

Figure 6.22. Poor sanitation in Ghana.

Source: https://cdn.modernghana.com/content__/640/457/623201951400_8dt2wkivvq_gh62.png.

CLOSER LOOK

FUTURE CHALLENGES IN WATER SUPPLY AND SANITATION

The future challenges in water supply and sanitation are increasingly becoming more complex as a result of rapid population growth and urbanization. With the expansion of the urban areas, the demand for clean water is on the increase, subjecting the available resources to unprecedented stress. The threat of water shortage looms in regions that are already experiencing scarce supplies. Any attempt at regulating the supply has to consider not only the quantity of available water but also its quality. Thus, innovative solutions must be used to protect water supplies from contamination and ensure safe delivery. Moreover, climate change compounds these issues through altered rainfall patterns and increased occurrences of intense weather phenomena. Thus, a future water supply and sanitation solution must be a multi-faceted one that balances sustainable means with regard to ecological equilibrium against the increasing demands of urban citizens.

In wastewater disposal and treatment, the future challenges also take the form of stakeholder engagement and technological adaptation. As conventional treatments may no longer be able to handle the increasing quantity and complexity of urban wastewaters, the exploration of advanced technology becomes a necessity. This includes recovering value from wastewater, as proposed by sanitation studies under the Circular Economy, where resources are transformed into valuable products. Such emphasis on transformation not only pushes for resource efficiency but also sustains economic models. The engagement of multiple actors, such as local governments, industries, and communities, in participatory management will likely make these interventions more efficient. Their engagement is vital to the fulfillment of sanitation standards and facilitating fair distribution of the benefits of improved wastewater management, thus cementing social equity's central role in new water policy.

Ultimately, sanitation, hygiene, and water supply remain an area of focus in the battle against future public health risks. As the world continues to grapple with the effects of inefficient sanitation systems, it is imperative that there is a heightened culture of education and health awareness of hygiene. Populations are heterogeneous in their access to safe sanitation methods, which can compound health disparities. Averting these disparities requires holistic sensitivity to the interconnectedness of water security, food security, and health in the context of urban agriculture transformations. Developing drought-resilient sanitation systems that are sensitive to community demands has the capacity to significantly enhance public health. Thus, having a high regard for comprehensive sanitation policy is pivotal in developing healthy communities as well as ensuring access to water resources in an increasingly exigent world.

SUMMARY

The acute need for effective water supply and sanitation facilities is paramount in fostering healthy communities. Effective management of water and sanitation resources could potentially drastically curtail the spread of waterborne diseases, encourage enhanced hygiene practices, and enhance health levels at large. Community education findings have documented disparities in access to safe drinking water and sanitation services, indicating that a sizeable percentage of populations persist in using poor and unsafe alternatives. For instance, while the majority of citizens in Ekosodin and BDPA use boreholes for water for consumption, the lack of proper sanitation facilities aggravates the health risk posed by inadequate WASH services, as the presented findings emphasize the urgent need for community-based intervention programs (Imarhiagbe et al., 2025). Consequently, greater access to clean water and sanitation can lead to better public health outcomes, reduced healthcare costs, and improved living for the residents.

Furthermore, findings from uMfolozi Local Municipality schools offer testimony to the complexities of provision of appropriate sanitation and hygiene practices among young people. Even though such schools exhibited some form of access to clean water, the structural challenges regarding the dependability of the supply of water and sanitation facilities remain a challenge. Reliance on diversified sources, for instance, municipal water, boreholes, and rainwater, presents challenges regarding constant access as well as quality assurance. Moreover, habits of hygiene, which greatly rely on handwashing facilities availability, were substandard in many of the schools, potentially undermining the well-being and health of the students (Lindokuhle et al., 2025). Improved infrastructure in such schools and more study programs on hygiene are crucial to improve health standards among students as they directly affect learning achievements and long-term community health.

Prioritizing water supply and sanitation facilities is critical in sustaining public health, particularly in vulnerable populations. Indicated by the inequalities identified across regions, collaborative action in enhancing water and sanitation facilities can address the underlying causes of the health disparities. Research-informed, community-led interventions, in turn, are important in addressing the problems effectively. Therefore, governments, NGOs, and local authorities must collaborate in establishing sustainable interventions to improve access to clean water, adequate sanitation, and hygiene education. By addressing these core needs, communities can construct cleaner and healthier settings that, besides leading to improved quality of life, contribute to the realization of overall developmental goals, particularly those founded on Sustainable Development Goals related to water and sanitation.

The critical examination of the supply and sanitation of water reveals some of the key issues that portray the necessity for effective management strategies at the community level. At the center of this analysis is the recognition of the character of water as a key resource that needs sustainable efforts on both the purification and supply sides. Effective water purification technologies, particularly those incorporating advanced technologies, provide clean water to communities and maintain natural reserves. As emphasized in various studies, the implementation of advanced methodologies in water treatment leads to improved public health results and also adds to broader environmental sustainability goals. Therefore, the imperative of communities is not only to provide access to water but to implement comprehensive water management programs that are aligned with long-term sustainability objectives, opening the door for healthier future generations.

Secondly, wastewater treatment is a pivotal element in maintaining environmental integrity through the maximization of energy recovery and agricultural production. It is much more than just an infrastructural necessity; it is an integral aspect of sustainable resource management. As noted, wastewater treatment also serves to prevent water wastage, ease pressure on dwindling freshwater resources, and convert organic waste into valuable products such as bio-methane and fertilizers for agricultural use (Rodr, 2023). Through the application of systematic approaches such as literature reviews to synthesize existing methodology, stakeholders can also appreciate the utility of wastewater management in preventive health infrastructure and its potential contribution to communities. Therefore, the combined focus on wastewater treatment in the sanitation discourse is used to increase overall water resource sustainability.

Another impelling shift in water quality management and monitoring is the integration of genetic faecal pollution diagnostics (GFPD) innovation. The use of nucleic acid-based methods like PCR and sequencing has transformed the identification and evaluation of microbial pollutants affecting health-related water quality (Demeter et al., 2023). Not only does this new science refine traditional water quality analysis, it also enhances the capability to trace sources of faecal pollution, providing a firm foundation for public health monitoring. Now with over 1,100 publications that highlight the diversity of GFPD's applications, it has been evident that these methods can be integrated with conventional techniques to give an integrated overview of microbial water safety. All these innovations underscore the symbiotic relationship between water supply, sanitation, and community health and demand an integrated approach to ensuring access to safe water and sanitation for all.

REFERENCES

1. Allen, L., Christian-Smith, J., Cohen, M. J., et al. (2010). *Clearing the Waters: A Focus on Water Quality Solutions.* https://core.ac.uk/download/75783230.pdf (accessed on 11th June 2025).
2. Angelakıs, A. N., Vuorinen, H. S., Nikolaidis, C., Juuti, P., Katko, T. S., Juuti, R. P., Zhang, J., et al. (2021). Water quality and life expectancy: Parallel courses in time. *Water, 13*, 752–752. https://doi.org/10.3390/w13060752 (accessed on 11th June 2025).
3. Bahri, A., Brissaud, F., & Drechsel, P. (2025). *Water Reuse in Africa: Challenges and Opportunities.* https://core.ac.uk/download/pdf/6764702.pdf (accessed on 11th June 2025).
4. Bartaula, R. (2016). *Performance Evaluation of Water and Wastewater Treatment Plant in Kathmandu Valley.* https://core.ac.uk/download/249960878.pdf (accessed on 11th June 2025).
5. Deffner, J., & Mazambani, C. (2010). Participatory empirical research on water and sanitation demand in central northern Namibia: A method for technology development with a user perspective. https://core.ac.uk/download/14526924.pdf (accessed on 11th June 2025).
6. Demeter, K., Linke, R., Ballesté, E., Reischer, G. H., Mayer, R., Vierheilig, J., Kolm, C., et al. (2023). Have genetic targets for fecal pollution diagnostics and source tracking revolutionized water quality analysis yet? *FEMS Microbiology Reviews, 47*. https://doi.org/10.1093/femsre/fuad028 (accessed on 11th June 2025).
7. Evans, B. E., Haller, L., & Hutton, G. (2004). Closing the sanitation gap: The case for better public funding of sanitation and hygiene.
8. Evans, B. E., Peal, A. J., & van der Voorden, C. (2010). *Hygiene and Sanitation Software: An Overview of Approaches.*
9. Fore, H. H. (2020). A wake-up call: COVID-19 and its impact on children's health and wellbeing. *The Lancet Global Health, 8*, e861–e862. https://doi.org/10.1016/s2214-109x(20)30238-2 (accessed on 11th June 2025).
10. Grimason, A., Lungu, K., & Morse, T. (2008). Ecological sanitation–Implementation, opportunities and challenges in Chikwawa. https://core.ac.uk/download/19610161.pdf (accessed on 11th June 2025).
11. Grimason, A., Morse, T., Nicholls, R., Smith, et al. (2008). Epidemiology of cryptosporidiosis in rural Malawi. https://core.ac.uk/download/19610159.pdf (accessed on 11th June 2025).
12. Imarhiagbe, E. E., Asemota, A. J., Erazua, E., Okafor, A. A., Gadimoh, P. E., Osamade, U. W., & Okpechukwu, E. M. (2025). Levels of water supply, sanitation, hygiene and health status of residents of two communities that share boundaries with a first-generation tertiary institution in Benin City, Edo State, Nigeria. *Journal of Applied Sciences and Environmental Management.* https://www.semanticscholar.org/paper/8cbeb29bdde42c7843f20befe757613634e1265b (accessed on 11th June 2025).
13. Justice, S. R., Smith, D. M., Tilsworth, T., et al. (1977). *Cold Climate Water/Wastewater Transportation and Treatment–A Bibliography: Completion Report.* https://core.ac.uk/download/162573813.pdf (accessed on 11th June 2025).
14. Magfhira, A., Kinasih, P., Salsabila, D., Marchella, E., & Fachrul, M. (2021). Domestic wastewater treatment with household-scale constructed wetland system using water fern plant (*Azolla pinnata*). *IOP Conference Series: Earth and Environmental Science, 894*. https://www.

semanticscholar.org/paper/83b768c8ed114d843a4e5ad968957cbe78e6257c (accessed on 11th June 2025).

15. Mahmud, I., & Mbuya, N. (2016). Water, sanitation, hygiene, and nutrition in Bangladesh: Can building toilets affect children's growth? https://core.ac.uk/download/75783689.pdf (accessed on 11th June 2025).

16. Mann, B. (2014). *Navigating the Water, Sanitation, And Hygiene (WASH) Sector: A Guide for Corporate Grantmakers*. https://core.ac.uk/download/71364948.pdf (accessed on 11th June 2025).

17. Marcy, A., Hadly, E., Sherratt, E., Garland, K., & Weisbecker, V. (2017). *Governance Frameworks for Wastewater Management*. https://core.ac.uk/download/96930789.pdf (accessed on 11th June 2025).

18. McBain, F., Tischbein, B., & Tsegai, D. (2013). *Water, Sanitation and Hygiene: The Missing Link with Agriculture*. https://www.econstor.eu/dspace/bitstream/10419/88321/1/773393722.pdf (accessed on 11th June 2025).

19. Radebe, L. C., Mokgobu, M. I., Molelekwa, G. F., & Mokoena, M. M. (2025). Assessment of the status of water, sanitation and hygiene (WASH) services at primary schools in uMfolozi Local Municipality, Kwa-Zulu Natal, South Africa. *International Journal of Environmental Research and Public Health, 22*. https://www.semanticscholar.org/paper/486c9dfd0b057fd61d725a1273ea2d9d4e1d8257 (accessed on 11th June 2025).

20. Sawhney, A., & Chanda, R. (2025). *Trade in Environmental Services: Opportunities and Constraints*. https://core.ac.uk/download/pdf/6604702.pdf (accessed on 11th June 2025).

21. Silva Rodríguez de San Miguel, J. A. (2023). Wastewater treatment and reuse for sustainable water resources management: A systematic literature review. *Sustainability, 15*, 10940–10940. https://doi.org/10.3390/su151410940 (accessed on 11th June 2025).

22. Sridhar, M., Okareh, O., & Mustapha, M. (2020). Assessment of knowledge, attitudes, and practices on water, sanitation, and hygiene in some selected LGAs in Kaduna State, Northwestern Nigeria. *Journal of Environmental and Public Health, 2020*. https://www.semanticscholar.org/paper/b780b47d6c70b090c00a9b9e1b1fffc06de92dc2 (accessed on 11th June 2025).

23. Titilawo, M. A., Josiah, C. G., Simeon, O. N., Ali, C. M., Ugwuocha, C. S., Ojediran, G. O., Titilawo, O. Y., et al. (2024). Physical quality and antibiotic susceptibility profile of *Escherichia coli* isolates from roof-harvested rainwater: A microcosm study. *Ife Journal of Science*. https://www.semanticscholar.org/paper/6c1aa2a20f5026c71987d1306ae32963bacc1f57 (accessed on 11th June 2025).

24. Yoshikawa, H., Wuermli, A. J., Britto, P. R., Dreyer, B. P., Leckman, J. F., Lye, S. J., Ponguta, L. A., et al. (2020). Effects of the global Coronavirus Disease-2019 pandemic on early childhood development: Short- and long-term risks and mitigating program and policy actions. *The Journal of Pediatrics, 223*, 188–193. https://doi.org/10.1016/j.jpeds.2020.05.020 (accessed on 11th June 2025).

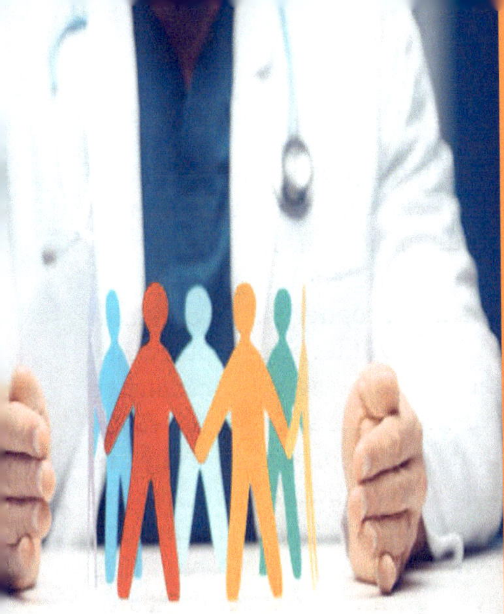

Chapter 7

COMMUNITY-BASED HEALTHCARE SYSTEMS

Contents

Introduction

Community-based health systems have emerged as major models for addressing health disparities and enhancing access to healthcare for populations. These systems are based on the belief that healthcare has to be offered in such a manner that is not only patient-focused but also embedded in the communities it serves. By applying the use of local resources and volunteers, community-based health programs create tailored services tailored to the native needs of diverse populations. Not only does this model strengthen the trust of health providers toward the community, but it also enables people to become active participants in their own health care. As observed through evidence based on history, such models can redefine healthcare paradigms significantly, emphasizing the role of non-governmental organizations (NGOs) and community health workers in improving health equity in underprivileged urban and rural communities (Riviere-Cinnamond et al., 2025). Interconnectedness of primary care and community health is necessary in order to ensure effective provision of healthcare. Primary care is the first contact with the healthcare system, offering prevention, diagnosis, and treatment services. Primary care is necessary in community health because it offers early intervention and continuity of care, hence averting complications brought about by undiagnosed disease. Moreover, primary care, when it is incorporated into community-based systems, adequately bridges the gaps in health care services by providing greater access. Integration results in a broader vision of health that incorporates social determinants, thus bridging the gap most felt by vulnerable populations. Removing transport, cost, and health literacy barriers is essential to achieving comprehensive community health plans (Lethbridge et al., 2011). In addition to primary care functions, NGOs play a very important role in health promotion activities of community-based programs. They are likely to fill gaps within government systems, particularly in underserved areas, by introducing innovative health programs and education programs. They mobilize community members through outreach and participation, empowering them to manage their own health. Furthermore, NGOs usually collaborate with local health authorities to try to achieve community-specific health indicators to ensure healthier and more sustainable health results. Overall, the contribution of non-profit organizations to healthcare not only enhances the service delivery but also supports broader public health goals of increasing access and equity in healthcare services throughout the population (Riviere-Cinnamond et al., 2025) (Figure 7.1).

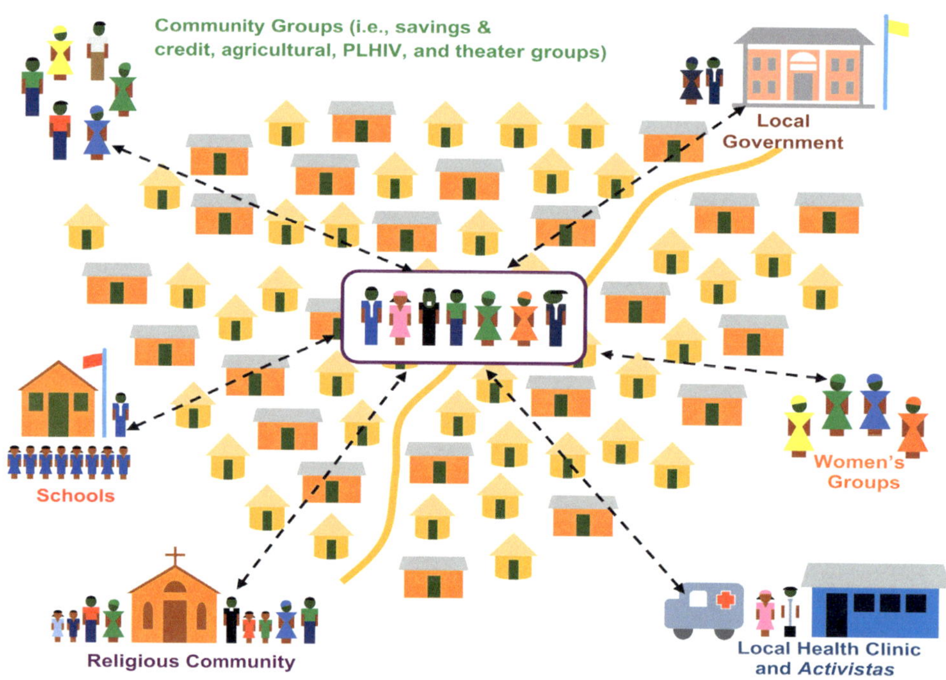

Figure 7.1. The community health system strengthening model.

https://www.researchgate.net/profile/Moriah-Ellen-2/publication/322960938/figure/fig1/AS:614036299341827@1523409070027/The-Community-Health-System-Strengthening-model-brings-together-people-from-existing.png.

Definition of Community-Based Healthcare Systems

An understanding of community-based healthcare systems can be defined as a strategy that emphasizes the delivery of health services at the community level and consolidating multiple services to promote access and general public health. The localized nature of these systems allows for provision with a chance for customizing care interventions according to local preferences and necessities. Engagement of community members in designing and delivering such health care services ensures a sense of responsibility and ownership, ultimately enhancing the effectiveness and sustainability of health promotion programs. By linking both public health services and clinical care within a community context, such systems aim to treat not only the more proximal issues of immediate health but also the social determinants of health that influence well-being. Toward this end, community-based healthcare systems are an apt model for enhancing healthcare provision, particularly in underprivileged regions where conventional healthcare infrastructures may not exist. Primary care as part of community-based healthcare systems is also a significant consideration. The primary care system is the entry point for people into healthcare services, providing comprehensive care that incorporates prevention, chronic disease management, and health education. It facilitates the scope of care continuity and long-term patient and health care provider relationships that are essential to good health management. Primary care physicians in most community-based systems collaborate with local agencies like NGOs and non-profits to extend their scope and develop service delivery. Such collaborations might involve scope consolidation, sharing, and outreach into community-based health programs with an integrated delivery of health. Integration of primary care in community settings not only improves health outcomes but also minimizes barriers to access, making the care more equitable and culturally responsive to populations with different backgrounds. Further, the role of non-profits and NGOs in systems of community-based healthcare is central to promoting health equity and addressing barriers to access. They tend to serve as a major impeller of resource mobilization, mobilizing the community and initiating focused interventions in healthcare directed at specific populations' requirements. One such NGO is Curamericas Global, Inc., whose objective is better maternal and neonatal healthcare through the formation of autonomous, community-led clinics in regions with inadequate healthcare facilities (Marley et al., 2015). By establishing local capacity and alliances with community stakeholders, these agencies contribute to the development of an interactive culture of healthcare that allows residents to actively participate in their own well-being. Additionally, where government resources may not be available, the contribution of NGOs can be instrumental in making healthcare systems efficient by identifying and leveraging points of improvement, ultimately resulting in an equitable healthcare system that serves multiple communities effectively (Riviere-Cinnamond et al., 2025).

Importance of Community Health in Overall Public Health

Community health forms a vital underpinning of general public health that links personal well-being with the dynamics of a community. By identifying the interdependence between them, communities can intervene to effectively address health disparities. Community health initiatives, for instance, are more likely to be collective approaches encouraging involvement by local residents in formulating health plans tailored to their specific needs. Such a participatory design not only empowers people but also increases the trust of public health systems, and this is more likely to lead to successful health results. The necessity to resolve community health is supported by the fact that effective interventions have proven to lead to precipitous reductions in communicable diseases, improved maternal and child health, and increased quality of life. Thus, the emphasis on community health is central to the attainment of universal health coverage and the provision of the benefits of advances in medicine to all members of a particular society. Access to medical care is among the key determinants of community health because access de facto determines whether individuals are able to gain necessary medical care. Furthermore, systematic barriers are prone to exclude marginalized populations from equal health care, worsening already existing inequalities in health. Community-based healthcare systems are crucial in overcoming these barriers by providing affordable and accessible services that are specifically designed to address the community's unique needs. These systems tend to combine primary care, preventive care, and health education, all of which serve to improve overall health within the community. Furthermore, the participation of non-profits and NGOs can be revolutionary in these initiatives, as they tend to bring valuable resources and support to resolve social determinants of health. By emphasizing expanding health care access, community health programs have the potential to make a tremendous difference in the general health situation of the population, allowing all people to thrive. Non-profit and NGO contributions to health promotion are priceless, particularly in low-resource settings. These types of organizations, in most instances, perform an essential bridging function between communities and health service providers, facilitating and allowing for the distribution of resources. They have an important role in designing health programs that are culturally relevant and that the local populace would find attractive, which is important for engendering community involvement. In addition, as with philanthropy in rapidly emerging economies like those in South East Asia, effective policy is required in order to maintain and promote philanthropic donations focused on serious social issues (Anand, 2014). Despite the challenges philanthropy has faced in such sectors, there is a good prospect for innovative collaborations between the non-profits and the local health system. Such collaborations have the capacity to enhance the community health interventions, thereby enhancing overall public health in general and ensuring that vulnerable populations receive the health care and assistance they need (Lavigne et al., 2013) (Figure 7.2).

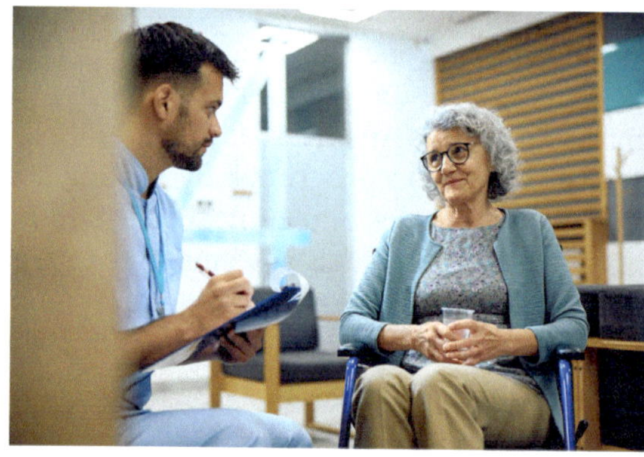

Figure 7.2. A healthcare professional consulting with an elderly patient as part of community health services.

Source: https://publichealth.tulane.edu/wp-content/uploads/sites/3/2020/05/why-community-health-is-important-for-public-health.jpg.

7.1. Types of Healthcare Systems

The diversity of healthcare systems worldwide reflects a range of sociocultural, economic, and political contexts, leading to the creation of various models. At a broad level, there are three general types of healthcare systems: the Beveridge Model, the Bismarck Model, and the National Health Insurance Model. The Beveridge Model, utilized by countries like the United Kingdom, is characterized by the provision and financing of healthcare by the government from tax revenue so that healthcare services are cost-free at the point of use. In contrast, the Bismarck Model, being used in countries like Germany and France implements an employer and employee contribution system, with a dual role of providing insurance, as well as fostering a competitive market among healthcare providers. These aspects bear a significant impact on community health indicators and primary care functions in terms of ensuring the maximum utilization of services, particularly among vulnerable populations. Community-based health systems have gained much popularity in the last few years as a strong tool in fighting health inequities, particularly in marginalized urban and rural communities. The systems concentrate on the integration of professional medical care with local resources to provide culturally sensitive care that resonates with diverse populations. They often introduce non-profits and NGOs to coordinate health education and outreach, which are essential in building trust within the community. These partnerships could facilitate the coexistence of both traditional and modern practices of healthcare, enhancing care accessibility. As noted in some research highlighting intercultural health practices, these community-based models not only increase access to allopathic care but also respect indigenous knowledge and health traditions, thus resulting in better health outcomes (Mignone et al., 2025). Health care services are usually hindered by numerous barriers, including economic, geographic, and cultural barriers. Rural populations, in most instances are heavily constrained by the unavailability of healthcare facilities and professionals, hence the call for innovative interventions. Health care models that are community-based have succeeded in addressing such constraints by providing authority to local health providers and employing mobile health centers to expand coverage. The application of feedback loops also guarantees that services provided are tailored to accommodate the specific needs of communities. Besides, the non-profits and NGOs also have an essential role to play in such settings, since they help pressure policy reform that is capable of promoting better resource allocation and funds for public health initiatives. This bottom-up healthcare model, besides guaranteeing equity and access, also ensures that policies become more responsive to local realities (Riviere-Cinnamond et al., 2025) (Figure 7.3).

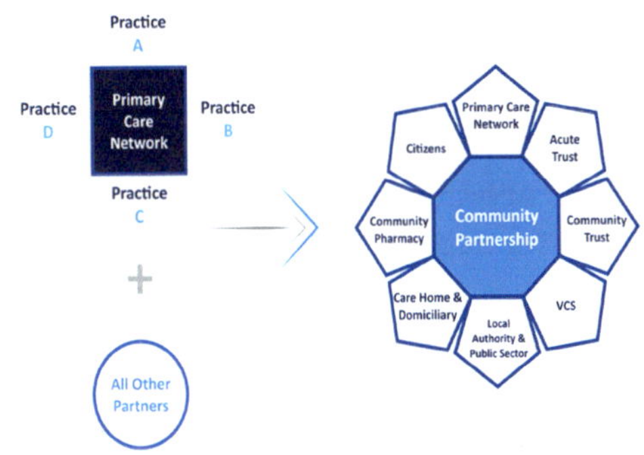

Figure 7.3. The different types of healthcare providers.

Source: https://media.licdn.com/dms/image/v2/D4E12AQHx707awjJWaQ/article-cover_image-shrink_720_1280/article-cover_image-shrink_720_1280/0/1689157357737?e=2147483647&v=beta&t=tWGv0O2-EqS7HpMOstRzzlN19PxZbuWOXK5fdQv9sgM.

7.1.1. Public Healthcare Systems

Public healthcare systems are fundamental to the facilitation of community health since they provide key services and allow care provision to the heterogenous population. Public healthcare systems tend to enhance accessibility and equity, so that individuals regardless of socioeconomic status receive medical care when they need it. The public healthcare model tends to be under government control, allowing for centralized financing and management of resources. This system can be applied to facilitate wide-scale health initiatives, immunization drives, and the establishment of primary health care networks. Community healthcare schemes are also a significant part of this system since they are more sensitive to local health requirements. With the utilization of community resources and collaboration with local stakeholders, public health systems can enhance the quality and efficiency of health care and a participatory system where patients are equal partners in their care. Despite the strengths of public health systems, there are many barriers which have the tendency to restrict access to essential services, particularly among marginalized populations. Insufficient finance, compromised healthcare infrastructure, and lack of human resources are some of the key obstacles to the performance of these systems. Moreover, social determinants of health such as poverty and education have the tendency to exacerbate health inequities. Evidence from a number of research studies shows that these barriers have differential effects on marginalized groups and consequently, on health outcomes (Owadara et al., 2025). For instance, involvement strategies in mental health care have been found to be successively mixed depending on whether public or private school settings are involved, offering evidence of differentials in the accessibility of treatment. Addressing these barriers will require addressing them on many fronts by uniting government agencies, health providers, and non-profit health-promotion agencies. Non-governmental organizations (NGOs) also help fund the public healthcare systems by complementing service gaps and advocating for policy changes in healthcare. NGOs are on the ground, with targeted interventions and outreach programs that target specific health conditions in the community. They are also flexible and have the ability to innovate, making them able to implement methods that are less feasible within bureaucratic public systems. Secondly, NGOs can spearhead the mobilization of resources, facilitate partnerships, and generate public health awareness of health issues, particularly in the event of stretched government budgets (Riviere-Cinnamond et al., 2025). Through connecting their activities to public health objectives, the organizations are able to achieve maximum effectiveness for the healthcare systems operating within the community while ensuring health equity in health services. Hence, there is a need for a collective response from all the stakeholders to drive the public healthcare agenda and improve health outcomes at the community level.

7.1.2. Private Healthcare Systems

In comprehending the intricate world of healthcare systems, private healthcare systems appear as individual entities that operate in tandem with public systems to provide medical care. Such systems tend to be profit-driven, separating them from the public systems that focus on welfare and community health. Private care generally offers more immediate access to care and greater options of specialized care, catering to those who have the means to pay from their pockets or through insurance policies. However, utilization of private systems raises concerns of access and equity, particularly among poorer segments of society. For the majority of cases, individuals are locked out, with enormous economic impediments to obtaining necessary health care, emphasizing the need for a comprehensive examination of how private systems operate as an integral part of overall health needs within the community (Bonica et al., 2017). Furthermore, the role of primary care within private health systems is significant but complex since it serves as the point of interaction with patients and the coordination of health resources. Primary care providers in private systems often must deal not only with medical disease, but also with extremely complicated insurance arrangements that might impact the patients experience and access to care. This scenario encourages disparities, whereby quality primary care is usually more accessible to those who have good insurance cover. Thus, individuals without such financial resources may be subjected to delays in getting preventative medicine or disease control for chronic conditions. Through this, the potential of primary care to transform and improve population health is thwarted, something that emphasizes a critical necessity for policy actions that can ensure inclusivity in healthcare delivery (Segura et al., 2020). Lastly, collaboration between private healthcare systems and non-profits or NGOs is also key to enhancing health and filling in service gaps. Non-profits usually step in and fill gaps by providing essential services to vulnerable populations where profit-based health systems cannot penetrate. By integrating community-focused programs with the private healthcare system, such companies can potentially encourage health literacy, provide preventive testing, and help manage chronic diseases in a way that would otherwise be unfeasible. This synergistic partnership is illustrative of the importance of intersectoral collaboration in enhancing health equity. An understanding of the limitations of private healthcare systems enables a well-informed debate concerning policy reform and community action initiatives that enable a better health for all individuals regardless of their socio-economic status (Bonica et al., 2017) (Figure 7.4).

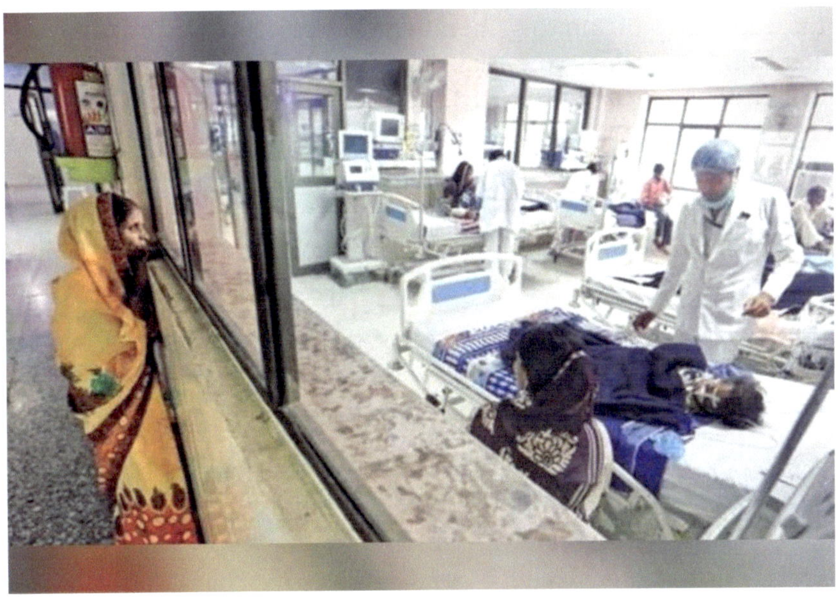

Figure 7.4. Private healthcare industry.

https://akm-img-a-in.tosshub.com/businesstoday/images/story/202007/hospital_660_140720073129.jpg.

7.1.3. Hybrid Healthcare Systems

In studying hybrid healthcare systems in relation to models of community-based healthcare, it is essential to comprehend their unique structures and working dynamics. Hybrid healthcare systems merge elements of the public and private healthcare systems with the goal of maximizing resources and broadening access to services. The model utilizes the strengths of the two sectors in yielding a wide range of services as well as a degree of financial adaptability. As the need for healthcare increases, particularly in underserved communities, hybrid systems answer visionary calls to address gaps in access and maximize comprehensive care delivery. Addressing the twin demands of function and reach, these systems focus on the integration of primary care services responsive to community needs and, therefore, building a stronger healthcare infrastructure as a whole. The main care in hybrid healthcare models is critical in enhancing community health outcomes. Primary care is a building block that not only addresses patient issues individually but also focuses on prevention and education. Primary care, working in a hybrid system, is able to coordinate referrals well, manage chronic conditions, and facilitate end-to-end care pathways. This integrated strategy enables healthcare workers to tackle social determinants of health, which are central to promoting general health equity. As indicated, strengthening democratic governance is directly able to influence healthcare access and effectiveness (N/A, 2022), and this reflects how hybrid systems can be useful in fostering sustainable health management strategies. Primary care integration in these systems, therefore, becomes central to closing gaps and maximizing health resources for community groups. However, despite their ensured advantages, hybrid healthcare systems are bound to experience numerous problems that can deter efficient functioning and implementation. Universal care for health services remains an ongoing difficulty, with socio-economic status, geographical location, and the supply of healthcare resources dominating the picture. Such challenges have the capability of limiting members of society from utilizing public and private healthcare provision to their optimal potential. Additionally, involvement by NGOs and non-profits plays a critical role in health promotion, such as the role of detecting gaps in service delivery through the provision of niche interventions and support. Their interventions can complement the hybrid healthcare model, for example, as seen from sustainable business models that address economic, environmental, and social factors (Shekarian et al., 2022). By addressing these problems in a collaborative way, hybrid health systems can work towards higher health accessibility and equity among the populations they serve (Figure 7.5).

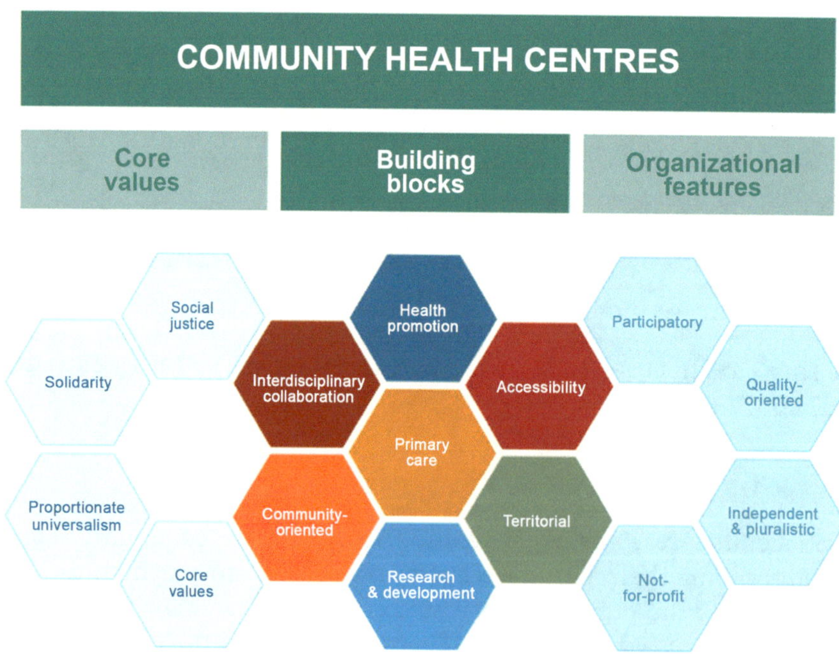

Figure 7.5. Context of community-based healthcare frameworks.

Source: https://transform-integratedcommunitycare.com/wp-content/uploads/2021/12/3.png.

7.2. Role of Primary Care in Community Health

The community health system's primary care role plays a key part in being the first point of contact for individuals receiving health care. Primary care practitioners are not only clinicians but also health educators whose practice operates on preventative therapy and long-term illness management. This progressive thinking guarantees a close liaison between health practitioners and the population, whereby interventions can be tailor-made to suit the individual demands of an area. Through constant interaction, primary care providers are able to identify and treat health disparities, ensuring equal treatment to vulnerable populations. Access, affordability, and continuity of care are central aspects of the model, performing a pivotal function in enhancing community health outcomes overall. By targeting these aspects, primary care is able to close gaps within wider healthcare systems and build up a culture of health awareness and self-management among members of the community.

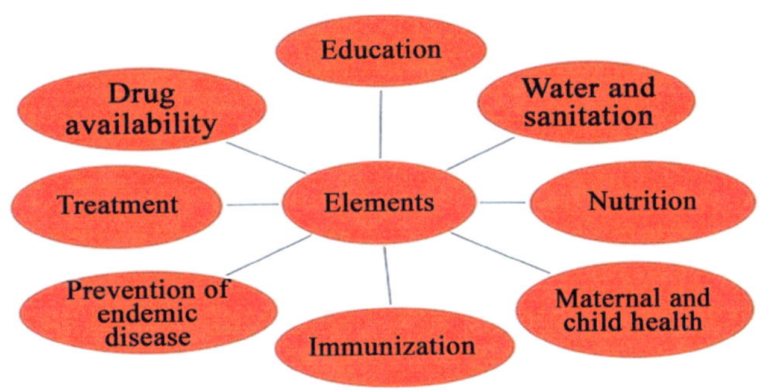

Figure 7.6. Elements of primary-health-care.

Source: https://nursingexercise.com/wp-content/uploads/2016/06/Primary-health-care-elements.jpg.

Community-based health systems also rely on coordination between the primary care providers and other actors such as non-profits and NGOs, which have important roles in sponsoring health activities. They broaden the scope of primary care by initiating programs that deal with specific areas of health issues, e.g., maternal and child health or control of chronic diseases. For example, the Lancet series on newborn survival highlights the crisis of high infant mortality in India, wherein 75% of deaths among infants are avoidable through better access to services and education (N/A, 2014). With their community position, non-profits and NGOs have the ability to apply training and resources to effect and thereby empower primary healthcare providers and improve service delivery. Such a collaborative organization enhances not only the strength of primary care but also community ownership of outcomes. Moreover, the incorporation of community health workers is an important approach to enhancing primary care in community-based healthcare systems. These workers act as bridges between members of the community and health providers, bridging gaps in accessing healthcare and ensuring that services are culturally adapted and respond to local needs. Evidence suggests that integrating community health workers (CHWs) in health delivery systems is better for improving equity and access, especially in marginalized groups. By having a good knowledge of local culture and beliefs about health, CHWs enhance participation and facilitate the utilization of primary care services (Riviere-Cinnamond et al., 2025). Their role is particularly vital in managing complex health issues, such as the relationship between animal and human health systems, which eventually leads to holistic health interventions. By such integration, primary care is made more holistic and effective, aligned with overall community health objectives, as well as generating an environment that is favorable to promoting health (Figure 7.6).

7.2.1. Definition and Importance of Primary Care

The delivery of primary care is a central component of community-based healthcare systems and serves as the first point of contact with health services that individuals access. Described as an integral, accessible form of care with a focus on long-term patient-practitioner relationships, primary care extends from mere treatment of acute illness and injury to the development of broad health and wellness. It is a key driver of chronic disease management, specialty service coordination, and prevention, all of which lead to healthier populations. Under patient-centered care, primary care clinicians establish patients' trust and motivate them to be self-accountable for their health, thereby improving health outcomes and quality of life. The relationship established by primary care also serves to reduce emergency room utilization and hospitalization, thus alleviating pressure on the health systems and enhancing the allocation of resources, which is essential in community-based environments where individualized attention is essential. Primary care plays not only a crucial role in individual health but also serves as a building block for public health initiatives. By working on social determinants of health and promoting equity, primary care can eliminate gaps in access to healthcare services disproportionately affecting marginalized groups. An effective primary care system can detect and solve race-, ethnicity-, and socioeconomic-status-related differences in health. Initiatives supported by such organizations as the Partnership for Healthy Outcomes have shown that it is achievable to enhance health access and outcomes using health provider-CBO partnerships, particularly among underserved populations (Miller et al., 2017). By integrating social services into primary care, these partnerships facilitate holistic solutions to health promotion and, subsequently, build community resilience as well as offering individualized care that responds to local needs. Furthermore, primary care is a pivotal element in the development of healthcare policy, which favors accessible and equitable services. The ongoing need to address racial and ethnic disparities emphasizes the requirement of bringing quality measures and strategic interventions into primary care facilities. Through the establishment of committees to collect data and evaluate health outcomes, healthcare systems can encourage targeted responses that provide for inclusivity (Alexander et al., 2009). This preventive approach not only enhances the quality of care but also encourages a setting in which patients are respected and heard. As community health systems further evolve, the role of primary care will remain supreme, driving initiatives that promote wellness and propel health equity across populations. By investing in primary care infrastructure, communities can establish robust health systems that can adequately deal with the many challenges of public health.

7.2.2. Impact of Primary Care on Health Outcomes

The role of primary care in bringing better health outcomes cannot be overstated, as it is the core of community-based healthcare systems. Not only does primary care facilitate easy access to basic health services, but it also provides continuity of care and coordination of various components of healthcare. This model ensures individuals get comprehensive and preventive treatment, which is of paramount significance in terms of early development and management of health problems. Through establishing a strong patient-provider relationship, primary care providers are better positioned to view their patients' individual health needs and thereby deliver more customized care. Moreover, as explained in Lethbridge et al. (2011), the realignment of health systems towards increased market orientation emphasizes the importance of having in place strong primary care services to balance accessibility and quality to improve overall health outcomes for diverse populations. In addition, primary care has far-reaching effects on not only individual health but also the community as a whole. Through emphases on public health education and prevention, primary care providers become agents for community action and empowerment. This proactive focus assists in tackling social determinants of health as well as easing impediments to healthcare access among marginalized groups. Integrated primary care programs that invest in ownership and community engagement are likely to cause significant improvements in health outcomes, thereby showcasing how integrated primary care can lead to healthier communities. This is once again reiterated by the pressing health concerns of nations like India, where highly focused intervention in newborn care demonstrates the significance of community engagement and effective service provision, as shown in N/A (2014). The emphasis on community engagement in primary care models not only contributes to better health outcomes but also to a more just health care system. The success of primary care as a force for enhanced health outcomes is often supported by working relationships among non-profits and NGOs. These organizations play a pivotal role in bridging gaps in primary care services, particularly in disadvantaged communities, by infusing resources and the expertise of specialists into healthcare delivery. By leveraging community resources and through partnership-building, non-profits can deliver creative health solutions that respond to specific population health needs. For instance, newborn care programs can have dramatic effects through community-based methods that encompass public awareness and training of health workers, as captured in N/A (2014). These partnerships specify the synergistic partnership between primary care and community agencies, together advancing the improvement of the health outcomes in tandem with combating the subtleties of health care access and equity across settings (Figure 7.7).

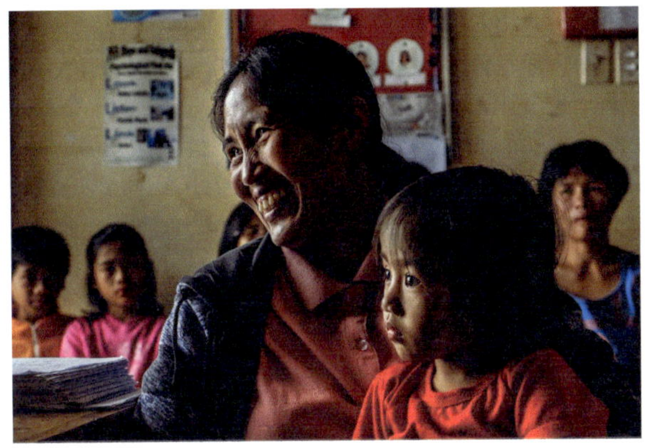

Figure 7.7. Impact of primary care on health outcomes.

Source: https://www.who.int/images/default-source/wpro/health-topic/primary-health-care/primary-health-care---ht.jpg?sfvrsn=8c78c416_4.

7.2.3. Integration of Primary Care with Community Resources

The integration of primary care and community resources is a key element in the creation of community-based healthcare systems. The integration enables a broader realization that health cannot be conceived within medicine alone, but that it must incorporate all the social determinants of health, which play a profound role in individual well-being. By filling the gap between healthcare providers and community resources, patients are provided with access to a wider array of support systems, such as mental health services, nutrition programs, and social services. This integrated model not only increases patient outcomes but also creates a sense of community, which provides resiliency against disparities in health. For instance, the combination of customary health practice and allopathic medicine may fulfill the particular cultural needs of diverse populations as requested in various intercultural health experiences detailed in Mignone et al. (2025). Additionally, NGOs and non-profits are key in facilitating the integration of primary care and community resources. They act as vital middlemen, typically deciding on local healthcare requirements and mobilizing resources accordingly. Such organizations usually provide critical services that complement primary care, such as preventive health education, outreach, and chronic disease management programs. By leveraging the networks available in communities, NGOs can extend access to healthcare from clinic walls to reach social barriers that an individual might have. As outlined in the literature, successful community-based initiatives are typically created through cooperative efforts that draw on the strengths of both formal and informal health systems, citing the necessity for meeting explicit community health requirements through innovative models and cooperative frameworks, as in Riviere-Cinnamond et al. (2025). Further, the sustainability of community-based health systems nearly entirely depends on solid partnerships between primary care providers and community assets. Effective integration not only improves service delivery but also fosters a culture of mutual accountability among stakeholders. Social service agencies, community leaders, and health providers need to work together to construct integrated care plans that address patients' different circumstances. For instance, food-insecure patients might need nutritional assistance programs in addition to standard medical care. Through the creation of collaboration and coordination mechanisms, community health systems are better positioned to address people's integrated needs, eventually allowing them to become more self-directed in managing their health. This model not only maximizes the delivery of primary care but also builds up the entire network of the community, so it becomes an impenetrable system that is addressing short-term health needs as well as long-term health promotion interventions.

7.3. Access to Healthcare Services

Access to health services is the final determinant of community and individual health status. Despite dramatic advances in medical technology and health-care delivery systems, disparities still exist and are often most prevalent among vulnerable populations. Economic status, geography, and system-based disparities are some of the determinants of unequal access, resulting in colossal health disparities. For most cases, the members of marginalized groups encounter barriers that undermine their access to necessary healthcare services, such as transport, cost considerations, and lack of health insurance. Structural disparities, as exemplified by social determinants like education and income, significantly influence an individual's ability to access healthcare services, as a report states. Overcoming such challenges is imperative to moving towards greater health equity and to making every population capable of attaining the best possible health outcomes. The role played by primary care in enhancing access to healthcare services cannot be overemphasized. Primary care systems strive to deliver integrated, accessible, and community-based services that address a wide range of health requirements. By being the point of contact first, primary care doctors are at the center of disease prevention, management of chronic diseases, and overall promotion of health. An efficient primary care system can stem the demand for emergency care, promoting a healthier, more sustainable healthcare model. On top of that, community health initiatives based on preventive medicine, education, and management of health resources empower individuals and families in impoverished communities. This systemic approach is also concordant with health expert recommendations emphasizing investment in primary care as a way to achieve better health outcomes and better access to healthcare for all (Abubakar et al., 2022). Non-profit and NGO organizations are also essential in filling gaps in access to healthcare, especially in low-resource settings. These organizations often coordinate community resources, offer grant funding, and supply innovative solutions to health problems in vulnerable populations. Through outreach programs, education, and direct service delivery, non-profits often deliver essential services to those who might otherwise lack them. They have been proven effective at solving designated public health problems and advocating for policy changes that ensure health equity. Through collaboration with governments and communities, these organizations can expand the scale and influence of public health interventions to include marginalized groups in the health access and delivery debate. The sustained effort of NGOs and non-profits is thus key to shaping a comprehensive community-based model of healthcare (N/A, 2022) (Figure 7.8).

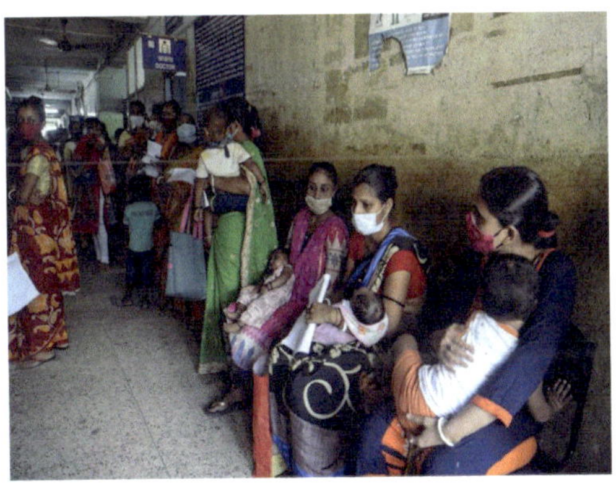

Figure 7.8. Access to healthcare.

Source: https://jansankalp.org/wp-content/uploads/2023/03/Access-to-healthcare-in-India-Issues-and-solutions-Jansankalp-Foundation.jpg.

7.3.1. Factors Influencing Access to Healthcare

Access to healthcare is heavily influenced by a group of social, economic, and geographic factors that create obstacles for marginalized populations. The most visible one may be socio-economic status, which dictates how much one can afford to pay for care, particularly where out-of-pocket expenses or transportation costs are the case. Individuals with lower incomes will, therefore, have healthcare as an afterthought to food and shelter, and thus treatment is postponed, and the condition gets worse. Moreover, geographical constraints are crucial; rural areas are usually lacking proper healthcare centers, compelling citizens to go miles and miles away to get even primary care. In such scenarios, healthcare systems like mobile health clinics provide innovative means of addressing this gap and raising access to healthcare among marginalized groups, leading to lowered reliance on emergency care and overall health equilibrium among such populations (Meghan et al., 2025). Cultural perceptions and health literacy are also determinants that directly affect the availability and access to care. Individuals' understanding of health threats and available services may determine their willingness to use care. As discussed in the context of background with respect to general health checks, individuals lacking knowledge or having inaccurate perceptions of healthcare systems may choose against necessary health services, which increases the rate of health inequalities. This behavior is most commonly observed among the immigrant group or ethnic minority group who may be distanced from the overall healthcare centers due to language disparities, other cultural beliefs, or previous negative experiences. It becomes the duty of healthcare professionals to formulate culturally sensitive care, acknowledging and accepting these different meanings for more involvement. Through addressing the information requirements and psychological resistance of heterogeneous communities, health organizations are able to enhance utilization of required services like preventive check-ups and disease screening, leading to increased health equity (Sommer et al., 2025). The roles played by non-profit organizations and NGOs in transcending healthcare access barriers cannot be overemphasized. Such organizations tend to plug important gaps by offering resources, education, and health promotion activities specifically suited to the needs of local populations. Mobile health clinics are an example of how non-profits use collaboration with local health systems to bring low-barrier services directly to where they are most needed, greatly expanding access for groups that have long been faced with barriers. Furthermore, NGOs are more likely to work towards increasing healthcare awareness and literacy in underprivileged groups, leading to an enlightened population that is better equipped to grasp the complexities of the health system. Most critically, they serve as important bridges between underprivileged communities and accessible health resources, thus playing a significant role in shaping health equity among populations (Meghan et al., 2025).

7.3.2. Geographic Disparities in Healthcare Access

Geographic health access variation generates significant challenges that have effects on population outcomes of health, particularly among rural and urban poor communities. Such variations typically result from the interaction among different factors, varying from economic limitations, infrastructure shortage, and cultural differences. For instance, the majority of rural populations suffer from shortages in healthcare facilities that result in inhabitants covering long distances to access even basic medical care. Not only does this increase the expense and duration of using health services, but it also adds to the existing health issues produced by the delay in intervention. As reported in some studies, effective community-based health systems can provide a solution to these disparities by gaining the trust of community leaders and breaking geographic and economic barriers to health delivery (McLaughlin et al., 2018). Besides, primary care's role increases in minimizing geographic disparities in health access. Primary care facilities can act as a point of first contact, enabling better management of one's health and early detection. In cases where specialist health facilities are limited in a given area, primary care workers can offer generic services that can minimize the impact of geographic remoteness. They form long-term friendships with patients, which is vital in remote communities where patient confidence in health systems may not be high. It is particularly important for older individuals or individuals with chronic conditions because their continued access to primary care can make a major difference to health outcomes. To effectively remedy these inequalities, community healthcare systems must place a priority on primary care as an initial foundation, employing outreach and engagement processes to serve hard-to-reach populations (Arens et al., 2023). Non-profit and NGO agencies play a vital role in the provision of equity in healthcare services access among marginalized populations. These agencies are likely to provide targeted interventions addressing particular geographic difficulties of specific populations. By partnering with members of the community, non-profits can modify their programs to meet the practical and cultural needs of the areas in which they are working. Examples include mobile clinics extending out into remote areas or partnerships with local leaders to assist with informing on available health care. Community-based health organizations have been described as successful in reducing geospatial disparities, demonstrated through their ability to engender trust and membership among underserved communities, thereby promoting equal access to healthcare (McLaughlin et al., 2018). Therefore, collaboration between government health systems and not-for-profit organizations is paramount to a broader approach to improving access to healthcare for everyone, especially in geographically remote communities (Figure 7.9).

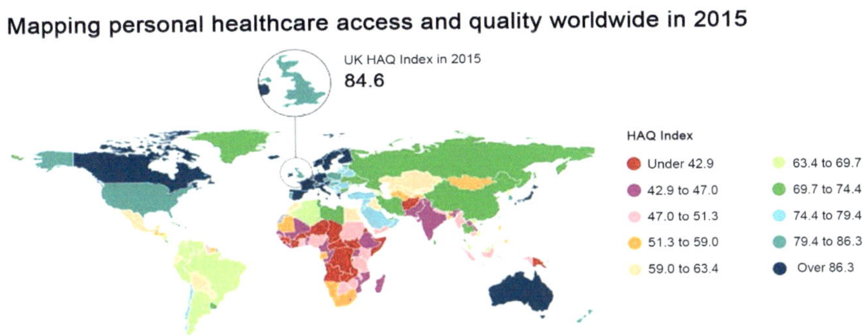

Figure 7.9. Geographic disparities in healthcare access.

Source: https://external-content.duckduckgo.com/iu/?u=https%3A%2F%2Fwww.lshtm.ac.uk%2Fsites%2Fdefault%2Ffiles%2FHealthcare%2520access %2520infographic%25202%2C%2520Lancet% 2520%26%2520IHME.JPG&f= 1&nofb=1&ipt= ce430 bfdd0fa8b45 fdb33e56d76a62a561 db89aeb7f239c25e6647f6f655674d.

7.3.3. Socioeconomic Factors Affecting Healthcare Access

Availability of healthcare services is significantly influenced by a variety of socioeconomic determinants that significantly influence individual and community health status. Furthermore, disparities in income, education, and occupation produce inequities that affect the accessibility of healthcare. Lower socioeconomic status individuals are more likely to face barriers such as not having insurance coverage, higher out-of-pocket costs, and limited access to transportation. Additionally, residents in underserved communities frequently encounter systemic barriers to care, including restricted availability of primary care and healthcare systems that lack the ability to serve the population (Bambra et al., 2018). Consequently, equity in health becomes a critical priority, requiring comprehensive approaches that address the social determinants of health and bridge the gap between socioeconomic status and healthcare access. Furthermore, the policy's role in stemming these disparities cannot be overstated. Effective public health policy must account for the socioeconomic determinants of health. For instance, initiatives that enhance education and economic security can enhance health literacy, which in turn means enhanced usage of healthcare services. Initiatives that familiarize people with seeking care among impoverished groups can also facilitate increased access to health services. These initiatives are supplemented by research that highlights the interdependence of socioeconomic status and health disparities, emphasizing the need for integrated interventions in order to achieve long-term health improvements among marginalized groups (Owadara et al., 2025). Non-governmental organizations and non-profit agencies often play a pivotal role in expanding access to healthcare in low-income populations where government assistance may be limited. By providing education, advocacy, and services specific to particular community health needs, these groups serve as valuable resources. Some are focused on reducing barriers to care by offering programs that provide transportation, financial assistance, or counseling, which can significantly improve access to care. These interagency partnerships can provide a foundation for an integrated model of health promotion and avoid leaving behind vulnerable populations. As observed with interventions in various settings, from schools, the constructive engagement of civil society can assist in attaining enhanced health promotion outcomes, ultimately reducing socioeconomic disparities in healthcare access (Bambra et al., 2018).

7.4. Barriers to Healthcare Services

Availability of health services is most often hindered by a plethora of barriers that most disproportionately affect marginalized groups. Socioeconomic issues, including low wages, limited education, and unemployment, are all significant roadblocks, creating a cycle of deprivation that restricts access to medical care. Members of such populations may struggle to find transportation to sites of care or may be geographically isolated in rural areas where there are shortages of healthcare workers. Moreover, cultural barriers like language and the unavailability of culturally competent care can exacerbate these issues and contribute to mistrust in the healthcare system. The outcome of such barriers is the resulting health disparities, which necessitate exploration into inclusive community-based health systems that are sensitive to the particular challenges presented by these groups. Yet another vital element of the obstacles to health care access is the inefficiencies in health care delivery systems. Bureaucratic obstacles and redundant services too frequently lead to delayed care, where patients spend extended periods of time waiting for appointments and treatments. Such delays most disproportionately affect vulnerable populations who can have their chronic conditions aggravated by the denial of access to punctual medical care. Furthermore, the fragmentation among disparate healthcare services—e.g., primary care, specialty care, and preventive care—is yet another obstacle that dissuades individuals from accessing care that they require. Having community-based healthcare systems can mitigate these inefficiencies by simplifying things, enhancing communication among providers, and providing a better-rounded emphasis on patient care that addresses physical, mental, and social health. Second, the potential role of NGOs and non-profits in bridging the gap between access to healthcare is vast.

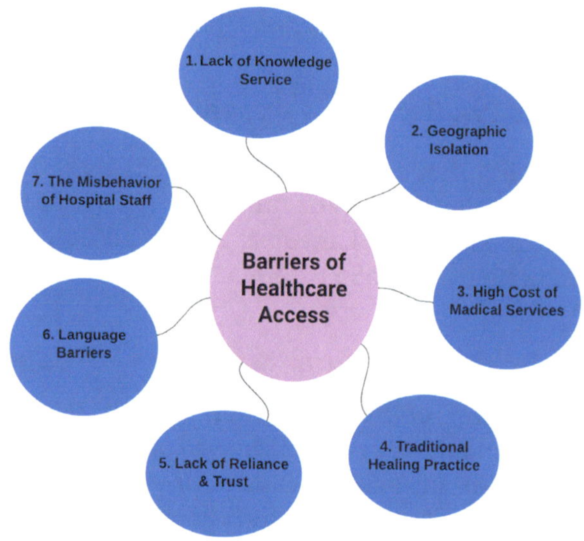
1. Lack of Knowledge Service
2. Geographic Isolation
3. High Cost of Madical Services
4. Traditional Healing Practice
5. Lack of Reliance & Trust
6. Language Barriers
7. The Misbehavior of Hospital Staff
Barriers of Healthcare Access

Figure 7.10. Barriers to healthcare services.

Source: https://www.researchgate.net/publication/373130775/figure/fig1/AS:11431281181614824@1692106994470/Barriers-to-healthcare-access.png.

These organizations are likely to be in the field, delivering grassroots services tailored to the population's needs and fostering trust and collaboration among community residents. By creating innovative health promotion interventions, they can help minimize most barriers, including financial capacity, educational deficits, and lack of awareness about available services. Most notably, instances of successful intercultural health practice demonstrate that integrating traditional and allopathic medicine can potentially expand access for indigenous and other culturally defined populations (Mignone et al., 2025). As demonstrated in a series of community-based health projects, the engagement with local knowledge and social networks maximizes the effectiveness of health interventions (Riviere-Cinnamond et al., 2025). Thus, promoting collaboration between public health institutions, NGOs, and target populations is very promising for dismantling barriers to healthcare (Figure 7.10).

7.4.1. Financial Barriers and Insurance Coverage

Financial constraints and insurance coverage are major barriers to the availability of healthcare services, especially in community-based healthcare systems. Most people, especially those of lower income, find it difficult to pay for routine care and emergency medical visits. The cost of health care out-of-pocket tends to generate financial pressure that makes families have to either sacrifice some medical care or some of their basic needs. This is exacerbated for the uninsured populations that rely on expensive interventions during times of health crises. Literature highlights that health risks pose an extreme threat to poor households' health and livelihoods; in situations of health shocks, the burden of cost rises further, even thrusting them into more poverty. Consequently, the lack of adequate insurance coverage and financial capacity strongly limits access to required healthcare services, illustrating an important barrier in the community-based healthcare system. Community-based health insurance (CBHI) schemes have been created as a credible solution to such financial barriers that seek to enhance the accessibility of healthcare to the vulnerable. Such initiatives aim to provide a safety net by pooling funds sourced from members of a community, thereby reducing the high cost associated with health care. CBHIs are typically characterized by their social administration, affordability, and emphasis on social solidarity—a central characteristic in economically downtrodden populations. Though less than 10 percent of developing countries' informal sector inhabitants enjoy health coverage through CBHIs, the sheer expansion of these schemes indicates their potential to break through systematic obstacles (Mignone et al., 2025). By recovering part of the health service costs, CBHIs can effectively limit out-of-pocket expenditures among members and facilitate ease in accessing health service provisions, thereby decreasing the burden on poor households. Nonetheless, the success of CBHIs is often hindered by several structural factors, such as poor management and minimal government support. The majority of schemes are plagued by resource mobilization problems, poor quality health services, and governance failures that undermine their sustainability. For example, while numerous community-based programs have been found to be crucial to bridging the gap between traditional and allopathic healthcare systems, often joined through intercultural health practices, they are plagued by funding issues that make them unsustainable (Mignone et al., 2025). The convergence of these financial barriers and insurance shortages exacerbates health inequalities, rendering innovative interventions and favorable policies critical in strengthening both community health programs and the overall healthcare system. Thus, overcoming these barriers is crucial in enhancing equitable access to healthcare in health facilities characterized by community predominance.

7.4.2. Cultural and Language Barriers

Cultural and language barriers significantly hinder communication and access to health care in community-based health systems. The barriers are likely to be caused by the misunderstanding between patients and health practitioners, leading to misdiagnosis, inappropriate treatment, and decreased patient satisfaction. Culturally competent care concerning local customs and beliefs about health is vital to indigenous communities and ethnic minorities. The Inter-American Development Bank highlights the importance of reconciling allopathic medical practices with the local health systems of the populations, demonstrating the potential inclusive approaches have to enhance access to healthcare. Incorporating traditional practice and respect for cultural context allows healthcare workers to better serve the communities, significantly enhancing health outcomes and community engagement (Mignone et al., 2025). Language barriers exacerbate the issues encountered in healthcare provision, especially in multicultural communities where there are several languages and dialects. Non-English speakers are usually unable to receive vital information regarding health services, and thus become more frustrated and less involved in their care. Language barriers have been countered by community-based health organizations by hiring bilingual personnel and using translation services to aid providers and patients in communicating. In rural and underserved populations, these organizations have proven that trust building among community leaders and the breaking of barriers—geographical, economic, cultural, and behavioral—can dramatically improve access to healthcare and healthcare outcomes. By tailoring interventions to the unique linguistic and cultural settings within which they are implemented, these organizations are the model response to how health equity can be promoted (McLaughlin et al., 2018). The role of non-profits and NGOs becomes particularly important in breaking down cultural and language barriers to healthcare. Non-profits can serve as critical go-betweens for healthcare systems and communities with whom they are contracted to provide service, bridging gaps with culturally appropriate care strategies. For instance, non-profits can set up community health worker programs, whereby locals are trained to enter the healthcare system and represent their populations well. By using credible community members who speak the local language and have knowledge of cultural nuances, health programs can be more effectively tailored to serve specific needs. Not only does this localized intervention facilitate more effective patient-provider relationships, but it also enables communities to take on more responsibility for their own health, ultimately contributing to the establishment of robust community-based health systems that can overcome these challenges (McLaughlin et al., 2018) (Figure 7.11).

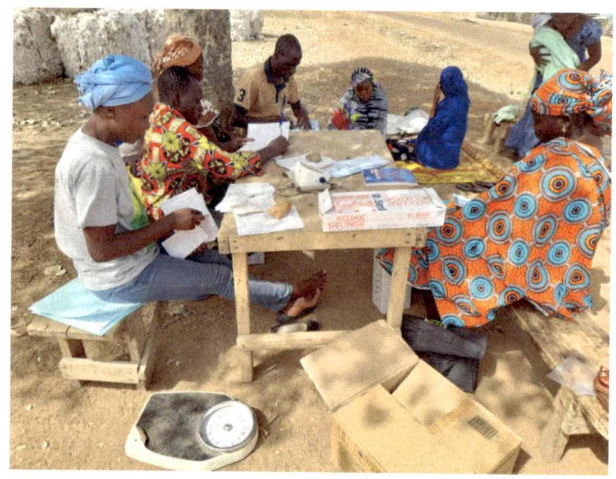

Figure 7.11. Access to healthcare services within community-based healthcare systems.

Source: https://upload.wikimedia.org/wikipedia/commons/8/88/Consultation_des_femmes_et_des_b%C3%A9b%C3%A9s.jpg.

7.4.3. Transportation and Logistical Challenges

In community-based healthcare systems, transport and logistics inefficiencies actually limit access to necessary health care. Well-established transport systems are essential in an effort to reach out to groups that are vulnerable, especially rural communities where access to health facilities might be far away. If transport systems are weak or non-existent, patients are postponed or fail to receive medical treatment altogether, further complicating health problems. The application of Community Health Worker (CHW) programs has been identified as one possible solution for these issues. Through leveraging local knowledge and trust, CHWs can serve as a bridge between the health care system and the community by educating and brokering access to care (Woldemariam et al., 2015). However, for such interventions to succeed, there has to be support in transport and supplies, which illustrates how transport infrastructure and successful community health programs have a co-dependent reliance. Furthermore, urban and rural settings have different transportation and logistical challenges that impact access to healthcare. In urban centers, traffic jams and poor public transportation may discourage citizens from accessing prompt care, whereas in rural environments, the environment tends to be deficient in road quality and connectivity. Studies have shown that empowerment efforts in urban cities, such as vocational training programs, have managed to incorporate community outreach approaches to overcome such challenges, whereas similar success on a large scale has not been recorded in rural environments (Learwellie et al., 2024). This disparity highlights a need for solutions tailored to the geographical limitations of each setting. Effective transportation and logistics must become a health policy priority in order to optimize program implementation, enabling both city and country dwellers to obtain necessary healthcare services without undue hindrance. In addition to route optimization to move, the engagement of non-profit organizations (NGOs) in the solution to logistical issues is necessary to facilitate programs of community health. NGOs often play a central function in designing and executing programs that most immediately compensate for lacking transportation infrastructure components, such as giving vehicles or organizing schemes of community transport. Besides, they can help in building collaboration with local governments to improve road access and transport services, which in turn improves the overall efficiency of healthcare delivery systems. The collaboration between community actors and NGOs enables collaboration in terms of resource and knowledge sharing, culminating in innovative solutions that can be adapted to specific local conditions (Woldemariam et al., 2015). Given that transportation and logistics are the foundations on which functional, successful community-based health systems are established, joint action by all parties is paramount in dismantling these barriers in order to improve healthcare accessibility and quality.

7.5. Role of Non-Profits in Health Promotion

Non-profit organizations have emerged as key players in health promotion, particularly in community-based healthcare systems. Their unique role is typically characterized by their ability to mobilize resources, tap into local expertise, and develop tailored interventions that address specific targeted health issues that are extremely prevalent in diverse populations. By incorporating the participation of community members, these organizations are extremely adept at defining issues that have been identified by various stakeholders, including chronic conditions, uninsurance, and variation in access to care. Apart from offering services, non-profits emphasize the people-focused element, which is essential in enabling cooperation and addressing mental and behavioral wellness concerns in communities. Such extensive engagement enables non-profits to identify and establish the most urgent health concerns in the target populations to ensure that the solutions being deployed are viable and effective in the immediate context (N/A, 2010). Non-profits, in particular, have an extremely crucial role to fulfill in health education and awareness, and act as vital intermediaries among communities and health systems. In their various programs, non-profits attempt to educate individuals about preventive measures, disease management, and health services available to them. Non-profit health educators often tailor their courses to consider the cultural determinants of health behaviors, thereby facilitating acceptance and participation from communities in health promotion efforts. This culturally sensitive approach can achieve extraordinary improvements in health outcomes, especially among vulnerable groups most impacted by disinformation. Non-profits also work closely with local health authorities and educational institutions, capitalizing on synergistic initiatives to drive coverage and establish the value of preventive health measures. Such partnerships not only maximize resources but also create an inter-sectional health promotion plan that is attuned to community needs and barriers to access (N/A, 2016). In addition, the agency of non-profits also involves advocating for systemic change within health systems. These non-profits can serve as chief advocates for marginalized people, getting their health concerns heard in policy and funding appropriations discussions. By focusing on health disparities in access and outcomes, non-profits aim to influence public policy and mobilize funding campaigns that focus on improving health services for low-income populations. This advocacy is particularly vital for susceptible groups such as children and women in tribal communities, where they are confronted with immense challenges in seeking healthcare. Not only do non-profits address present health conditions, but they also seek long-term solutions to structural inequalities, demonstrating their inherent worth as actors in health promotion and the creation of equitable health systems. Based on this, they are key to the achievement of broader public health goals and the promotion of overall community well-being (N/A, 2016) (Figure 7.12).

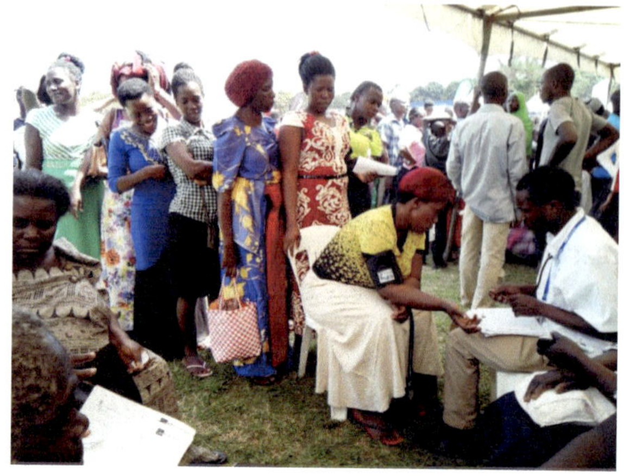

Figure 7.12. Role of non-profits in health promotion.

Source: https://mod.or.ug/wp-content/uploads/2020/08/4-1-768x576.jpg.

7.5.1. Overview of Non-Profit Organizations in Healthcare

Non-profit organizations are a key component of the health care setting by bridging service gaps and accessing vulnerable populations with critical care. Non-profits also develop as a response to direct health needs, providing services that cannot be provided by for-profit agencies and public health systems. Non-profits can present as community health centers, advocacy organizations, and educational institutions with a focus on prevention and health promotion. Their mission-driven approach emphasizes community engagement and cooperation with local stakeholders, serving to create a more integrated health care delivery system. For instance, efforts to build coordinated medical home networks, as seen in N/A (2008), emphasize the importance of cooperation among healthcare providers, government, and local organizations as a method of effectively meeting the health needs of the underserved. These models illustrate the ways through which non-profits can efficiently contribute to integrated care while enhancing community health improvement. An important aspect of healthcare non-profits is that they are able to advocate for policies favoring access and equity to care. They generally serve as intermediaries between policymakers and the population, ensuring that the interests of marginalized populations are represented and heard appropriately. This ground-level lobbying is most critical in the context of rising healthcare costs and disproportionate access to essential services. Non-profits tend to research and do needs assessments that enable them to better understand the issues with which their constituents are grappling, which can inform policy recommendations and systemic reform. For example, programs like Sun Devils Together at Arizona State University, as quoted in N/A (2020), meet student homelessness by raising awareness and coordinating resources, thus demonstrating how non-profits can deal with multifaceted social issues that shape outcomes in health. By fostering a context for partnership among stakeholders, non-profits are significant actors in policymaking choices that enhance public health. Moreover, non-profit organizations have a unique position in bridging gaps in healthcare access, particularly for at-risk populations that may have significant barriers to obtaining care. Such barriers may involve economic considerations, transport issues, and cultural factors that result in communication failures between physicians and patients. By providing affordable or free services and outreach activities specifically tailored to meet the diverse needs of their populations, non-profits reduce healthcare disparities. They often employ targeted interventions such as mobile clinics, health promotion campaigns, and preventive screenings. These efforts not only provide more access to required healthcare services but also educate individuals on information about their health decisions. This community-oriented program focuses in turn on generating improved health outcomes and healthier citizens and culture, demonstrating the critical role non-profits play in the overall healthcare continuum.

7.5.2. Programs and Initiatives Led by Non-Profits

Non-profit agencies are at the forefront of the delivery of community-initiated healthcare programs that address the unique health requirements of various segments of society. Concentrating on projects that involve preventive medicine, education on health, and access to health care, non-profit agencies fill significant gaps lacking in state networks of healthcare. Thus, non-profits attempt to fill the gap between conventional systems of health and culture-specific care that appeals to native populations. As discussed in Mignone et al. (2025), there have also been effective intercultural health models in some countries that bring into focus the importance of integrating allopathic and traditional methods of healing. It not only widens the access to care but also empowers the community by validating their cultural practices, hence encouraging a sense of ownership and engagement in health interventions. Focusing on particular health concerns within underprivileged communities is another key initiative area for non-profits, particularly in early childhood development and nutrition. Programs like Nourishing Our Future show the impact made by initiative-based interventions aimed at addressing malnourishment within risk groups, such as infants in urban slums. Through the concentration on the child 0-36 months, the program targets the window of opportunity for healthy growth and brain development. Non-profits, though occasionally starved for cash, collaborate with the government and donors to expand their scope and influence. These are the associations that serve to build upon existing systems, for instance, government-supported midday meals, and work towards encouraging an integrated systems approach to health that aims to position nutrition at the core of the new paradigm of total well-being, as emphasized in N/A (2011). Further, the non-profit advocacy also plays an important role in raising awareness on healthcare disparities and pushing for policies to promote health equity. Through mobilization of the community and stakeholders, these non-profits put the concerns of access to healthcare services, as well as concerns with vulnerable groups, into the limelight. Their work typically consists of activism for policy change directed at dismantling system barriers, which may include a lack of funding for community health centers or socioeconomic status barriers. Non-profit work not only pressures certain advances in community health but also instills a culture of activism that allows people to speak about their health needs. By implementing such multi-faceted interventions, non-profits ensure community-based healthcare systems are more responsive and robust to the intricate needs of the populations they address.

7.5.3. Collaboration Between Non-Profits and Community Stakeholders

Cooperation between non-profits and community stakeholders has a pivotal role in setting up healthcare systems based in the community. Non-profits act as the bridge between healthcare services and poor communities by knowing the particular health needs and advocating for the appropriate resources. Such cooperative actions not only strengthen the communities but also guarantee ownership by local stakeholders. Because they work closely with various stakeholders, including local governments and community leaders, they are able to design tailored health programs that are both relevant at the local level and accessible. Such a responsive model not just caters to basic health needs but also to overall social determinants of health, which, by extension, enhance the overall health of members of the community. By maximizing the capacities of diverse stakeholders, non-profits can potentially contribute significantly to achieving sustainable health outcomes and supporting policy reform that promotes health equity and access. The success of collaborations relies on intentional partnerships among non-profits and public stakeholders, particularly within the context of Federally Qualified Health Centers (FQHCs). As highlighted in existing research, administrators in these centers grapple with numerous issues in their application of ineffective strategic management and planning methods. Nonetheless, by the use of insights from diverse stakeholders in the community, non-profits can establish and surmount the issues that interfere with their effectiveness. Data gathered from semi-structured interviews among Texas FQHC decision-makers showed the greatest need for enhanced leadership abilities and collaborative partnerships. These alliances can help create long-term solutions that strengthen organizational culture and, eventually, financial stability and growth in the health sector. This alliance provides an environment where health programs can flourish, driving positive influences on service provision and patient' care. Further, the pursuit of shared value can also reinforce alliances between non-profits and local stakeholders in the healthcare sector. While firms recognize the value of addressing unmet healthcare needs in low- and middle-income populations, they can reconcile their business with the interests of community health. In doing so, there is a symbiotic relationship established where the needs of community health are addressed and corporations achieve competitive advantage in markets expanding worldwide. When shared value values are applied to non-profits, they can develop innovative partnerships that activate resources and skills from the private sector. All such alliances not only enhance the range and effectiveness of healthcare programs but also promote community involvement in health-promoting efforts. Thus, this cooperation between non-profits and the community ultimately forms a robust community-based health system promoting health equity and accessibility for all (Figure 7.13).

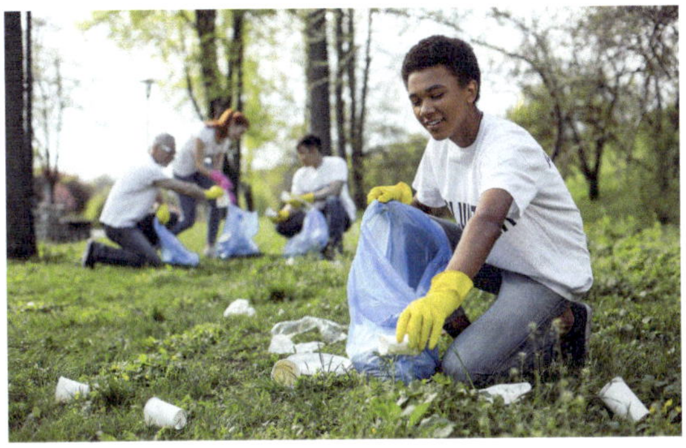

Figure 7.13. Non-profits and community stakeholders.

Source: https://i0.wp.com/bendrelocationservices.com/wp-content/uploads/2020/11/GIving-to-Nonprofits.jpg?resize=1080%2C675&ssl=1.

7.6. Role of NGOs in Health Promotion

Non-governmental organizations (NGOs) play the most crucial role in health promotion in community-based healthcare systems, usually filling up gaps that are created within public health infrastructure. Relying on local knowledge and resources, NGOs are optimally placed to provide context-specific programs of health depending upon local needs. NGOs tend to be engaged in key activities such as health education, disease prevention, and basic healthcare delivery services, particularly in poverty-stricken regions. The impact of such organizations can be profound, as they foster community participation and enhance the likelihood of health interventions being culturally sensitive and responsive. Moreover, NGOs act as a force for health equity, pushing for policy change based on interventions addressing social determinants of health and translating into improved population-level health outcomes. Their work within community health settings is significant, particularly where government support is minimal or absent, thereby enhancing the sustainability of interventions for health promotion (N/A, 2022). The role played by NGOs in health promotion is also heightened by the capability of NGOs to form alliances with stakeholders. Their work together with local authorities, healthcare providers, and community leaders, allows NGOs to harmonize their work towards broader public health goals. This cross-sector model has the potential to create synergies, amplifying the impact of health promotion interventions. NGOs, for instance, mobilize resources and skills, closing the access gap for services including immunization, maternal healthcare, and nutrition. They also have an important role to play in conducting studies and gathering evidence, which can be utilized in designing evidence-based interventions and determining priority issues in community health. This evidence-based approach is crucial in an effort to secure support and funding from national as well as international donors, thereby guaranteeing sustained health programs. NGOs, therefore, not only contribute to short-term health impacts but play a considerable role in shaping long-term health policy and strategy in the subject communities (Abubakar et al., 2022). Significantly, the role of NGOs in promoting health extends beyond their provision of direct health services; they also intervene at the systemic level to remove obstacles to healthcare access facing vulnerable populations. Poverty, illiteracy, and cultural stigmatization are all important obstacles to access to healthcare, and NGOs are likely to work against these issues by mobilizing and empowering communities. By creating awareness and educating people about health-related issues, NGOs empower people with the knowledge required to make appropriate health choices. In addition, NGOs advocate policies of improved access to health, which ultimately lead to universal coverage. Advocacy by them also goes further to address socio-political barriers that prevent equal access to health, and therefore, they are included in a comprehensive strategy for health promotion in communities. Therefore, the incorporation of

NGOs into community health models not only enhances current health results but also sets a foundation for change on a systemic level and increases the quality of life among the overall population (N/A, 2022) (Figure 7.14).

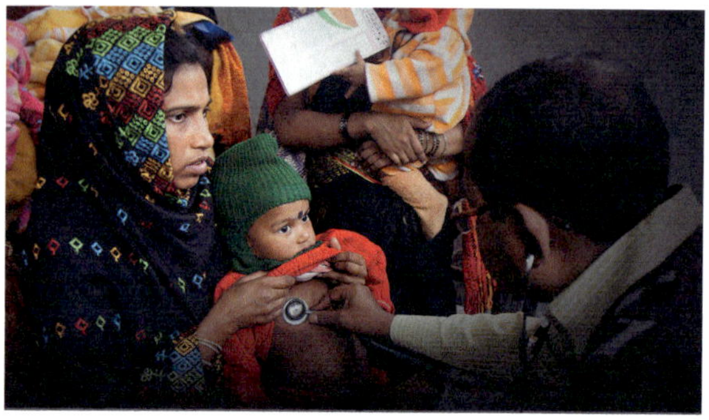

Figure 7.14. NGOs in health promotion.

Source: https://give.do/blog/wp-content/uploads/2021/12/Main-Banner-3.jpg.

7.6.1. Definition and Function of NGOs in Healthcare

NGOs play a pivotal role in healthcare, particularly in systems that are based on the community, where there is a need for equal access and effective health promotion. Since they are independent entities operating outside the government sector, NGOs are inclined to address inequalities in health by supplying services that are not well addressed by public health. Their activities typically encompass various activities that range from direct service delivery, education for health, and promotion to advocacy for policy change. For instance, community-based initiatives led by NGOs can mobilize local resources and facilitate involvement, enabling communities to set their specific health needs and solutions that best fit their environments. Active participation is crucial to developing health literacy and enabling people, thus facilitating improved health outcomes in line with the broader goals of community-based healthcare systems. Also, NGOs' working systems highlight how they can innovate and adjust, especially in responding to local health demands. Unlike ordinary government organizations, NGOs can easily shift their strategies and methods towards new health crises or alterations in the needs of society, rendering them invaluable resources. Through grassroots approaches, they tend to fill gaps left by public services, especially in marginalized communities. The majority of NGOs have managed to implement programs that integrate traditional health practices with allopathic medicine, an indication of which may be observed in various intercultural health experiences documented across Latin America (Mignone et al., 2025). Integration serves to provide a comprehensive perspective on health with emphasis on the significance of cultural competency in healthcare provision and the facilitation of the accessibility of health services to groups. Other than program implementation and service delivery, NGOs are also key promoters of system transformation in health administration. They play a role in bringing people's concerns to the fore about their health through awareness, thereby making policy discussions more active. NGOs are involved in ensuring more representative health policies that are specifically addressed to marginalized groups by consulting with the local government and other stakeholders. The impact of these organizations is best realized in rural communities, where they often act as a liaison between the community and national health systems, such as in community-based animal health projects where NGOs facilitate the incorporation of local health workers into national systems (Riviere-Cinnamond et al., 2025). Such efforts not only enhance the provision of services but also ensure that health interventions are sustainable, culturally sensitive, and responsive to the unique needs of diverse populations.

7.6.2. Case Studies of Successful NGO Interventions

NGO work in community-based health interventions can be explained by numerous case studies that illustrate their impact on public health indicators. For instance, in most regions of the world, NGOs have managed to integrate healthcare services with nutrition and sanitation programs, addressing the root causes of health problems rather than symptoms. These combined approaches have been seen to fight poverty and disease more efficiently, according to a report bringing together experience from 17 countries. The results of the case studies confirm the necessity of concerted action in addressing health-related challenges in an integrated fashion, thus permitting sustainable gains in health in communities (N/A, 2011). This approach has established a precedent for all future interventions, noting that health spending through comprehensive approaches is necessary in an effort to achieve long-term development goals. The response to the HIV/AIDS pandemic is yet another applicable case study that demonstrates successful NGO interventions. Programs and projects funded by donors have supported local NGOs, religious groups, and community-based organizations in playing central roles in combating HIV/AIDS through targeted interventions and investments. These community groups have been facilitated by such organizations as the Global Fund and PEPFAR, valuing their unique ability to extend to communities and meet localized requirements effectively. With HIV/AIDS expenditure reaching an all-time high of $6.1 billion in 2004 from $1 billion in 2000, local groups have been instrumental in delivering services directly to clients. Their deep and long-term knowledge of grassroots environments has enabled them to mobilize groundbreaking interventions that are necessary for enhancing health, proving local NGOs to be priceless partners in effectively resolving public health crises (Cornman et al., 2005). Furthermore, successful case studies illustrate how NGOs not only deliver vital health care but also enhance community resilience and empowerment. By involving local communities in planning and implementing health interventions, NGOs create a sense of ownership and agency among the communities. This approach fosters sustainable health behavior and makes interventions culturally acceptable and specific. Maternal and child health programs, for example, have been enhanced by integrating local women in education and outreach. The resultant mobilization of the community has, as a consequence, created increased access to and quality of healthcare. Such joint initiatives not only enhance the efficiency of healthcare plans but also provide the groundwork for long-term health promotion programs, upholding the value of NGOs in reengineering the field of community health.

7.6.3. Challenges Faced by NGOs in Health Promotion

The health promotion environment is more complicated, particularly for community-oriented NGOs, given the multiplicity of healthcare systems in most countries. One of the biggest challenges that such organizations bring, for example, is the fragmentation of healthcare systems, which can lead to inefficiency and duplicated efforts. Most countries, as quoted by an all-encompassing report looking into health in Latin America, have multiform healthcare structures that will automatically stifle concerted health promotion activities. For NGOs, operating within these fragmented systems often means not only vying for money but also requiring a refined understanding of local health needs and politics in order to execute effective programs (Calderon et al., 2019). As such, this poor policymaking can curtail the potential of NGOs to contribute to better community health, again necessitating coordination and integration among different sectors of health. Financial constraints are another serious challenge confronting NGOs working in health promotion. Lack of certainty in funding can limit the scope of programming and prevent work on current projects, since it is difficult to achieve sustainable health outcomes. As presented in a number of case studies, NGOs rely on external funding sources, which can be unreliable and based on political or economic changes (N/A, 2011). This financial uncertainty, aside from weakening the development and implementation of health programs, affects staff morale and turnover as well. Without assured financial support, NGOs can sacrifice their operations, with the eventual effect on their ability to act on pressing health issues in communities. While NGOs grapple with these financial concerns, the need for innovative finance mechanisms and partnerships becomes increasingly urgent in a bid to sustain their health promotion program. Further, the challenge of cultural competency poses serious challenges for NGOs in mobilizing diverse communities for health promotion. Effective health interventions are contingent on a realization of people's popular culture beliefs, practices, and social forces that could be quite different even within an adjoining geographic region. NGOs subsequently must take time and funds to establish trust and appropriate relations with community individuals in order to foster acceptance and participation in health programs. This culturally based approach is vital, particularly where there is customary practice and resistance to external influences (N/A, 2011). By neglecting to acknowledge and include these cultural considerations, NGOs risk alienating the very people whom they aim to assist, illustrating the importance of culturally sensitive health promotion practice in achieving successful and worthwhile community outcomes (Figure 7.15).

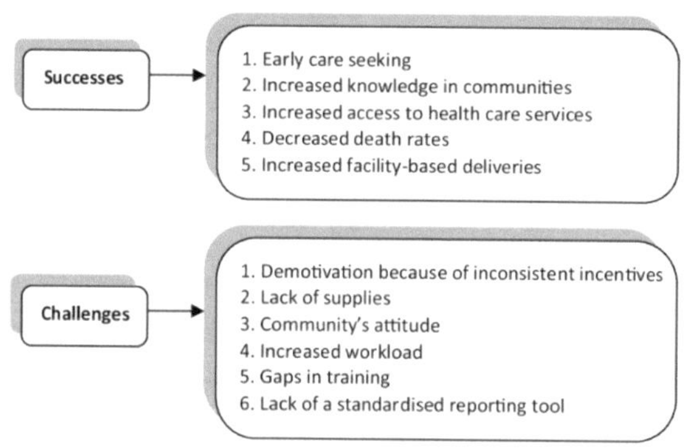

Figure 7.15. Challenges faced by NGOs in health promotion.

Source: https://www.researchgate.net/publication/323400129/figure/fig2/AS:614036370620441@1523409087551/Perceived-successes-and-challenges-in-health-promotion.png.

CLOSER LOOK

FUTURE OF COMMUNITY-BASED HEALTHCARE SYSTEMS

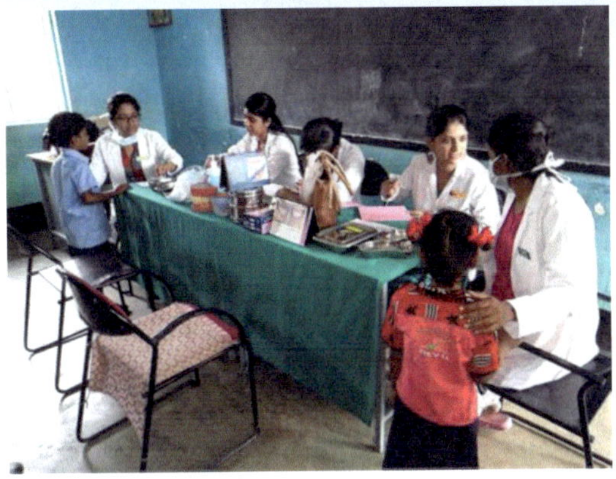

The future of the community health care systems is likely to become increasingly important in addressing the multifaceted issues of different populations. An important aspect of this evolution is the integration of traditional and new approaches to health, particularly for marginalized groups such as indigenous people. For instance, the vital function of intercultural health models that bridge traditional knowledge with allopathic medicine stresses best practices from regions like Suriname and Ecuador to show that effective health systems can enhance accessibility and effectiveness by being attentive to cultural values and norms. Such strategies not only enhance community trust but also ensure the provision of culturally competent healthcare, allowing practitioners to gain knowledge and address the unique health needs of the diverse communities, thus opening doors for more equitable healthcare practice. As further models of community-based healthcare are evolved, technological innovation and data sharing are also likely to play a major role. One of the hopeful developments is the merging of health information systems that allow communities to take ownership of their health. With the application of technology to facilitate better service delivery, health professionals can improve monitoring of trends in community health, enhance communications among stakeholders, and provide intervention where most needed. For example, community engagement encourages a participatory setting where citizens are involved in health decision-making, which is critical in the face of major challenges like maternal and child health. Community ownership drives both the delivery of services and ensuring that healthcare systems are responsive to people's needs and preferences. In addition, the function of NGOs and non-profits in health promotion is assuming a much more significant role within community health care systems. These groups play a critical role in plugging gaps in conventional healthcare systems, especially in settings where resources are limited. Non-profits tend to introduce scalable programs that attack defined health emergencies, i.e., newborn mortality, which is still disproportionately high in countries such as India. With collective partnership with community stakeholders, these agencies fashion outcome-specific interventions that are efficient in mobilizing resources for disease prevention and health promotion. Thus, the future of healthcare systems at the community level will be based on greater collaboration among NGOs, governmental institutions, and community organizations to bring about a more integral strategy to health that focuses on accessibility, equity, and cultural competence.

SUMMARY

Community-based health care systems' implementation is an urgent shift towards extensive health services encompassing all segments. It is particularly relevant to the case of increasing economic disparities and access limitations, noted in certain research. For instance, Southeast Asian emerging economies have grappled with containing escalating levels of wealth alongside deep-seated poverty, highlighting the need for targeted health interventions to manage the inequalities. The public policy-philanthropy interface remains essential in shaping the effectiveness of these mechanisms, underpinning the role of community engagement in establishing resilience and flexibility within healthcare systems (Anand, 2014). With community contribution increasing in its role in health promotion, there is an ever-growing likelihood for sustained health improvement. The role of primary care in community health also cannot be overemphasized. Primary care is the first line of defense for access to healthcare, delivering preventive and routine care that is necessary for early detection of health disparities. Primary care also builds relationships between healthcare professionals and community members, establishing trust and boosting participation. Functional primary care systems ensure that marginalized populations, frequently disadvantaged by the conventional models of healthcare delivery, are given due attention and intervention. The establishment of health franchises, as evident in the examples of CFWshops in Kenya and Mi Farmacita Nacional in Mexico, is a clear demonstration of how integrated service delivery can enhance access to healthcare and ultimately lead to an improvement in the health status of vulnerable populations (Sankar et al., 2009). These models demonstrate the necessity of adapting strategies in primary care so that local needs can be addressed while enhancing the welfare of communities. Finally, the coordination of non-profits, NGOs, and government agencies is crucial in successful health promotion and overcoming obstacles that constrain access to care. By pooling resources, sharing information, and designing targeted interventions, these institutions play a key role in advancing community health programs. Their ability to adapt and utilize health program strategies to the local context is essential, especially against the backdrop of emerging public health challenges exacerbated by social inequalities. Given that they traverse numerous different healthcare settings, their nonprofits must exercise reflective practices that assess the effectiveness of their program strategies to optimize their contribution to community health outcomes. The future of healthcare relies on leveraging these shared efforts to develop systems that not only respond but also act proactively to enhance health equity and community resilience.

In exploring the world of community-based healthcare systems, it is essential to recognize the diverse types and their individual contributions to public health. These types of systems tend to emphasize care within localized areas and are developed to address unique community needs and thus increase patient involvement and reinforce confidence. Notably, these systems may range from public health programs to private non-profit institutions, but all of them would play their part in contributing to equal access to health care. Implementation of primary care within such systems is necessary as it is the first line of defense against taking care of health problems. Through preventive care and health education, primary care could significantly improve community health results. This multi-disciplinary approach calls for a deep understanding of existing systems and their potential to handle the complexities of delivering healthcare across varying settings. The role of primary care in community health cannot be overemphasized, especially in the context of considerations around accessibility and health equity. Primary care providers are key intermediaries between patients and the broader healthcare system, often navigating barriers of cost, transportation, and cultural competencies that may deter individuals from appearing for critical care. In longitudinal, integrated care, primary care providers can identify and mitigate social determinants of health that create disparities within diverse populations. Besides, as systems become mature by embracing technological innovation, telehealth care, and community outreach programs, they are successful in bridging gaps of access and participation. Finally, in keeping primary care central, it is essential for facilitating health literacy and preventing chronic illness, which endorses the entire system of community-based health care. Non-profit agencies and NGOs are also central to health promotion, often intervening by filling the gaps left by traditional systems of health care. Such organizations tend to focus on underserved populations, emphasizing public education, awareness campaigns, and direct service delivery that aim to promote healthy lifestyles. The role of such organizations in preventing public health problems—such as infectious diseases and chronic diseases—has been noted by a number of research studies. Non-profit-initiated community programs can provide examples of care that illustrate how communities can shape the health of populations, particularly in low-resource settings. As discussed in analyzing health care systems, it is essential to understand how community resources and access to health care relate and affect each other in an effort to come up with effective public health policies. On this note, synergic action on the basis of the aggregate strengths of both public and non-profit sectors can revolutionize community health outcomes (Aarestrup et al., 2015; Bonica et al., 2017).

REFERENCES

1. Aarestrup, A., Ahuja, V., Aidara-Kane, A., Zumla, A., Allegranzi, B., Allegranzi, B., et al. (2015). Exploring the evidence base for national and regional policy interventions to combat resistance. https://core.ac.uk/download/36779210.pdf (accessed on 11th June 2025).
2. Abdulmalik, J., Aguocha, C., Eaton, J., et al. (2020). *Partnership for the Implementation of Mental Health Policy in Nigeria: A Case Study of the Comprehensive Community Mental Health Programmer in Benue State.* https://core.ac.uk/download/293755543.pdf (accessed on 11th June 2025).
3. Abubakar, I., Dalglish, S. L., Angell, B., Sanuade, O. A., Abímbọ́lá, Ṣ., Adamu, A. L., Adetifa, I., et al. (2022). The Lancet Nigeria Commission: Investing in health and the future of the nation. *The Lancet, 399*, 1155–1200. https://doi.org/10.1016/s0140-6736(21)02488-0 (accessed on 11th June 2025).
4. Anand, P. U. (2014). Levers for change: Philanthropy in select South East Asian countries. https://core.ac.uk/download/75781680.pdf (accessed on 11th June 2025).
5. Arens, K. (2023). Healthcare innovation: Challenges and strategies for developing a financially sustainable health insurance product for the senior market in collaboration with Advance Care. https://core.ac.uk/download/614522028.pdf (accessed on 11th June 2025).
6. Bambra, C., Forster, T., & Kentikelenis, A. (2018). *Health Inequalities in Europe: Setting the Stage for Progressive Policy Action.* https://core.ac.uk/download/199426311.pdf (accessed on 11th June 2025).
7. Bonica, M. (2017). *Healthcare Management Primer.* https://core.ac.uk/download/215509297.pdf (accessed on 11th June 2025).
8. Calderon, M., Gallagher, M., Haque, S., et al. (2019). *A Comprehensive Analysis on The Healthcare Systems in Latin America.* https://core.ac.uk/download/286731467.pdf (accessed on 11th June 2025).
9. Cornman, H., Grimm, C. D., & Rana, S. (2005). *Engaging Local Non-Governmental Organizations (NGOs) in the Response to HIV/AIDS.* https://core.ac.uk/download/72048685.pdf (accessed on 11th June 2025).
10. Green, A. R., Betancourt, J. R., & King, R. R. (2009). Improving quality and achieving equity: A guide for hospital leaders. https://core.ac.uk/download/71352207.pdf (accessed on 11th June 2025).
11. Lavigne, M., & Vargas, L. H. (2013). *Social Protection Systems in Latin America and the Caribbean: Jamaica.* https://core.ac.uk/download/38672365.pdf (accessed on 11th June 2025).
12. Learwellie, B. A. (2024). *Analyzing Youth Empowerment Programs and Their Impact in Urban and Rural Liberia.* https://core.ac.uk/download/619721931.pdf (accessed on 11th June 2025).
13. Lethbridge, J. (2011). *A Parallel Approach to Analysis of Costs/Benefits and Efficiency Changes Resulting from Privatization of Health Services.* https://core.ac.uk/download/6179016.pdf (accessed on 11th June 2025).
14. Marley, P., & NC DOCKS at Appalachian State University. (2015). *Procedures of Nongovernmental Organizations and Social Entrepreneurship in International Development: Two Case Studies.* https://core.ac.uk/download/345081926.pdf (accessed on 11th June 2025).

15. McLaughlin, C., Rosqueta, K., & Hobble, R. (2018). *Community-Based Approaches to Health: How Engaging Local Community Members Can Transform the Health of Hard-To-Reach Populations.* https://core.ac.uk/download/480183399.pdf (accessed on 11th June 2025).

16. Mignone, J., O'Neill, J., & Bartlett, J. (2025). *Best Practices in Intercultural Health.* https://core.ac.uk/download/pdf/6394130.pdf (accessed on 11th June 2025).

17. Miller, E., Line, L., & Nath, T. (2017). *Working Together Toward Better Health Outcomes.* https://core.ac.uk/download/86445047.pdf (accessed on 11th June 2025).

18. O'Neill, M., Redelmeier, R. J., Michalski, C. A., Macaraeg, R., Gans, M., Schoffel, A., Diemert, L. M., et al. (2025). Implementation and evaluation of a novel community-based urban mobile health clinic in Toronto, Ontario. *Canadian Journal of Public Health = Revue Canadienne de Santé Publique.* https://www.semanticscholar.org/paper/7d22c0f8b2ebc55dd3f794f86d8221597bb8dc68 (accessed on 11th June 2025).

19. Owadara, F. O. (2025). A survey of the implementation of participation strategies to enhance inclusive workplaces in the public and private educational systems in Lagos State. https://core.ac.uk/download/644030553.pdf (accessed on 11th June 2025).

20. Peterson, K., Rehrig, M., Stamp, M., & Kim, S. (2012). *Competing by Saving Lives: How Pharmaceutical and Medical Device Companies Create Shared Value in Global Health.* https://core.ac.uk/download/71359569.pdf (accessed on 11th June 2025).

21. Riviere-Cinnamond, A. (2025). Animal health policy and practice: Scaling-up community-based animal health systems, lessons from human health. https://core.ac.uk/download/pdf/7055421.pdf (accessed on 11th June 2025).

22. Sankar, R. (2009). Study of health franchises in resource limited settings. https://core.ac.uk/download/4421890.pdf (accessed on 11th June 2025).

23. Segura, G., & Pastor, M. (2020). *No Going Back: Policies for an Equitable and Inclusive Los Angeles.* https://core.ac.uk/download/480184928.pdf (accessed on 11th June 2025).

24. Shekarian, E., Ijadi, B., Zare, A., & Majava, J. (2022). Sustainable supply chain management: A comprehensive systematic review of industrial practices. *Sustainability, 14*, 7892–7892. https://doi.org/10.3390/su14137892 (accessed on 11th June 2025).

25. Sommer, I., Harlfinger, J., Toromanova, A., Affengruber, L., Dobrescu, A., Klerings, I., Griebler, U., et al. (2025). Stakeholders' perceptions and experiences of factors influencing the commissioning, delivery, and uptake of general health checks: A qualitative evidence synthesis. *The Cochrane Database of Systematic Reviews, 3*, CD014796. https://www.semanticscholar.org/paper/889c2cfa0f77bdfd96fd7139e2e7c14fd66d27b3 (accessed on 11th June 2025).

26. Tabor, S. R. (2025). *Community-Based Health Insurance and Social Protection Policy.* https://core.ac.uk/download/pdf/6314326.pdf (accessed on 11th June 2025).

27. Taylor, E. (2023). *Improving Strategic Management Planning in Non-Profit Organizations: Federally Qualified Health Centers.* https://core.ac.uk/download/595325293.pdf (accessed on 11th June 2025).

28. Woldemariam, A. T., Maeda, A., Dahn, B., Lu, C., Von Glahn, D., Perry, H., & Vosburg, K. (2015). *Strengthening Primary Health Care Through Community Health Workers: Investment Case and Financing Recommendations.* https://core.ac.uk/download/75761404.pdf (accessed on 11th June 2025).

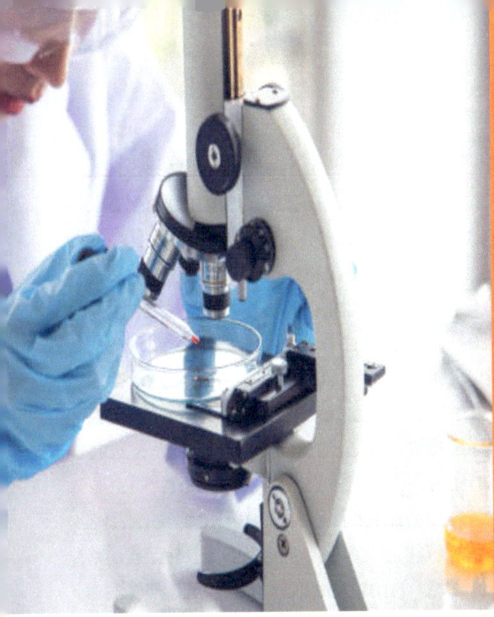

Chapter 8

EPIDEMIOLOGY AND PUBLIC HEALTH RESEARCH

Contents

Introduction

Epidemiology is the fundamental foundation of public health research, enabling researchers and practitioners to scientifically explore the determinants and distribution of health-related events among populations. Epidemiology essentially examines the trend of disease transmission, who gets affected, and the social determinants of health outcomes. This is especially significant for public health practitioners tasked with managing responses to acute health concerns, as information regarding the incidence, prevalence, and mortality patterns provides essential context for successful intervention. Through analysis of both quantitative and qualitative aspects of health data, epidemiologists enable stakeholders to obtain valuable perspectives to solve health disparities and improve population health overall. Furthermore, the introduction of new methods of data collection has revolutionized the field to provide more precise estimates and quicker response to public health emergencies, thus overall improved ability to protect community health. Incidence and prevalence are applied as basic principles to explain the complexity of public health. Incidence refers to the rate of newly developed disease cases in a time frame, and it reflects patterns of disease emergence and transmission. Prevalence, however, is the total number of cases, and it provides information on the population's disease burden. These distinctions assist public health professionals in determining the effect of health interventions and efficient utilization of resources. The incorporation of high-quality epidemiological data can ground decision-making initiatives, especially during public health crises. As seen in existing literature, challenges in information collection, such as accessing timely and reliable data, can significantly undermine response initiatives; however, data collection of population health data remains imperative in ensuring adequate planning and resource allocation under such circumstances, as seen in Checchi et al. (2017). Conducting community health evaluations is a practical application of epidemiology, connecting theory and practice. Evaluations involve collecting and analyzing data for the determination of a community's health needs and issues to ultimately inform public health interventions. Evaluation typically involves several methodologies, including surveys, focus groups, and screenings, to accurately obtain data on the health status of communities. As illustrated in recent training courses, for instance, the Disaster Preparedness and Response Training, understanding epidemiological methods is important in a bid to effectively apply rapid needs assessments in disaster settings (N/A). These methods allow public health practitioners to obtain vital information that informs interventions on addressing emerging health threats and enhancing community resilience to counter public health crises. Incorporating these findings into public health policy not only confirms the relevance of epidemiology but also enhances health and preparedness in communities (Figure 8.1).

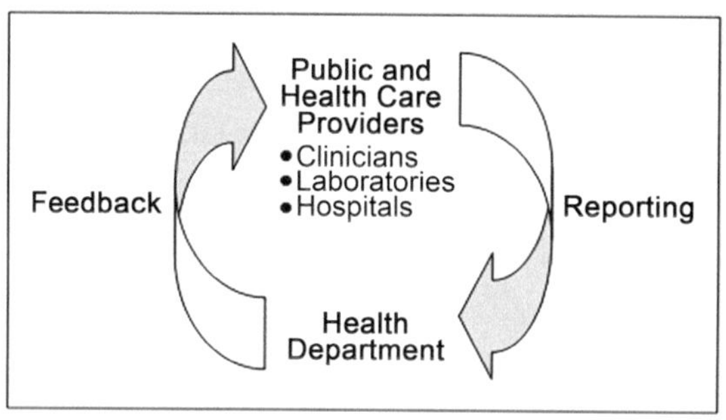

Figure 8.1. Epidemiology and public health.

Source: https://archive.cdc.gov/www_cdc_gov/csels/dsepd/ss1978/lesson1/section4_html_files/Figure1.3a.png.

Definition and Importance of Epidemiology

Epidemiology is the research into how often diseases affect populations and what causes such trends. It is a root science that forms the basis for investigation and public health programs. By researching determinants and distribution of states of health, epidemiologists aim to discover the hidden reasons and risk factors behind health discrepancies. This discipline draws on various quantitative and qualitative methods to collect data, which subsequently informs interventions that can reduce disease incidence, prevalence, and mortality. In effect, epidemiology provides the key information necessary to detect public health problems and ultimately inform effective means of enhancing the health of populations. In addition to tracking disease occurrences, epidemiology is of utmost importance in designing preventive interventions and policy. For instance, through analysis of information from specific groups, epidemiologists can reveal vulnerable populations and environmental factors associated with disease conditions. This information becomes important when dealing with public health emergencies, as it aids in resource allocation and the setting of specific interventions. Additionally, understanding disease transmission through epidemiologic research allows public health officials to make informed responses to health threats. These research findings are invaluable in creating health advisories and guidelines that ultimately ensure community well-being and health. The information gathered can also identify the effectiveness of existing health programs, and hence advance public policies further. Research shows that epidemiology has enormous implications for the healthcare and environmental management industries. For instance, estimation of temperature-mortality rates due to ischemic heart disease in various cities is a representation of the necessity to make public health interventions place-specific to mitigate climate change, an observation that stands out in research conducted across Chinese cities. This evidence-based practice not only supports forecasting of looming health crises but also determines the necessity of place-specific interventions that are based on regional climatic diversity (Armstrong et al., 2012). In the same way, in geriatric oncology, identifying how age-related aspects affect the outcome of surgery through careful evaluation can make a big difference in treatment strategies and patient results. This interaction between epidemiology and specialized areas of public health strengthens the discipline's role in providing solutions to intricate health issues and improving population health by providing evidence-based decision-making (Lampugnani et al., 2017).

Historical Context and Development

The epidemiologic historical context paints the picture of a discipline shaped by vast scientific and public health progress. From the very beginning, the field evolved after epidemics and individuals like John Snow laid down a foundation with diligent data gathering and analysis in the 19th-century cholera epidemics. His work proved the importance of identifying incidence and prevalence as elementary principles that direct public health interventions. Over time, the practices expanded to encompass statistical practices and a broader recognition of social determinants of health. This shift is a move in the direction of a more evolved understanding of disease processes, progressing ultimately to a comprehensive community health assessment considering not just biological variables, but also socio-economic status and environmental determinants that contribute to public health outcomes. As the discipline progressed, so did the methods of data gathering and analysis for public health studies. Progress in epidemiologic tools and techniques has facilitated the development of a solid understanding of disease patterns and epidemics. Modern epidemiology employs sophisticated statistical analysis and geographic information systems (GIS) to visualize and analyze data, which leads to more effective public health interventions. Moreover, technology interfacing, such as electronic health records and mobile health software, enables real-time data collection that enhances the ability to monitor disease prevalence and incidence. This route mirrors the necessity of continuous innovation in public health research so that practitioners are able to address emerging health concerns and to mitigate both acute public health emergencies and their chronic sequelae. The recent global health crises, particularly the COVID-19 pandemic, have placed the critical role of epidemiology in the face of public health emergencies into sharp relief. The unprecedented scale of the pandemic necessitated the rapid and unrelenting collection of data efforts, marking a new era in the history of public health research. For instance, over 40,000 patients of COVID-19 were admitted to the hospitals in the city of New

York as of April 28, 2020, and had an urgent need for full epidemiological data regarding the clinical course and outcome of the infected persons. These examples illustrate how previous traditions of epidemiology are being applied to meet existing challenges and demonstrate the field's flexibility and versatility. The lessons learned through these experiences will certainly guide future public health policies and strategies, further illustrating the value of well-established historical context in shaping current research and practice.

Role of Epidemiology in Public Health

The role of epidemiology is public health-oriented, aimed at providing the basis for studying causes and distributions of disease in populations. By analyzing the occurrence and prevalence of health conditions, epidemiologists are able to establish risk factors and guide morbidity and mortality reduction measures across different populations. For instance, through meticulous data gathering and analysis, epidemiologists can ascertain the role of socio-economic status, environmental exposure, and behavioral factors in health inequalities. Such science-inclined methodology comes into play particularly during public health emergencies, when rapid measurements of disease spread can guide intervention efforts.

The importance of getting such information accurately becomes critical in the creation of registries to track patient outcomes, as in N/A (2020). By accurately identifying health trends, epidemiology not only directs short-term intervention but also directs health policy development in the long run. Furthermore, successful community health assessments largely depend on epidemiologic methods. These enable public health agencies to gather and interpret data regarding community needs and hazards to health. With the use of quantitative and qualitative data gathering, such as focus groups and surveys, epidemiologists can paint an overall picture of a population's health environment. This data is crucial when dealing with specific health concerns, such as infectious disease outbreaks, chronic illness, or environmental health hazards. With the use of surveillance data, vulnerable populations can be targeted and targeted health interventions created. Overcoming the challenges of Alzheimer's disease and related dementias (ADRDs) among underrepresented ethnoracial groups raises the issue of the intersection of epidemiological research and community health assessment. Directed research is essential to enhance understanding and ensure equitable health interventions, as described in Ganesh et al. (2018). In addition, the application of epidemiology does not stop with the evaluation of individual health; it is essential in resolving public health emergencies. During epidemic or pandemic situations, the timely collection and interpretation of epidemiological information are important for effective containment. Epidemiological models are used far and wide by public health officials for forecasting disease spread patterns and in administering vaccines. Forecasting is important to plan resource allocation, public education, and preventive intervention to avert mass health crises. As demonstrated by recent experience with global pandemics, harmonizing epidemiologic data with health policy decisions can have significant consequences for population health outcomes. The advances outlined in N/A (2020) for data analysis and registry management underscore this imperative, emphasizing ongoing innovation and collaboration within the field. In general, epidemiology is a useful model for strengthening public health efforts and healthier populations in the end (Figure 8.2).

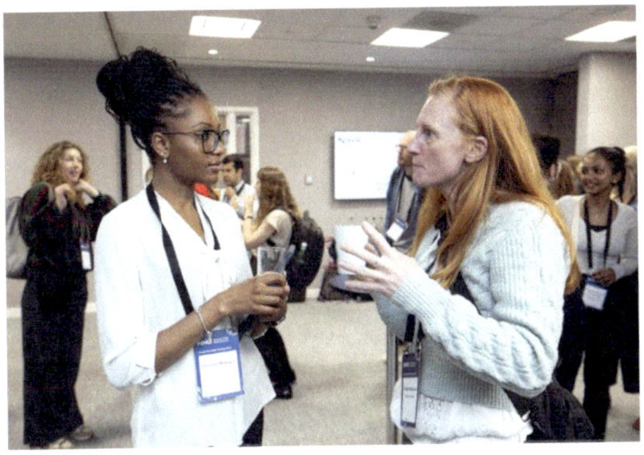

Figure 8.2. Public health professionals networking during a research conference event.

Source: https://sphr.nihr.ac.uk/wp-content/uploads/resized/2024/10/day2-082-e1728483262173-768x512-c-center.jpg.

8.1. Basics of Incidence and Prevalence

Understanding the incidence and prevalence is central to epidemiology and public health research. Incidence is defined as the number of new cases of a disease within a specified period of time among a specific population. Public health planners need this measure in order to be able to ascertain the risk of disease and to implement timely interventions. By measuring the incidence rate, scientists can identify emerging health issues and track their progression. In measuring tuberculosis among children in the Philippines, for instance, scientists recorded a weighted prevalence rate of 6.4%, with some locations reporting much higher rates, illustrating the application of incidence to guide targeted strategies in medicine. Furthermore, the following incidence allows for the measurement of the effectiveness of preventative measures and allocation of healthcare resources to areas where larger numbers of new cases have arisen, ultimately informing public health practice and policy. Prevalence, however, encompasses the total number of cases—new and existing—that are present in a population during a specific time. This can be a significant step to assess the disease burden as a whole, as it reflects the impact health conditions have on a population. Prevalence rates advise policymakers of the extent of healthcare needs and demands for resources. For example, high prevalence rates of pulmonary disease in specific populations could indicate environmental health issues or disparate access to healthcare. Prevalence analysis is part of community health assessment because it determines population-at-risk and social determinants that are the drivers of health. Accessibility to health facilities has been revealed to be a key driver in isolated communities, determining the prevalence level and the demand for individual outreach programs is thus amplified to minimize health disparity and promote the general well-being of the populace. The connection between incidence and prevalence is crucial to the comprehensive public health approach. Incidence may quantify the rate of disease spread, but prevalence offers a quantification of the overall impact on society. This type of distinction is essential in the instance of public health emergencies, when rapid response mechanisms have to be established to reduce disease spread and its impact on health. For instance, by virtue of extreme temperature oscillations, studies have proved the existence of non-linear associations between environmental conditions and ischemic heart disease mortality rates, proving the need for context-specific health responses as a function of prevailing conditions. The acknowledgment of the interplay between incidence and prevalence allows public health professionals to formulate evidence-based strategies sensitive to the competing needs of divergent populations. Effective public health programs rely on good data collection systems that report incidence in addition to prevalence, giving a firm basis for responding to health problems within communities and thereby establishing resilience in public health systems (Figure 8.3).

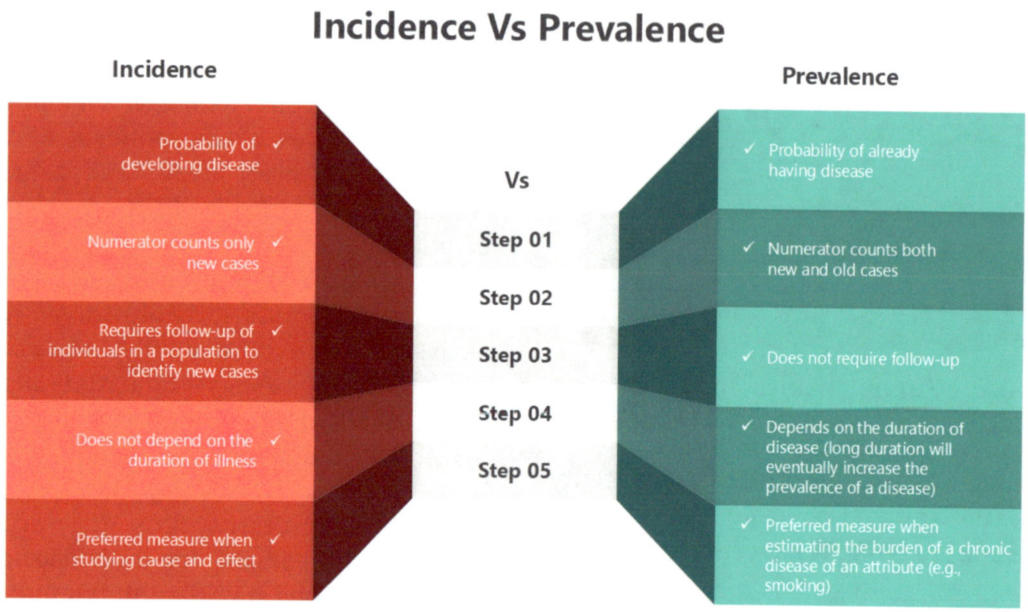

Figure 8.3. Incidence-vs-prevalence.

Source: https://www.slideegg.com/image/multi-slide/73322/501115-incidence-vs-prevalence-01.png.

8.1.1. Definitions of Incidence and Prevalence

Incidence and prevalence are fundamental terms in epidemiology and public health research that provide critical measures of disease dynamics in populations. Incidence is the number of new cases of a disease in a population over a defined period of time. This measure is crucial to assess the risk of disease transmission since it allows researchers to track emerging threats to health and to invest resources in an optimal manner. For instance, understanding the prevalence of healthcare-associated infections (HAIs) in hospital settings can guide interventions to reduce transmission rates and improve patient safety. Monitoring trend incidence thus benefits public health. It helps identify vulnerable populations and offer necessary preventive interventions in a timely manner, thereby solidifying its role in community health assessments and healthcare decision-making (Mullings et al., 2019). Conversely, prevalence measures the total number of new and existing cases present in a population at one point in time. It is a snapshot of the general burden of disease, which is important in estimating the need for healthcare services and the development of effective health policies. Prevalence is particularly useful in the context of chronic disease, where the diseases persist for a long duration and therefore have implications on healthcare planning and resource utilization. For example, the knowledge of the prevalence of conditions such as diabetes would allow health authorities to plan resource allocation in preventive and treatment programs. Through the illumination of disease burden, prevalence data can inform initiatives towards alleviating health inequities, enhancing community health outcomes, and resource distribution (Brodbelt et al., 2014). Incidence and prevalence measurements, although distinct, provide an overall view of public health problems. They serve complementary roles in epidemiologic research, supporting the determination of health trends and informing disease management and prevention policy. Because incidence captures the dynamics of disease development, prevalence reflects the broader impacts of diseases on a community's health. This complementarity enables policymakers to create interventions for addressing both acute and chronic demands, enabling responses to public health emergencies effectively. A grasp of these definitions and how they are implemented is imperative to the conduct of robust community health assessment and data collection to facilitate evidence-based interventions in managing health crises and improving overall public health outcomes (Mullings et al., 2019; Brodbelt et al., 2014) (Figure 8.4).

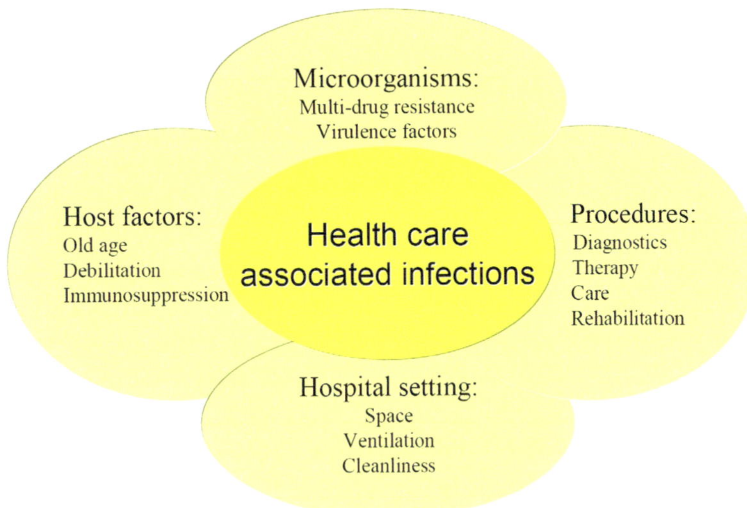

Figure 8.4. Factors determining healthcare-associated infections.

Source: https://www.researchgate.net/profile/Hans-Kolmos/publication/221925213/figure/fig4/AS:668677443690514@1536436534912/Factors-determining-health-care-associated-infections.png.

8.1.2. Calculation Methods and Formulas

In the field of epidemiology, understanding calculation methods and formulas is pivotal for analyzing data related to public health. These methods form the foundation for computing crucial metrics such as incidence, prevalence, and mortality rates. Incidence refers to the number of new cases of a disease within a specified population over a given timeframe, while prevalence measures both new and existing cases at a certain point. To calculate incidence, researchers frequently employ the formula: Incidence Rate = (Number of New Cases / Total Population at Risk) × 1000, making it possible to standardize data between various populations. With this quantitative approach, public health professionals can track disease trends and allocate resources effectively, ultimately improving disease prevention strategies and intervention programs in the targeted communities. Death rates, yet another key calculation in epidemiology, are indicators of health outcomes and health care system effectiveness. Using formulas like Mortality Rate = (Number of Deaths / Total Population) × 1000, scientists can come up with insightful findings concerning the effects of diseases on populations in the long run. The calculations necessarily demand accurate data collection procedures, such as health records and vital statistics, in order to guarantee reliability and accuracy. The Whitehall

II cohort study is an example of the necessity for rigorous data analysis, showing the impact of exercise on diabetes incidence and mortality rates among research subjects (Yerramalla et al., 2019). These epidemiological studies emphasize the necessity of applying reasonable calculations to guide health policy and improve public health interventions aimed at recognized needs in community health. Also, having the response to public health emergencies involve applying calculation methods that are founded on newly emerging data from rapid assessment and surveillance systems. In outbreak or crisis situations, faster data compilation and processing are needed in a bid to develop timely responses. With formulas such as Attack Rate = (Number of Cases / Total Population at Risk) × 100, infectious disease transmission is readily computed by epidemiologists, and high-risk groups for intervention are readily identified. Background to studies of ataxia-telangiectasia (A-T) is as vivid an illustration as any of how careful analysis of genetic susceptibility informs cancer mortality and public health policy (Swift, 2001). Finally, efficient calculation tools and formulas are key in developing evidence-based interventions that help mitigate urgent public health concerns while improving resilience among communities in times of emergencies.

8.1.3. Importance of Understanding These Metrics

Public health measures, i.e., incidence, prevalence, and mortality rate, are essential for public health decision-making and planning. These are important indicators of disease burden and overall community health status. For instance, incidence rates inform health authorities about the number of new cases within a population over a specified period, allowing targeted intervention efforts. Conversely, prevalence rates provide a broader overview by indicating to what degree a disease is widespread at a specific time point, and that affects policy formulation for health and the allocation of resources. Death rates, indicating the number of deaths induced by diseases, are most relevant to determining the intensity of health issues in populations. Combined, these metrics provide a quantitative basis for the evaluation of health programs and responsiveness to emerging health concerns, indicating their applicability in epidemiology and public health research. Moreover, they are not used only for situational awareness; they form the basis for conducting comprehensive community health assessments. Successful measurements rely on having recent data reflecting the local health concerns and population makeup. As stressed in various modules of training, e.g., in Disaster Preparedness and Response Training Course, awareness of the above steps enables health professionals to make rapid needs assessments and develop appropriate responses to disaster. The integration of incidence and prevalence data in assessments enhances detection of vulnerable groups and the appropriate systems of service delivery. Without such a good grasp of these measures, health professionals would be poorly equipped to counter pressing public health issues, ultimately precluding their ability to deliver timely and effective measures, particularly during times of emergency. Finally, an evidence-based reaction to public health emergencies demands a solid grasp of these measures for effective data gathering and analysis. For instance, the problems emphasized on data quality and accessibility during crises indicate the importance of standardized methods in metric evaluation, as emphasized in Checchi et al. (2017). An integrating framework can facilitate a timely and coordinated response, saving lives. Also, as emphasized in capacity building initiatives, like those issues raised in (N/A), capacity development in epidemiological methods among health workers enhances the ability to manage complex health emergencies. Strong indicators allow health authorities to target intervention at the most severe and prevalent health issues, ensuring that the resources are directed where they are needed most. Thus, knowing such metrics in public health is critical to both timely response and long-term health benefits.

8.2. Understanding Mortality Rates

Knowledge of mortality rates is at the core of epidemiology and public health research since they provide important insights into populations' overall well-being. Death rates are measured by the number of deaths that occur within an established population over a defined time period, often per 1,000 or per 100,000 individuals. Mortality rates can provide various stakeholders with insights into the burden imposed by disease and disparities in health across communities. Through the investigation of death rates, health officials can identify high-risk groups and areas that need targeted interventions. Also, death statistics may serve as an indicator for evaluating the effectiveness of health policy and programs. From the perspective of mortality analysis, a more comprehensive understanding of the determinants of death can be obtained, enabling the construction of targeted strategies to prevent preventable deaths. During public health emergencies, the need for accurate mortality statistics is even more critical. During crises, i.e., disasters or war, ordinary mortality rates not only may be a distortion of actual deaths, but also specialized methods of data collection must be used. The character of disaster epidemiology reinforces the necessity of involving epidemiologic techniques in disaster management. This integration allows for systematic collection of data relating to health outcomes and risk determinants during emergencies, thus allowing vulnerable populations to be managed and provided for better. Continuous tracking of mortality during disasters is necessary for decision-making within relief interventions and distribution of resources, thus enhancing the resiliency and recovery of affected communities following disasters. Additionally, reliable mortality data also play a significant role in responding to longer-term public health objectives, particularly the struggle against systemic health inequities. Analysis of mortality sheds more light on socioeconomic status, geographic, and access differentials, forming a master plan for interventions in health. For instance, (Checchi et al., 2017) accentuates the importance of obtaining quality health information in evolving emergencies as a means of ensuring that the humanitarian interventions are appropriately targeted. Furthermore, having a robust framework for data gathering that includes community health surveys is crucial to transforming public health strategies over time. This emphasis on death in the broader context of studies on health can lead to policy making based on data that addresses underlying determinants of health, as evidenced by (N/A). In the end, death rates are at the heart of creating healthier populations and averting avoidable deaths in both every day and crisis public health contexts (Figure 8.5).

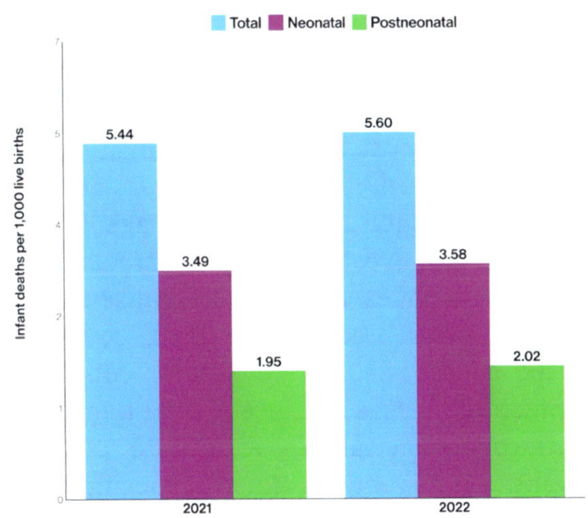

Figure 8.5. Mortality rates.

Source: https://i.abcnewsfe.com/a/d8bd8dfa-3a44-46f8-8a87-f63af73e9015/Infant_Mortality_v02_dnl_1698838479261_hpEmbed_1x1.jpg.

8.2.1. Definition and Types of Mortality Rates

It is essential for public health studies to know mortality rates because it provides information about the determinants of death risks and causes of death in a population. Mortality rates can be defined simply as measures that depict the number of deaths in a population over a certain period, typically calculated per 1,000 or 100,000 individuals. These rates not only reflect a community's health and longevity but are also essential indicators through which epidemiologists and public health administrators may witness trends and aberrations in the health experiences of diverse populations. The decomposition of mortality rates may differ and permit targeted intervention that responds to health inequities and health improvement, especially among risk populations as indicated in research in aging and the health care situation of the geriatric population (Lampugnane et al., 2017). Among the most commonly applied forms of mortality rates in epidemiology are crude mortality rates, age-specific mortality rates, and cause-specific mortality rates. The crude death rate provides a broad picture of a region by calculating deaths total and then dividing the outcome by the population total, thus one of the simplest and most straightforward measures. Age-specific death rates provide more accurate results by categorizing deaths in age groups, which is useful in establishing the impact of age on health outcomes. Furthermore, cause-specific mortality rates break down death counts by specific causes, i.e., cardiovascular conditions or infectious diseases, thereby enabling public health professionals to formulate effective preventive interventions aimed at specific health hazards of populations. Full data for such rates are important, especially in the formulation of public health policy and reactions to new emerging health crises (Armstrong et al., 2012). Mortality rate application can also be seen in other public health indicators, particularly when calculating mortality impacts of environmental factors, such as heat and cold temperatures, on specific diseases. For instance, research has documented how extreme heat and low temperatures, respectively, can significantly raise mortality rates of ischemic heart disease in Chinese cities. Results indicated discrete patterns of mortality regarding temperature extremes, which mirror variances according to regional climatic conditions. Observations obtained through such analyses underscore the importance of integrating mortality rate data into wider epidemiological studies, further facilitating public health responses to climate change and health crises. Through extensive gathering and processing of mortality rate statistics, public health researchers can not only document patterns of disease but also guide evidence-based interventions to enhance public health outcomes and minimize mortality hazards in diverse populations (Armstrong et al., 2012).

8.2.2. Factors Influencing Mortality Rates

The determinants of mortality are multifaceted and include a myriad of social, economic, and environmental determinants that together determine public health outcomes. Socioeconomic status is a vital one; those with lower income levels have more limited access to good-quality healthcare and therefore greater mortality from avoidable disease. Education also has a related measure, health literacy, which influences health behaviors and health service uptake. For instance, individuals with higher education are likely to utilize healthcare services more effectively, such as preventing mortality. It is thus imperative to understand the impact of socioeconomic factors on health outcomes, in order to create targeted interventions that can reduce mortality rates among different populations. Environmental factors also significantly determine the rate of mortality, particularly in developing nations where a lack of proper waste management and pollution results in adverse health effects. As indicated in Atnkut et al. (2025), poor solid waste management can lead to increased exposure to harmful substances, with ill effects on health among communities. Poor disposal of trash in or around inhabited areas or bodies of water can lead to the spread of infectious diseases, thus increasing mortality risks. Furthermore, airborne as well as waterborne contaminants exacerbate pre-existing diseases, particularly for vulnerable populations such as children and the elderly. Intervention of such environmental determinants by strong public health policy and community action is critical in diminishing their contribution to mortality. Finally, demographic determinants such as age and gender are also central to the determination of mortality rates. Evidence indicates that elderly people are more prone to death due to chronic illness burden and loss of physiological reserve. Furthermore, gender disparities typically result in mortality rate variations; for example, maternal health issues disproportionately affect females in the majority of regions, as indicated in Onak et al. (2024). All these demographic factors must be considered in public health surveillance and epidemiological studies to formulate more effective interventions. With the integration of demographic variables into socioeconomic and environmental contexts, public health professionals could potentially design comprehensive responses to reduce mortality rates and improve health equity (Figure 8.6).

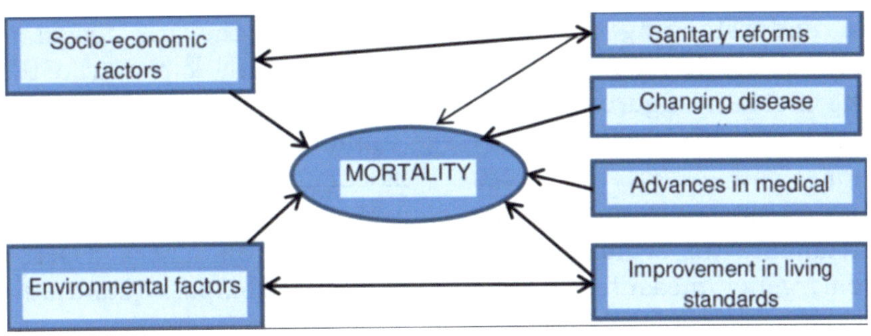

Figure 8.6. Factors influencing mortality rates.

Source: https://www.researchgate.net/profile/Muazu-Shamaki/publication/353556626/figure/fig2/AS:1050946561912833@1627576594422/A-Model-of-factors-affecting-mortality-level-Source-Adapted-from-Barrett-1992.png.

8.2.3. Implications of Mortality Data in Public Health

The interpretation of mortality data has important public health implications, which have policy and resource-allocating consequences. Public health practitioners can understand the priority health risks in a population through knowledge of mortality rates, thereby targeting interventions at high-risk groups. For instance, mortality data on cervical cancer can reflect significant health inequalities, particularly through incidence rate analysis by varying population groups and geographical areas. Greater understanding of these disparities can mobilize efforts to increase access to preventive interventions, such as HPV vaccination and screening programs, that in the end will reduce the burden of this preventable disease in high-risk populations, illustrating the strength of data in public health planning (Ul et al., 2025). Moreover, death rates are an essential feedback mechanism on the effectiveness of public health interventions. Through the uniform collection and analysis of data regarding mortality patterns by varying health conditions, researchers can establish the impact of measures instituted, such as increased access to healthcare and community health assessment. For example, the reported timely analysis of acute kidney injury (AKI) reveals high-priority public health needs, particularly in Latin America, where enormous gaps in the delivery of healthcare services exist. Findings from research indicated that AKI resulted in high morbidity and mortality, which suggests that dedicated research and intervention are required to prevent its contribution to public health outcomes (Jose et al., 2025). Thus, the utilization of mortality data can guide and inform more evidence-based and rational decisions, which can enhance public health readiness and response. In addressing public health emergencies, the implications of mortality data become more vital. Timely and accurate data collection becomes crucial during outbreaks or crises, where understanding mortality patterns can inform strategic responses. For instance, analyzing mortality figures in real-time can help public health officials identify at-risk populations and direct resources where they are needed most. Additionally, this data can be instrumental in evaluating the effectiveness of emergency measures against communicable and non-communicable diseases alike. By establishing a robust infrastructure for data collection and sharing in times of emergencies, public health practitioners are not only able to improve the speed of their responses but also leverage the information obtained to inform longer-term health system strengthening and resilience efforts. Ultimately, mortality information emerges as a basis for evidence-based public health practice to bolster population health outcomes in the long term.

8.3. Conducting Community Health Assessments

For effective management of public health conditions, community health assessment is the foundation. Community health assessments are organized evaluations of the health status, needs, and resources of the community, culminating in a thorough understanding of local health issues. No measure of participation by the people can be overemphasized, as involvement of the people in the assessment process ensures the development of relevant health issues as well as the suitability of interventions. Such participatory methodology ensures the development of trust as well as the utilization of culturally specific health measures, thus strengthening the utility of the assessment findings. Suppose public health professionals can conceptualize their work based on good empirical evidence, as noted in studies like the one that investigates oral cancer in East Africa. In that case, they can design interventions that are more likely to penetrate the population and deliver sustainable health results enhancement (Aminu et al., 2025). The methodologies applied in community health assessment are of top priority to ensure the right data gathering and interpretation. These assessments are most likely to encompass quantitative and qualitative data gathering strategies, like surveys, focus groups, and health screenings. Utilizing tested models like the Centers for Disease Control and Prevention's (CDC) Assessment Protocol, public health professionals can systematically gather applicable data regarding health indicators, demographic factors, and social determinants of health. Further, as the recent studies on influenza surveillance in wastewater matrices showed, new techniques are available to access information that will mirror the general status of health within the community (Dlamini et al., 2024). Public health officials can determine trends, disparities, and future health threats by analyzing such information, so it is essential that the applied methods are strong and reactive to the specific situation of the community under assessment. Following data collection and analysis, the next is the interpretation of the findings into actionable public health actions. The dissemination of the findings of the assessment to stakeholders, including community leaders, clinicians, and policymakers, is vital in facilitating collaboration and mobilizing resources for the implementation of interventions that are suggested. In addition, setting measures to track and evaluate the impacts of the interventions ensures continued improvement and responsiveness to emerging health needs. For instance, the definition of specific risk factors, say, Toombak consumption in oral cancer diagnosis, will inform particular educational campaigns and preventive interventions in society (Aminu et al., 2025). Finally, conducting intensive community health evaluations builds the groundwork for an anticipatory, evidence-based public health response that enhances public health outcomes and resilience against future public health emergencies (Figure 8.7).

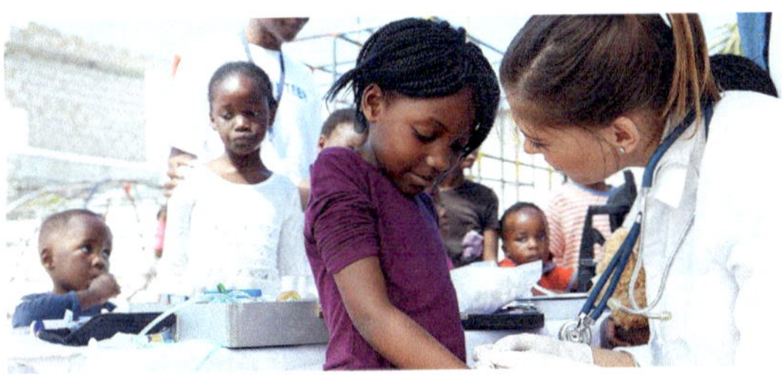

Figure 8.7. Hospitals demonstrate practical application of the community health assessment tool.

Source: https://www.aha.org/sites/default/files/styles/900x400/public/2018-06/social-determinants-900x400.jpg?itok=EvFNc_Sn.

8.3.1. Purpose and Objectives of Community Health Assessments

Community health assessments are fundamental instruments in public health studies, allowing healthcare practitioners and policymakers to ascertain the health issues and needs within specific populations. The key role of assessments is to provide a comprehensive description of local health status, risk factors, and intervention resources. Conducting these assessments in a systematic manner aids in the establishment of health disparities and prioritization of what should be addressed. Without these evidence-based observations, effective interventions would be out of reach, susceptible to resulting in wasted resources or ineffective strategies. Community health assessments are in the tradition of values that epidemiology holds dear, centered on the interaction between population health needs and particular health strategies. In such situations, information collected can be applied to inform the development of public health efforts, particularly aimed at improving outcomes and eliminating existing health disparities in communities. Community health assessment purposes extend beyond data collection; they are designed to involve communities and create ownership of health promotion programs. As part of the assessment, members of the community have the opportunity to apprise public health officials of cultural factors, barriers to care access, and other nuances affecting outcomes. Also, these measurements enable the identification of key stakeholders within the community, which facilitates collective action for improved health services and results. Engaging different members of the community not only enriches the data but also helps in the development of capacity and trust within the community. As public health infrastructures strive to address the shifting health demands of populations, community health assessments present themselves as key avenues for ethical consideration, community participation, and sustainable interventions, thereby becoming more pertinent in the evolving public health landscape. In the end, community health assessments provide a medium for continuous assessment and optimization of localized and systemic health outcomes. With changing health needs and arising public health challenges, such reviews from time to time would be necessary to keep the assessments up to date and relevant in the current health situation. In addition, data collected from these assessments can contribute to evidence-based policy changes and budgeting, particularly for low- and middle-income nations with documented health disparities. For example, data from the evaluation of community health can be used to inform the needed health system reforms in order to achieve equitable and quality care, as evidenced by Margaret et al. (2018). Thus, the objectives of these assessments are not only to gather data but also to construct the resilience of communities and enhance the quality of health systems in responding to their own particular needs, ultimately doing so to achieve better health outcomes for all.

8.3.2. Key Components of a Health Assessment

Systematic health assessment is a critical public health research tool because it is the foundation for understanding population health needs and developing successful interventions. Health assessment is a multifaceted process to collect, analyze, and interpret information about a population's health status. Essential components are demographic data, which provide insight into the population's structure, vital rates such as birth and death rates, and health indicators such as disease prevalence and incidence rates (e.g., influenza, cervical cancer). Familiarity with these components is essential in creating effective public health policy and appropriate resource allocation. The structured gathering of health information allows researchers and practitioners to identify disparities in health and prioritize interventions targeting the focused needs of the community, promoting improved health outcomes and health equity. Moreover, the methodology used in health assessments is the most important factor in their effectiveness and validity. Effective data collection tools such as quantitative questionnaires, qualitative interviews, and observational measures allow accurate determination of the health issues affecting the community. Application of strict sampling techniques ensures the gathered data are representative of the total population, thereby leading to strong and generalizable results. In a rural Bangladeshi study on cervical cancer prevention, for instance, a cross-sectional design facilitated the identification of principal risk factors like prevalence of HPV and limited access to care (Taher, 2024). Secondly, incorporating community participation into the assessment process will increase participation levels and help yield more profound insights into the sociopolitical and cultural determinants of health. Such holistic approaches are critical to solving public health crises and enhancing the overall health of communities. Finally, using the outcome of health assessments in influencing public health interventions can impact health outcomes profoundly. Effective translation of information into action not only includes the identification of health needs but also the design of targeted intervention strategies to address those needs.

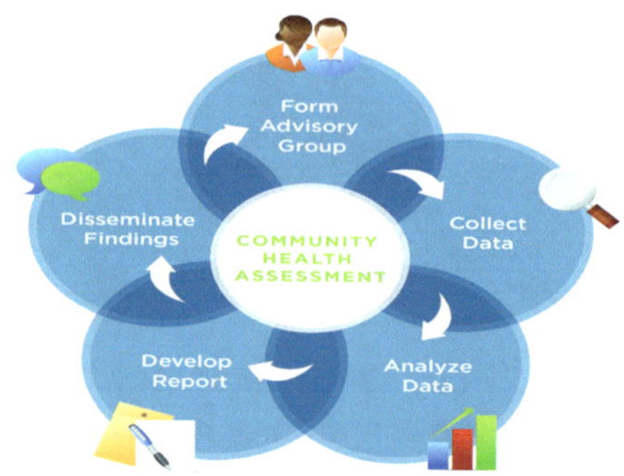
Form Advisory Group
Collect Data
Analyze Data
Develop Report
Disseminate Findings
COMMUNITY HEALTH ASSESSMENT

Figure 8.8. Components of community health assessment.

Source: https://nursingexercise.com/wp-content/uploads/2019/03/Community-health-assessment.jpg.

For example, the use of wastewater surveillance to monitor influenza virus circulation is an excellent innovation for complementing traditional approaches in disease surveillance, as indicated in recent systematic reviews (Dlamini et al., 2024). Using assessment data in executing interventions for education campaigns and prevention can lead to heightened awareness and participation of communities in health interventions. Moreover, continuous evaluation and adaptation of the interventions keep them relevant and effective in addressing emerging public health issues. Lastly, integrating holistic health assessments in public health systems is essential in building a strong health system in place to address present and future public health problems (Figure 8.8).

8.3.3. Stakeholder Involvement and Engagement

Stakeholder active participation is core to the practice of epidemiology and public health research, particularly with the presence of high-level health issues that disproportionately affect targeted populations. By involving members of the community, clinicians, and lawmakers, public health action can have input from a very diverse set of perspectives and capacities. This collaboration not only enhances the accuracy of data collection and analysis but also supports the identification of the unique needs and issues of various communities. For instance, the environmental justice movement identifies the necessity of engaging marginalized communities exposed to environmental pollution. Engagement is significant in the development of evidence-based interventions that are specific and intended to lessen health disparities and attain health equity (Association, 2001). Consequently, stakeholder engagement makes the research environment more representative, and this can enhance the effectiveness of measures to address both current and future public health emergencies. Secondly, having stakeholder input in community health assessments allows for broader awareness of drivers influencing health outcomes. By employing insights gained from grassroot stakeholders, researchers can unveil underlying social determinants of health that may not be unveiled using traditional epidemiological methods. These insights are particularly pertinent in cases where it is known that knowledge gaps regarding the health status of particular populations, such as those with undiagnosed dementia (Aldus et al., 2020), are present. Involving stakeholders at all stages of the research process ensures the integration of the community's concerns and priorities in study design, implementation, and reporting of findings. Doing this through a stakeholder approach ultimately makes public health research more applicable and meaningful in practical settings, ensuring that interventions will be embraced by the very people they are intended to target. In addition, stakeholder involvement is a critical vehicle of establishing trust and facilitating communication between the research community and those groups under research. Prudent strategies of engagement can constrain skepticism and increase community acceptance of public health interventions. When stakeholders feel confident that they are heard and their opinions are valued, they are most likely to engage positively in health promotion programs and adhere to interventions recommended. This trust is particularly critical in the face of public health emergencies when speed of response is necessary. By creating open communication and co-ownership of health program initiatives, public health investigators can mobilize community resources and enhance intervention sustainability. Therefore, investing in stakeholder dialogue not only enhances epidemiologic inquiry but also allows communities to respond as a whole for improved health.

8.4. Data Collection Methods in Public Health Research

Methods of data collection in public health research are vital for grasping the health dynamics of populations and informing effective interventions. Data collection methods can be broadly divided into qualitative and quantitative methods, each playing different roles in research design. Qualitative methods like focus groups and interviews offer depth and context, uncovering underlying behaviors, beliefs, and motivations that could be missed by quantitative data. Conversely, quantitative techniques like surveys and epidemiological studies allow for the collection of numerical data that may be statistically analyzed to determine trends, associations, and correlations. The union of the two approaches usually enhances study findings, e.g., disease research on such conditions as respiratory syncytial virus (RSV), where qualitative depth and quantitative solidity are merged in an attempt to present a complete picture of public health issues (Floriana et al., 2025).

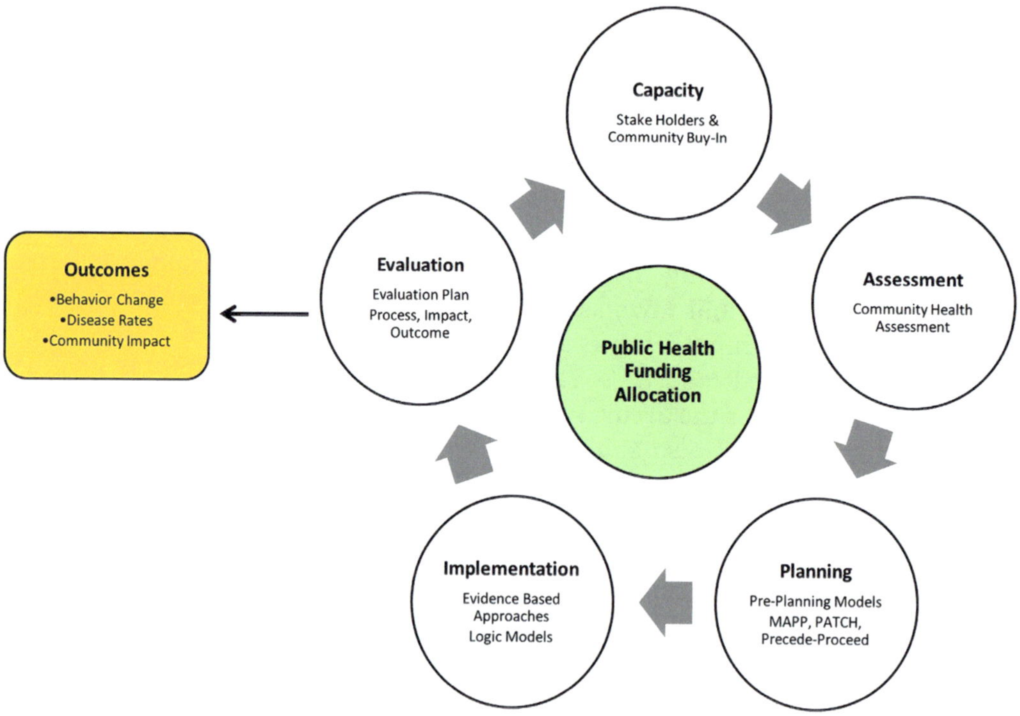

Figure 8.9. Data collection and management in public health.

Source: https://library.fiveable.me/_next/image?url=https%3A%2F%2Fstorage.googleapis.com%2Fstatic.prod.fiveable.me%2Fsearch-images%252F%2522Survey_and_questionnaire_design_in_public_health_research%253A_data_collection_validity_reliability_pilot_testing.%2522-fpubh-05-00192-g001.jpg&w=1080&q=75.

In public health, the effectiveness of data collection depends not only on the methods applied but also on the appropriateness of these methods to the target population. For instance, case-control studies can be particularly helpful when one is examining the outcome of illness in relation to specific risk factors, such as pneumonia in children under the age of five. With the use of systematic random sampling and the application of structured questionnaires, it is possible for researchers to effectively measure the occurrence of diseases and the respective demographic variables, such as immunization status and birth weight. The data thus gathered will be representative of the population, hence the validity of the research results. Add to that, the statistical analysis itself, done by means of the likes of chi-square tests, supports the connection of identified factors to health outcomes, an antecedent to evidence-based public health interventions (Meirawati et al., 2024). Lastly, the determination and execution of data collection methods in public health research have a substantial influence on the excellence of epidemiological evidence as well as the excellence of public health programs. As new public health challenges emerge, researchers must employ advanced data collection methods attuned to the emerging health problems and population dynamics. Disease outbreak surveillance and monitoring of health trends constitute the centerpiece of this approach. Opening up such systems for representing groups such as elderly people in the case of RSV highlights the critical importance of representative data collection in informing on-time public health interventions. By advocating for an integrated data collection strategy, public health professionals will be able to better anticipate and address the requirements of diverse populations, thus making health interventions equitable and effective in disease burden mitigation (Floriana et al., 2025) (Figure 8.9).

8.4.1. Quantitative vs. Qualitative Data Collection

In public health and epidemiology studies, the distinction between quantitative and qualitative data gathering is significant for guiding intervention and policy. Quantitative data uses measurable figures such that researchers are able to quantify in numbers phenomena of health, such as incidence, prevalence, and mortality. One can use this method to ascertain patterns and relationships, which can be analyzed statistically to produce generalized results that can be applied in broader situations. But while quantitative approaches provide a robust evidence-based platform for measuring the trend in health, they will disregard contextual factors that significantly impact a person's experience and the consequent health outcomes. The researcher must therefore consider accommodating qualitative data, which provides richer insight into people's lived experience in a community, hence a richer interpretation of quantitative outcomes. Qualitative data collection addresses the limitations of quantitative methodology by exploring the subjective nature of health issues. Procedures such as interviews, focus groups, and ethnographies focus on participants' opinions, experiences, and perceptions of illness and health. Rich narrative data provide background information that quantifiable figures cannot offer, revealing intricacies that can inform health behavior, service access, and utilization of resources. For instance, knowledge of community perception of vaccination can shed light on obstacles that are not clear when only vaccination rates are analyzed. In addition, qualitative methodology can be used to inform the construction of culturally sensitive health interventions designed for certain groups therefore, whereas the quantifiable data will describe the what and how many, qualitative data provides essential information on the why, noting the complexity of engagement in public health settings. Finally, the blending of qualitative and quantitative data in public health studies can lead to more effective programming and decision-making. Data triangulation is achievable through a mixed-methods approach, as it brings together the strengths of both research designs to provide an elaborate picture of what public health issues are all about. During public health emergencies, such as outbreaks or natural disasters, both quantitative information—morbidity and mortality rates—and qualitative data on individuals' experiences and feelings can be used for determining an appropriate response to emergencies. Furthermore, as recent literature suggests, an urgent need for methodological innovation aimed at the specificity of gathering health data in the context of humanitarian crises is real. Through a systematic data collection method with both quantitative and qualitative elements, public health professionals can better answer the multifaceted problems of vulnerable populations, such as children affected by disasters, and offer more responsive and efficient health interventions (Checchi et al., 2017; Mansourian et al., 2020).

8.4.2. Surveys, Interviews, and Focus Groups

Use of interviews, surveys, and focus groups is an essential method used in public health research, providing in-depth information regarding the needs of community health. These qualitative study methods allow researchers to engage respondents directly, accessing their opinions and experiences that quantitative data might not capture. For instance, community survey research can be helpful in establishing the prevalence and burden of specific health problems, for instance, substance abuse, which has been linked with a wide range of comorbidities, including sleep disorders, as indicated by public health literature. Through these approaches, researchers can gain greater insight into the social determinants that influence health to inform interventions that are community-responsive and culturally appropriate. This qualitative data is pivotal in the response to public health emergencies, as it recognizes gaps and areas of necessity that must be met urgently, thereby informing policy and resource allocation. Key informant interviews and focus groups also enable deeper discussion among stakeholders, with researchers being able to explore complex health issues from multiple perspectives. For example, the Research Education and Community Health (REACH) coalition places a high value on incorporating qualitative data from focus groups to hear community voices during the health assessment process. By actively hearing from community members, public health practitioners are ideally suited to learn their needs, challenges, and aspirations, which would result in more effective program development and implementation. The collective process of such strategies is used to establish increased community trust and participation, engendering a spirit of communal ownership for public health initiatives. It is through such a continuous loop of feedback harvesting and re-tuning of strategies that public health programs are perhaps revolutionizing, targeting the root causes of health disparities in populations.

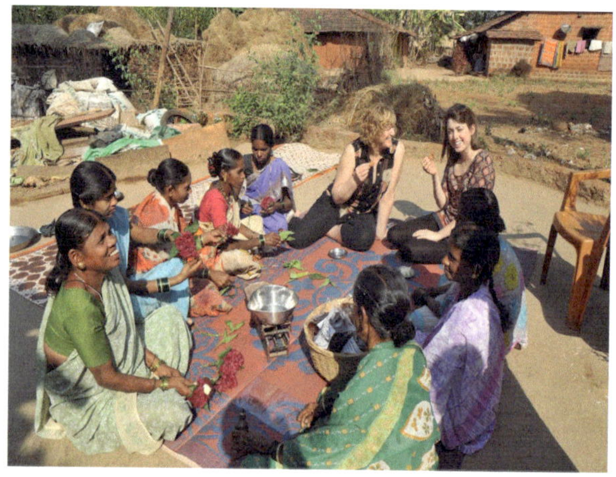

Figure 8.10. Rural empowerment and community health (REACH).

Source: https://walawalkarhospital.com/wp-content/uploads/2016/07/4.jpg.

Practically speaking, the use of surveys, interviews, and focus groups in public health research provides an integrated context for understanding community health dynamics. As observed from the Galveston County health survey, qualitative data can pinpoint entrenched problems, such as the lingering effects of crises, such as the COVID-19 pandemic, on youth mental health. By integrating existing data sources with direct experience from the public, researchers can identify prevailing health trends and emerging issues requiring intervention. Such points of information are critical in developing targeted action plans since they reveal trends in resource usage and behavior patterns that may not be captured by quantitative indicators. Therefore, surveys, interviews, and focus groups are crucial in evaluating public health issues but also in positively informing future policies on health that seek to advance the well-being and resilience of the community, thereby increasing public health outcomes in diverse populations (Figure 8.10).

8.4.3. Ethical Considerations in Data Collection

The most important ethical concerns regarding data collection in public health research are the nature of the health information, which is personal. The rights and autonomy of study participants must be prioritized by researchers through the obtention of informed consent, which clearly spells out the intent, risks, and benefits of the research. This safeguards the participants as well as the integrity of the study. Besides, ethical principles dictate that data collection operations be done with confidentiality and respect for privacy and in a way that personal identifiers are removed or anonymized to protect people against harm or discrimination. Failure to observe such ethical guidelines not only erodes public confidence in health research but also warrants severe legal sanctions against researchers and involved institutions in the misuse of data collection operations. In epidemiology, the ethical data collection must also be sensitive to connotations of social determinants of health. It is ethically incumbent upon researchers to consider the influence of socio-economic status, race, and geography on the results of studies. There is an ethical obligation to be respectful, and vulnerable populations must not be over-represented or exploited in studies. Instead, representation and inclusion of various demographic groups in data gathering processes are most vital to the achievement of equitable public health outcomes. This emphasizes the importance of involving communities in the research agenda so as to secure collaborations that empower voices at the local level and allow improved understanding of trends in health. By prioritizing such ethical issues over others, researchers can maximize the relevance and applicability of their research outcomes to public health programs, thereby informing relevant interventions that really address community needs. Technology, particularly artificial intelligence (AI) and big data analytics, raises new ethical issues in data collection. While these technologies open up new frontiers for public health research development, they also open up challenges in the data privacy, security, and algorithmic bias fronts. As noted in Adefemi et al. (2023), implementing AI in public health policy necessitates close monitoring to prevent hazards because of weak data governance frameworks. Ethical norms have to be modified to be able to accommodate the rapid rate of improvement in data collection methods so that utilization of AI is aligned with core ethical principles such as beneficence, non-maleficence, and justice. Scholars must engage with stakeholders when developing open protocols that not only protect the privacy of the individual but also make data use accountable. By anticipatory attention to these ethical concerns, the public health community can capitalize on technological innovation and maintain public trust and adherence to ethical research standards.

8.5. Data Analysis Techniques in Public Health Research

In research in public health, data analysis methods play a key role in the interpretation of intricate data and in providing bases for informed decision-making. Statistical methods, such as descriptive and inferential methods, are among the key methods. Descriptive statistics summarize core features of health data, revealing patterns and trends in disease occurrences among communities. Inferential statistics, on the other hand, enable researchers to make predictions and inferences based on sampled data. It is where these methods meet that is of ultimate importance in assessing public health concerns, such as disease incidence and prevalence. By using these statistical methods, researchers are able to identify trends, potential outbreaks, and where intervention will be required, allowing for effective public health interventions aimed at improving the health of communities. The second important element of public health data analysis is the use of geographic information systems (GIS). GIS technology facilitates spatial data analysis and visualization, demonstrating the interaction between geographic points, socio-economic status, and environmental conditions with health outcomes. This spatial analysis is particularly useful for disease distribution and appropriate resource targeting. For instance, foodborne disease outbreak analysis entails taking into account pathogen data along the various stages of the food chain. With the analytic tools described in discussions between food safety scientists and policymakers, researchers can assess how changes in consumption and production patterns influence disease risk and economic effects (Anonymous et al., 2025). This interdisciplinary approach not only enhances the robustness of public health data but also informs policy and practice to encourage positive health interventions. Lastly, technological advancement also reinforces methods employed in public health research, particularly through diagnostic assay advances. Molecular assays have transformed the detection and characterization of infectious diseases, and this is an outstanding example of how data analysis approaches improve to keep pace with new public health issues. For instance, molecular surveillance of Trichomonas vaginalis infection has transformed opinions and unveiled the prevalence of the disease among diverse populations, necessitating additional screening efforts (Munson et al., 2016). Such a shift in testing, coupled with successful data analytics, facilitates a thorough understanding of disease transmission dynamics and associated health implications. The arrival of new technologies and new analytical approaches underlines the requirement for continuous adaptation in data analysis methods to ensure that public health research can effectively respond to continuously changing epidemiological trends and public health emergencies (Figure 8.11).

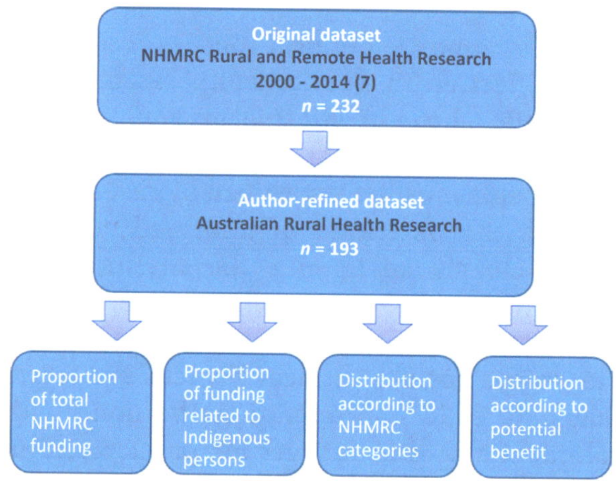

Figure 8.11. Data analysis techniques in public health research.

Source: https://www.researchgate.net/publication/324269559/figure/fig1/AS:612605345398784@1523067904230/Overview-of-data-analysis-method.png.

8.5.1. Statistical Methods for Data Analysis

In epidemiology and public health science, it is critical to have a background in statistical procedures to analyze data. Statistical procedures allow scientists to measure incidence, prevalence, and mortality by quantifiable rates, and these provide scientists with insights into matters of public health. For instance, for chronic diseases such as Chronic Obstructive

Pulmonary Disease (COPD), statistical rates like age-standardized mortality and incidence rates are helpful to characterize trends and patterns over time. Likewise, comparison of these rates with causative risk factors—e.g., smoking and air pollution—gives a clearer disease burden and helps in formulating effective health policies against these causes. With extended statistical analyses, researchers can identify vulnerable groups and ascertain the impact of interventions, thereby linking public health programs to the Sustainable Development Goals outlined in global health agendas (Naeem et al., 2025). Moreover, good data analysis extends beyond mere descriptive statistics; it comprises multivariable models that account for the multifaceted interplay between several health determinants. For example, HIV rates in adolescents and adults in Rakai, Uganda, were analyzed using logistic generalized estimating equations (GEE) and Poisson generalized linear models (GLM) to identify associations between individual and community-level factors. By employing this nuanced approach, researchers are able to examine the impact of interventions like antiretroviral therapy (ART) and voluntary medical male circumcision (VMMC) on health outcomes within specific populations. Through investigating health event trends and correlates, such higher-level statistical methods enable researchers to make actionable findings, informing targeted public health interventions capable of effectively minimizing disease burden among populations (Grilo et al., 2025). Ultimately, the application of rigorous statistical methods within public health research not only enhances validity in findings but also supports evidence-based decision-making. During periods of public health emergencies, immediate data analysis, with speed and accuracy, becomes imperative. Scientists must quickly make sense of trends within the data in order to inform real-time response, direct resource allocation, and shape public health messaging. The integration of real-time data collection and analysis methods allows public health officials to adapt strategies dynamically as they respond to the emergent aspects of health crises. To that purpose, statistical competence is not merely a mental exercise but also a critical skill by which public health practitioners are able to make sense of complexity and achieve better health outcomes for various populations (Naeem et al., 2025; S Grilo et al., 2025) (Figure 8.12).

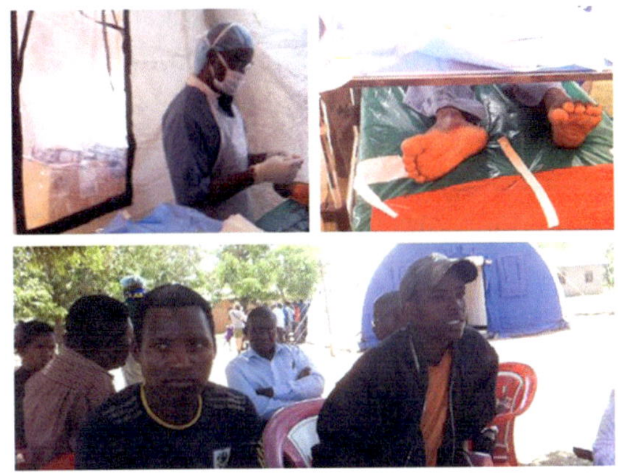

Figure 8.12. Voluntary medical male circumcision in the field.

Source: https://www.intrahealth.org/sites/default/files/styles/max_width_800/public/vital-images/2014-10-15-VMMCHeaderImage_0.jpg?itok=-V6nBRuD.

8.5.2. Software Tools for Data Analysis

In public health research and epidemiology, the application of data analysis software is most crucial in offering evidence for effective interventions and making decisions. The software tools enable the measurement of incidence, prevalence, and death rates, which are important markers for an understanding of public health dynamics. The transition from traditional methods to advanced software products has facilitated more intricate manipulation of data and presentation, all in aid of real-time response to public health emergencies. Software packages SAS, SPSS, and R present advanced statistical capability for the identification of patterns and trends in massive data sets. This technological innovation enhances the ability to generate sound insights from data, something essential in crises when decision-making within an expedient timeline can significantly influence population health outcomes. Furthermore, methods employed in public health research for data collection have also evolved with software development. Electronic data collection systems, such as mobile applications and web surveys, have made it easier to collect health data from diverse populations. These instruments not only increase the efficiency of the data acquisition process but also the quality and accuracy of the information obtained. In settings where there is a need for humanitarian intervention, as much research has shown in recent times, the challenges in data collection in crisis settings raise the importance of well-established analytical tools. Such software programs have the ability to cross logistical barriers, and it becomes feasible to have current health information even in the worst of conditions. Being able to effectively analyze such data allows public health practitioners to respond proactively to current health issues that might originate, thereby improving community health assessments and interventions. The integration of geospatial analysis in computer packages has also revolutionized public health research even more by allowing the examination of geographic disparities in health in datasets. For example, studies on the impact of proximity to healthcare facilities on the incidence of disease have had significant correlations that can be utilized to inform the allocation of resources. As demonstrated in a recent study, analysis of tuberculosis incidence among children living in geographically isolated populations was utilized to demonstrate the way in which access barriers affect outcomes. Geospatial-capable data analysis software enables researchers to spatialize such disparities, leading outreach activities to underserved areas. These are essential in the management of complex public health emergencies in which demographic and spatial elements are intertwined. Effective use of software to process data not only enables one to comprehend its health patterns but also plays an important role in developing strategic public health interventions, thereby ultimately enhancing the resilience of population health (Figure 8.13).

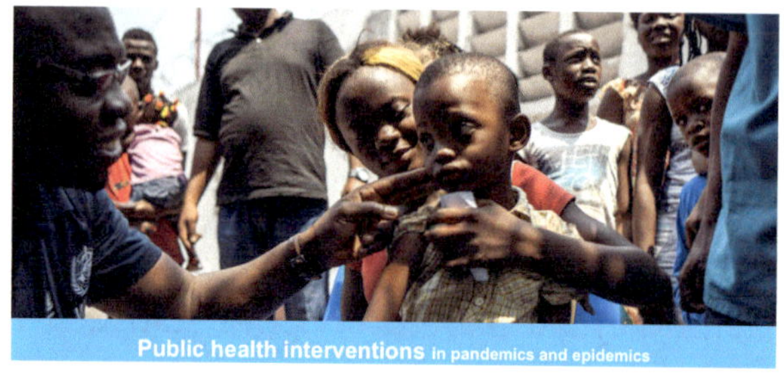

Figure 8.13. Public health interventions and strategies.

Source: https://openwho-public.s3.openhpicloud.de/courses/7lxpM2JVSfswmhKttUZM2L/visual_v3.png.

8.5.3. Interpreting and Presenting Data Findings

Presenting and interpreting findings of data is a critical public health research component, particularly in addressing the frequency and mortality rates of such diseases as oral cancer and HIV/AIDS. Presentation relies on presenting empirical evidence effectively using various presentations such as graphs, tables, and thematic overviews. The worth of graphical aids not only helps to explain but also identifies significant trends that can be less than obvious in unanalyzed data. One such is the result from a scoping review of oral cancer in East Africa, indicating differences in awareness levels, which could easily be represented using comparative bar charts identifying the gaps between populations and professional groups. These visual representations are intended to emphasize the urgency of targeted interventions, thus facilitating an even greater awareness of public health issues that require immediate attention and resources (Aminu et al., 2025). Secondarily, interpretation of data must be situated in the socioecological model to account for the numerous variables that shape health outcomes. For example, the pattern analysis of HIV/AIDS trends among Filipinos shows how age, sex, and occupational exposure, which are demographic variables, dominate epidemiological patterns. It aids researchers in identifying risk groups by employing this approach and designing preventive interventions accordingly. Longitudinal data analysis uncovers time trends, establishing the importance of temporal associations to infer public health policy. The findings indicate that community-based interventions for target groups are crucial because one-size-fits-all approaches may overlook essential dimensions of social dynamics. Hence, effective presentation of the findings enables the stakeholders to comprehend the importance of target interventions for multifaceted communities (Montegrico et al., 2024). Lastly, effective interpretation and presentation of the data should adhere to ethical standards for public health research. This entails ensuring that the outcomes presented truly reflect the information and are free from bias, thereby establishing stakeholder and affected community confidence. Use of comprehensive reviews and systematic reviews allows a robust argument about findings and recommendations. For example, the research by the review of East African oral cancer research warrants urgent public health action towards stopping Toombak consumption, which is a cancer risk factor. Formulating such calls through strategic communication, for instance, policy briefs and community workshops, enhances the effectiveness of the research findings. By this, public health professionals can initiate resources and promote community engagement, eventually leading to improved health outcomes for all at-risk populations (Aminu et al., 2025).

8.6. Addressing Public Health Emergencies

In managing public health emergencies, knowing the incidence and prevalence of a given condition helps in ensuring the best intervention measures are adopted. The information helps public health workers and scientists to allocate resources effectively and intervene in a timely manner. For instance, acute kidney injury (AKI) is a new emerging public health problem in nations such as Mexico, where studies have established a prevalence rate of 35% in hospital inpatients, with resulting mortality rates up to 36% (Jose et al., 2025). Detection of such important health crises calls for a coordinated effort from healthcare providers, policymakers, and community organizations to enhance patient outcomes and reduce mortality. Failure to handle such emergencies can result in enhanced morbidity and overburdened healthcare systems, ultimately eroding public trust and the effectiveness of future health initiatives. Moreover, management of public health crises entails inclusive community health reviews to detect precise risk factors affecting disease transmission. For instance, in Uganda, HIV incidence in adolescents and young adults by a decade had been decreased by large margins due to strategic public health programming, such as the expanded access to antiretroviral therapy (ART) and voluntary medical male circumcision (VMMC) (Grilo et al., 2025). These community-level interventions addressed not only individual health but also helped to create broader societal awareness and support. Through the use of community information in public health emergency measurement, stakeholders are able to inform evidence-based prevention and optimize health resources. Communities are more likely to engage actively in health promotion programs when they are informed and engaged. Quality data collection and analysis are essential in guiding responses to public health emergencies.

Reliability of data is the foundation of effective surveillance systems and health interventions. Good data collection enables continuous monitoring of disease patterns, and this helps public health practitioners respond actively to emerging threats.

For AKI in Mexico, systematic reviews and meta-analyses have presented key epidemiological results that must be tackled across various levels of care (Jose et al., 2025). Similarly, the Rakai Community Cohort Study points to the necessity of constant monitoring of data to uncover information on HIV dynamics among communities. This integrated approach to data collection and analysis not only informs emergency response strategy but also builds the groundwork for preventive action that minimizes future public health crises. Continuous institutionalization of strict research in public health practice enhances overall community emergency resilience (Figure 8.14).

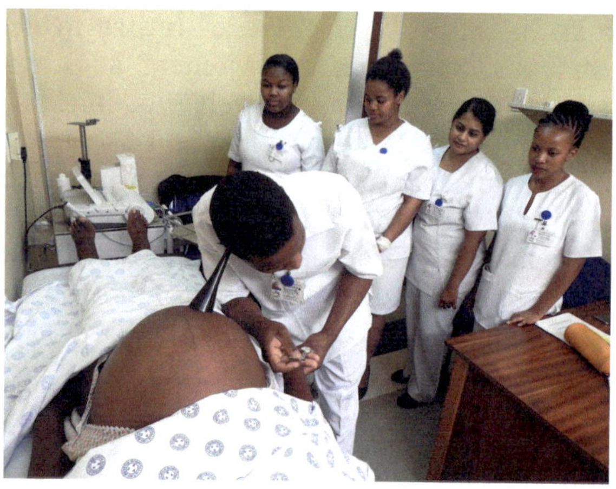

Figure 8.14. Same-day antiretroviral therapy (ART) initiation in pregnancy.

Source: https://icap.columbia.edu/tools_resources/same-day-antiretroviral-therapy-art-initiation-in-pregnancy-is-not-associated-with-viral-suppression-or-engagement-in-care-a-cohort-study/.

8.6.1. Definition and Types of Public Health Emergencies

Public health emergencies are serious events that necessitate early interventions by health authorities, governments, and communities. The emergencies usually result from infectious disease outbreaks, natural or human-made disasters, or sudden spikes in health indicators above baseline levels. The World Health Organization (WHO) categorizes public health emergencies as risks that present an imminent threat to health and, therefore, the need for immediate interventions to mitigate their impact on populations. Such emergencies can come in various forms, such as epidemics, natural disasters, bioterrorism, and pandemics. It is important to differentiate among various categories of emergencies in a bid to develop effective prevention and response measures, since the nature of each public health emergency could play a significant role in the effectiveness of interventions. Among the broad categories of public health crises, infectious disease outbreaks are unique owing to their high potential for transmission and mortality rates. The current COVID-19 pandemic is a prime example of a public health crisis that required the deployment of global health authorities and activation of resources to put containment in place in a timely manner. These interventions involved contact tracing and community health surveys where epidemiologists gathered data on incidence and prevalence to inform public health interventions. Practice guidelines laid out in international guidance documents, such as the management of severe acute respiratory infection, underscore the absolute necessity of solid surveillance and prompt intervention in stemming the disease transmission (Organization, 2020). Such measures are of supreme relevance in countering the present public health menace as well as potential future outbreaks. Apart from infectious disease hazards, non-infectious emergencies such as environmental disasters and natural disasters also make big contributions to public health. Natural disasters like industrial explosions, floods, and hurricanes can cause large-scale injuries and fatalities and thus require complex disaster relief processes. Non-infectious emergencies typically exacerbate existing health inequalities, and public health researchers must conduct comprehensive community surveys to identify vulnerabilities. Data collection methods during the aftermath are important in determining health outcomes and the implementation of interventions needed. For instance, public health authorities can employ geographic information systems (GIS) to analyze spatial data in health service accessibility and environmental health hazards. The effectiveness of such assessments has a direct bearing on how communities prepare for and respond to pending emergencies, thus demonstrating the interconnectedness of epidemiological research and public health practice (Zeppenfeld et al., 2022).

8.6.2. Response Strategies and Protocols

Effective response strategies and protocols are at the forefront of public health crisis control, ensuring speedy and coordinated action in alleviating adverse health impacts. Strategic management of public health is concerned with putting in place effective structures that provide guidance when making decisions under pressure. One essential component of these frameworks is the identification of key stakeholders, for instance, local health authorities, community organizations, and healthcare providers who must coordinate and work together effectively to implement response actions. For instance, during health emergencies such as infectious disease outbreaks, these coordination activities draw on real-time data and data analysis to facilitate interventions. Early detection and timely response not only reduce incidence rates but also enhance the general resilience of the community in responding to health threats. In this light, incorporating existing management theories, such as those highlighted by the Resource-based Theory and Porter Diamond Theory, can inform the development of effective mechanisms of response (Amico et al., 2024). In rural settings, understanding the different epidemiological profiles of populations is crucial to the successful adaptation of response protocols. A recent piece of research on valvular heart disease (VHD) has highlighted the different presentations and management needs in such areas, which could easily be overlooked by urban-prejudiced health infrastructure. By way of community health screening and proactive assessment, public health practitioners can identify the populations at risk and apply evidence-based interventions aimed at solving discovered health issues. The lack of pertinent and comprehensive data from rural communities makes the need for individually tailored data collection and analysis methods, as well as response strategies, even more imperative. Engagement of the local populations not only enhances the relevance of health interventions but also promotes ownership and sustainability. Such localized efforts can lead to the establishment of effective response systems for addressing unique rural health needs and thereby closing the gaps in public health surveillance and response (Amico et al., 2024). Besides, strategic planning is necessary to ensure the activation of response mechanisms that appropriately respond to the nuances of public health emergencies. This necessity is best exemplified in the recent study on the management of tuberculosis (TB) in Kenya through the engagement between strategic management and effective health interventions. The development of standard operating plans backed by comprehensive training and resource planning is essential to ensure consistency in TB case-finding activities and overall public health programs. Notably, mobilizing multidisciplinary technical teams and building interagency collaborative networks can enhance community outreach and improve service delivery, particularly for vulnerable and marginalized groups. In the context of emerging new health issues, enhancing response systems through the integration of technological advancements in gathering and analyzing data will be essential in public health systems. These enhancements guarantee more responsive and effective processes, consequently leading to better health outcomes across populations (Angala et al., 2024) (Figure 8.15).

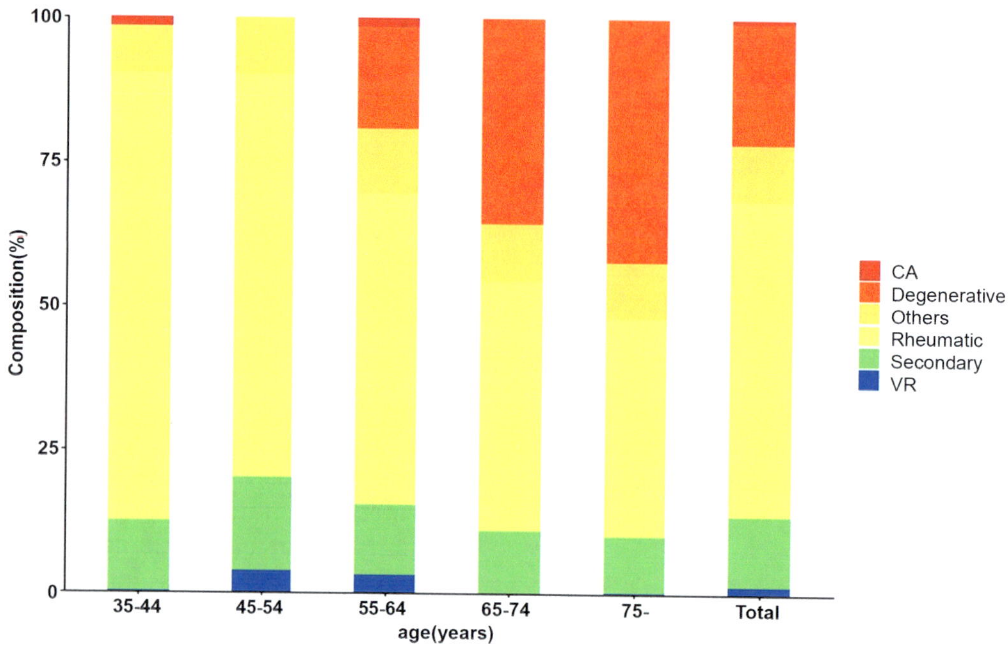

Figure 8.15. Etiology of valvular heart disease.

Source: https://media.springernature.com/lw685/springer-static/image/art%3A10.1186%2Fs12872-021-02154-8/MediaObjects/12872_2021_2154_Fig1_HTML.png.

8.6.3. Role of Communication in Emergency Management

Effective communication plays a central role in emergency management, especially during public health emergencies when information release can mean the difference between life and death. An effective communication strategy helps to provide accurate information about the nature and extent of the emergency to communities. Through the integration of incidence, prevalence, and mortality data, emergency management practitioners can design their messaging across groups, addressing specific vulnerabilities and needs of the targeted groups. For instance, when there is an outbreak, public health officials must be able to relay important information on measures of prevention, symptoms, and available healthcare facilities. Such collective effort can minimize panic and disorientation, establishing confidence between the authority and the people (Association AL, 2001). Furthermore, emergency communication is also made easier by established protocols and technologies, which enable agencies and stakeholders to share information in a timely fashion, as necessary for effective decision-making and resource allocation. Community engagement during emergencies strongly relies on the efficacy of communication efforts. When vulnerable groups are integrated into the communication process, opportunities for compliance with public health measures significantly increase. Emergency managers will need to work to produce culturally appropriate and accessible messages, which involves an understanding of the dynamics of the community and the barriers to communication. Where air pollution, as it is seen, disproportionately affects low-income and minority ethnic communities in cities, outreach is essential (Association AL, 2001). Using several channels of communication such as social media, local media, and community organizations, public health officials can reach a large population. Regular updates not only inform the public well but also allow individuals to practice preventive measures, thereby leading to enhanced public health responses in case of emergencies. Finally, the role played by communication in achieving effective management of incidents encompasses not only crisis response in emergencies but also post-emergency planning and evaluation. Engaging communities in conversation after an emergency may yield a good source of information concerning the experience with communication approaches employed. This reflective process allows public health professionals to identify gaps in information delivery and areas for improvement in future preparedness plans. Open communication with stakeholders and public health practitioners also aids in developing best practices in data collection and analysis to ensure that lessons learned are adequately addressed. Through this loop of feedback, emergency management will be able to improve and fortify its response, creating a resilient public health structure that is capable of responding well to future events.

CLOSER LOOK

DIVISIONS OF EPIDEMIOLOGY

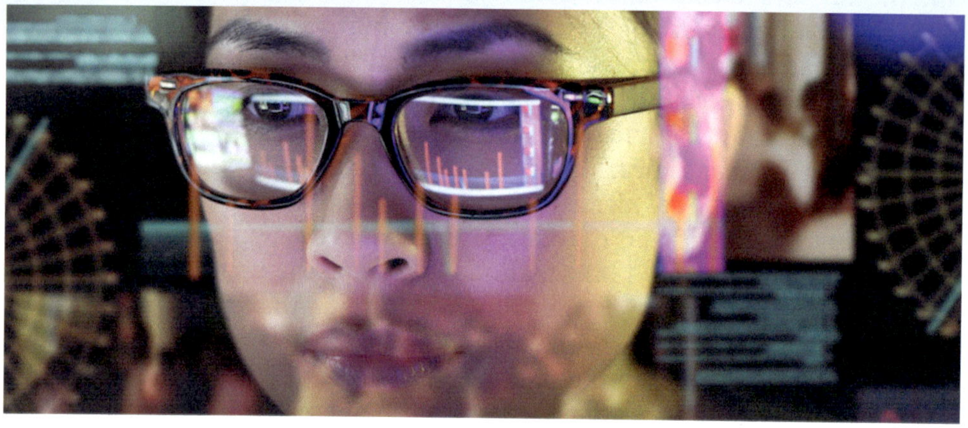

Figure 8.16. Researcher analyzing complex health data for epidemiological insights.

Source: https://www.mayo.edu/research/departments-divisions/quantitative-health-sciences/divisions/epidemiology/overview.

Divisions of Epidemiology refer to the various branches or subdisciplines within the field that examine various aspects of disease and health across populations. Divisions are used to help researchers and public health practitioners understand the distribution, causes, and prevention of diseases. Descriptive Epidemiology is one of the largest divisions and discusses the "who, what, when, and where" of disease patterns. It is the collection and analysis of data to identify trends and risk groups that serves as the foundation for further study.

Another central branch is Analytical Epidemiology, focused on "how and why" disease occurs. It utilizes comparative studies—cohort, case-control, and randomized trials—to study causal relationships between exposures and health problems. This branch is crucial to determine risk factors and validate the effectiveness of interventions. Clinical Epidemiology applies these principles to patient management and decision-making in the clinical setting, making medical practices evidence-based and sensitive to population demands.

Field Epidemiology consists of on-the-scene public health investigations during emergencies or outbreaks. Field epidemiologists are typically sent out to identify sources of disease and interrupt transmission in the early stages. Molecular and Genetic Epidemiology is a more recent discipline that examines the interaction of genetic susceptibility and environmental exposures to disease occurrence, using molecular biology methods to uncover disease mechanisms. Social Epidemiology examines how social structure and behavior and inequalities influence the health outcomes of populations.

These all subdivisions collectively facilitate a clear view of health at individual and population levels, which improves planning, prevention, and response actions in public health.

SUMMARY

Public health and epidemiology studies are core fields of inquiry that provide crucial data for determining trends in health and responses to community needs. Incidence, prevalence, and mortality rates analysis provide researchers and policymakers with significant information about disease burden. Studies, such as those on acute kidney injury (AKI) in Mexico, show the importance of integrated data collection methods that can be applied for the purpose of specific interventions toward the prevention of health emergencies (Jose et al., 2025). Through the systematic analysis of trends and determinants of health events, public health practitioners are capable of establishing measures that target vulnerable populations and improve health outcomes at a general level. Therefore, continued focus on epidemiological studies is essential to enhance readiness for and response to public health emergencies. In addition, conducting community health assessments is an essential component in developing effective public health policy. By conducting such assessments, practitioners can gather qualitative and quantitative data about health needs, preferences, and barriers in specific populations. For instance, emerging trends in the incidence of HIV in the Philippines suggest that groups such as overseas workers and sex workers require focused preventive interventions (Montegrico et al., 2024). Public health research involving community participation fosters a culture of participation in which interventions are locally relevant and accessible. This participation is required for promoting health equity, as well as for enabling communities to solve arising health challenges together. Lastly, addressing public health crises demands the intersection of efficient data collection mechanisms and meticulous analysis. Utilization of multiple data sources offers insights into health dynamics and is applied in decision-making by the stakeholders. Scholars identify that clinical evidence determines the interventions and emphasize the need for training healthcare professionals who can apply epidemiological information (Montegrico et al., 2024). Therefore, investing in public health research and evidence-based practice is essential to making our health systems resilient for future crises. Investing resources in this vital work helps us build resilient communities that can transcend health inequities and attain sustainable health gains.

Epidemiology has a central role in public health research, particularly with regard to the concepts of incidence, prevalence, and mortality. These are vital in assessing the state of health of populations and informing public health intervention and planning. Incidence refers to the frequency of new cases of disease over a period, while prevalence refers to the total number of cases at a point in time, leading to the disease burden. Mortality is concerned with the death rates caused by diseases, which are essential for assessing the impact of public health programs. These indicators need to be measurably quantified and processed to enable efficient resource deployment as well as track health outcomes in the long term. As highlighted in earlier evidence, public health information quality is of utmost importance but remains hindered by various context-specific challenges that need to be addressed to allow for enhanced public health research outcomes (Checchi et al., 2017). Community health assessment is an essential public health research phase that allows researchers to identify the health needs and resources in specific populations. These assessments incorporate data collection methods that might involve surveys, interviews, and focus groups to capture a general snapshot of the health environment of the community. Through the assessment of determinants of health such as socioeconomic status, healthcare access, and risk behavior factors, public health practitioners are able to design interventions specifically designed to meet the special needs of the community. Effective community health assessment is the foundation for the design of targeted public health interventions and mobilizing stakeholders to achieve collaborative outcomes. Further, the use of multiple data collection methods ensures credibility and reliability of results, and thus improves health outcomes in populations (N/A). Public health crises require prompt and concerted intervention to prevent the impact on health and the loss of resources. Central to this is the application of robust systems for surveillance and data collection that provide timely intelligence about health trends during disasters. These systems enable public health practitioners to grasp the scale of the emergency, deploy required resources, and determine the impact of intervention. The Disaster Preparedness and Response Training Course shows that competency in swift needs assessments and disaster surveillance methodologies must be developed. This targeted training of health workers supports improved public health emergency awareness and enhances the ability to respond effectively. Through the integration of such training elements into public health practice, community resilience as a whole to public health emergencies can be improved, and crisis preparation can be increased (N/A).

REFERENCES

1. Adefemi, A., Ukpoju, E. A., Adekoya, O., Abatan, A., & Adegbite, A. O. (2023). Artificial intelligence in environmental health and public safety: A comprehensive review of USA strategies. *World Journal of Advanced Research and Reviews*. https://www.semanticscholar.org/paper/2d4b99d56bac1454d7801e337b7a1b47beff6a49 (accessed on 11th June 2025).
2. Aldus, C., Arthur, A., Brayne, C., et al. (2020). Undiagnosed dementia in primary care: A record linkage study. https://core.ac.uk/download/305118448.pdf (accessed on 11th June 2025).
3. American Lung Association. (2001). *Urban Air Pollution and Health Inequities: A Workshop Report*. https://core.ac.uk/download/323074325.pdf (accessed on 11th June 2025).
4. Amico, M. A., Busi, G., Vannini, M., Bruscoli, F., Marchionni, N., Boccanelli, A., & Carrabba, N. (2024). PREVASC: Prospective registry of epidemiology of valve disease in asymptomatic Italian subjects. *European Journal of Preventive Cardiology*. https://www.semanticscholar.org/paper/20f61ef140a7c2387088b102886cfc60aa25ffe8 (accessed on 11th June 2025).
5. Aminu, K., Aladelusi, T. O., Adisa, A., Ezeagu, C. N., Salami, A., Nwafor, J., Uwambaye, P., et al. (2025). Epidemiology, literacy, risk factors, and clinical status of oral cancer in East Africa: A scoping review. *PLOS ONE, 20*. https://www.semanticscholar.org/paper/ab1fe497decdbb3438c8190f337203fbda180ab3 (accessed on 11th June 2025).
6. Angala, P., Abongo, B., & Masinde, D. (2024). An assessment on the application of the Porter Diamond Model aspects within tuberculosis treatment healthcare facilities in Nairobi County, Kenya. *The International Journal of Business & Management*. https://www.semanticscholar.org/paper/d204691d84890f51b071191a2015795dfff78a71 (accessed on 11th June 2025).
7. Anonymous, Jensen, H. H., & Unnevehr, L. J. (2025). *Tracking Foodborne Pathogens from Farm to Table: Data Needs to Evaluate Control Options*. https://core.ac.uk/download/pdf/6551081.pdf (accessed on 11th June 2025).
8. Armstrong, B., Guo, Y., Jaakkola, J. J. K., et al. (2012). Extremely cold and hot temperatures increase the risk of ischemic heart disease mortality: Epidemiological evidence from China.
9. Atnkut, B., Nigussie, A., Kumera, B., Tsega, A., Tiruneh, F., Minale, W. K., Anemut, F., et al. (2025). Factors influencing solid waste management practices and challenges in Awi Administrative Zone, Northwestern Ethiopia. *BioMed Research International, 2025*. https://www.semanticscholar.org/paper/4d3fc79f04c31910596964bb4259836031d17d40 (accessed on 11th June 2025).
10. Babulal, G. M., Quiroz, Y. T., Albensi, B. C., Arenaza-Urquijo, E. M., Astell, A., Babiloni, C., Bahar-Fuchs, A., et al. (2018). Perspectives on ethnic and racial disparities in Alzheimer's disease and related dementias: Update and areas of immediate need. *Alzheimer's & Dementia, 15*, 292–312. https://doi.org/10.1016/j.jalz.2018.09.009 (accessed on 11th June 2025).
11. Brodbelt, D. C., Church, D. B., McGreevy, P. D., et al. (2014). Approaches to canine health surveillance. https://core.ac.uk/download/36777547.pdf (accessed on 11th June 2025).
12. Checchi, F., Polonsky, J., Prudhon, C., et al. (2017). Public health information in crisis-affected populations: A review of methods and their use for advocacy and action. https://core.ac.uk/download/96626534.pdf (accessed on 11th June 2025).

13. Condray, R., & Devine, K. (2017). *Behavioral and Mental Health in Nevada*. https://digitalscholarship.unlv.edu/cgi/viewcontent.cgi?article=1057&context=social_health_nevada_reports (accessed on 11th June 2025).

14. Croisant, S. P., Bohn, K., Pennel, C., Tumilty, E., Hallmark, C., & Tobon, P. (2025). 261 Driving community health and mental health programming through collaborative, ongoing community health needs assessments. Journal of Clinical and Translational Science, 9, 80–81. https://www.semanticscholar.org/paper/0f18e771107a973e9a180ca22d700071bd59f20d (accessed on 11th June 2025).

15. Cummings, M. J., Baldwin, M. R., Abrams, D., Jacobson, S. D., Meyer, B. J., Balough, E. M., Aaron, J. G., et al. (2020). Epidemiology, clinical course, and outcomes of critically ill adults with COVID-19 in New York City: A prospective cohort study. *The Lancet, 395*, 1763–1770. https://doi.org/10.1016/s0140-6736(20)31189-2 (accessed on 11th June 2025).

16. D'Ambrosio, F., Lomazzi, M., Moore, M., Maida, A., Ricciardi, R., Munno, L., Lettieri, M., et al. (2025). Addressing the underestimated burden of RSV in older adults in Europe: Epidemiology, surveillance gaps, and public health implications. *Vaccines*. https://www.semanticscholar.org/paper/67981945b24184f9c5aafd56da0de02ed0425801 (accessed on 11th June 2025).

17. Dlamini, M., Msolo, L., Ebomah, K. E., Nontongana, N., & Okoh, A. I. (2024). A systematic review on the incidence of influenza viruses in wastewater matrices: Implications for public health. *PLOS ONE, 19*. https://www.semanticscholar.org/paper/cb718695b745e075e30de59f7c458d9d9f8b3df9 (accessed on 11th June 2025)

18. Frerks, G., Huber, D., Klot, J., M'Boup, et al. (2010). *HIV/AIDS, Security and Conflict: New Realities, New Responses*. https://core.ac.uk/download/pdf/29237791.pdf (accessed on 11th June 2025).

19. Gostin, L. O., Hardcastle, L. E., Jacobson, P. D., et al. (2011). *Restoring Health to Health Reform: Integrating Medicine and Public Health to Advance the Population's Wellbeing*. https://core.ac.uk/download/70374138.pdf (accessed on 11th June 2025).

20. Grilo, S., Thompson, J., Chen, I., Nalugoda, F., Lutalo, T., Wei, Y., Spindler, E., et al. (2025). Declines in HIV incidence and prevalence and predictors among adolescents and young adults: An observational cohort study, Rakai, Uganda, 2005–2020. medRxiv: The Preprint Server for Health Sciences. https://www.semanticscholar.org/paper/10fd499140105c77af2b37a6d0f8e14f1dda128c (accessed on 11th June 2025).

21. Kruk, M. E., Gage, A., Arsenault, C., Jordan, K., Leslie, H. H., Roder-DeWan, S., Adeyi, O., et al. (2018). High-quality health systems in the Sustainable Development Goals era: Time for a revolution. *The Lancet Global Health, 6*, e1196–e1252. https://doi.org/10.1016/s2214-109x(18)30386-3 (accessed on 11th June 2025).

22. Lampugnale, C. A. (2017). *Surgical Assessment of The Geriatric Oncology Patient*. https://open.bu.edu/bitstream/2144/26707/5/Lampugnale_bu_0017N_13146.pdf (accessed on 11th June 2025).

23. Mansourian, H. (2020). *Measuring Separation of Children from Their Usual Caregivers in Humanitarian Contexts: The Case for A Holistic Approach to Measurement, With Implications for Practice*. https://core.ac.uk/download/287655156.pdf (accessed on 11th June 2025).

24. Meirawati, D., & Priyani, T. (2024). Factors related to the incidence of pneumonia in toddlers at Karangrejo Metro Utara Community Health Center. *Journal Kesehatan Metro Sai Wawai*.

https://www.semanticscholar.org/paper/32a06c64f5580e3c2c7dbab38e3744d2a4f4ca3c (accessed on 11th June 2025).

25. Montegrico, J., Lee, J., & De Los Santos, J. A. A. (2024). A 13-year trend analysis of HIV epidemiology in the Philippines (2010 to 2022). *Journal of Community Health Nursing, 41*, 226–240. https://www.semanticscholar.org/paper/c17e00607fc67952fded37b589f001c2d7ead49c (accessed on 11th June 2025).

26. Mullings, A., McFarland, A., Leanord, A., Ross, E., Mason, H., Reilly, J., Ritchie, L., et al. (2019). How do we evaluate the cost of nosocomial infection? The ECONI protocol: An incidence study with nested case-control evaluating cost and quality of life. https://core.ac.uk/download/293866892.pdf (accessed on 11th June 2025)

27. Munson, E., Munson, K. L., & Napierala, M. (2016). *Update on Laboratory Diagnosis and Epidemiology of Trichomonas Vaginalis: You Can Teach An "Old" Dog "New" Trichs*. https://core.ac.uk/download/213085579.pdf (accessed on 11th June 2025).

28. Naeem, S., Wang, F., Mubarak, R., Shen, H., Li, X., Mommers, I., Hussain, S. R., et al. (2025). Mapping the global distribution, risk factors, and temporal trends of COPD incidence and mortality (1990–2021): Ecological analysis. BMC Medicine, 23. https://www.semanticscholar.org/paper/282e527dbf6c76e3973f581203ebe26ad9752ea3 (accessed on 11th June 2025).

29. Onak, E. T. T., Odongo, A., & Kariuki, J. G. (2024). Sociocultural factors influencing utilization of reproductive health services in selected South Sudan public health facilities. *International Journal of Community Medicine and Public Health*. https://www.semanticscholar.org/paper/9a6e14334fc3c28f92d6bdbef18ea4647ae330d7 (accessed on 11th June 2025).

30. Swift, M. (2001). Public health burden of cancer in ataxia-telangiectasia heterozygotes. *Journal of the National Cancer Institute, 93(2)*, 84–85. https://www.semanticscholar.org/paper/493004ed22e654545256ac2501715b591f1d9245 (accessed on 11th June 2025).

31. Taher, A. A. M. A. (2024). Major risk factor for cervical cancer in rural area: How to reduce its incidence along mortality rate. *IAR Journal of Medicine and Surgery Research*. https://www.semanticscholar.org/paper/a8b89bcbcdcad3a69d49cf32f5dcf91595d5273c (accessed on 11th June 2025).

32. Ul, R., Amin, B. T., Bakhtiar, S. M., & Ul Islam, S. (2025). Advances and challenges in cervical cancer: From molecular mechanisms and global epidemiology to innovative therapies and prevention strategies. Cancer Control: Journal of the Moffitt Cancer Center, 32. https://www.semanticscholar.org/paper/2527ce58b2a872dbb376d73d6874fafbf3e02fbc (accessed on 11th June 2025).

33. World Health Organization. (2020). Clinical management of severe acute respiratory infection (SARI) when COVID-19 disease is suspected. Interim guidance. Pediatria I Medycyna Rodzinna, 16, 9–26. https://doi.org/10.15557/pimr.2020.0003 (accessed on 11th June 2025).

34. Yerramalla, M. S., Fayosse, A., Dugravot, A., Tabák, Á., Kivimäki, M., Singh-Manoux, A., & Sabia, S. (2019). Association of moderate and vigorous physical activity with incidence of type 2 diabetes and subsequent mortality: 27 year follow-up of the Whitehall II study. *Diabetologia, 63*, 537–548. https://www.semanticscholar.org/paper/7439df629f31fecccf41e5df3a2bc25fba715825 (accessed on 11th June 2025).

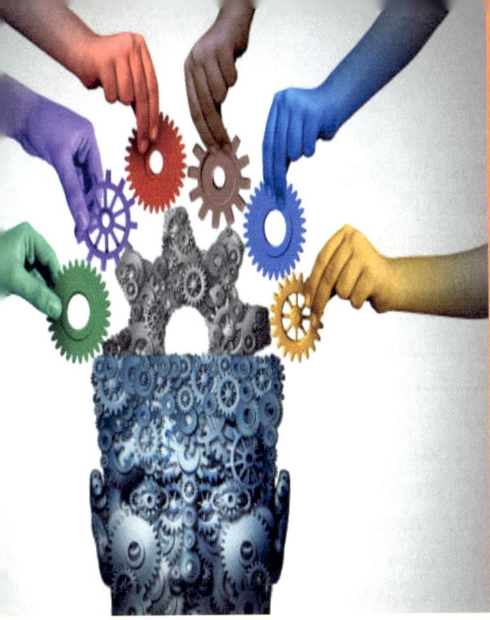

Chapter 9

MENTAL HEALTH IN THE COMMUNITY

Contents

Introduction

Conceptualizing mental health is a multi-dimensional task that is increasingly falling into place, particularly in the context of community health. Mental health is emotional, psychological, and social well-being, which impacts how individuals think, feel, and act. In contrast, mental illness refers to diagnosable disorders that include alterations in thinking, mood, or behavior that significantly impact daily functioning. While society continues to grapple with the long-term effects of the COVID-19 pandemic, there has been a sharp rise in mental health issues that have driven the need for effective community-based interventions. Fulfilling these needs entails a multipronged approach that involves understanding individual experiences around mental illness but is also actively involved in promoting mental wellness and resilience in community settings. Promoting mental health literacy lies at the core of constructing supportive environments and eliminating the stigmatization of mental illness. As noted by the current evidence, the psychological effects of the COVID-19 pandemic have manifested as instances of various mental health conditions, further corroborating the urgency for community-based mental health care. It is documented that individuals have experienced higher levels of depression, anxiety, and stress as a result of social isolation, economic uncertainty, and poor health (Giorgi et al., 2020). This demographic shift represents a turning point for the delivery of community-based mental health services and in-home interventions. Such services may range from resilience training sessions to peer support networks aimed at establishing connections among individuals and bridging gaps in access to mental health care. Fostering a culture of compassion and understanding, communities may become protective factors that deter the escalation of mental health issues, eventually enhancing the lives of those affected. In addition to promoting mental well-being, an integral component of maintaining mental health within the community is countering the stigma generally associated with mental illness. Stigma can deter treatment seeking, increase feelings of isolation, and perpetuate undesired attitudes in society toward mental health (Hossain et al., 2020). Stigma reduction must be multifaceted, incorporating education, advocacy, and direct community engagement. Through providing a stronger voice to those who have experiences, communities can desensitize their people from myths and facilitate an atmosphere of acceptance. It is essential that mental health campaigns be made to address diverse populations, hence ensuring inclusivity. Thus, discussing mental health in the community not only improves the welfare of individuals but also helps in building a resilient society that can tolerate crises as well as conform to times of growth (Figure 9.1).

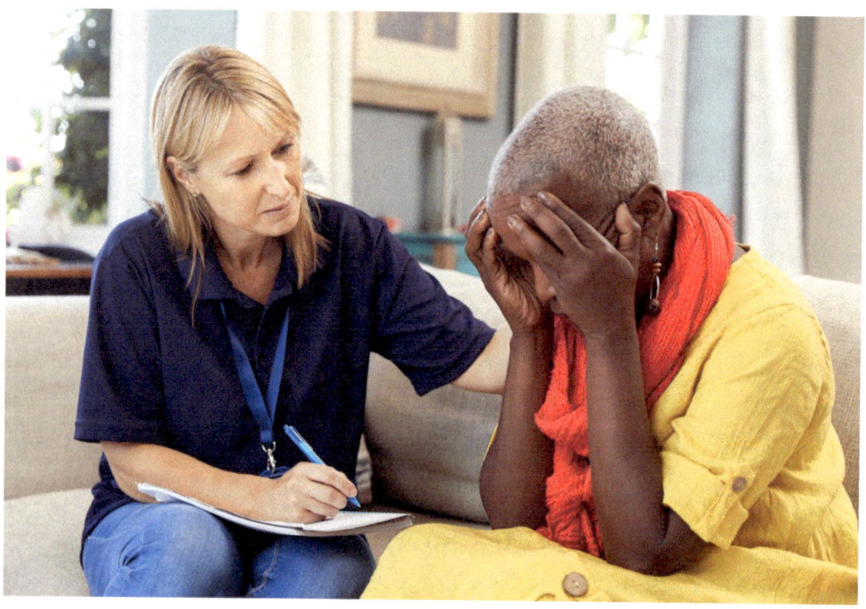

Figure 9.1. Community-mental-health.

Source: https://www.awaresociety.bc.ca/wp-content/uploads/2021/09/Community-Mental-Health-1280x854.jpg.

Definition of Mental Health

Mental health is a complex interplay of psychological, emotional, and social well-being that essentially dictates the way individuals think, feel, and act. Furthermore, mental health also has an important role in dictating how one copes with stress, relates to others, and makes significant life decisions. The World Health Organization has defined mental health as a state where individuals can fulfill their potential, can cope with life's usual stresses, can work effectively, and can contribute positively to society. This is a change of focus to emphasize wellness and resilience over the mere lack of mental illness. It stresses the need to take preventive actions in order to attain mental stability, which, as part of community schemes of health, can help build an environment supporting overall psychological well-being. Community-based mental health services play a vital role in defining and promoting mental health by integrating local support mechanisms and resources. Their importance exists in their coverage and ability to meet the particular needs of respective populations. By prioritizing prevention and intervention at the initial stages, community programs are able to act on mental health issues while they are not as severe. Programs that provide education, low-cost counseling, and peer support networks are a must. They serve as preventatives and means of developing resilience in communities because individuals learn and assist one another in shared experiences. Besides, these services incline to place emphasis on cultural appropriateness, ensuring that practice in mental health is according to the values and experience of community members to ensure effective engagement and effectiveness. The development of ideas such as moral injury shows the advancement in the understanding of mental health, particularly in specific populations such as military members. Since the stress resulting from behavior that is antithetical to one's moral standards, moral injury illustrates that mental illness can result from influences outside of the traditional social psychological frameworks. As research in the area is further developed, it is illustrated that mental illness cannot be cut off from the social and cultural contexts within which it occurs, as reflected in studies of the impact of trauma on soldiers and civilian reintegration. Furthermore, the recognition of moral injury necessitates the bridging of the gap between extant mental health interventions and the unique presentation of individuals experiencing moral dilemmas. This stretching of mental health necessitates a holistic strategy that synthesizes disparate experiences and narratives, thus promoting expansive understanding in community contexts (Claudia et al., 2019; Brandon et al., 2019) (Figure 9.2).

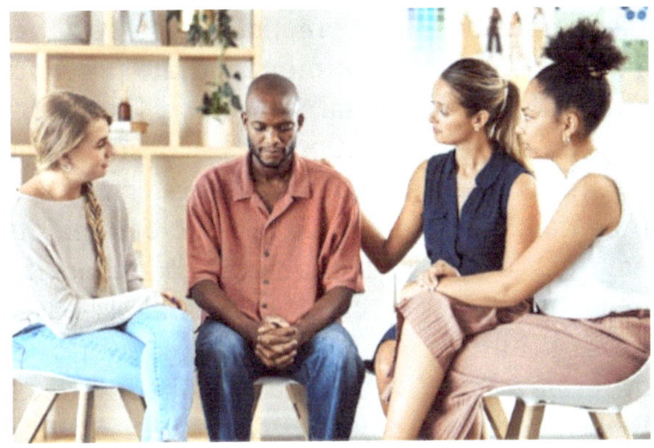

Figure 9.2. Support group session providing emotional care and community-based mental health assistance.

Source: https://external-content.duckduckgo.com/iu/?u=https%3A%2F%2Fimg.freepik.com%2Fpremium-photo%2Fgroup-therapy-support-mental-health-community-comfort-sad-black-man-with-anxiety- depression-stress-diversity -friends-women-people-c ounseling- psychology-trust-meeting-help_590464-85077.jpg&f= 1&nofb=1&ipt=ab0f58e5541667ca13479b0a48adbcf51db 9ea0e4816049d ff5413ef1a7fc761.

Importance of Mental Health in the Community

The importance of mental health among the community cannot be overstressed, particularly in recent years, given the challenges of the COVID-19 pandemic. The pandemic has fueled an increased rate of mental illnesses, particularly among children and youth, who are being subjected to unprecedented levels of pressure and stress as witnessed by teachers across Ontario. Teachers have indicated a notable rise in mental health problems among learners, which has led to urgent questions about their ability to engage constructively with the curriculum despite experiencing psychological pain. Detection of such challenges highlights the need for inclusive community support systems prioritizing mental health literacy among teachers and caregivers. By giving them the data and tools necessary to understand and manage mental illness, societies can cultivate environments that promote resilience and emotional well-being. This focus on treatment and education can be considered an essential step to addressing the long-term effects of mental illness on individuals and community health as a whole. In addition to enhancing mental health literacy, enabling community-based mental health service accessibility is critical in addressing the diverse needs of people with mental health problems. Organizational-led programs, such as career and technical student organizations (CTSOs), are the leading locations for youth involvement in mental health awareness. These programs not only equip students with the authority to recognize early warning signs of mental illness but also provide them with opportunities for leadership that can promote greater civic engagement. The involvement of youth in these programs highlights proactive means through which communities can become involved in constructing support networks that not only consider intervention but also prevention. By developing resilience through the establishment of supportive peer environments, community mental health services can offset dangers posed by mental illnesses among varied populations, ultimately adding to increased overall community well-being and integration. De-stigmatization of mental illness is also a critical element in the promotion of community-level mental wellness. Stigmatization has the effect of causing individuals to feel stigmatized and avoid seeking help for their mental illness. Community initiatives to make individuals more knowledgeable about mental illness issues and treatment-seeking as a norm can promote greater open discussion in society. Producing materials, such as mental health manuals aimed at teachers, is designed to enhance education on mental illness symptoms and intervention. The resources also address the discomfort teachers can experience with talking about mental illness among students, a concern in numerous studies. By fostering spaces that promote understanding and empathy, society can break down the stigmas that act as hindrances for people to access the important systems of support. In doing so, this emphasis on de-stigmatization not only promotes the affected but also mobilizes community cohesion, strengthening the collective resilience against mental illness that occurs.

9.1. Understanding Mental Health

Mental health encompasses a broad spectrum of variables that result in both mental wellness and the presence of mental illness. Mental health is not just defined by the lack of mental disorders, but also by emotional balance, flexibility, and stress tolerance. An integrated approach acknowledges that individuals' mental health is influenced by a multifaceted set of contextual circumstances, including economic, social, and environmental factors. For marginalized groups, such as gay, bisexual, and other men who have sex with men (GBMSM), the influences are particularly powerful. Syndemics theory, which provides us with insight into the interrelatedness of more than one negative health outcome within social contexts, teaches us about the particular problems these individuals face. This suggests that social stigmatization and isolation can exacerbate mental illness, and that interventions must address both the mental illness and structural factors underpinning it (Ferlatte et al., 2020). Promoting mental well-being and resilience is about building interventions within communities that are enabling and ones that develop support networks. Community cohesion is a crucial aspect of enhancing mental health outcomes since people benefit from the ability to identify with others who share similar experiences and concerns. Effective community programs are likely to be based on salutogenic approaches, which emphasize strengths and assets within communities rather than deficits. Activities in such programs may involve mental health education, peer support groups, and skills-building workshops designed to enhance coping and resilience. By encouraging environments where individuals feel accepted and supported, communities can reduce cases of negative mental health outcomes and enhance the resilience of their members. Such programs are crucial in mitigating the ill effects of stigma and discrimination, which have been demonstrated to be linked with poor health outcomes among marginalized populations (N/A, 2023). To become effective in understanding and addressing mental health at the community level, stigma reduction along with mental health promotion needs to be adopted. Stigma not just discourages individuals from coming out for assistance but also sustains adverse health outcomes and solitude. Public campaigns that work against myths of mental illness and offer individual experiences of recovery can be a game-changer. School programs that include demystifying mental health issues and fostering empathy can facilitate increased acceptance for the affected. Furthermore, community interventions that ensure a collaboration between social and mental health professionals and local residents can assist in fashioning approaches that appeal especially well to target populations. By positioning mental health goals within broader social justice movements and community resources, stakeholders can construct a culture of support that optimizes mental health and resilience across diverse community landscapes (Ferlatte et al., 2020; N/A, 2023) (Figure 9.3).

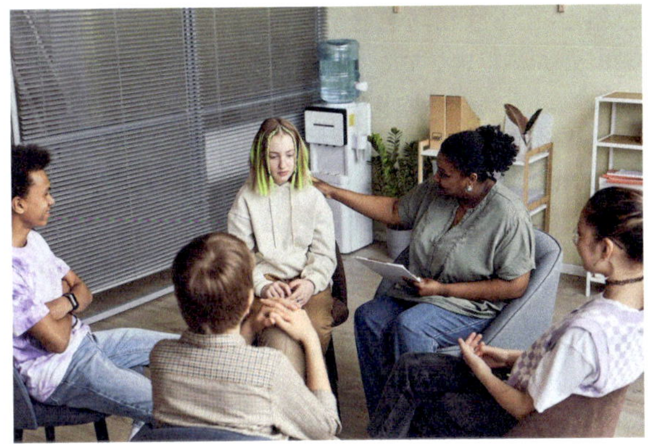

Figure 9.3. Mental health.

Source: https://external-content.duckduckgo.com/iu/?u=https%3A%2F%2Fopenminds.org.au%2Fwp-content%2Fuploads%2F2022%2F12%2Fmental-health-support.jpeg&f=1&nofb=1&ipt=f8682879b278983a0187b20e43ab85954de31f8f3cdb641c6876da9637175018.

9.1.1. Components of Mental Health

Mental health contains a number of different components that have a great bearing on the general well-being of a person within a population. These are elements such as emotional, psychological, and social factors that indicate how a person thinks, feels, and behaves during daily life. Regulation of emotions, self-awareness, and healthy relationships are core elements that lead to mental well-being. It is important to identify such factors, particularly in the case of such contemporary challenges as the COVID-19 pandemic, which has sped up mental illness issues among such sensitive groups as children and adolescents. Educators, for instance, have reported a great increase in mental health issues among students, necessitating an urgent need for a proper comprehension of emotional health in an attempt to construct amiable learning environments to counteract the challenges. Meeting these requirements effectively translates to the necessity of higher mental health literacy among members in the community, especially those in roles that overlap with youths, e.g., teachers (Robinson et al., 2024). Social relationships and community engagement are major components of mental health since they provide individuals with a feeling of belonging and purpose. The social relationships formed in communities not only enhance resilience but also act as protective factors against mental illness. Community-level social interaction and peer support-based interventions can strongly mitigate loneliness, typically experienced by individuals with mental disorders. Shared models such as the Health Extension: Advocacy, Research, and Teaching (HEART) Initiative prove strong local input and community organization integration to address complex behavioral health issues. By leveraging partnerships and trust that already exist within communities, such models optimize capacity to address mental health needs comprehensively, demonstrating how collaboration can be used effectively to develop resilience and promote mental well-being (Condie et al., 2024). Building connectedness in community structures thus benefits not only individual mental health but collective well-being as well.

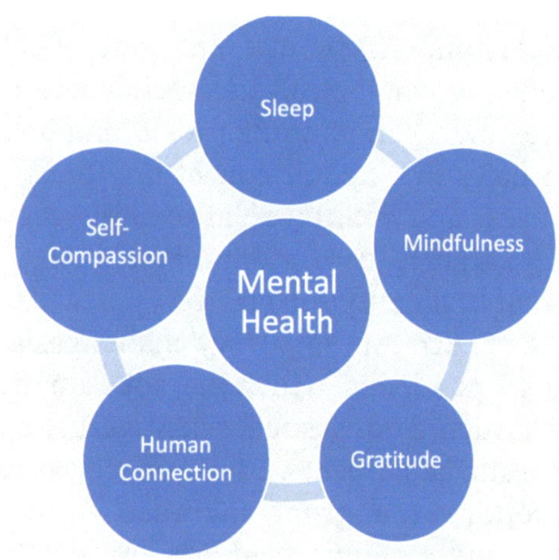

Figure 9.4. Elements-of-mental-health.

Source: https://i0.wp.com/wallacekpond.com/wp-content/uploads/2022/12/Five-Elements-of-Mental-Health.png?fit=1631%2C1402&ssl=1.

Moreover, mental health promotion encompasses an active strategy with education and intervention methods that address varied population requirements. Mental health literacy is a significant vehicle within this goal, permitting individuals to recognize the indicators of mental health issues and seek the appropriate assistance. Resource production, such as the production of mental health handbooks for instructors, provides an excellent instance of the effort to provide members of the community with the required information and tools. These resources can potentially facilitate early intervention and identification, and help recognize mental health conditions prior to them being more severe. The educational activities can also empower individuals and communities in taking healthier lifestyles, engaging in positive dialogues regarding mental health, and resisting stigma on mental illness. By creating places with an emphasis on understanding and accessibility of mental health care, communities will be able to maximize their capacity for resilience while building a supportive culture and environment of awareness for mental illness (Robinson et al., 2024) (Figure 9.4).

9.1.2. Factors Influencing Mental Health

A number of factors play a major role in mental health, from biological, psychological, social, to environmental factors. Biological factors include genetic predispositions, neurochemical imbalances, and physical illness. Mental illnesses such as schizophrenia or bipolar disorder are typically hereditary in nature, meaning family history leads a person to be at increased risk. Psychological factors like personality, coping strategies, and trauma histories also play a very important role in one's mental health status. For instance, an individual with high resilience will likely be able to manage stress, hence reducing the risk of mental illness. The knowledge of these factors underlies successful community-based interventions for mental health that focus on promoting well-being. Social determinants also shed more light on the intricacy of mental health disorders, highlighting the essential use of community and interpersonal relationships. Socioeconomic status, education, and access to medical care have considerable impacts on mental health. Low-income families can experience additional stressors in terms of economic instability and are prone to mental health problems. Social interactions, such as social support networks, are now seen as important determinants for mental health. Interventions that encourage community involvement, such as the Walking for Wellness program, illustrate the ways in which participation in a group activity can enhance interpersonal connections and establish emotional support. Making room for connection and support, communities can establish an environment of care for mental health and resilience that models the complexity of mental well-being. Stigma related to mental illness continues to inhibit seeking help, resulting in harmful mental health consequences. Misconceptions and social stereotypes about mental illness might deter individuals from accessing pertinent services, and they remain isolated, with conditions worsening further. As highlighted in other initiatives, community-based interventions are important for the reduction of stigma. For example, promoting candid openness about mental illness can facilitate a supportive atmosphere. Moreover, initiatives like the C-Card program aim not only to provide essential health care but also to combat widespread myths about sexual health and mental well-being in teenagers. Thus, stigma reduction through targeted intervention at the community level is central to increasing the effectiveness of mental health promotion programs and to motivating people to seek help without fear of retaliation.

9.1.3. Differences Between Mental Health and Mental Illness

The differentiation between mental health and mental illness is crucial in building an inclusive understanding of well-being within community settings. Mental health is a state of being where an individual's emotional, psychological, and social well-being determines their mode of thought, feeling, and behavior. It includes the capacity to cope with stress, be social with others, and make choices. In contrast, mental illness is diagnosed disorders that disrupt a person's thinking, feeling, or behavior, such as anxiety disorders, depression, bipolar disorder, and schizophrenia. Mental health can fluctuate according to what goes on in someone's life, while mental illnesses are long-standing, requiring professional assistance and treatment. Grasping this distinction provides the foundation for encouraging good mental health, enabling people to learn to be resilient and cope with stressors so that they can promote positive outcomes within their social contexts and relationships. In the community context, an appreciation of mental health and mental illness differences can greatly contribute to the efficacy of interventions. Community-oriented mental health services can be modified to address both needs simultaneously by promoting mental wellness and providing services for the mentally ill. An illustration would be mental health literacy programs in community centers that will allow individuals to take charge of checking their mental well-being and seek help when necessary. As found through recent studies, the majority of educators indicate that they are not adequately prepared to handle mental problems within their classrooms due to a lack of training and self-efficacy. The development of resources, such as handbooks on mental health, aims to address this gap, equipping community leaders and teachers with the knowledge necessary to foster settings conducive to mental health (Robinson et al., 2024). The effects of ignoring the differences between mental health and mental illness can lead to serious public health outcomes, particularly among vulnerable groups, such as children and adolescents. Scientific findings indicate that untreated mental health conditions can become severe mental illness and result in tremendous costs to society, including lost productivity and increased care costs (Eichner et al., 2009). Particularly, one out of five children has psychiatric symptoms each year, but fewer than 20% of them are treated. Prioritizing education about mental health and mental illness, communities can institute early intervention techniques that promote resilience and treat prospective mental health problems before they become fully-fledged. This double-pronged approach places more importance on stigma reduction systems that enable individuals to seek help without fear or misinterpretation of their situations, leading to healthier communities (Figure 9.5).

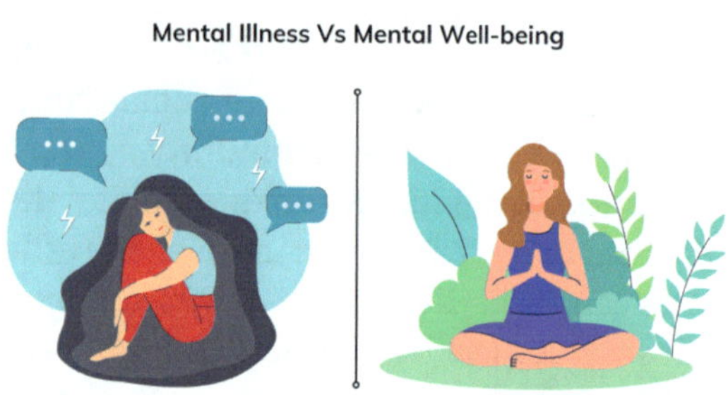

Figure 9.5. Differences between mental health and mental illness.

Source: https://external-content.duckduckgo.com/iu/?u=https%3A%2F%2Fvisitmhp.com%2Fwp-content%2Fuploads%2F2022%2F01%2 Fdifference- between-mental-health-and-mental-illness-788x443.png&f= 1&nofb= 1&ipt= 7fb9c3e57564b12daf1c 1854a2fa09f1b6d7 b6b1ec7d3ec6633cec28d4d043d0.

9.2. Understanding Mental Illness

Identification and understanding of mental illness are key components within the broader discussion regarding mental health within society. Mental illness represents a wide range of diseases, such as anxiety, depression, bipolar disorder, and schizophrenia, each with unique difficulties for the individual and for society at large. An important aspect of this knowledge is the recognition that mental health exceeds the absence of illness but constitutes a dynamic relationship between emotional, psychological, and social functioning. Rising mental health illnesses among communities and particularly among youth and children underscore the necessity to integrate mental health literacy into community systems. As explained in the teachers' report of struggling to address mental health in students, there is a necessity for inclusive models that prepare one with the capacity to recognize and deal with mental health crises efficiently (Robinson et al., 2024). Such frameworks can break down myths and provide an enhanced support environment for those dealing with mental health problems. The educational framework plays a core role in shaping knowledge and perception regarding mental illness, particularly regarding the care that teachers provide to students. This contact is gaining importance, especially against the background of growing mental health challenges for the younger generations, driven further by such crisis events as the COVID-19 pandemic. Notably, educators report feeling inadequate in assisting students with mental illness due to a lack of training and mental health competencies. As noted in earlier research, the system has moved from treatment to preventive care, with an oversight of preparing educators to aid students in resilience and well-being (McCartie et al., 2018). Plugging this gap calls for the imposition of specific education resources, such as handbooks developed to enhance mental health literacy and provide pragmatic recommendations for teachers, ultimately benefiting both teachers and pupils. Community mental health services offer essential pillars in promoting the understanding and management of mental illness. These services target a holistic model as well, not just the individual with mental health issues but the support networks surrounding them, including families, schools, and communities. Expanding mental health services and interventions is a means of empowering communities to enhance mental health and resilience within their populations. Besides, through programs aimed at breaking stigma, these services facilitate the creation of a culture in which individuals will be empowered to seek help without the threat of stigmatization. The effective collaboration of community resources with educational programs has the potential to lead to greater awareness and understanding of mental illness, enabling all members of the community to contribute positively to mental health concerns, ultimately fostering a more united and empathetic social tissue (Robinson et al., 2024; McCartie et al., 2018).

9.2.1. Common Types of Mental Illnesses

One of the most prevalent conditions of mental illness is anxiety disorders, which include such conditions as social anxiety disorder, panic disorder, and generalized anxiety disorder. Symptoms for such conditions are typically manifested in the form of excessive worry, fear, or anxiety that will easily compromise everyday functioning. Within the community environment, the impact of anxiety disorders can lead to increased health care utilization and decreased productivity, which ultimately places a burden on community resources. Besides, anxiety disorders frequently co-occur with other mental illnesses, such as depression, which makes their effects more severe for individuals affected as well as populations. Being aware of the nature of such disorders is instrumental in promoting mental well-being and resilience among population areas, considering that early detection and treatment can greatly improve the outcome for individuals affected. Mood disorders, particularly depression and bipolar disorder, are another significant category of mental illness encountered among population groups. Depression is characterized by prolonged episodes of sadness, hopelessness, and loss of interest in activities formerly enjoyed, interfering with people's physical and emotional well-being. Bipolar disorder, however, involves mood shifting, from mania to depression, interfering with individuals' functioning in their lives on a personal and professional level. Stigma towards mood disorders results in people finding it hard to access help, thereby worsening their conditions as well as limiting interventions at the community level. Treatment of the disorders through community-based care not only alleviates suffering for the individual but also makes education and awareness more possible and establishes a mental health recovery-friendly climate. Substance use disorders (SUDs) are increasingly being embraced as a major mental health condition, affecting millions of members of communities. SUDs comprise a spectrum of alcohol and illicit drug-related issues, which can have physical, psychological, and social consequences, from homelessness to imprisonment.

The effects of these disorders extend beyond the individual to have wide-ranging implications for families and larger social networks. Effective intervention approaches, like improving access to evidence-based treatment and the application of harm reduction practices, are crucial in addressing the multifaceted nature of SUDs. By tackling the community-based elements, though, both the individual and systemic determinants of substance use can be tackled, ultimately improving public health overall. Initiatives that promote treatment innovation and prevention will also be key in minimizing the impact of SUDs as well as building resilience in affected communities (Wallman-Stokes et al., 2015; Robinson et al., 2024) (Figure 9.6).

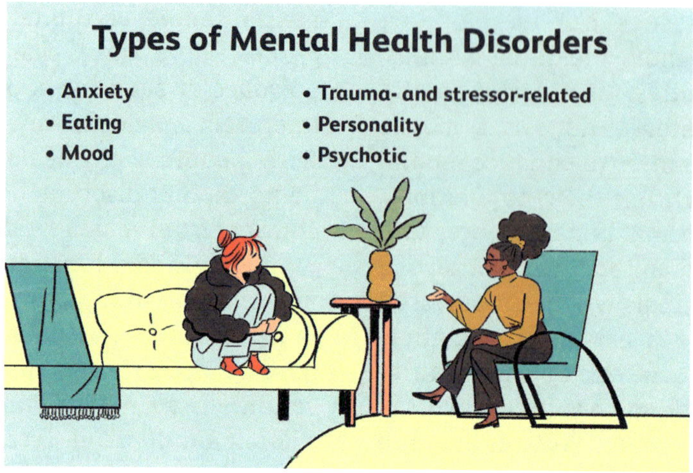
Types of Mental Health Disorders
• Anxiety
• Eating
• Mood
• Trauma- and stressor-related
• Personality
• Psychotic

Figure 9.6. Common types of mental illnesses.

Source: https://external-content.duckduckgo.com/iu/?u=https%3A%2F%2Fwww.verywellhealth.com%2Fthmb%2FHMdLiI9VgLkCJo5u5SPqL2Qbwig%3D%2F1500x1000%2Ffilters%3Ano_upscale()%3Amax_bytes(150000)%3Astrip_icc()%2Ftop-mental-health-disorders-a-mental-illness-list-5210092_final-90ba5c61e17e40ccb2e6023354ef9827.jpg&f=1&nofb=1&ipt=90cacb9941cc172eb1b062ba4f3a1267dbd2c8f45cca5470f6cdbedaabc6e6be.

9.2.2. Symptoms and Diagnosis of Mental Illnesses

Identification of mental illness relies on the occurrence of certain symptoms, which vary for different disorders. Mental illnesses occur in a myriad of ways, including disturbances in mood, cognitive impairment, and behavioral problems. For instance, anxiety disorders commonly appear as worrying or fearing excessively to an extent that it interferes with daily functioning, while depressive disorders could be characterized by constant sadness, loss of interest or pleasure in activities, or changes in appetite or sleep. Mental illness, in its nature, demands a careful and systematic evaluation procedure. The diagnoses typically come after application of diagnostic standards stipulated in the Diagnostic and Statistical Manual of Mental Disorders (DSM-5) in order to ensure that mental illnesses are accurately determined according to standardized symptom profiles. The systematic procedure ensures differentiation from normal emotional responses, an essential element for effective treatment and intervention procedures. Screening for mental illnesses is vital for early recognition and intervention, especially in the face of their prevalence and potential impact on quality of life. Community-based mental health services play a central role in this initiative by providing accessible screening tools and resources that allow for early detection. Mental health workers are trained to recognize a broad range of symptoms, from minor to severe presentations. Moreover, there is greater emphasis on employing trauma-informed care to treat individuals whose symptoms might have been brought about by prior negative experiences. With the identification of the relationship between trauma and mental illness, medical practitioners are able to formulate tailor-made interventions to address symptoms along with causes. These combined approaches are important in promoting resilience and providing long-term mental well-being within societies, hence reducing the stigma of seeking help for mental health problems. The new literature calls for understanding the intersection between childhood adversity and mental health outcomes. Traumatic experiences in early life have been shown to alter neurodevelopmental mechanisms, leading to increased susceptibility to various mental health disorders in adulthood. As highlighted in trauma-informed care frameworks, addressing these early experiences can significantly improve health trajectories and promote resilience among affected individuals. With nearly half of American children experiencing at least one traumatic event, mental health professionals must prioritize strategies that integrate this understanding into their diagnostic processes. Incorporating systematic screening in pediatric care, where early detection can trigger early support services, could drastically stem long-term mental illness. As a nation, fostering sensitivity for the impact of childhood adversity not only increases diagnosis but also the efficacy of mental health interventions towards creating a gateway for healthier generations to thrive (N/A, 2023; James et al., 2021) (Figure 9.7).

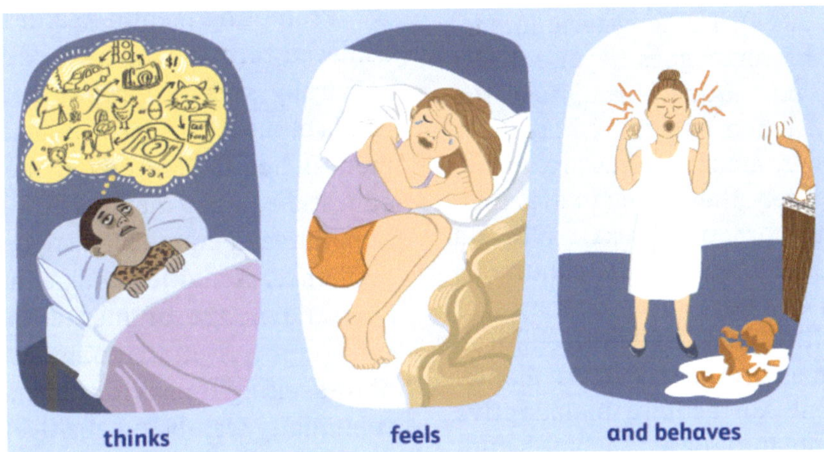

Figure 9.7. Symptoms of mental illnesses.

Source: https://www.verywellmind.com/thmb/u_YyxyiUz6qeT5AtcsF41O42ngY=/1500x0/filters:no_upscale():max_bytes(150000):strip_icc()/definition-of-mental-illness-4587855-v1-cd7f9f37c61c49099ac8ede282db1e73.png.

9.2.3. Impact of Mental Illness on Individuals and Families

The impact of mental illness on the family and individuals is extensive and multidimensional, extending to emotional stability, relationships with others, and life patterns. Individuals with mental illness typically exhibit a constellation of disabling signs and symptoms like anxiety, depression, and impairment of intellect, which disable them in the course of their daily lives. This disturbance impacts not just the individual but also alters the dynamics of families, with relatives struggling to understand and show support for victims. The 2008 National Mental Health Policy calls for recovery-oriented approaches that promote early detection and treatment and reiterate the imperative of re-establishing individual functionality and community involvement as the foundation of mental health reform, thus developing a supportive environment that fosters resilience and mental wellness in all (N/A). Families, burdened with the mental illness struggles of their members, typically experience a difficult scenario riddled with emotional tensions and social stigmas. The threat of being judged or discriminated against can lead to the creation of a state of isolation, effectively closing off access to vital support systems. Moreover, family members may also develop caregiver burnout as they strive to provide emotional and practical support, which can also lead to their own mental health conditions.

Interventions that address the education of family groups regarding mental illness and its influence can significantly decrease stigma and create a facilitating domestic environment. The function of community involvement is highlighted within research relating to public awareness campaigns' effectiveness, showing that empowering communities with educated involvement can enhance support groups, ultimately having beneficial implications for those with mental illnesses and their families (Braybrook et al., 2013). The long-term impact of mental illness, however, goes beyond direct family members, resonating throughout the larger community. When patients whose lives have been touched by mental illness are unable to integrate into society, their own families then feel the impact in the form of financial strain and decreased social engagement. These conditions can establish intergenerational patterns of mental illness within families since children who develop up in environments where mental illness is prevalent can acquire maladaptive coping styles. Community-based mental health care is, therefore, a critical aspect in building resilience and assisting families in attaining mental health. By the focus on diminishing stigma and enhancing access to community resources, these programs foster supportive communal environments that recognize the collective responsibility of mental health care, ultimately transforming society's views and facilitating recovery (N/A, 2023).

9.3. Promoting Mental Wellness

Promoting mental health in communities is a multifaceted strategy that considers the unique social and cultural context of people. Mental health services that are culturally sensitive and attuned to local traditions will likely enhance the uptake and impact of interventions considerably. Inclusive approaches, such as the blending of psychological support with customary and acceptable practices, not only reduce stigma but also enhance the nurturing social climate of individuals with mental illness. Research has proven that well-specified interventions, like the Cameroon Baptist Convention Health Services, efficiently improved the coping abilities of participants and reduced symptoms of mental illness by as much as 25% after a period of one year (Nganyu, 2025).

Promoting mental health is therefore best achieved through community mobilization and culturally specific programs sensitive to the needs of the local populace, leading to improved mental health. Moreover, mental well-being education among members of the community is imperative in minimizing stigma and promoting resilience. Activities that enhance awareness and knowledge of mental health problems can empower individuals to be involved in help-seeking behavior, ultimately affecting community well-being positively. An interesting study conducted in Indonesia demonstrated that participatory mental health education significantly enhanced mental disorder awareness and sympathy among members of the community and health cadres (Mulyani et al., 2025).

Participants reported a greater desire to engage with people who are affected by mental illness and to share their new knowledge with their social network. These learning programs counteract stigma and misconceptions regarding mental illness, creating a ripple effect that results in a tolerant and accepting society. By educating, communities can develop a culture of mental health, resulting in well-being. Finally, the development of resilience is a critical factor in promoting mental health in community settings. Programs that help develop coping skills, emotional regulation, and interpersonal support systems can allow individuals to improve their ability to manage life's challenges. The integration of resilience-building strategies into community mental health interventions can allow individuals not only to cope with existing mental illness but to prevent future complications. This emphasis on resilience is reflected in findings from community-based interventions, where the building of emotional well-being was found to increase participants' abilities to cope (Nganyu, 2025). With the provision of practical resilience tools to members of the community, we create a platform for long-lasting mental health that can thrive even in the face of adversity. Lastly, improving mental health among populations entails an integrated approach that entails education, cultural sensitivity, and building resilience (Figure 9.8).

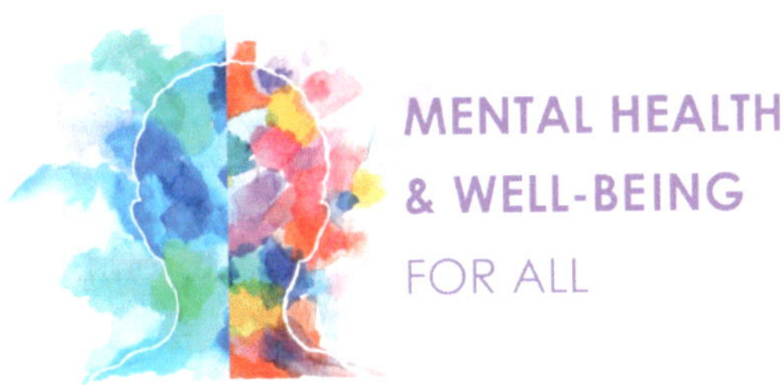

Figure 9.8. Mental health and well-being.

Source: https://external-content.duckduckgo.com/iu/?u=https%3A%2F%2Fburnabyschools.ca%2Fwp-content%2 Fuploads %2F2019%2F04%2F Mental HealthWell-beingforAll_graphic.png&f= 1&nofb= 1&ipt=095470b55220166e c482280447 e6a8984a59d0c5f4fd2b1d5 e0280f0429d7dcb.

9.3.1. Strategies for Enhancing Mental Wellness

Developing mental well-being within communities needs a multi-pronged approach that incorporates prevention, education, and support systems to create resilience. An education system , with the priority of mental health, is needed, particularly at schools and in workplaces. For instance, creating curricula that emphasize emotional intelligence and stress management allows individuals to cope with problems in life efficiently. Such learning programs not only deliver required mental health services but also establish a well-being culture that promotes peer support and community engagement. Also, making training sessions available to teachers and employers on recognizing and responding to mental health issues is essential. These training programs promote an awareness of how to care for troubled individuals and create safety-promoting settings that enhance mental well-being, as put forth by the consensus statement on maximizing well-being in schools (Bishop et al., 2019).

Other than education, improving mental well-being also requires programs that are community-oriented and focused on early intervention and supporting vulnerable groups. Community groups are also responsible for making available mental health resources and services on the basis of specific demographic needs. Early intervention in the progression of mental illness, particularly in children and adolescents, has been shown to be followed by changes for the better as well as recovery (Eichner et al., 2009). This can be brought about through cooperation with schools, health workers, and local groups so that screening programs can be carried out and immediate intervention can be provided. Secondly, giving family-oriented resources fosters mental health with inclusive practices so that all can take an active role in interventions and discussions. By combined action by communities to reduce stigma around mental illness, communities empower individuals to seek assistance and build resilience, and the community as a whole becomes mentally healthier.

Lastly, promoting mental well-being within communities requires physical health programs to be put together with mental health programs. Studies indicate that physical health has a great influence on mental well-being, which means the approach should be holistic in nature and consider both at the same time. Community sports programs, well-being seminars, and nutritional education are not only beneficial to physical health but also to mental health, as they reduce stress and improve mood. Coordination between mental health professionals and physical health advocates is therefore important when creating programs that consider these interrelations. Further, creating active living environments such as safe recreational facilities and parks has the potential to create social settings for connection and support networks. Incorporating physical health into programs of mental well-being, treating mental illness is effective in communities (Eichner et al., 2009).

9.3.2. Role of Lifestyle Choices in Mental Health

The interaction between mental health and lifestyle is central to developing resilience and improving well-being in populations. The regular engagement in physical activity is typically linked with lower anxiety and depression since it reflects the physiological and psychological effects of exercise on mental health. By incorporating a balanced diet rich in nutrients, individuals can aid their mood and mental performance since some vitamins and minerals are crucial to the production and moderation of neurotransmitters. In addition, sleep is critical in aiding emotional control and overall mental well-being; sleeping deprivation can exacerbate underlying mental disease, creating a cycle of increasing illness. Therefore, community programs that inform individuals about healthy ways of living not only allow them to make informed choices but also result in the reduction of the prevalence of mental disorders (Robinson et al., 2024). Also, social relationships play a significant role in influencing mental health outcomes, necessitating the establishment of healthy relationships in community setups. Those with healthy social relationships experience a greater sense of belonging and self-worth, which can serve to mitigate the effects of stress and anxiety. Social isolation, conversely, can trigger or increase mental illness, highlighting the worth of promoting an open community setting. Engagement in group activity or support networks can provide those with vital emotional resources, bolstering resilience and coping abilities. Through implementing community-based mental health care that encourages peer support and interaction, local communities are able to radically reduce the stigma surrounding mental illness as well as simultaneously counteract the vulnerability that is created by isolation (Mostafa et al., 2023). For that reason, placing the greatest priority on the value of social well-being as part of an overall framework provides a route toward increased mental health success. In recognition of the critical overlapping areas between lifestyle choices and mental health, community programs also need to emphasize mental health literacy. Many individuals, including teachers, may lack the essential knowledge to recognize mental health problems or utilize useful coping strategies (Robinson et al., 2024). Through the creation of material that educates individuals on the importance of their life choices, including diet, exercise, sleep, and social interaction, communities can enable citizens to enhance their mental health in an active way. Workshops, educational speeches, and the sharing of educational resources can be employed to de-stigmatize mental illness and promote healthy lifestyle behaviors. Lastly, promoting mental health literacy along with the adoption of a healthy lifestyle generates an empowered populace that prioritizes mental wellness and develops resilience against mental illness and, as such, transforms the complexion of mental health care at the community level (Figure 9.9).

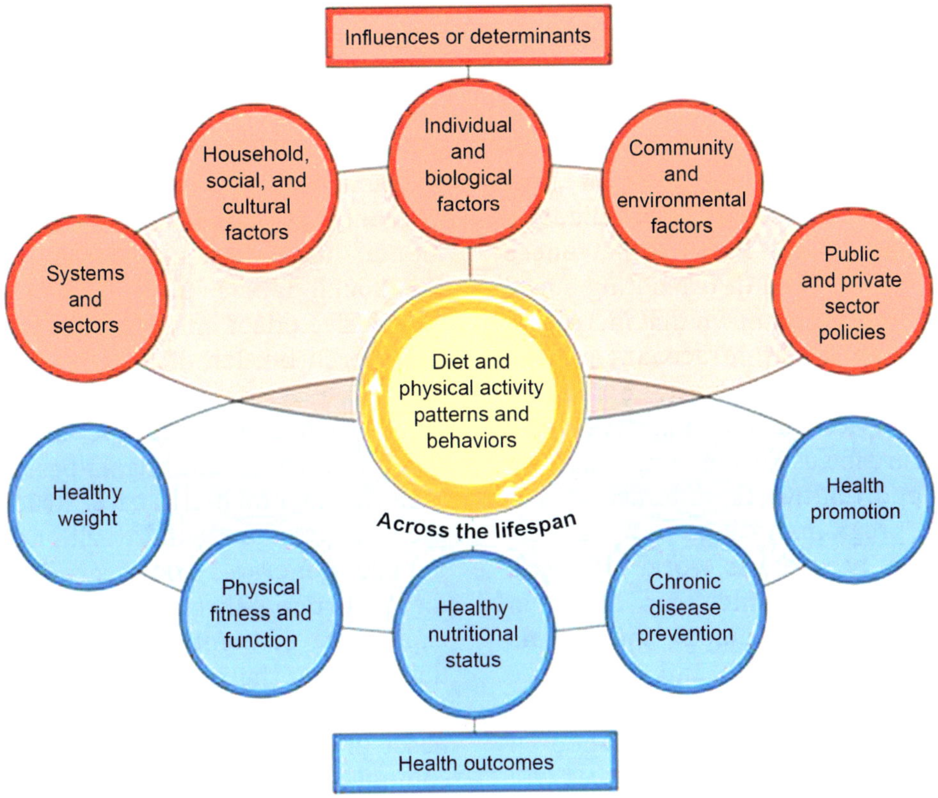

Figure 9.9. Role of lifestyle choices in mental health.

Source: https://sleck.net/wp-content/uploads/2020/12/image002.jpg.

9.3.3. Importance of Social Support Networks

Social support networks also act as significant influences in the promotion of mental health, particularly in community settings. Such networks, which typically consist of family, friends, peers, and community institutions, provide emotional resources, instrumental aid, and a sense of belonging. Robust social support within vulnerable populations, such as young adults surviving the risks of mental illness, has been found to be associated with improved psychological functioning as well as increased resilience. Research has revealed that individuals with good social connections are less likely to experience distress and anxiety and more likely to have overall better well-being. Building such networks is thus important for creating an environment that will promote good mental health, especially with the rising trends of mental illness triggered by challenges like socioeconomic stressors and the pandemic's legacy of COVID-19 (Abbasi et al., 2022). The addition of family involvement in treatment interventions, therefore, functions to highlight the importance of networks of support in mental health treatment. Families are key to the recovery process since acceptance and understanding on their behalf can really cut down the stigma often wrapped around mental illness. Community-based models, such as the Centers for Psychosocial Care (CAPS), promote the inclusion of families in the treatment process, leveraging their potential as a therapeutic support system. When family members are engaged in the recovery process, they can help reinforce coping skills, increase compliance with treatment, and contribute to building resilience in individuals with mental illness. As noted in various studies, some of which include the experiences provided by practitioners who work with CAPS, the collaborative intervention between families and mental health services assists in validating and legitimizing users' living experiences (Randemark et al., 2014). In promoting social networks of support, it is known that increasing mental health also needs to account for the broader context of the community. Community mental health services must aim at developing programs that are inclusive in nature and assist in creating opportunities for interaction and support. Such programs include peer support groups, community wellness workshops, and mentorship programs, which can assist in developing relationships among individuals affected by mental illnesses and emphasize teamwork and mutual support. Moreover, reducing stigma through minimizing taboo on conversations concerning mental illnesses will assist in developing an inclusive community setting. By proactively nurturing such nurturing environments, communities not only enhance the mental health outcomes of individuals but also the broader resilience of society, opening the door towards a holistic treatment of mental wellness which is centered around interconnectedness and collective healing (Abbasi et al., 2022).

9.4. Building Resilience

Resilience, or the ability to react favorably when faced with hardship, is a key component of mental health in community environments. Building resilience can do a great deal to minimize the danger brought about by mental health disorders and encourage recovery in already affected individuals. Community intervention is central to this process because it provides support environments that promote resilience through resources, social interactions, and collective experiences. Through participation in community activities, individuals are likely to feel a sense of belonging that underpins their coping. Communal support can be crucial, especially for individuals with stigma related to mental illness. Thus, enhancing resilience not only enhances individual outcomes on mental health but also helps in reinforcing the social fabric, ultimately resulting in a cumulative effect on public health by reducing the overall burden of mental illness. Building resilience at the individual and community levels also highlights the urgent need to remove structural and stigma-based obstacles to receiving mental health care. Structural stigma, according to the Mental Health Commission of Canada, generates healthcare inequities that disproportionately affect individuals with lived experience of mental health issues and thus detract from their capacity to build resilience. Finding and removing such obstacles is at the heart of enhancing mental well-being among communities. Winning strategies can include training health professionals on cultural competence and equipping them with skills in communicating effectively with individuals who suffer from stigma. Such system changes enable people to receive care without being discriminatorily locked out, and hence open the doors for the process of resilience and promoting access to mental health as a key community outcome. Moreover, community resilience is enhanced when individuals have the knowledge and skills for emotional management and self-care. Mindfulness, stress, and coping curricula play a central role in enhancing mental health and illness knowledge. Support groups and workshops are also vehicles for knowledge sharing, where individuals learn and exercise resilience practices together. The integration of these strategies in community mental health interventions provides a level on which self-efficacy is dominant, enabling people to advocate for themselves and collaborate. Communities are not only capable of de-stigmatizing mental illness through awareness and knowledge but can also enable people to employ their strengths in resilience development that may result in community mental health (Figure 9.10).

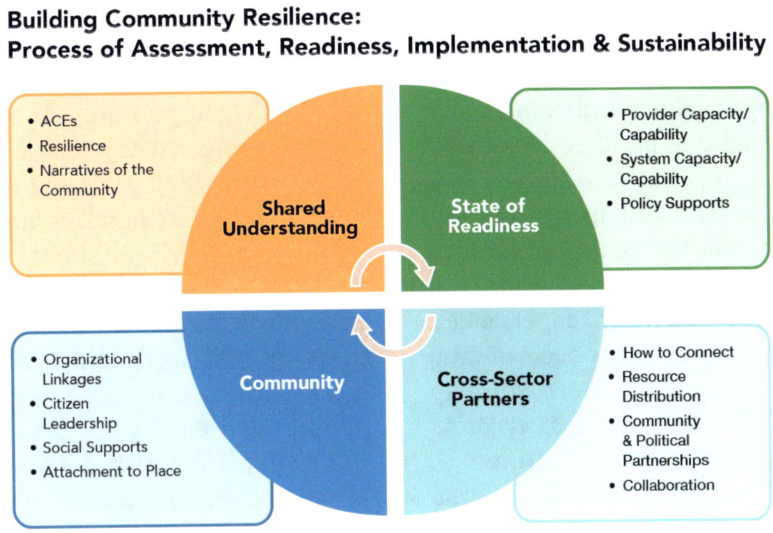

Figure 9.10. Center for community resilience.

Source: https://ccr.publichealth.gwu.edu/sites/g/files/zaxdzs4361/files/2022-05/case-study-graphics-1.png.

9.4.1. Definition and Significance of Resilience

Resilience, or the ability to bounce back from hardship and learn how to cope with adversity, is key to maintaining mental health and well-being in populations. It is the person's ability to bounce back from setbacks while growing stronger as a result of having experienced hardship. In mental health, resilience is most critical, as is evidenced by its relevance to schools. As the COVID-19 pandemic has magnified mental health concerns among students, instructors are now increasingly recognizing the significance of fostering resilience in their curricula to further encourage not only academic success but emotional growth as well. Through the offering of students with resilience-building skills, classrooms are an environment where students can become more skilled at bouncing over obstacles and reaching out for help when needed, hence cultivating a culture of support within the broader community (Robinson et al., 2024). The impact of resilience transcends individual skills; it glances back on the social configuration within which mental health is constructed. Community-based mental health initiatives increasingly emphasize resilience as a fundamental component in mitigating mental health disorders. These initiatives recognize that resilience can be cultivated through supportive relationships, community engagement, and access to resources. By promoting an understanding of resilience, mental health services can empower individuals to respond proactively to life's challenges. The Positive Psychology framework, embraced by teachers and mental health professionals alike, provides a roadmap to the development of resilience through directed strategies and interventions. These interventions not only stress treatment but also work towards enhancing mental well-being by preventing mental illnesses from arising by fostering community resilience (McCartie et al., 2018). Moreover, the value of resilience in mental health conversation demands an understanding of the stigma traditionally associated with mental illness. Resilience-valuing communities create environments in which individuals are able to speak of vulnerabilities without the fear of judgment. By promoting greater mental health literacy among teachers and community members, it is achievable to build conversation about mental well-being that normalizes talk regarding mental health challenges. Resilient communities deconstruct stigma in advance by building awareness, understanding, and acceptance of diverse mental health experiences. As teaching aids, such as the proposed mental health handbook, prepare teachers to help students effectively, they also serve as triggers for broader community activities aimed at promoting resilience and reducing stigma (Robinson et al., 2024). Resilience thus emerges as a cornerstone of not only individual recovery but also the development of inclusive and empathetic communities.

9.4.2. Techniques for Developing Resilience

Resilience is a key component of mental health, particularly in community settings where individuals face adversity. Another helpful way to foster resilience is through developing healthy social connections. Research indicates that social support is a good barrier to stress and increased well-being. Communities that center on relationship building—be they social networks, support groups, or community activities—create environments where individuals feel understood and appreciated. This sense of belonging diminishes loneliness and makes people more at ease to disclose their experiences, which in turn may encourage more effective coping. Furthermore, mental health-centered awareness programs can make it acceptable to talk about adversity, which has been seen to de-stigmatize mental illness and encourage help-seeking. These social marketing campaigns aim to heighten community awareness and responsiveness to mental health crises, thus ultimately contributing to a more resilient population (Braybrook et al., 2012). An additional key strategy for promoting resilience is the inclusion of skills-building workshops on emotional regulation and problem-solving skills. Such workshops equip community members with tangible strategies to deal effectively with stressors as well as make sound decisions in challenging moments. When people acquire cognitive-behavioral coping techniques during difficult times, they are better equipped to deal with life's difficulties, which overall improves their mental well-being. These skill-building interventions are especially helpful for young people who are in the process of establishing their identities and coping styles. Nonprofit organizations in communities can organize these workshops so more people become aware and more are likely to participate. By targeting proactive strategies to foster resilience, communities can establish a context in which individuals not only endure but are able to flourish even in difficult situations and enjoy long-term mental health (Abdullaev et al., 2018). Incorporating mindfulness and self-care practice into community programs is another effective way to foster resilience. Mindfulness meditation has been shown to reduce anxiety and depression levels and enhance overall emotional well-being. By providing accessible resources such as mindfulness training, yoga exercises, or mental health initiatives, organizations can introduce individuals to engaging in self-care, hence building emotional and psychological resilience. They enable individuals to get in touch with their emotional responses and feel they are responsible for their thoughts and emotions. In addition, the inclusion of mindfulness exercises in community mental health interventions has been shown to reduce the stigma around mental illness because they provide open and honest conversations regarding emotional states. This approach, in general, not only supports individuals in their pursuit of resilience but also strengthens community ties, creating an empathy and compassion culture (Braybrook et al., 2012).

9.4.3. Role of Community in Fostering Resilience

The role of community in fostering resilience is at the heart of mental health progress and prevention of mental illness. Resilient communities create environments that facilitate social support, foster interdependence, and evoke a sense of belonging, all of which are critical to mental health. If citizens perceive their communities as supportive, they are more apt to use resources that foster resilience, such as mental health services, recreation, and support groups. Moreover, community cohesion can counteract stressors by providing citizens with a support network of relationships that assist them in coping during difficult times. In this regard, communities can also act as buffers against mental illness by promoting civic involvement and collaborations, which result in individual and collective resiliency. Through mutual experience and mutual support, communities can help people better endure harm and create a common ethos of wellness. Working to reduce stigma surrounding mental illness in building a vibrant community further emphasizes resilience. Stigmatization can be a barrier to seeking assistance from others, augmenting feelings of shame and isolation. Mental health initiatives in making people aware and accepting of mental health issues can help minimize such stigmas and enable open discussions of mental health. Education campaigns, workshops conducted in communities, and peer support programs are crucial in establishing an environment where mental health is freely discussed and brought to the forefront. As evidenced through studies on recovery stigma and addiction, building group membership and social support is essential in modifying individual experiences of mental health challenges. By establishing a sense of belonging within groups, people can feel empowered, belong, and be resilient and ultimately enhance their capacity to thrive in the face of challenges (Parker-Grewe et al., 2017). Besides, community interventions based on collective approaches make an incredible contribution towards strengthening resilience. As communities come together to establish systems and engage in mental health activities, they form an enabling infrastructure for responding to both individual and community requirements. Mental health screening programs, workshops, and access to resources must be actively engaging community members in planning and program implementation.

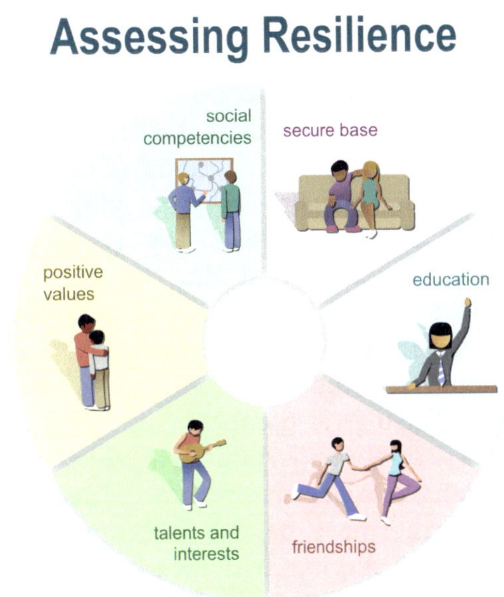

Figure 9.11. Fostering resilience.

Source: https://content.iriss.org.uk/fosteringresilience/images/diagram_large.gif.

This collaborative approach not only ensures the usability of the services provided but also ensures ownership by members of the community. As suggested in suicide prevention strategies, engagement of community resources and the reinforcement of protective factors are imperative (Wang et al., 2023). Through collaborative action, stakeholders in the community, including local organizations, health practitioners, and individuals, can positively influence mental well-being, decelerate mental health disorder rates, and enhance resilience within the community at large (Figure 9.11).

9.5. Community-Based Mental Health Services

In mental health, community-based services offer a great link in making care accessible and enhancing resilience among individuals with mental health conditions. They meet the local population's specific needs through a diverse array of resources that may include preventive interventions, management of crisis situations, and ongoing support. For instance, career and technical student organizations (CTSOs) can contribute significantly to improving mental health in schools. CTSOs engage students in activities that reveal the risk factors of psychological distress as well as build protective factors that enhance resilience. Such a strategy not only empowers students to advocate for mental health but also gives them the leadership skills that lead to career opportunities in mental health professions, as seen through efforts (Beck et al., 2022). Furthermore, pairing community-based mental health services with local organizations further enhances their efficacy. A good case in point here is the Health Extension: Advocacy, Research, and Teaching (HEART) Initiative, which harmoniously combines members of the community and various stakeholders in combating substance use disorders. This initiative is a good representation of a culture of collaboration, embracing the application of an interdisciplinary team along with community-based participatory research (CBPR) in tailoring interventions to rural populations' unique needs. The ability of community-based services to organize resources effectively and draw on community trust underscores the value of local partnerships in coping with challenging behavioral health crises, providing a model for successful shared resilience and support that can be applied across other contexts (Condie et al., 2024). Community-based mental health services also have an essential role in combating societal stigma surrounding mental illness. By developing environments in which mental health is conveniently discussed, such services can contribute significantly to implementing cultural shifts that lead to seeking help becoming the norm. Interventions that promote good mental health engage individuals in conversation freely, dispelling myths and stereotypes related to mental health. School and community programs involving peer-based interventions can contribute significantly to attitude shifts and the stigma linked with such illnesses, since younger generations learn to appreciate assisting others.

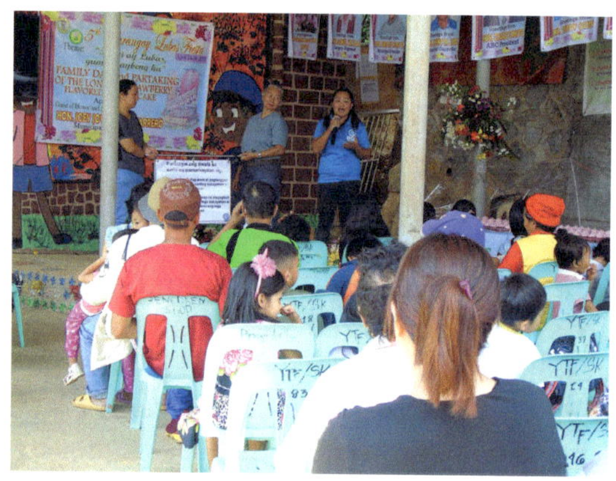

Figure 9.12. Community-based mental health program (CBMHP).

Source: https://external-content.duckduckgo.com/iu/?u=https%3A%2F%2Fwww.pmhacci.com%2Fwp-content%2Fuploads%2F2022%2F06%2FLubas.jpg&f=1&nofb=1&ipt=2441f54d58618bf4af0f2e601e7 2b754af8f838f96e75d512aa961dbd9f5bd79.

Thus, the complementarity of advocacy and education in community-based care not only enhances the mental well-being of individuals but also yields a more supportive climate that respects recovery and resilience and leads to healthier communities overall (Figure 9.12).

9.5.1. Types of Community Mental Health Services

Community mental health programs play a critical role in delivering mental health care via an integrated system designed to benefit individuals across a range of settings. Community mental health programs comprise a range of interventions, including outpatient therapy, crisis intervention, and community support programs. Outpatient therapy provides individuals with access to mental health practitioners who tailor treatment interventions to meet their individual needs, building resilience and coping skills. Crisis intervention services are most valuable to those experiencing acute mental health crises, stabilizing and supporting them immediately, and averting a resolution into more severe states. Also, community support programs—such as peer counseling and support groups—offer full-service settings that encourage social connectedness and mutual understanding, central components in the prevention of mental health stigma and facilitation of the help-seeking behavior of individuals. Special groups, like children and adolescents and disenfranchised populations, require specialized community mental health care in order to properly address their individualized needs. Child-focused services, for instance, are more likely to emphasize prevention and early intervention since it has been observed that mental health disorders recognized later in life tend to start as untreated issues during childhood. A public health approach to children's mental health becomes increasingly relevant, as it focuses on early identification, so too does it highlight the need for coordinated systems of care in schools and communities (Eichner et al., 2009). Similarly, there are disenfranchised groups that have specific barriers to receiving mental health care, necessitating culturally responsive services that promote equal access and awareness. Such population-focused interventions tackle the systemic inequalities and foster resilience, thus enhancing mental wellness and overall health in the community. Reducing stigma is a vital aspect of community mental health care because it directly influences the readiness of individuals to access treatment. Community education campaigns aim to raise people's awareness and normalize discussions on the issues of mental health, a step that lessens concomitant stigma against mental illness. The Movember Foundation's collaboration with the Centre for Men's Health is a direct reflection of this emphasis on research into successful mental health promotion and early intervention among boys and men specifically (Gough et al., 2015). Such schemes allow for honest conversation, thereby encouraging a culture in which individuals take responsibility for their mental health. Also, stigma reduction plays a crucial role in organizational policies and practices in mental health services in the community in such a way that not only are individuals provided with the care they require, but they are also valued and respected during the recovery process.

9.5.2. Benefits of Community-Based Interventions

Community-based programs are central elements in addressing mental health needs in various populations. With a focus on prevention and early intervention, these interventions have the ultimate goal of maximizing general well-being at the community level. School programs, for example, utilize the unique environment to foster emotional resilience and social competency among adolescents. The implementation of systems such as social-emotional learning (SEL) and peer-support systems not only increases educational engagement but also decreases levels of depression and anxiety, ultimately decreasing the prevalence of mental illness among this group. In addition, community-based interventions are plausible and within one's grasp, whereby individuals receive the assistance they need within more localized settings, thereby improving engagement and participation in mental health care (Dimitra et al., 2025). The effectiveness of community mental health programs often relies on culturally appropriate designs that resonate with the specific needs and histories of local communities. For instance, the Cameroon Baptist Convention Health Services Community-Based Health Program demonstrates highly promising outcomes with the blending of evidence-based psychological interventions with locally accepted practices. The outcome of this program reveals a clear improvement in participants' mental health status and coping mechanisms, establishing a 25% decrease in symptom severity over one year. These findings support the notion that integrating traditional clinical practice with local indigenous cultural practices not only recruits participants but also reduces stigma for mental health. These tailored interventions reflect an important shift towards integrating mental health care into broader community health strategies, promoting holistic wellness among diverse groups (Nganyu, 2025). Ultimately, the benefits of community-based interventions extend beyond individual improvement to foster systemic change in mental health perceptions and support structures. These initiatives often cultivate a sense of belonging and community engagement, which are essential for combating stigma associated with mental illness. Through an emphasis on participatory and collaborative approaches, programs enlist collective action and advocacy, challenging communities to put mental health on their agendas. Reducing stigma and encouraging open talk about mental health can greatly increase help-seeking behavior, with interventions occurring earlier and outcomes improving. With an increasing global population embracing such an integrated practice, the holistic options for enhancing mental well-being and resilience become increasingly attractive, necessitating stakeholders to advocate further for the enhancement of community-based mental health services (Dimitra et al., 2025; Nganyu, 2025) (Figure 9.13).

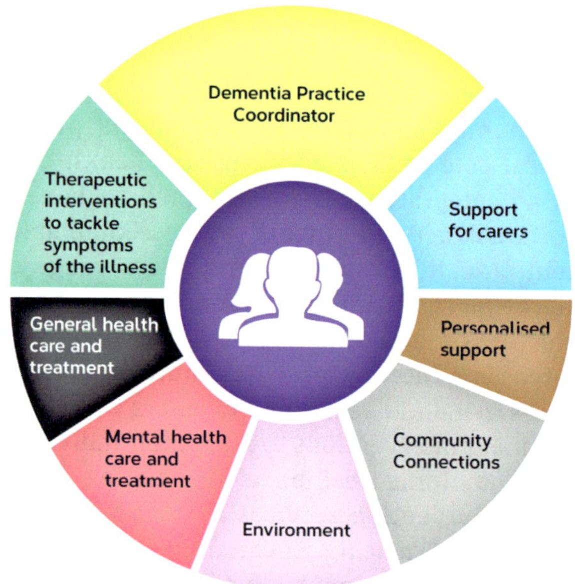

Figure 9.13. Model of community support.

Source: https://www.alzscot.org/sites/default/files/images/0002/1753/8_Pillars_Model-01.png.

9.5.3. Challenges Faced by Community Mental Health Services

Mental health community services are also severely tasked with providing proper care for individuals suffering from mental illness. The significant issue is that mental illness still has a negative perception, and this serves as a barrier to individuals availing themselves of care. The stigma leads to isolation, stigmatization, and a lack of awareness in communities and even within the healthcare system. This is compounded by a lack of adequate financing and resources for mental health treatment, which undermines their ability to provide effective care. Many individuals with mental illness are not provided with the treatment that they require, elevating the serious service deficit. As stated, about 10% of children have mental conditions resulting in impairment, but less than 20% are treated (Eichner et al., 2009). Therefore, the stigma issue is entangled with systemic barriers to the success of community mental health interventions. A lack of professionals who can respond to various mental health needs is another primary challenge the community mental health services are encountering. Educators and service providers most frequently report they are inadequately prepared to assist individuals who have mental health problems due to a lack of training and education on appropriate responses (Robinson et al., 2024). Thus, this lack of mental health literacy among the most critical stakeholders leads to prolonged avenues for early detection and intervention. Without a strong essential knowledge of mental health, school teachers and community workers would avoid discussions on mental health or not recognize when a person is distressed. This is even more critical in the rising mental health challenges post-COVID-19, where there is a greater need for staff trained in mental health. Closing this gap requires not just better training and education courses but also ongoing professional development in order to build confidence among mental health care providers. Lastly, to a certain extent, community mental health services are too often beset by issues of access and resource allocation. People in underserved communities, particularly those living in low-income communities or in rural communities, quite frequently have geographical and socioeconomic factors restricting their access to mental health treatment. Transportation barriers, lack of proximate facilities, and limited resources significantly contribute to sustaining disparities in mental health service receipt. Present-day circumstances indicate that a majority of communities are not sufficiently equipped to provide for the needs presented to them, significantly because of categorical underfunding of mental health infrastructure and services. Proper access to care is especially essential for children and youth because premature diagnosis and treatment can make mental illness worse (Eichner et al., 2009). Thus, the need for a fair and strategic approach to managing resources among community mental health services is most crucial so that all individuals can be given the opportunity to receive proper care.

9.6. Stigma Reduction Strategies

Stigma relating to mental health must be confronted in an effort to foster a more accepting and supportive community culture. Effective stigma reduction is often integrated with education-based interventions that challenge myths of mental illness. For instance, awareness campaigns targeting exposure to services such as Employee Assistance Programs (EAPs) can enhance the knowledge base of mental illness among both health professionals and the broader public. By means of activities such as the Plan-Do-Study-Act cycle to facilitate educational presentations, stakeholders can efficiently highlight the benefits of EAP services. Other than rendering the process less enigmatic, it also discusses the confidentiality bestowed on such resources, which would eventually result in a radical decrease in stigma. As greater knowledge of mental health services is raised, so does the potential that individuals will step forward to receive assistance without concern of stigma or discrimination (Gould et al., 2023). Another potentially effective way to decrease stigma is to get youth involved in mental health advocacy through career technical education classes. Student participation in programs, such as career and technical student organizations (CTSOs), allows them to play an active role in promoting mental well-being among their communities. Youth-defined activities that raise awareness of risk and protective factors for psychological distress are used in these programs to foster peer-to-peer support and openness when it comes to discussing mental health matters. Research shows that participation in CTSOs can serve to offset the disadvantages faced by young people, providing an outlet for leadership and engagement. Moreover, by inspiring students to initiate mental health campaigns, these organizations can build a generation that values mental health and thus reduce stigmatizing attitudes prevalent in their environments (Beck et al., 2022). Community-based therapies specifically tailored to reduce stigma can also significantly enhance public awareness and acceptance of mental illness. These therapies most commonly adopt a multiple strategy using media campaigns, public hearings, and alliances with influential community opinion leaders to counteract and disassemble negative stereotypes. Through focusing on stories of recovery and resilience, these campaigns are able to humanize mental health challenges, calling for sympathy and compassion among citizens.

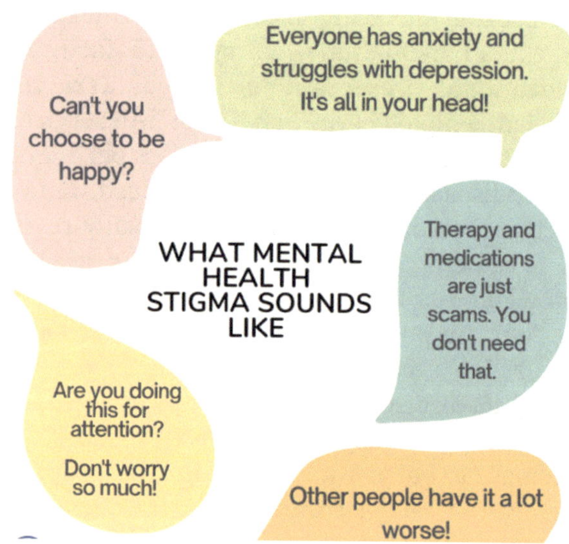

Figure 9.14. Stigma reduction.

Source: https://cccmedscoalition.org/wp-content/uploads/2023/02/What-MentAL-Health-Stigma-Sounds-Like-1024x1024.png.

Also, working with community groups can be applied to hold workshops and seminars that educate participants about the realities of mental illness, as well as supporting environments. In combination, these steps help to create an environment in which individuals are motivated to come forward and receive assistance, while interpersonal relationships are increased, and stigma attached to mental health disorders in community settings is decreased (Figure 9.14).

9.6.1. Understanding Stigma and Its Effects

Mental illness stigma has deeply ingrained effects, not only for individuals immediately affected but also for society in general. Stigma is manifested in a variety of ways, including social exclusion, discrimination, and negative stereotyping, which reinforce a vicious cycle of exclusion and distress. Once individuals are stigmatised, they come to internalise these negative attitudes themselves, leading to low self-esteem and exacerbation of mental health issues. With unemployment, for example, research has highlighted the degree to which the dual pressures of economic hardship and loss of identity lead to dramatic deterioration in mental health. The evidence of the unemployed in Bradford speaks to how, not only do the material challenges pose a risk to welfare, but the loss of a valued social status can drive the sense of insufficiency and despair that accompanies individuals being excluded from their society (Giuntoli et al., 2011). Understanding the social contexts of stigma can help in the development of successful interventions to counteract it. In the majority of marginalized populations, stigma becomes entangled with other health problems, creating an impact referred to as syndemics. A study examining the health outcomes among gay, bisexual, and other men who have sex with men (GBMSM) revealed that stigma and discrimination account for the conglomeration of negative health outcomes, including poor mental health (Ferlatte et al., 2020). Through the recognition that the presence of stigma is central to these syndemic settings, mental health care in community environments can structure interventions to eliminate the very social determinants fueling stigma. These teachings will be critical in building resilience and promoting mental well-being in community environments. Moreover, reducing stigma is crucial in enhancing the availability of mental health services. Where individuals feel stigmatized in seeking help, they will be more resistant to receiving community-based mental health services and thereby further isolate themselves from needed assistance. Education and awareness programs are the most successful method of reducing stigma and developing a mental health culture that recognizes mental health as integral to general health. Implementation of community-driven programs that focus on personal narrative and shared experience can break destructive, stigmatizing generalizations and develop respect and empathy. Finally, stigma reduction not only encourages the mental health of the individual but also a more accepting society in which people feel empowered to come forward and be in supportive relationships without fear of stigma.

9.6.2. Effective Strategies for Reducing Stigma

Stigma removal against mental illness is most crucial in creating support within communities and enhancing access to necessary services. The most impactful action is engaging community outreach programs where the force of aggregation of knowledge is utilized to break myths related to mental illness. Such programs encourage open discussion about mental health and allow individuals to share their experiences and learn from one another. Through the promotion of empathy and understanding, communities are able to dismantle harmful stereotypes and fill the void with stories of recovery and resilience. Community involvement not only builds resilience in social support but also sustains a sense of community, reaffirming that mental health is a shared effort. These shows are valuable venues for making it possible for the proper discussion of mental illness and reducing the feelings of isolation for so many, thereby producing environments favorable to healing and growth (Taliana et al., 2023). Educating healthcare workers and community leaders to be sensitive to their own biases against mental illness is a necessary stigma reduction activity. By engendering awareness and understanding of mental health issues, these individuals can, in fact, serve as change agents in their own neighborhoods. To illustrate, the use of Employee Assistance Programs (EAPs) in hospitals has been effective not only in promoting mental wellness but also in curbing stigma among medical staff themselves. One of the projects was aimed at nurse practitioners and demonstrated that an educational intervention increased awareness of EAP services while also dispelling myths surrounding their use. This strategy empowered health providers to seek assistance without stigma, illustrating how educated providers can influence community attitudes towards mental health services. Thus, engaging medical professionals in stigma reduction training enhances their ability to turn into effective role models by fostering an environment of acceptance (Gould et al., 2023). Stigma reduction in school and work environments through education interventions also plays a great part in reducing stigma by providing information on mental health, illness, and available resources. The activities can be delivered as workshops, seminars, or merely informal discussions aimed at engaging diverse audiences. By talking about mental health in an open way and incorporating evidence-based practices, such programs can de-stigmatize mental illness and generate hope among those affected. Peer support groups can be introduced in schools in which students are encouraged to share their experiences and challenges concerning mental health, thereby creating safe spaces to cultivate understanding and resilience. Similarly, workplace mental health training can equip employees and employers with the skills to establish inclusive workspaces that prioritize mental well-being. Through such initiatives, communities can build supportive networks that actively reduce stigma and prompt people to seek help, fostering a comprehensive approach to mental health that notices and validates the experience of all (Taliana et al., 2023) (Figure 9.15).

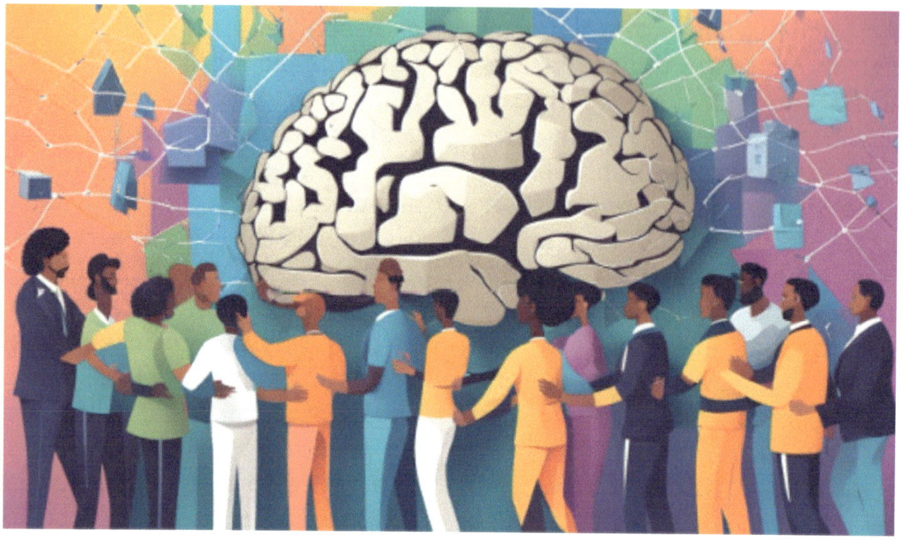

Figure 9.15. Effective strategies to fight bipolar disorder stigma.

Source: https://external-content.duckduckgo.com/iu/?u=https%3A%2F%2Fimages.squarespace-cdn.com%2Fcontent%2Fv1%2F6366ee2084b1c1355a31b927%2F08be0257-f865-448d-b8c1-1309126844fe%2F4.jpg%3Fformat%3D1500w&f=1&nofb=1&ipt=5aa7b0fbdca764ff0ec934f5942cc9a6c 63584d692fc2bfe95cd979d18fdb8da.

9.6.3. Role of Education and Awareness in Stigma Reduction

Education and awareness form the core drivers within the multifaceted process of stigmatization elimination regarding mental health. By educating individuals regarding mental illnesses, common myths can be refuted, enabling communities to form a more compassionate understanding of mental ailments. Secondly, awareness campaigns that center on personal stories and lived experiences have the potential to profoundly humanize individuals suffering from mental disorders to a point where empathy and fear would decline. It is particularly important in the college years, in which statistics indicate that a majority of students experience distress but do not access help due to stigma—few as an estimated 11% of those with diagnosable disorders access professional care (Vogel, Wade, & Hackler, 2007). Hence, a systematic educational strategy can serve as a bridge, bridging the treatment desire with a welcoming environment, essentially lowering barriers to mental health treatment (Halvorson et al., 2015). The educational function extends beyond raising awareness; it involves equipping individuals with knowledge that they can apply to action on mental health and coping. Training that involves the learning of efficient skills of emotional management and stress reduction can equip individuals to carry out self-help interventions themselves, diminishing the burden on community mental health care. Education-focused interventions such as these can foster resilience that allows individuals to manage adversity without succumbing to stigma. For instance, community-level interventions involving educational modules for early warning signs of mental illness have the potential to empower individuals with proactive help-seeking skills. Education integration within mental health services has been reported to increase community knowledge of mental illness and decrease discriminatory attitudes, thus being consistent with the global objective of improving mental well-being (Imperiale et al., 2016). Stigma reduction is also contingent upon the flexibility of education programs to multiple cultural contexts and sensitivity to the diverse factors influencing individuals' help-seeking behaviors. Such a context can illuminate how gender roles, cultural beliefs, and societal norms influence perceptions of mental health. For example, certain cultural communities may possess old-timey perceptions of opposing open discussion of emotional suffering, which creates ingrained stigma. By embedding culturally appropriate tools and resources in educational projects, it is possible for stakeholders to engage with communities that are diverse more effectively. Beyond the promotion of mental health literacy, this also promotes discussions on the complexities entailed in stigma around mental health. Responsive and inclusive education programs, therefore, must be capable of empowering all stakeholders in a community to embrace debates on mental health and promote an increased sense of understanding of the environment (Imperiale et al., 2016).

CLOSER LOOK

IMPORTANCE OF COMMUNITY INVOLVEMENT IN MENTAL HEALTH

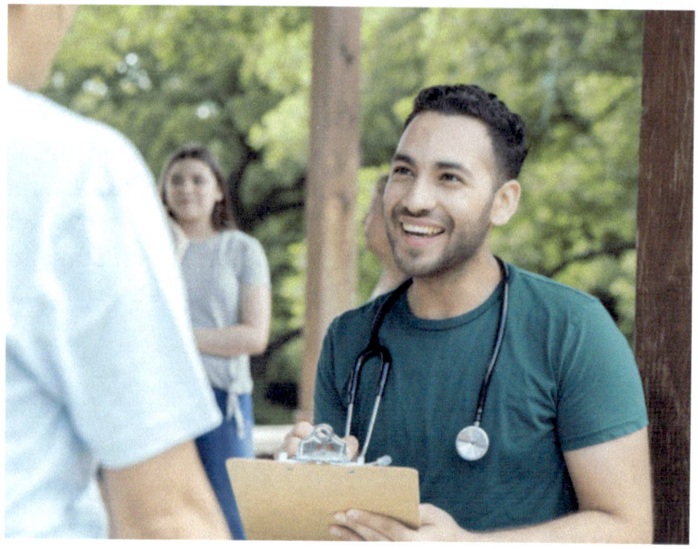

Figure 9.16. Community health worker engaging with a patient during an outdoor medical outreach.

Source: https://kenosiscenter.com/wp-content/uploads/2023/08/unnamed-2-1-1024x768.png.

Community involvement is crucial in addressing mental health issues through the development of supportive ecosystems that foster well-being and resilience. By uniting around issues of mental health, people develop support networks that can isolate feelings of isolation and stigma often attached to mental illness. By this coming together, mental health issues are brought to the fore, and honest dialogue is fostered that is critical to public education. Including community members in mental health activities makes them more aware and appreciative of mental health, and thereby society is more informed. This also impacts policies and resources in the community to empower the communities to tailor mental health interventions and services that are tailored to the needs of various populations and, therefore, inclusive and effective in addressing mental health. Besides, community-based mental health treatment plays a vital role in encouraging recovery by delivering support and resources to the individuals themselves. In case such services are included in their close-by community, then the neighborhood makes it more convenient for those who need assistance, i.e., overcoming major barriers that usually dissuade treatment from occurring, including lack of transport and access. Community-based engagement signifies that these treatments are not merely a response but also preventive, promoting resilience and early intervention. The participants in community mental health programs become members of healthy environments, in which they can share their experiences and acquire coping mechanisms. From active participation, belonging, and purpose are created. Lastly, from the collaborative strategy towards mental health programs, communities can establish sustainable structures that reinforce social welfare, yet fight the then-pervasive stigma about mental illness. Stigma reduction around mental health is inextricably tied to community engagement. Stigma has the power to be an enormous block to receiving help, most often keeping people from seeking the treatment and help they deserve. When communities become engaged in mental health advocacy, it's possible to dispel myths and encourage a more empathetic narrative. This involves not just awareness campaigns, but also the establishment of supportive communities that enable people to be in a position to narrate their own experience and stories without fearing stigmatization. Successful stigma-reduction requires the collaboration of diverse stakeholders, including local authorities, health care workers, and community organizations, to establish an inclusive setting celebrating the experiences of people with mental illness. Hence, both collaborative efforts in terms of community engagement and active reduction of stigma are required to create a society that prioritizes mental health and treats it equally.

SUMMARY

The study of mental health in the community reveals the multifaceted nature of mental illness and the paramount significance of understanding its various aspects. Ultimately, mental health issues have to be dealt with through a process that entails not only care at the level of the individual but also systemic interventions that are engendering resilience and wellness at the community level. Applying the staggering statistics of mental illness, such as one in five children having psychiatric symptoms annually, highlights the essential need for broad efforts that emphasize prevention and early intervention. By pursuing a public health strategy that includes understanding mental illness and promoting mental well-being, communities are in the best position to address the public health problem of untreated mental disorders, truly diminishing the staggering burden of disability and lost productivity that comes with these diseases (Eichner et al., 2009). Beyond the multidimensional comprehension of mental health, community-based interventions are also the way to deliver the best care. By participating in neighborhood activities that promote supportive networks, we can disarticulate the stigma and silence related to mental health, and create open discourse about mental health. Such a focus on being connected with the community not only promotes a sense of belonging but also develops a robust buffer against life stressors, which otherwise would be harmful to psychological well-being. Strategies of advocacy and education are central to empowering communities to seek assistance without the risk of stigma, enhancing access to existing mental health services. The success of these models in diverse cultural contexts also highlights the adaptability and relevance of community-based interventions to improving mental health and resilience (Taliana et al., 2023). Ultimately, unrelenting commitment to enhancing mental health in populations has to involve the participation of all parties, including policymakers, healthcare practitioners, and even the population itself. Future initiatives aimed at solving the mental health crisis will benefit from innovative strategies that integrate elements of successful models while upholding values of inclusivity and cultural responsiveness. Moving forward, it is essential that we do everything we can to pursue the implementation of comprehensive mental health services and interventions that address the unique needs of our populations. Through establishing environments that not only support individuals with mental illness but also enhance mental well-being, we will establish a strong foundation for healthier communities. The vision to move forward in mental health is not an overreacting response to challenges of today but is a visionary plan for tomorrow, where emotional and psychological well-being are natural features of life in communities (Eichner et al., 2009; Taliana et al., 2023).

It is also essential to understand the complexity of mental health and mental illness to foster a sense of community responsibility of support. Since mental illness manifests itself in invisible problems that can be faced by individuals at any age, popular belief is that everyone's business is mental health. This phrase emphasizes that it is everyone's business to recognize and resolve issues of mental health within communities. Furthermore, research indicates that there is a high prevalence of mental health problems among students in universities, pointing to the significance of mental health as a public health matter. Education and awareness programs can negate such challenges by equipping members of society with the necessary information to support one another in an appropriate manner, reiterating that mental health is a component of overall well-being that should be taken into consideration and action by everyone (Carter et al., 2017). Inculcating mental well-being and resilience has to be accomplished through a thorough understanding of the numerous factors that determine the mental health outcomes. Through a strengths-based practice, communities can encourage individuals to build resilience through self-improvement and collaboration. Community-based mental health services and interventions have an active role in this regard, involving a tailored method addressing the specific needs of the diverse population. Such interventions can enable making resources accessible, essential in the development of mental well-being, and eliminating the negative effects of mental disorders. Coalition efforts of mental health professionals, community agencies, and individuals must work together to create dynamic support systems that empower people without, at the same time, eliminating stigma attached to mental illness (Carter et al., 2018). Secondly, stigma reduction programs are crucial in mobilizing communities to acceptance and understanding. These efforts can include, for instance, public awareness campaigns, education, and normalizing talking about mental health in daily conversations. The aim is to create an environment where individuals feel free to relate their experiences with mental health problems without facing stigma or discrimination. By creating an open culture, communities can make individuals with such problems interact and form support groups that provide emotional and functional support. Lastly, stigma reduction is crucial in the broader context of mental health, as the embracing of diversity in mental health experience results in healthier, more diverse communities with well-being at the center for all (Carter et al., 2017).

REFERENCES

1. Abbasi, M. T., Rameez, S., Tahir, A. T., Usman, R., Islam, A., & Munazza. (2022). Students' health and well-being project, Pakistan. *Journal of Pakistan Psychiatric Society*. https://www.semanticscholar.org/paper/f77bc6a9392de27f9ae461ce0965bbf5b9c548f0 (accessed on 11th June 2025).
2. Abdullaev, T., Bhavaraju, R., Byrne, E., Citro, et al. (2018). *TB Stigma–Measurement Guidance*. https://core.ac.uk/download/287580942.pdf (accessed on 11th June 2025).
3. Beck, C., Loera, G., Nakamoto, J., et al. (2022). A qualitative study: Examining students' involvement in a career and technical student organizations and practicing and promoting mental wellness. https://core.ac.uk/download/543685820.pdf (accessed on 11th June 2025).
4. Bishop, J., Forrest, K., Hu, W., et al. (2019). Medical student wellbeing–a consensus statement from Australia and New Zealand. https://core.ac.uk/download/237216994.pdf (accessed on 11th June 2025).
5. Braybrook, D., Robertson, S., & Robinson, M. (2012). *Evaluation of the Choose Life North Lanarkshire Awareness Programmer: Final Report*. https://core.ac.uk/download/29018946.pdf (accessed on 11th June 2025).
6. Carter, M. A., & Francis, A. (2017). *The Inaugural Australasian Mental Health and Higher Education Conference 2017: Conference Information and Book of Abstracts*. https://core.ac.uk/download/303783308.pdf (accessed on 11th June 2025).
7. Condie, A. W., Judd, H., Keady, T., et al. (2024). Cooperative Extension's role in addressing the opioid overdose crisis: Best practices from the HEART Initiative model. https://core.ac.uk/download/617838652.pdf (accessed on 11th June 2025).
8. Cross, R. M., Kinsella, K., & South, J. (2011). *An Evaluation of the C-Card Scheme in Bradford District*. https://core.ac.uk/download/29018944.pdf (accessed on 11th June 2025).
9. Duffee, J. H., Szilagyi, M., Forkey, H., & Kelly, E. T. (2021). Trauma-informed care in child health systems. *Pediatrics, 148*. https://doi.org/10.1542/peds.2021-052579 (accessed on 11th June 2025).
10. Eichner, J. C. (2009). *Early Childhood Mental Health: A Public Health Approach*. https://core.ac.uk/download/12206650.pdf (accessed on 11th June 2025).
11. Ferlatte, O., Flowers, P., Frankis, J., Gilbert, et al. (2020). Informing theoretical development of salutogenic, asset-based health improvement to reduce syndics among gay, bisexual and other men who have sex with men: Empirical evidence from secondary analysis of multi-national, online cross-sectional surveys. https://core.ac.uk/download/293867764.pdf (accessed on 11th June 2025).
12. Giorgi, G., Lecca, L. I., Alessio, F., Finstad, G. L., Bondanini, G., Lulli, L. G., Arcangeli, G., et al. (2020). COVID-19-related mental health effects in the workplace: A narrative review. *International Journal of Environmental Research and Public Health, 17*, 7857–7857. https://doi.org/10.3390/ijerph17217857 (accessed on 11th June 2025).
13. Giuntoli, G., Karban, K., Kisella, K., et al. (2011). *Mental Health, Resilience and the Recession in Bradford*. https://core.ac.uk/download/29018948.pdf (accessed on 11th June 2025).

14. Giuntoli, G., Kinsella, K., & South, J. (2013). *An Evaluation of the Walking for Wellness Project and the Befriender Role.* https://core.ac.uk/download/29018943.pdf (accessed on 11th June 2025).

15. Gough, B., Hanna, E., Raine, G., et al. (2015). *Promoting Mental Health and Wellbeing with Men and Boys: What Works?* https://core.ac.uk/download/30267232.pdf (accessed on 11th June 2025).

16. Gould, S. (2023). *A Quality Improvement Project to Increase Awareness and Utilization of Employee Assistance Program Services Among Healthcare Providers.* https://core.ac.uk/download/597009069.pdf (accessed on 11th June 2025).

17. Griffin, B. J., Purcell, N., Burkman, K., Litz, B. T., Bryan, C. J., Schmitz, M., Villierme, C., et al. (2019). Moral injury: An integrative review. *Journal of Traumatic Stress, 32*, 350–362. https://doi.org/10.1002/jts.22362 (accessed on 11th June 2025).

18. Halvorson, M. D. (2015). *Impact of Culture on Stigma Related to Help-Seeking Behavior in College Students.* https://core.ac.uk/download/211332523.pdf (accessed on 11th June 2025).

19. Hocking, B. (2025). *A Life Without Stigma.* https://core.ac.uk/download/pdf/30676353.pdf (accessed on 11th June 2025).

20. Hossain, M. M., Tasnim, S., Sultana, A., Faizah, F., Mazumder, H., Zou, L., McKyer, E. L. J., et al. (2020). Epidemiology of mental health problems in COVID-19: A review. *F1000Research, 9*, 636–636. https://doi.org/10.12688/f1000research.24457.1 (accessed on 11th June 2025).

21. Imperiale, M. G., Perera, E., & White, R. G. (2016). The capabilities approach: Fostering contexts for enhancing mental health and wellbeing across the globe. https://core.ac.uk/download/42370416.pdf (accessed on 11th June 2025).

22. Katsarou, D. V., Kougioumtzis, G., Efthymiou, E., Sofologi, M., & Mantsos, E. (2025). School-based mental health interventions for adolescents: Supporting typically developing students and students with neurodevelopmental disorders. *Review of Clinical Pharmacology and Pharmacokinetics–International Edition.* https://www.semanticscholar.org/paper/1d27d750ebd201d433eaaf57369a84e81f466b23 (accessed on 11th June 2025).

23. McCartie, L. (2018). *A Junior Educator's Guide to Proactively Promoting Mental Health And Well-Being Through Resilience.* https://core.ac.uk/download/160475436.pdf (accessed on 11th June 2025).

24. Mostafa, M. (2023). *From the Arab World to the United States of America: The Wellness of Arab Graduate Women Studying in the U.S.* https://core.ac.uk/download/603960668.pdf (accessed on 11th June 2025).

25. Mulyani, A., & Hardiyanti, T. (2025). Community-based mental health education for reducing stigma and improving knowledge in Batujajar Timur Village, West Bandung. *Indonesian Journal of Community Development.* https://www.semanticscholar.org/paper/dc415091dbad854132e23e7d30f5d0021632a382 (accessed on 11th June 2025).

26. Nganyu, G. N. (2025). An evaluation of the mental health component of the Cameroon Baptist Convention Health Services' community-based health program: A quasi-experimental study. *Greener Journal of Social Sciences.* https://www.semanticscholar.org/paper/01b51768b253b90dc5754cf9156b1012b5e519b6 (accessed on 11th June 2025).

27. Ojo, S., Okoye, T. O., Olaniyi, S. A., Ofochukwu, V. C., Obi, M. O., Nwokolo, A., Okeke-Moffatt, C., et al. (2024). Ensuring continuity of care: Effective strategies for the post-hospitalization transition of psychiatric patients in a family medicine outpatient clinic. *Cureus, 16*. https://www.semanticscholar.org/paper/3cf420b960f385b3ae2104336cd106ae24688b17 (accessed on 11th June 2025).

28. Parker-Grewe, T. (2017). *Fostering Awareness, Inclusivity, And Self-Efficacy: Facing Social and Internalized Recovery Stigma*. https://core.ac.uk/download/200292693.pdf (accessed on 11th June 2025).

29. Randemark, N. F. R., & Barros, S. (2014). The family in therapeutic design of users of CAPS: Representations of health professionals. *Journal of Nursing UFPE Online, 8*, 1956–1964. https://www.semanticscholar.org/paper/c72bcd3d923dc552fb6e27dae279f4a7819e737b (accessed on 11th June 2025).

30. Reardon, C. L., Hainline, B., Aron, C. M., Baron, D., Baum, A., Bindra, A., Budgett, R., et al. (2019). Mental health in elite athletes: International Olympic Committee consensus statement (2019). *British Journal of Sports Medicine, 53*, 667–699. https://doi.org/10.1136/bjsports-2019-100715 (accessed on 11th June 2025).

31. Robinson, M. (2024). *Supporting Mental Health Education in Ontario Secondary Schools: A Cross-Curricular Handbook for Ontario Secondary Teachers*. https://core.ac.uk/download/604185245.pdf (accessed on 11th June 2025).

32. Ta, U. (2023). Overcoming structural inequity in healthcare for people living with substance use issues and mental illness. *International Journal of Integrated Care*. https://www.semanticscholar.org/paper/d0856615e46d9504a2de7321067459c666f75c9d (accessed on 11th June 2025).

33. Taliana, L. (2023). *The Role of Community Engagement in Promoting Mental Wellness*. https://core.ac.uk/download/596259226.pdf (accessed on 11th June 2025).

34. Wallman-Stokes, C., Bechtolsheimer, G., Appel, J., Gable, J., Chiu, J., Rosqueta, K., & Hobble, R. (2015). *Lifting the Burden of Addiction: Philanthropic Opportunities to Address Substance Use Disorders in the United States*. https://core.ac.uk/download/75783859.pdf (accessed on 11th June 2025).

35. Wang, F. (2023). *Suicide Prevention: A Must-Do Task*. https://core.ac.uk/download/578764267.pdf (accessed on 11th June 2025).

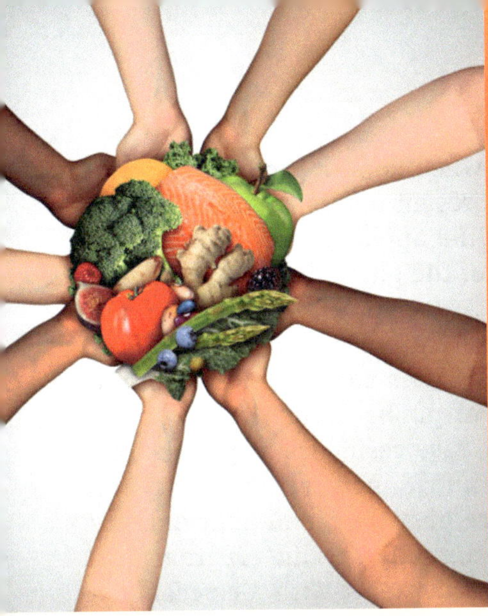

Chapter 10

ENHANCING COMMUNITY AND PUBLIC HEALTH THROUGH NUTRITIONAL STRATEGIES

Contents

Introduction

The incorporation of nutritional strategies into public health systems has become more of a requirement in the control of chronic illnesses and promoting community welfare. As lifestyle-related disorders such as obesity, diabetes, and cardiovascular illnesses have risen in prevalence, there has been a further need for integrated nutrition strategies. Through the adoption of eating habits as a central element of health promotion, communities are better able to address such prevalent conditions. Nutrition is an essential element in disease prevention because research has established the ability of dietary intervention to achieve remarkable health improvement among populations. Through nutrition education and resources, public health programs can foster a culture of wellness with the inclusion of healthy patterns of food consumption and informed food choices, increasing the well-being of all individuals and lowering the costs of diet-related disease care. In recent years, the term probiotics has become increasingly popular as a promising element of nutritional regimens aimed at enhancing public health. Probiotics are live microorganisms that, when administered in adequate numbers, have a health-improving effect on the host, and they represent a very powerful tool for fighting a broad spectrum of diseases. With the changes in diets, the application of probiotics in daily nutrition has acquired the power to improve the well-being of the gut, enhance the immune system, and treat mental diseases. The International Scientific Association for Probiotics and Prebiotics explains the importance of a precise definition and application of probiotics to help consumers effectively. Coverage of this emerging field not only educates communities regarding making educated food choices but also becomes a valuable part of public health action as they seek out multifaceted solutions to increase the well-being and disease resilience of populations. Furthermore, improving community health through evidence-based nutrition interventions requires a multidisciplinary intervention that includes dietitians, healthcare providers, and policymakers. To be effective, these initiatives require, at a fundamental level, community-specific programs that meet local dietary habits and food choices. Tailoring its approach in accordance with socioeconomic determinants of health, such as food access and cultural dietary habits, makes this more effective. Public health interventions can make health advice easier to adhere to and improve participation in wellness programs by adapting nutritional strategies to specific requirements for different groups of people. Engaging communities to tailor these strategies has the ability to induce long-term behavioral change, which ultimately results in a healthier population. Thus, the inclusion of targeted nutritional strategies is one such opportunity to enhance community and public health effectively (Figure 10.1).

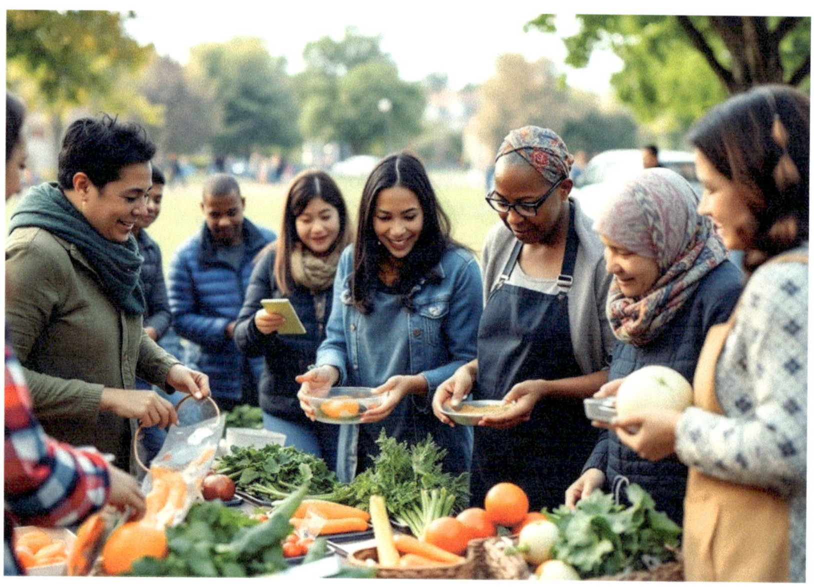

Figure 10.1. Promoting public health nutrition community strategies.

Source: https://drzam.com/wp-content/uploads/2025/04/promoting-public-health-nutrition-community-strategies-jhl.jpg.

Definition of Community and Public Health

The intersection of community and public health is essential to understanding how public action can result in improved health. Community health is the product of a specific set of people's health, and in most circumstances, it is dictated by environmental, socio-economic, and cultural factors. Effective community health programs take these dynamics into account and attempt to counteract them using evidence-based measures. A critical component is active engagement by community members in problem definition and solution conceptualization, creating a sense of ownership and empowerment. For instance, within the Market district of South Belfast, Queen's Communities and Place (QCAP) and the Market Development Association (MDA) collaborated to engage residents in discussions illuminating their personalized issues related to drug use and the need for targeted education programs (Arago´n et al., 2023). In the development of participatory methods, such initiatives can ensure that health policies are effective and relevant. Public health, however, encompasses bigger actions to safeguard and promote the health of populations. It includes enforcing policies, prevention activities, and health education that are oriented to lower health hazards and improve health equity on a population scale. Public health professionals assess the effectiveness of various interventions and make them dynamic based on epidemiological evidence and population feedback. More especially against the background of the COVID-19 pandemic, the expansion of telemedicine services demonstrated how public health initiatives are ready to address pressing healthcare needs while increasing equity and access (Chen et al., 2023). By integrating technology into the provision of healthcare, public health systems can access underserved populations more effectively, thereby decreasing health disparities. This broad framework indicates the need for harmonized methods involving public health understanding and community expertise. Public and community health strengthening necessitates a vision that engages nutritional strategies in the promotion of public health outcomes. Nutrition is crucial in its influence on community health because diet patterns shape the prevalence of disease as well as the quality of health. Community-based nutritional education programs have the potential to enable individuals to make informed decisions that result in healthier living, which ultimately reduces the chronic disease burden. For instance, programs developed jointly with local institutions tend to align with community concerns and preferences, making them more effective. Similarly, the availability of healthy foods is also critical and needs to be addressed alongside educational efforts. Achieving food equity falls into line not only with public health objectives but also with building community resilience and cohesion. Therefore, effective improvement of community and public health through nutrition is contingent upon the coming together of educational efforts, available resources, and active participation of community members in planning health interventions (Figure 10.2).

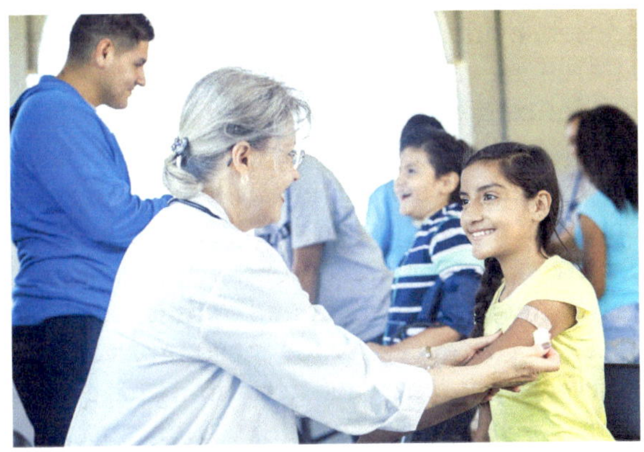

Figure 10.2. Healthcare provider administering vaccination to a child during a community health event.

Source: https://images.aspen.edu/wp/uploads/2020/01/GettyImages-545353282-scaled.jpg.

Importance of Nutrition in Health Outcomes

The contribution of nutrition towards influencing health outcomes cannot be overstated, given that it is inextricably linked to the well-being of the individual and population. Poor nutritional intake can lead to a variety of chronic diseases, including obesity, diabetes, and cardiovascular disease, that disproportionately affect the most vulnerable populations. As noted by recent research, lower-income groups, particularly among Latinos and African Americans, have poor access to healthy nutrition, thereby exposing them to more adverse health conditions than those of their higher-income counterparts. Thus, while addressing public health, one should not just consider dietary lifestyles but also the overall socio-economic determinants that control these lifestyles. By putting nutrition education and healthy food availability at the center of these populations, we can begin to close the disparity gap in health and create healthier results in diverse populations (Bowie et al., 2004). In addition, integrating nutrition into public health activities encourages healthy eating patterns from childhood, especially in children. Evidence indicates that well-nourished children are more able to perform successfully academically and socially, and ultimately as healthy adults. With the introduction of school and childcare center nutritional programs, communities can provide children with access to nutrients that are essential for maximum growth and development and optimal cognitive function. The necessity for these interventions is further apparent when accounting for cyclical poverty's role in continuing poor nutrition. Thus, policymakers are urged to consider a comprehensive approach, such as improving access to fruit and vegetables and nutrition education, for achieving a healthier future for all children (Garrett et al., 2020). Last but not least, the future capacity of effective nutritional approaches is not only found in short-term health gains but also in fostering a culture of well-being within communities. Through recognizing and overcoming barriers to healthy eating, such as economic constraints and a shortage in health food access, it is more evident that certain interventions are capable of inducing long-term change. Projects designed to enhance local assets, such as farmers' markets in a specific area and community gardens, are not only capable of providing fresh foods but also of educating the public about healthy choices. These programs not only lower the incidence of diet-related diseases but also empower people to manage their health results. While we keep looking for the link between nutrition and public health, it is clear that with a unified effort, drastic changes can be achieved, ultimately producing a healthier, more just society (Bowie et al., 2004).

Overview of Nutritional Strategies

A complete examination of nutrition interventions illustrates the multifaceted approaches that must be utilized in an effort to enhance community and public health. Child care and health system integration is among the most important approaches that focus on reducing health disparities among low-income children. Existing research indicates that poor, African American, and Latino children are likely to experience significant difficulties in obtaining health care and have significantly poorer health status compared to their middle-class counterparts. By employing targeted programs—like increasing health care and health education funding—communities are able to make the health playing field more even. Not only can these programs potentially improve children's health, but they can also act with ease in targeting the neediest populations, identifying the importance of well-designed support systems based on policy and professional recommendations (Bowie et al., 2004). The other crucial nutrition strategy is in promoting the farming practices of smallholder farmers. This strategy, in the main part, addresses raising food production to be both consumed at home and sold in the market and, consequently, directly affects nutritional outcomes. The smallholder value chain approach highlights three main channels: improved nutrition from home consumption, better income from the sale of agricultural produce, and better income through local purchase schemes. Through involving smallholder farmers, communities can offer a more stable supply of nutritious foods that can alleviate food insecurity and enhance diets. Apart from this, these strategies demand filling important gaps in agricultural-nutrition linkages knowledge to maximize them in serving public health maximally (Dorp et al., 2025). Not only do these strategies enhance local economies, but they also allow communities to be masters of their nutritional welfare. Lastly, having nutritional education programs is a key to developing healthier food intake in communities. The educational programs play a crucial role in eliminating prevalent conditions such as obesity and dietary diseases. With individuals educated on what they should consume, the programs can promote the consumption of food that is nutrient-rich and avoid the use of processed foods that are high in sugars and fats.

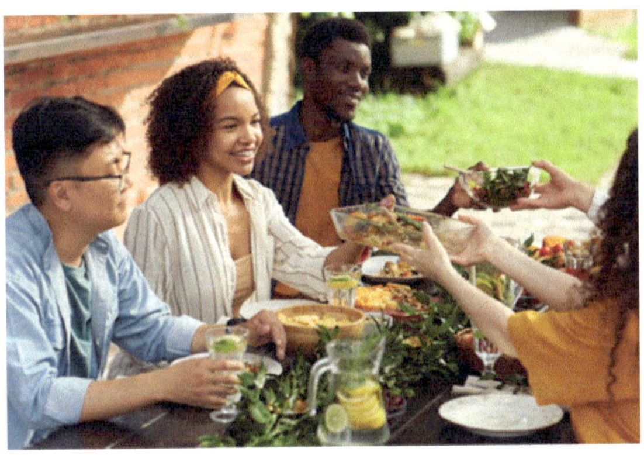

Figure 10.3. Nutrition in the health sector.

Source: https://ugc.futurelearn.com/uploads/images/50/3e/regular_503eedfa-335d-4361-84e7-9d1f37b83870.png.

Encouraging community participation via workshops, cooking courses, and accessible information has been shown to enhance knowledge as well as generate behavior change in nutrition. With communities learning more about their nutritional needs, the chances of embracing healthy lifestyles become higher, subsequently contributing to improved public health levels. By continuing to support these education programs, communities have enhanced opportunities towards instilling a culture that emphasizes educated dietary choices and healthy living (Figure 10.3).

10.1. The Role of Nutrition in Public Health

Nutrition plays an important role in the arena of public health because it influences the overall well-being and quality of life of communities and individuals. Nutrition and its relationship with health are evident in the prevalence of diet-related diseases, such as obesity, diabetes, and cardiovascular diseases. Individuals with limited access to nutritious foods often encounter a multitude of health issues, which create a disease-economic struggle cycle. Addressing these problems requires a comprehensive strategy that not only encompasses nutrition education but also environmental modification of food environments. An understanding of the etiology of food access allows public health programs to better craft their programs to serve the needs of at-risk populations and promote healthier food consumption habits that can have a profound impact on community health outcomes (Mikkelsen et al., 2007). Public health nutrition strategies also emphasize the importance of culturally suitable foods to trigger acceptance and participation of communities. When food programs are designed with local communities' input and preferences, they stand a greater likelihood of success in achieving sustainable changes in diet. Community setting-based interventions can respond to healthy eating barriers specific to multicultural settings, rendering health promotion more acceptable and accessible. For instance, the utilization of local food resources and promotion of local foods can assist in nutritional enhancement as well as economic sustainability. All these programs not only improve health but also increase social relationships within the community, creating a high-level social investment in public health results (Garrett et al., 2020). Last but not least, the implementation of public policies that promote nutrition-based programs is important in the long term for enhancing community health. Collaborations between local governments, health agencies, and community organizations can lead to effective policies that increase access to healthy foods and reduce disparities concerning the availability of food. Programs that increase food literacy, such as cooking classes or nutrition workshops, can empower individuals with the knowledge and skills needed to make smart dietary choices and influence the general public's health environment. Since health leaders in public communities recognize that nutrition is a central part, it is more necessary to advocate for policy that supports food security and accessibility so that all communities will be able to have the resources to encourage optimum health (Mikkelsen et al., 2007) (Figure 10.4).

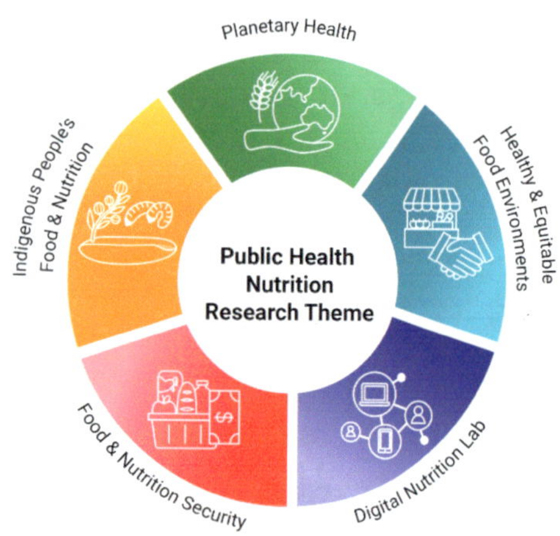

Figure 10.4. Public health nutrition research.

Source: https://www.monash.edu/__data/assets/image/0008/3374396/overview-diagram-circular-whitelines.png.

10.1.1. Impact of Diet on Chronic Diseases

The relationship between diet and chronic disease is increasingly recognized as the key to public health. Diet is a key driver of the development and exacerbation of obesity, diabetes, cardiovascular disease, and high blood pressure. Chronic diseases are interdependent, with one condition promoting another to produce a mesh of health issues that reinforce one another. For example, an unhealthy diet with high amounts of processed food, sugars, and fatty foods increases the risk of obesity, one of the most common risk factors for type 2 diabetes. Moreover, an unhealthy diet can lead to inflammation and insulin resistance, adding to health issues. Disrupting such eating patterns through interventions that take place within communities can promote healthier citizens who are less vulnerable to chronic diseases, thus enhancing public health in general. Healthy dietary improvement strategies should consider the environmental and socioeconomic determinants of unhealthy nutrition, particularly in vulnerable groups. Social and economic gradients in access to healthy foods through diets usually underlie increased rates of chronic disease in disadvantaged communities. Healthy behavior promotion programs, such as state-level policy to enhance nutrition in child care and schools, have been promising in controlling childhood obesity as well as chronic diseases. These programs focus on creating enabling environments that enable people to make healthier lifestyle choices. By implementing such actions at the level of the community, public health agencies can respond not only to short-term nutritional needs but also contribute to long-term health improvement by reducing the social and economic costs arising from chronic disease, as cited in recent studies (N/A, 2009). In addition, there is a need to determine the unique problem that specific segments, such as HIV-positive individuals, experience with increased vulnerability to chronic diseases.

While advances in medical treatment allow these individuals to live longer, the danger of secondary complications like diabetes and hypertension is enhanced. This example underlines the need for individualized nutritional therapy and support services aimed at addressing health and social disparities, particularly in low-income African American women. Project THANKS demonstrates the value of incorporating a socio-ecological model into this plan by addressing individual, social, and environmental requirements. Such efforts not only seek to enhance eating habits but also empower communities to minimize adverse health outcomes linked with chronic diseases (Amutah et al., 2015). Prioritizing these targeted nutritional interventions is essential in order to enhance community well-being and provide equal access to wellness resources.

10.1.2. Nutritional Disparities in Different Communities

Nutritional disparities among different populations pose a significant public health problem. Economic constraints tend to restrict the availability of healthy food, particularly for poor communities, which can lead to reliance on low-cost foods with high calorie density but are largely nutrient-poor. For instance, families that reside in food deserts usually have poor access to fresh fruits and vegetables and, therefore, perpetuate poor diets with corresponding higher rates of malnutrition. The World Health Organization emphasizes that malnutrition is detrimental to child health and development, and efforts are needed for targeted interventions to eliminate these gaps. Interventions that promote maternal nutrition, as evidenced by the Mamta nutrition program in Pakistan, demonstrate how fortified foods can catalyze children's nutritional status improvement and break cycles of malnutrition, demonstrating the scope for strategic programming in nutrition to bridge these gaps (Hussain et al., 2025). Moreover, the role of community and infrastructural planning in nutritional disparity must not be underemphasized. Urban green spaces such as community gardens can provide solid foundations in food-insecure areas.

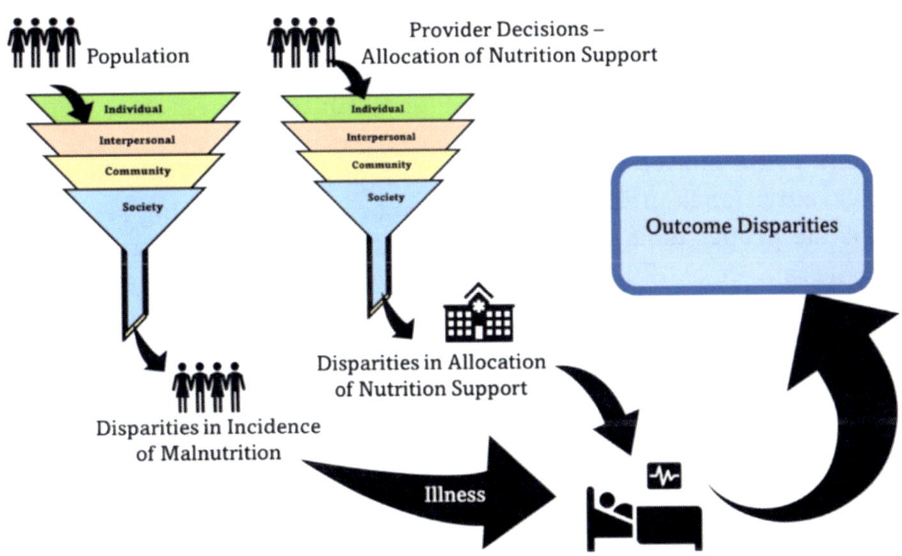

Figure 10.5. Disparities and differential allocation of nutritional therapies.

Source: https://media.springernature.com/lw1200/springer-static/image/art%3A10.1007%2Fs40137-024-00417-9/MediaObjects/40137_2024_417_Fig3_HTML.png.

Green infrastructure for eating adds to the contribution of fresh food but is also a contributor to community involvement and social cohesion, with resultant better overall health and well-being. Evidently, urban green spaces are of great importance in terms of having a strong correlation with improved health outcomes, particularly for those cities under high environmental stress (Russo, 2024). Access to such spaces is thus pivotal in supporting nutritional equity because they can neutralize the effects of socioeconomic disparities and promote healthy living among different populations. Nutritional inequalities thus need to be controlled via a mix of education and infrastructure measures. Nutrition education is a critical part of empowering communities to make healthy food selections, particularly where there may be limited health literacy. Through guided outreach and assistance, people are able to become adept at selecting healthier choices and using available food sources more efficiently. Aiding this educational aspect with initiatives aimed at increasing access to healthful foods, such as by subsidizing farmers' markets or through partnerships with food banks, can also help improve community nutrition. Lastly, a complete understanding of the unique challenges posed by different communities is needed to create effective nutritional interventions, offering all groups the proper tools to achieve optimal health (Hussain et al., 2025; Russo, 2024) (Figure 10.5).

10.1.3. Importance of Nutrition Education

Nutrition education plays a fundamental role in influencing food habits, thus impacting public and community health outcomes significantly. Nutrition education equips individuals with information on nutrition science, enabling them to make informed, healthy food choices informed by an awareness of the health impacts of their eating patterns. Nutrition education is crucial in the control of chronic lifestyle diseases prevalent in most communities, such as obesity and diabetes. For instance, nutrition education programs that instruct on whole foods instead of processed foods can provide better health outcomes. Additionally, with the inclusion of culturally relevant nutritional knowledge, the population is more likely to embrace these lessons, making long-standing changes in dietary habits that honor health and heritage. In this case, the issue is not only providing information but empowering individuals to make more informed decisions that resonate within their cultures, a critical element of effective nutrition education. Nutrition education is also rendered more critical since it can empower communities to take charge of their health. Involvement of community members in nutrition education programs enhances their capacity to make informed decisions regarding food buying, meal planning, and food preparation. Through the development of food databases and meal planning competencies, nutrition education not only enhances the health of individuals but also reinforces the resilience of communities against food insecurity. The fact that such empowerment has been evidenced, manifesting itself through grassroots movements demanding policy changes to improve access to healthy food, is significant. For example, as documented in capacity strengthening research to respond to food security program needs, effective training in nutrition can induce generalized improvement in line with the objectives of ensuring accessibility and adequacy of food (Msuya et al., 2025). Nutrition education is thus a catalyst for broader community health intervention in terms of individual empowerment as well as group advocacy. Last, incorporating nutrition education into public health policy is essential for the improvement of community health and the prevention of diet-related diseases. It offers a process of formation through which individuals can acquire critical skills and knowledge to make healthy choices within a complex food system.

In addition, sustainable dietary modifications—nurtured by appropriately designed education programs—fight against the global epidemic of malnutrition, including undernutrition and overnutrition. As highlighted by nutrition counseling advocacy groups, well-educated communities are more likely to overcome the hurdles of food deserts and unhealthy food marketing. Thus, by acknowledging the importance of nutrition education, public health policies can better address systemic challenges to healthy eating and enable initiatives that lead to food accessibility equity, creating healthier populations (Garrett et al., 2020).

10.2. Community-Based Nutritional Programs

Community-based nutrition interventions have become increasingly important strategies in public health promotion and the alleviation of nutritional inadequacies, particularly among vulnerable groups. These interventions tend to be community-oriented, with the planning and implementation of the interventions involving the participation of the community. There is evidence that access to nutritious foods has a very significant effect on dietary consumption patterns, particularly among low-income individuals. Through the identification of healthy food access barriers and engagement of residents in the process of creating solutions, such programs not only promote nutritional enhancement but also a stronger sense of community. Through nutrition workshops, food preparation demonstrations, and local procurement, community-based programs empower others to make healthy choices regarding their diet, responding to the pressing concern of food insecurity and the resultant health threats (Mikkelsen et al., 2007). In addition, the success of community-based nutrition interventions is frequently dependent on their capacity to build upon existing local infrastructure and information, inducing lasting long-term effects. Partnerships with local farmers and entrepreneurs benefit the local economy in addition to improving food security and nutrition choices. Programs may also integrate culturally applicable practices and foods, thus building ownership and pride among participants. Notably, studies have confirmed that active participants in such community programs among residents are more likely to adopt healthy eating habits, and encourage their families and larger community social networks to follow suit. Moreover, regular review and revision of such programs guarantee that they remain effective and sensitive to changing community needs and priorities (Garrett et al., 2020).

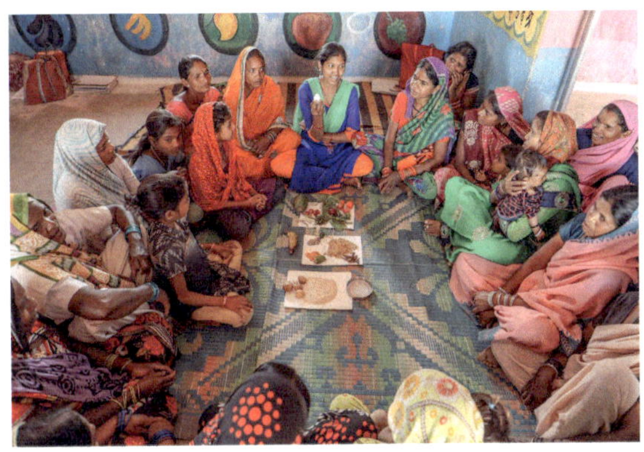

Figure 10.6. Community-based nutrition programs.

Source: https://poshan.ifpri.info/files/2020/04/OFM.jpg.

In short, the positive effects of neighborhood-based nutrition programs extend beyond improved consumption habits; they also favor broader public health goals. In reaching explicitly targeted obstacles to wholesome consumption and implementing grassroots interventions, these programs can enhance physical and mental well-being in communities disproportionately impacted by food insecurity and associated health disparities. Thus, they remain an important area for additional research, policy-making, and funding. By emphasizing collective approaches that engage residents, community-based food programs set the stage for healthy, health-conscious communities that are capable of sustaining healthy behaviors in the long term (Mikkelsen et al., 2007) (Figure 10.6).

10.2.1. Examples of Successful Community Programs

Innovative community programs have been shown to have the potential to enhance public health through targeted nutritional interventions. A prime example is the STRETCH Initiative, a community program that makes use of a community-based solution to address food insecurity by promoting access to nutritious foods. The initiative allows residents of the community to take charge of their nutritional well-being by establishing community farms and farmers' markets. The program not only creates a culture of health consumption but also encourages social coherence between participants, thereby addressing several facets of health equity. Besides, integration of nutrition and cooking skills educational workshops provides essential knowledge for members in a community to make well-informed dietary choices, which ultimately contributes to improved health conditions and reduction of diet-related diseases, as is consistent with the overall strategies discussed in the assessment of successful public health programs (Ugwu et al., 2025). Another great program is the development of disaster-resilient village projects in Surakarta, focusing on environmental health and nutrition. This intervention has integrated sanitation improvements and water quality monitoring with education on nutrition, emphasizing the connection between clean environments and food. By improving infrastructure and good eating habits, the program has recorded a significant decline in diet and water-borne diseases. As an example, better sanitation conditions and the availability of safe drinking water have helped decrease disease transmission rates, and nutrition education helps inform members of the community about the benefits of eating a balanced diet. The combination of these elements reveals how the promotion of environmental health by community programs can have serious effects on the resilience of public health (Subarno et al., 2025). Finally, the success of community programs will rest on their ability to engage local populations and address specific health concerns with innovative strategies. The lessons learned from these programs highlight the importance of collaboration between health organizations, local institutions, and community members. Programs like the STRETCH Initiative and disaster-resilient villages set the stage for potential intervention, showing how empowering contexts can be used to create sustained improvements in health. Both methods emphasize empowerment and participation in public health interventions, particularly since communities are confronted with the issues of food security and health inequity. Policy makers and practitioners can further develop efficient nutritional policies that enhance the well-being of the individual and community through drawing on these lessons obtained (Ugwu et al., 2025; Subarno et al., 2025).

10.2.2. Role of Local Organizations in Promoting Nutrition

Local organizations play an important role in nutrition promotion as they serve as connecting links between society members and facilities and support systems tailored to enhance their food habits. Being well-acquainted with the particular cultural and socioeconomic features of their residents, local organizations are able to more effectively apply strategies that are acceptable and effective locally. Through the organization of workshops, nutrition education, and the encouragement of community gardens, such organizations empower communities and families to take charge of their health. They encourage communities where healthy eating is not only accessible but also culturally acceptable, and they work to change food-related community values and norms. With collaborations with governments and businesses at the local level, such organizations receive more resources at their disposal, hence a healthier community. This participatory process shows how local organizations are at the forefront of propelling public health initiatives towards improving nutrition. Besides, local organizations played a vital role in fighting the odds that low-income people face while attempting to get access to healthy food. They advocate policy changes that improve food equity so that all people gain equal opportunities for a healthy life, regardless of their level of income. For instance, by means of public consultation, local authorities can implement helpful interventions for promoting healthy eating and exercise, particularly in areas that are designated as food deserts. These interventions, in addition to mitigating the adverse effects of poor eating habits, also give a sense of belonging and collective responsibility to the community members. Through best practice profiling and the sharing of success stories, local institutions inspire other groups of people to adopt similar approaches, pushing the power of localized intervention in responding to public health challenges. This advocacy and support facilitate a healthy food environment, contributing substantially to improved health outcomes among different groups of people (Burns et al., 2009). In addition to advocacy and education activities, local organizations play a key role in establishing networks that enhance partnership among stakeholders in the health sector. Through partnership with schools, health professionals, and the government, they can adopt a coordinated approach to advancing nutrition at all levels. Networks facilitate the sharing of resources, experience, and knowledge, hence ensuring that the impact of each initiative is maximized. Besides, local organizations also serve as reporting and feedback structures at the local level, essential for identifying future health needs and responding accordingly. As highlighted through various reports, like the DRA Project Report No. 11-0, the collective strength of these networks can lead to systematic change that targets health equity and builds community resilience (Birnbaum et al., 2011). In the end, collaborative efforts leveraged through community organizations provide a firm foundation for enduring change in food practices, which reinforces the public health system in communities as a whole (Figure 10.7).

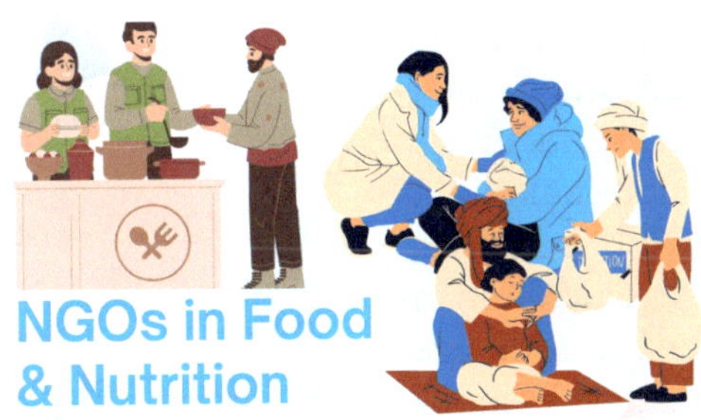

Figure 10.7. NGO-in-food-and-nutrition.

Source: https://ngofeed.com/blog/wp-content/uploads/2024/07/ngo-in-food-and-nutrition.jpg.

10.2.3. Strategies for Community Engagement

Successful community participation is essential to guarantee the successful development and implementation of nutritional interventions for enhancing public health. One of the main approaches is developing partnerships with indigenous organizations familiar with the local needs and traits of their communities. These partnerships serve to build a synergy in which resources can be shared and expertise transferred. For instance, the community-based organization can provide insight into cultural food preferences so that diet interventions are effective as well as culturally appropriate. This is in line with evidence demonstrating how businesses can leverage community insights to create competitive advantage as well as enrich lives, since the report emphasizes opportunity in emerging markets to develop strategies enhancing community well-being (Wendel et al., 2012). Such collaborations are critical in designing focused strategies that resonate with the members within the community, thereby increasing participation and fostering long-term health benefits. Creating open forums for discussion is also a critical way of enhancing community participation in nutrition efforts. Public forums, town meetings, and focus group discussions may be effective forums for exchanging ideas and concerns regarding nutrition issues. These opportunities for engagement enable community members to speak to their needs and experiences, which can actually inform program development and implementation. Democratization of engagement and decentralization of decision-making become a necessary consideration to guarantee that all voices have an opportunity to be heard, especially those of underrepresented groups. An example here is the Buffalo, New York public school food system, in which just transition traits facilitate a more inclusive process of decision-making in food issues (Gilbert et al., 2018). In this setting, where community members engage actively in debate, trust develops, and interventions are supported more widely. Educational workshops and outreach initiatives are an active approach to community participation in nutritional health. By scheduling interactive sessions in which members can learn about nutrition, cooking, and meal planning, a practical knowledge of healthy eating can be obtained. Regional foods can also be emphasized in these workshops to encourage greater exposure and consumption of healthier foods. Furthermore, local agricultural resources being included in these learning activities may help bridge the loop between agriculture, food preparation, and health. As demonstrated by community-based initiatives, educational interventions can truly extend well beyond information exchange, provoking change within the community and promoting healthier living. Lastly, the synergistic interdependency of education and participation ensures that members of a community are not merely passive recipients but active participants in their health process, hence enhancing community ownership and sustainability of nutrition strategies.

10.3. Policy Interventions for Nutritional Improvement

Policy measures to improve nutrition are one of the main policies in combating public health problems caused by poor eating habits. Governments and agencies are increasingly recognizing the need for holistic strategies that cover in a broad-based manner the determinants of nutritional deficiency and diet-related illness. Interventions may range from controls over food marketing, particularly to children, to the offering of subsidies on better foods. Such interventions, once effective, not only foster more wholesome food intake habits among communities but also serve towards the eradication of the prevalence of diet-related chronic diseases, for the sake of enhancing community well-being. Moreover, the creation of education programs that serve to improve nutritional competence is essential to empowering informed consumer decisions, ultimately building an eating culture that is healthful and nutritionally beneficial within communities. In addition to education initiatives, structural changes in the food system are essential to enhancing nutrition outcomes. Such policies as the establishment of community gardens, promotion of farmers markets, and increasing access to fresh fruit and vegetables are essential in solving food deserts—areas with limited access to healthy, affordable foods. Such policy measures can fill the nutrient gap experienced by the most vulnerable and enhance the local economy by supporting small-scale food producers and farmers. In addition, incorporating nutrition education into public campaigns can enhance the message to provide individuals with adequate information to make improved food choices. As established by results from numerous research institutions, such as community-based approaches to address local food preferences and barriers, can result in sustained nutritional health improvement at the population level (Garrett et al., 2020).

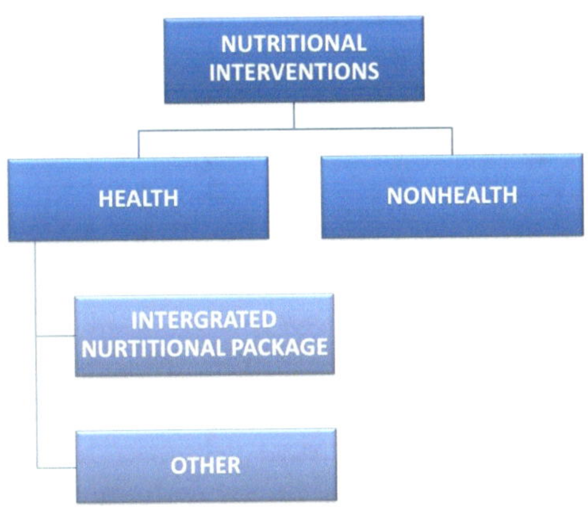

Figure 10.8. Policy interventions for nutritional.

Source: https://external-content.duckduckgo.com/iu/?u=http%3A%2F%2 Fimage.slidesharecdn.com%2Fnutritionalinterventions-111026081039-phpapp01%2F95%2Fnutritional-interventions-4-728.jpg%3Fcb%3D1319617768&f=1&nofb= 1&ipt=61c2ca855310bb07d24da84d57e637100cdfcf9ce6e3fca9f55724f165a99d72.

Last, the increasing awareness of child obesity as a new emerging public health issue has led to interventions specifically for children. School physical activity policies, regulation of food sales in schools, and family nutritional programs are all significant factors that affect children's eating habits. By establishing an environment that supports healthy eating and physical activity, communities can help prevent the risk of obesity and its related health issues. Public-private collaborations, like the alliance between the CPRC and the NICHQ, illustrate the potential of collaboration in addressing this epidemic (Murphy et al., 2008). Emphasizing a shared responsibility among the stakeholders—parents, schools, and policymakers—will be essential in disseminating sustained efforts towards better nutrition for generations to come. Through these multi-dimensional interventions, policy interventions can be potent agents in enhancing community and public health outcomes (Figure 10.8).

10.3.1. Government Regulations on Food Marketing

The food advertising government regulations are vital to promoting public health, particularly children's dietary health. Children are likely to be targeted by pushy marketing tactics that favor unhealthy foods, and it becomes essential to have regulatory systems in place to guarantee that such risks are curbed. By establishing rules that define how food companies can advertise their products, such as restricting advertisements to children, governments can limit childhood obesity and the health issues that accompany it. Good rules will revolutionize the food industry, compelling businesses to develop improved alternatives while making sure that responsible marketing is carried out that puts the health of the individuals first before profits. Government policies, therefore, serve as a stimulus to creating a healthier food environment essential in facilitating the well-being of populations and mitigating health disparities among vulnerable populations (Cabrera et al., 2017). Further, the policies encompass more than advertisement limitation; they entail broader public health interventions in the context of healthy eating behaviors. Numerous states have begun adopting policies that not only limit food marketing to children but also institute overall measures to encourage healthy behavior across different sectors, including schools and healthcare. For instance, measures may include nutritional guidelines for schools to offer children healthy food so that the negative effects caused by the aggressive marketing of unhealthy foods are reversed. Through establishing a healthy decision-making-supportive culture, the policies can have a profound impact on population levels of childhood obesity and health.

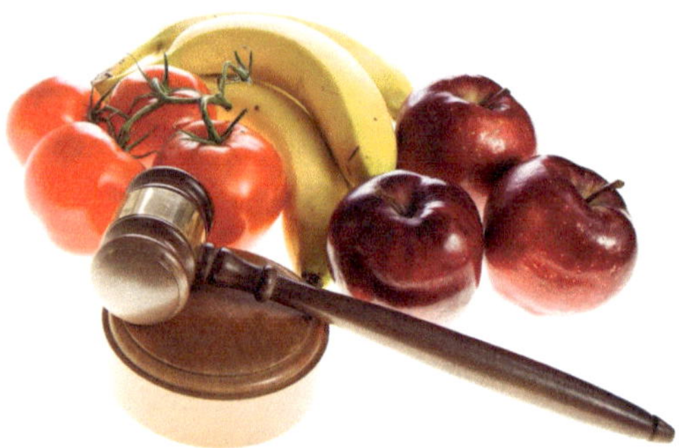

Figure 10.9. Food laws and regulation.

Source: https://hmhub.in/wp-content/uploads/2017/12/Food-laws-e1514207541417.jpg.

The interaction between education and regulation is key to changing population norms around healthy eating as well as instilling healthy habits in children in the long term (N/A, 2009). Beyond reducing childhood obesity, government regulation of food marketing can also target identified socio-environmental determinants that inform food choices. Both socioeconomic and physical access to healthy food in neighborhoods are such determinants. Through their study, regulatory bodies can develop targeted strategies aimed at enhancing access to affordable and healthy food sources, particularly in low-income communities. Community empowerment through better food marketing policies can guarantee healthier dietary habits and hold corporations accountable for their role in public health. Therefore, government intervention plays a vital role in transforming the food system to meet wider public health ends to eventually ensure community welfare and a healthier tomorrow for everyone (Cabrera et al., 2017) (Figure 10.9).

10.3.2. Subsidies for Healthy Food Options

The utilization of subsidies on healthy foods is a critical aspect in the advancement of public and community health. Subsidies reduce the price of purchasing healthy foods, primarily fruits and vegetables, and have the potential to greatly increase access for low-income communities that primarily face economic hardship to consume healthy foods. Evidence indicates that these financial rewards have the potential to promote healthier eating and reduced rates of chronic disease associated with a poor diet. Furthermore, as discussed in relevant studies, effective interventions generally highlight improved availability of healthier food by supporting community-based initiatives that are best tailored to local demands. Such schemes demonstrate the efficacy of subsidies as economic tools, as well as vehicles for changing the healthiness of environments and behaviors of vulnerable groups and eventually bridging the gaps in health status that currently exist across socio-economic lines (Bowie et al., 2004). In addition, the impact of healthy food subsidies extends beyond the individual purchaser to induce the public health gains of declining obesity rates. Current evidence has established strong relationships between increased consumption of fruits and vegetables and decreased prevalence of diet-related diseases, such as obesity and diabetes. Targeted analysis of policy interventions reveals that food-bowl subsidies for healthy foods can precipitate agricultural transformation to grow more nutrient-dense crops rather than commodity crops that lead to poor eating patterns. This change serves not only the public health, but also ensures economic viability in the local food sectors. The probable benefits of such a policy are immense, as local economies and community health will thrive, and the acute issue of obesity and the associated healthcare costs will be reduced (Garson et al., 2009). In addition to the direct health benefits, strategic subsidy targeting for healthy foods can enhance community resilience through the support of local food systems. Encouraging local production and consumption not only enhances access but also stimulates investment in community-based farming schemes that already serve marginalized populations. By cultivating a network of local farmers and businesses committed to offering healthy options, communities can foster a community interest in health consequences. Such an integrated approach encourages an ecological idea of food systems in which economic interests support public health goals. Therefore, properly constructed subsidy programs can build sustainable models that not only cut through the immediate barriers to healthy eating but also promote the social fabric of populations by placing health as a shared goal (Bowie et al., 2004).

10.3.3. Implementation of Nutrition Labeling

Implementation of nutrition labeling is a key action for enhancing public health and facilitating the adoption of healthy eating choices by the populace. Accurate nutrition labeling provides the consumer with valuable information concerning the nutritional content of food items, thereby making informed choices. Such an action is especially relevant in low-income groups, where current and credible nutrition data might be substantially limited. By adopting well-framed and detailed labeling policies, local governments are able to encourage healthier diets and, in the process, address diet-related disparities in health in such areas. As highlighted in Burns et al. (2009), effective nutrition labeling policy must be developed and implemented with involvement from meaningful participation at the community level, and interventions need to be very specific in addressing the particular needs of local communities. In addition, the role of nutrition labels in preventing obesity and chronic diseases cannot be overstressed. With growing consumption of processed foods, there is a critical need for ingredient declaration and caloric labeling. Nutrition labels become an educational tool, pointing consumers towards healthier foods, ultimately reducing the incidence of obesity as well as attendant health risks. Besides, the consistency of information communicated through standardized labeling makes complex nutrition information less of an enigma, more comprehensible to a multicultural society. The initiative mentioned in Burns et al. (2009) highlights the importance of promoting healthy consumption by way of such actions, particularly among deprived sections where nutritional information may be less prevalent. Aside from their role of informing consumers, nutrition labels also have a pivotal role in shaping the practice and policy of the food industry. By establishing strict labeling requirements, policymakers encourage producers to make food products more nutritious, leading to an increased healthy trend across the market. This strategic initiative not only helps in advocating healthier food habits among consumers but also serves as a ground where healthy food options become the standard and not the alternative. In order to be able to implement such modifications, food safety standards and labeling rules have to undergo radical changes, as shown by. Having a separate body to oversee food safety and enforcement against labeling mandates can also enhance the public health impacts of nutrition labeling as a tool, ultimately resulting in healthier communities (Figure 10.10).

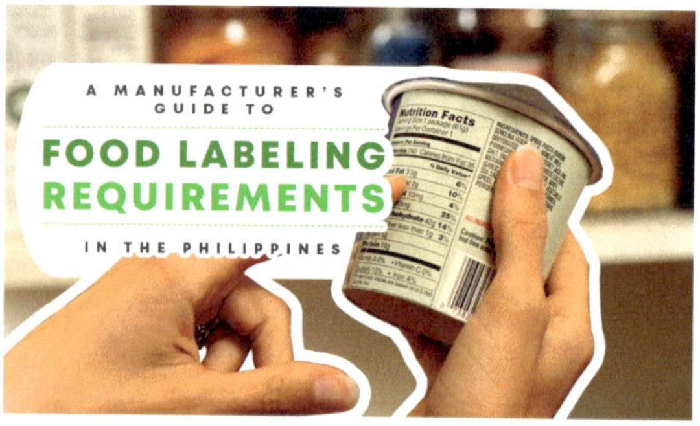
A MANUFACTURER'S GUIDE TO
FOOD LABELING REQUIREMENTS
IN THE PHILIPPINES
Nutrition Facts

Figure 10.10. Food-labeling.

Source: https://www.elixirphil.com/wp-content/uploads/2021/01/Food-Labeling.jpg.

10.4. The Importance of Access to Healthy Foods

The availability of healthy food is one of the fundamental determinants of enhancing public health as well as the' overall status of communities. Healthy food influences eating choices, mainly among low-income families who may have limited means. When neighborhoods have stores and markets offering fresh fruits, vegetables, and whole grains, citizens tend to eat healthier. The access has a culture in which healthy food options become not just a luxury but a routine aspect of everyday life. Such changes have tremendous impacts on public health outcomes, eradicating the possibility of having chronic diseases such as obesity, diabetes, and heart disease, which are prevalent in communities with lower food access. Therefore, food deserts and expanding access to healthy foods must be given priority in an effort to create healthier communities. Interventions aimed at the expansion of health food availability have been shown to yield important advantages to both individuals and families. The programs that involve local farmers and community-supported agriculture have been shown to have beneficial impacts on nutrition. By incorporating a smallholder value chain strategy, towns can double their production and simultaneously provide nutritious food to the most vulnerable. This model not only reinforces local economies but also empowers residents by providing them with an arsenal of fresh vegetables and fruits, which are essential for good health (Dorp et al., 2025). As additional families become empowered to access these resources, inequities in nutrition and health can start to decrease, ultimately making the entire society more equitable. Institutionalizing programs that finance these community-level interventions is vital to making such changes last. Additional research on food access and its significance reiterates the need for policy change to allow healthy eating habits among populations at risk. Studies indicate that poor families struggle to find healthy food, primarily due to price and the lack of neighborhood grocery stores (Mikkelsen et al., 2007).

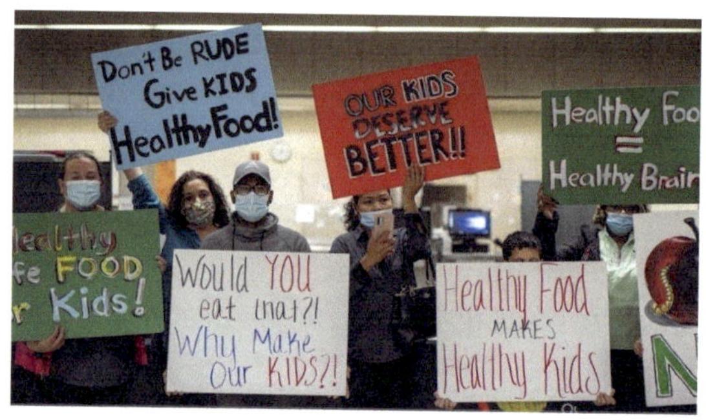
Don't Be RUDE Give KIDS Healthy Food!
OUR KIDS DESERVE BETTER!!
Healthy Foo = Healthy Brair
Would YOU eat that?! Why Make Our KIDS?!
Healthy Food MAKES Healthy Kids
Kids!

Figure 10.11. Improve school food for our children's health and well-being.

Source: https://external-content.duckduckgo.com/iu/?u=https%3A%2F%2Fassets.change.org%2Fphotos%2F8%2Fzi%2Fry%2FuozirYFuRnGXpQc-1600x900-noPad.jpg%3F1694747331&f=1&nofb=1&ipt=9a583e93279b891de3c3f60329c6ea18b87087d436ba19f5f2974ae1e035eff4.

Policymakers can enhance access with efficient interventions by grasping such disparities and developing healthier environment approaches. Interventions such as subsidies of fresh produce, incentives to local stores to offer healthier options, and community garden plots can fill gaps in food availability with great efficiency. By assigning high priority to putting these programs into practice, public health workers can become a key agent for community health, reduce health care costs, and improve the quality of life for residents. The value of access to healthy food thus goes beyond personal choices; it involves wider systemic changes that are able to change communities (Figure 10.11).

10.4.1. Food Deserts and Their Impact on Health

Food deserts with the limited supply of healthy food and food that is within their affordability, particularly, have a significant impact on public health, particularly among the poor. Residents within these neighborhoods primarily obtain their food from convenience stores and fast-food chains that offer predominantly unhealthy and processed foods. The limited access leads to poor food choices, which contribute to the development of numerous diseases, including obesity, diabetes, and cardiovascular diseases. Studies have established that food desert environments reinforce health inequities, and for this reason, the need for community-based interventions is well-established. By increasing access to points of healthy food, communities are able to promote better nutrition and, subsequently, better health outcomes. Specifically, initiatives that increase transportation to farmers' markets and supermarkets or establish local food production can directly counteract the disadvantages of living in a food desert, promoting an overall culture of health and wellness. The challenge of addressing food deserts is further exacerbated by structural factors impacting the availability of food and consumer options. Policy initiatives addressing healthy eating and exercise—like those enshrined in 2007–08 proposals—have sought to achieve healthier community planning and increased access to healthy food. However, despite these efforts, persistent public health disparities remain prevalent, with poorer families facing extra barriers in accessing healthy food. The research identifies a concerning relationship between socioeconomic status and the quality of diet as the occupants of low-income homes are exposed to a minimal variety of nutrients needed for adequate health, and in turn, produce long-lasting adverse outcomes. Clearly, thus, systemic reforms are required in order to yield sustained outcomes that cut across localities, enrich food environments across all sections, and reduce health inequities. Lastly, the deeply seated issue of food deserts needs a more inclusive solution that integrates both upstream and direct approaches. Policymakers should prioritize strategic program development that takes into account the unique needs of low-income families. Recent evaluations of food and nutrition policy have revealed that new approaches that entail life-course thinking may effectively curb such deeply seated inequalities. By addressing the multifaceted challenge of accessing food—considering transportation, socio-economic barriers, and community participation—these strategies hold the potential to construct lasting change. By concerted effort, only that combines health, policy, and community assets, we can expect to enhance public health through enhanced nutritional availability, eventually setting the stage for healthier, more resilient communities.

10.4.2. Strategies to Improve Food Access

Confronted by this intricate issue of food access, guaranteeing a healthy population, particularly among poor communities, is crucial. One viable method is to increase the accessibility of healthy foods through community-based initiatives. Local food systems in the form of community gardens and cooperative grocery stores can enhance access significantly while promoting sustainability and food sovereignty. These not only provide fresh produce but also a sense of community and belonging. Furthermore, research indicates that improved access to nutritious food has a positive effect on the diets of families, particularly for those families that have children. For example, understanding the extent to which environmental factors determine food accessibility allows for strategic local policy interventions that encourage healthy foods. This intervention is consistent with new research and policy interest that aims to tackle the issue of food deserts and healthy consumption, particularly for disadvantaged populations (Mikkelsen et al., 2007). Another essential approach is education and outreach programs that empower people with the knowledge necessary to consume healthier foods. Nutrition education programs may be delivered through schools, community centers, and other outreach programs, exploring the importance of a balanced diet and the long-term effects of nutritional health. By engaging members of the community in hands-on cooking, low-cost meal planning methods, and learning about accessible local resources, such programs are able to reduce barriers to accessing healthy food. In addition, collaboration with local organizations and sharing educational materials can maximize community engagement and participation. As nutritional literacy rises, individuals are more apt to try healthier foods, effectively changing the food environment in underserved populations. Developing these educational strategies is critical for the creation of sustainable health outcomes within communities (Mikkelsen et al., 2007). Merging policy-level interventions offers a second tier of effectiveness in improving food access. Policymakers are able to have a strong impact by backing equal food environment reform initiatives, such as rewarding grocery stores for opening up stores within low-access areas or subsidizing healthy fruits and vegetables through public programs. This policy not only enhances access but also ensures that affordability does not limit healthy meals. Broader initiatives, including those taken by organizations like the Alliance of Bioversity International and the International Center for Tropical Agriculture, emphasize the role of research-based policies in ensuring local food systems. Involvement of stakeholders at all levels, starting from farmers to consumers, ensures cooperation and integrated solutions to food access issues. Ultimately, an integration of grassroots activism with systemic policy changes can dramatically alter access to food and, consequently, effectively enhance community and public health (Figure 10.12).

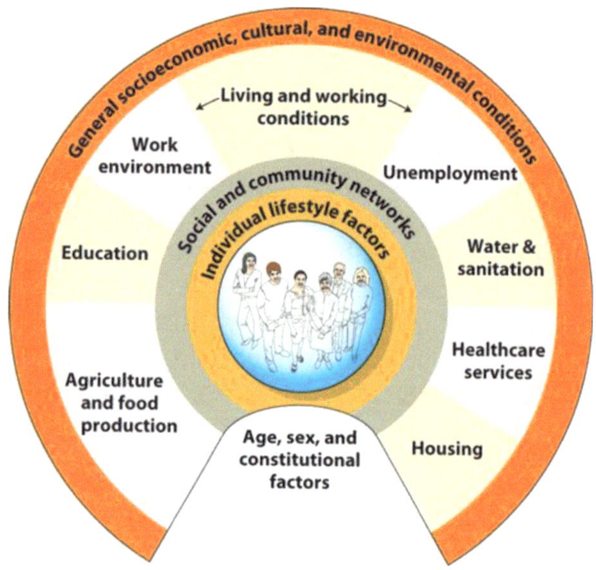

Figure 10.12. National goals for nutrition and health.

Source: https://spscc.pressbooks.pub/app/uploads/sites/9/2020/07/image12-6.jpeg.

10.4.3. Role of Transportation in Food Accessibility

Transportation is key to food access, serving as the lifeline linking food producers and consumers. When transportation infrastructure is functioning well, communities are able to have a steady supply of diversified foods, particularly in cities where food deserts prevail. Inadequate transportation infrastructure can restrict access to fresh fruits and vegetables, leading to the consumption of processed foods, which are less nutritious. As a result, this shortage can exacerbate issues of malnutrition and diet-related health problems. An integrated approach emphasizing the expansion of transportation infrastructure, particularly for rural and poor urban populations, is essential for maximizing food access and supporting public health initiatives. Optimizing these networks not only supports efficient food distribution but also stimulates the consumption of more healthful foods, essential to enhancing community nutrition and overall health. Also, the impact of transportation on the availability of food is not just a matter of basic logistics but also impacts economic profitability for regional farmers and food businesses. Efficient transport can lower the costs of food distribution, allowing regional producers access to broader markets and fostering a healthy regional economy. The development of secure and reliable transport systems has the capacity to empower small-scale farmers by providing them with an expanded market, which in turn encourages the production of diverse and healthy food varieties. Additionally, where transport becomes economically viable, individuals are able to access less expensive food, hence easier access to healthy food. As observed in research on biofortified foods, which are designed to combat nutritional inadequacy, success in these interventions hinges primarily on efficient transport to reach the most vulnerable (Lungelo, 2024). Investing in transport infrastructure, then, is not merely an issue of operational necessity but also a strategic decision to improve public health through improved access to food. Sustainability in transport systems is also more pressing than ever in addressing the issue of food accessibility. Because climate change imperils agricultural production, sustainable modes of transport reduce the carbon footprint of food delivery without undermining the accessibility of good foods. Partnerships such as food hubs and CSA programs often incorporate sustainable transport modalities as a means of connecting consumers and producers directly, thereby enhancing food security. By developing these connections through innovative transportation options, communities can promote not just access to fresh food but also local economies and resilience. This interconnectedness is the motivation for an integrated food systems strategy that looks at transportation infrastructure optimized for accessibility and sustainability. Lastly, the role of transportation in bringing food to the table is essential in realizing the public health goals associated with improved nutrition, in line with enhancing the well-being in communities (Editor, 2024).

10.5. Nutrition Education and Awareness

In public health, nutrition education and awareness are key considerations in influencing the dietary practices and health conditions of populations. Individuals who have adequate nutrition knowledge use food to their advantage for their overall well-being. Through education on key nutrients and their roles in the body, holistic programs can enable individuals to appreciate the value of balanced diets. This empowerment is particularly critical in the context of rising obesity and diet-related disease, where general nutrition education can be a prevention measure. Further, the encouragement of nutritional awareness also provides for personal development, but enhances the community's resilience to food insecurity and malnutrition as well. As communities are educated about healthier diets, the possibility of improving public health becomes more likely. Proper nutrition education programs need to be executed through partnerships between various stakeholders, including schools, healthcare providers, and community organizations. Through these partnerships, they can draw upon their resources and skills to develop curricula that are specific to the needs of various groups of people. Applying culturally competent materials and methods, these programs will be attractive to people and make the information more practical and applicable. In addition, public health campaigns can also be coordinated with these educational programs to reinforce outreach, utilizing media such as social media, workshops, and community events to push more community engagement. As emphasized in the model put forward by the Alliance of Bioversity International and International Center for Tropical Agriculture (CIAT), there is a requirement to assess and refine educational methods to adapt to changing needs and demands within communities so that the impact of nutrition education interventions can be optimized (Garrett et al., 2020). Also, holistic approaches that combine nutrition education with practical uses—such as cooking instruction, gardening programs, and local food systems—can significantly bolster the effectiveness of awareness activities. These experiential learning opportunities allow the mastery of knowledge through the practical application of food preparation and local foods. By establishing a supportive setting and encouraging collaboration between local growers, health workers, and educators, communities can increase the accessibility and quality of healthy food. These interventions not only impart useful skills but also engender a sense of ownership among communities over what they eat, which may translate into sustainable changes in diet. In the backdrop of the importance of enhancing capacity, as it is determined in literature as a reaction to food security, integrating nutrition education into local contexts can provide a foundation for better living and ultimately lead to improved public health indicators (Msuya et al., 2025) (Figure 10.13).

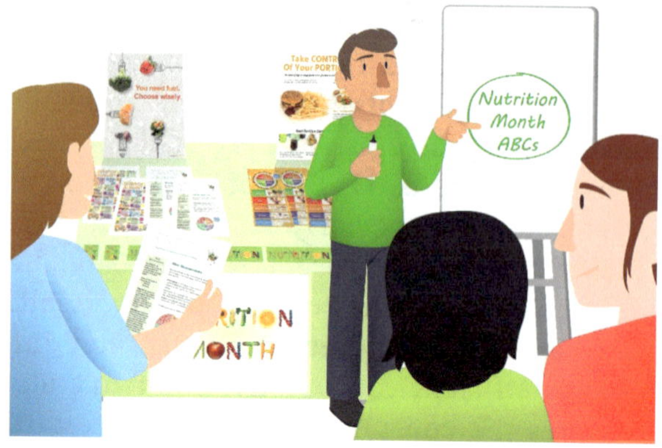

Figure 10.13. Nutrition education and awareness.

Source: https://external-content.duckduckgo.com/iu/?u=http%3A%2F%2Fnews.nutritioneducationstore.com%2Fwp-content%2Fuploads%2F2016% 2F03%2FDisplay-2.jpg&f=1&nofb=1&ipt=4d87fadd2b0fa93a771b1fd724b2c2d3a5faa5 d1d3d944cdc03d014d20aa595e.

10.5.1. Importance of Nutritional Literacy

The significance of nutritional literacy cannot be overstated, particularly when considering its role in enhancing public health outcomes. Nutritional literacy empowers individuals to make informed food choices that directly impact their overall health. When communities possess a strong understanding of nutrition, they are better equipped to identify healthy food options, interpret food labels, and recognize the implications of their dietary choices. This awareness is crucial in managing chronic diseases with robust lifestyle and dietary habits, such as diabetes, obesity, and cardiovascular conditions. Additionally, by fostering nutritional literacy, communities can combat health disparities that predominantly affect low-income and minority groups that typically experience deprivation of access to healthy foods as well as education. According to research supported by the Robert

Wood Johnson Foundation, improving the health of vulnerable children calls for activities that emphasize nutritional education, thereby creating the tremendous demand for enhanced literacy activities in the populations (Bowie et al., 2004). Public health programs incorporating nutritional education improve not just individual health but also population health. An educated populace can inform the dialogue on food security and facilitate peer-to-peer nutrition initiatives. Once individuals understand the connection between nutrition and health, they become advocates for healthy food environments within their community, beginning in schools and in local markets. This shift in awareness can catalyze increased demand for health food and food access innovation. For instance, efforts to improve local food systems are more effective in reaching the nutritionally vulnerable. Further, including culturally relevant nutrition education provides different populations with the ability to gain healthy habits that fit their culture and values. These efforts align with evidence that indicates the necessity of inclusive public health nutrition interventions (Nagujja et al., 2025). Lastly, improved nutritional literacy is the cornerstone for sustained public health benefits. Better-informed communities will tend to have healthier diets, which in turn will have long-term beneficial health impacts. Not only is the trickle-down effect of increased nutritional literacy experienced at the individual level, but it also extends to the household and eventually the community at large. As educated citizens advocate for nutrition education and access to healthy foods via policy, things on the systemic level can be adjusted, leading to healthier environments overall. Thus, integrating nutrition literacy into community-based health programs not only battles existing nutritional inequalities but also creates a resistance to future public health challenges. There is no doubt that enhancing nutritional literacy is a key strategy in the advancement of health equity and general welfare for everyone in a particular community (Bowie et al., 2004).

10.5.2. Programs Targeting Schools and Families

As a response to the critical issue of child nutritional disparity, school and family programs make a valuable contribution to enhancing public and community health. They aim to establish healthier food habits from a young age, sometimes in partnership with local schools to integrate nutrition education into school curricula. By promoting cooking classes, workshops, and gardens, such initiatives teach families how to make healthy food choices and equip them with the capability to do so. Having schools involved benefits young children with reinforced messages about nutrition, both in school and at home, positively reinforcing healthy behaviors and improving long-term health outcomes. These strategies address both the acute nutritional needs and set the stage for a lifetime of healthy habits and therefore represent integral components of community health plans aimed at reducing childhood obesity as well as the myriad accompanying diseases. School and family programs are also supported by targeted interventions which target underserved populations. Research has shown that children from lower-income levels often face significant barriers to access to healthy food sources, reinforcing health inequalities. Efforts are now underway to bridge this gap through expanded access to healthy food sources in neighborhoods. For instance, food stamp programs and neighborhood connections with local farmers can significantly increase access to fresh fruits and vegetables in such neighborhoods where these food sources are scarce. According to widespread studies on food availability and its impacts on poor households, enhancing such nutritional demands through extra efforts is the first step in rendering healthy and equitable results for every child, as mentioned in findings reviewed in Mikkelsen et al. (2007). Updated recently, the feasibility of such school and family-led nutrition programs is the determining factor for their long-term sustainability. While initiating such schemes requires careful planning and investment in resources, the impact can be immense if well done. Interplay among stakeholders in the society—health workers, educators, and local governments—results in a better-balanced approach towards improving the health of children. Organization-supported efforts, like those receiving support from the Robert Wood Johnson

Foundation, aim to develop combined systems that not only emphasize nutrition education but also leverage child care and health infrastructures that already exist. By reaching vulnerable populations, these interventions can change the landscape of child health, as shown by their capacity to reach those with the greatest obstacles to receiving healthcare and accessing healthy food options, as discussed in Bowie et al. (2004). Establishing strategies for these programs to be resilient and adaptable will enable communities to sustain the momentum required for healthier generations.

10.5.3. Use of Technology in Nutrition Education

In the recent past, the use of technology in nutrition education has increasingly been at the core of conveying key dietary information to diverse groups. Online platforms like mobile applications and interactive sites offer personalized study materials that are addressed to specific dietary needs and preferences. A case in point is customized food tracking applications that allow users to engage with their nutritional goals, thereby enhancing their ability to monitor dietary intake and make rational choices. Parallel technology facilitates nutrition education by providing evidence-based content that can be used in meal preparation and cooking techniques. With time, the tools may be even more developed, making their use more intuitive and interactive with user patterns, hence enhancing eating habits for the community. Technology also facilitates improved access to nutrition education for underprivileged populations. Telecommunications equipment, such as webinars and online workshops, enables remote or low-access populations to participate in educational opportunities that otherwise would be lost. Such improvements are valuable for mitigating health disparities, particularly where underserved populations exist, which are at risk of being underserved by in-person nutrition counseling.

The ability to serve more people through these internet platforms offers an efficient mechanism for disseminating necessary knowledge about food sources, cooking methods, and nutritional science. By putting equal access to nutrition education first, technology fortifies the community's overall public health and empowers efforts to improve eating habits and health indicators. Moreover, the analytical capability of technology enables the systematic assessment of nutrition educators' intervention effects. Through data analysis and feedback loops, participants' progress can be tracked by educators, and educational content can be altered based on real-time outputs. These measurements provide a better understanding of the needs of the community, allowing education strategy refinement to be continuous. For example, trend data on dietary food consumption habits as revealed through tracking nutrition apps can be utilized for purpose-specific education in specific regions. Such evidence-based approaches, with support from accurate data collection, enable nutrition educators to develop effective community programs directly for addressing public health problems. In this context, technology is not only a learning medium but also a crucial tool for continuous upgrading of nutritional strategies towards improving the health of people in communities (Figure 10.14).

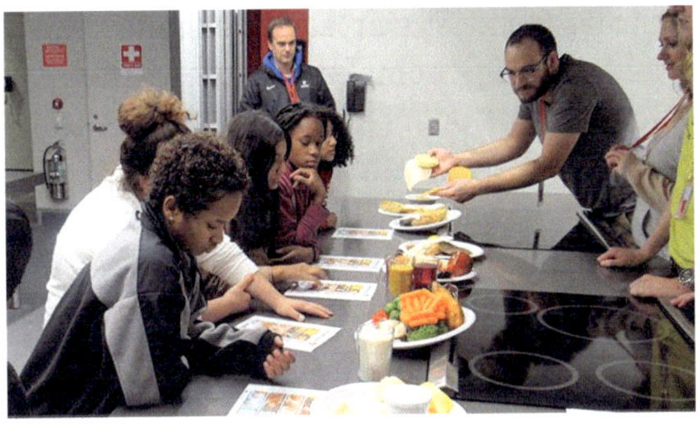

Figure 10.14. Med students cook up community nutrition education.

Source: https://extern al-content.duckduckgo.com/iu/?u=https%3A%2F%2Fwww.unmc.edu%2Fnewsroom%2Fwp-content%2Fuploads%2F2018%2F12%2FNutrition1219.jpg&f=1&nofb=1&ipt=aaab1831c4d1582 0513c00ac9c481b3 0fd04d471f4cfe 85a87 80723fbf810ff5.

10.6. Collaboration Between Stakeholders

There must be strong stakeholder partnership to enhance the health of the community and the public through diet. Different stakeholders, including corporations, non-profit organizations, healthcare workers, and local governments, must come together with a purpose of fulfilling common goals and creating cooperative programs. Through intersectoral partnerships, communities can collaborate their resources, expertise, and networks to develop comprehensive solutions. Stakeholders can develop interventions that are targeted to the needs of their populations so that nutritional strategies are actionable and tailored to a population's traditions and culture. The partnership process not only raises participation from stakeholders but also facilitates more effective implementation, as stakeholders feel more invested in the process when they take part in planning. Healthy partnerships must include conscious partnership and open communication between stakeholders. Common vision and joint responsibility development is necessary since they facilitate a collective effort towards community health objectives. Utilizing toolkits like those developed in the Healthy Eating Active Living Convergence Partnership fortifies the process by offering stakeholders structures and strategies to enable healthy environments. These tools serve as a blueprint for the coordination of stakeholders' efforts in a manner that best responds to the intersection of nutrition and public health. Therefore, a collective approach to creating and sustaining partnerships between stakeholders can ensure maximum effectiveness of nutritional interventions within the community. In addition, ongoing testing and fine-tuning of collaboration activities are also necessary for their effectiveness and sustainability. Regular evaluations by stakeholders help them know the results of their actions and areas of improvement. Dissemination of information and knowledge between partners promotes openness and confidence and deepens the ties in the partnership. Guidelines from thorough analysis, like the ones presented in the State of Health Equity Movement report, are useful in streamlining collective approaches. Through prioritizing stakeholder working relationships and ensuring that the evaluation is dynamic, communities can be sure that their nutrition interventions are current and responsive to the evolving public health setting, ultimately enhancing health outcomes and equity.

10.6.1. Role of Healthcare Providers in Nutrition

The healthcare workers play a pivotal role in the nutritional scenario in both public and community health. Using their professional expertise, such workers will be tasked with establishing nutritional deficiencies and guiding patients on the need for balanced feeding. This training outreach is paramount in coming up with healthier lifestyles since most individuals will never make the appropriate food choices because they lack proper information. By adding nutrition counseling to routine health assessments, practitioners can address particular health ailments, such as obesity and diabetes, that are most frequently brought about by unhealthy habits. Additionally, health professionals can join forces with community organizations to promote large-scale nutritional education initiatives that resonate with various populations, ultimately culminating in reduced health disparities and improved overall community health outcomes. Strategies employing the expertise of healthcare providers ensure that nutritional advice is evidence-based and culturally sensitive, maximizing impact in various population environments. Healthcare providers' roles are not confined to patient-to-provider interaction; they play a pivotal role in shaping nutritional policy and interventions at the population level. For example, health professionals provide feedback on public health campaigns favoring better food environments, such as campaigns for the availability of fresh fruits and vegetables in low-income communities.

Their involvement in food systems debates in policy guarantees that public health activities are steered based on the best food security and nutrition practices. As advocates, such as in this role, providers can apply data and research evidence to inform policy reforms that not only encourage healthier eating but also tackle systemic factors that drive malnutrition and obesity. Such initiatives can be paralleled with initiatives seen in large-scale projects such as that created in partnership between the CPRC and NICHQ, which aims to fight childhood obesity by involving healthcare providers in community interventions (Murphy et al., 2008). This inclusive model points to the critical role that healthcare providers play in influencing individual and collective health status. Further, integration of a nutrition-oriented framework in healthcare facilities can lead to enhanced health literacy among members of the public. The medical practitioners can arrange workshops, cooking classes, and nutrition seminars to enable individuals to make healthier food choices and understand how eating impacts long-term health. Collaboration between healthcare providers and community-based organizations has the potential to yield innovative strategies that address the individual nutritional needs of target populations. For instance, attempts to engage the private sector in helping to strengthen health through local food systems can reinforce community support and trust, addressing both nutritional needs and economic development. As observed in Chile, where there is promotion of the private sector's alignment with social responsibility initiatives, these collaborations can bring considerable gains to public health outcomes for communities (Grindle et al., 2014). The collaborative leadership of healthcare providers in the areas of nutritional education and campaigning is therefore core to improving individual and public health through successful nutritional interventions (Figure 10.15).

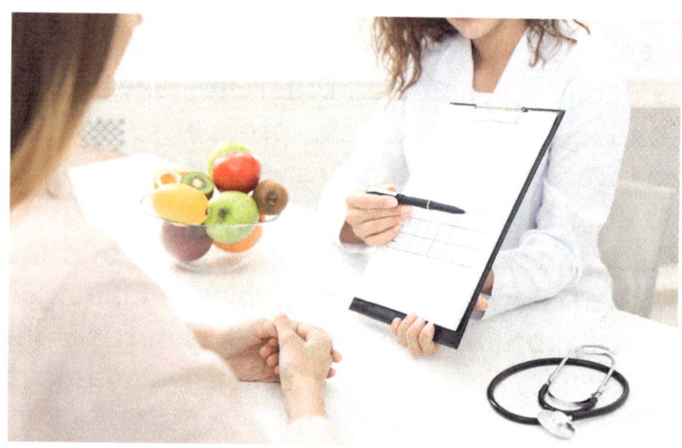

Figure 10.15. Role of healthcare providers in nutrition.

Source: https://postgraduateeducation.hms.harvard.edu/sites/default/files/PGME/01.05.2022_The%20Role%20Of.jpg.

10.6.2. Partnerships Between Public Health and Private Sectors

The coordination of public efforts with private capacity is an innovative model of enhancing community health, particularly in nutritional intervention. Public health organizations are constrained by resources, yet they have the financial, technological, and logistical resources to aid in government efforts. A win-win collaboration can leverage these capacities by having common goals in terms of enhancing nutritional status. Successful cooperation is also apparent in joint ventures involving private firms in the manufacturing and provision of healthy foods, which demonstrate how innovation from the private sector has the potential to address public health challenges appropriately. Energy created in such cooperation translates into more sustainable health interventions, and therefore to reciprocal gains for both industries and society as a whole through projecting more holistic improvements in diet. Besides, the evolution of private sector and public health partnerships must prioritize creating shared value, where business and social interests intersect. Shared value, defined by Harvard's Michael Porter, clarifies how private firms can achieve competitive advantage while benefiting society's challenges, such as poor nutrition. In such a setting as Chile, where private sector input in social advancement is being questioned, companies have the capacity to push compliance above its bare minimum and actively participate in public health initiatives. Implementing industry-initiated nutritional programs not only adds to the company's image but also generates confidence and goodwill among people. These collaborations are fundamental to addressing access, quality, and affordability of healthy food issues, eventually resulting in public health indicators and healthier citizens. Additionally, effective coordination between private enterprise and public health policy makers can enhance the effect of nutrition-oriented policies through evidence-based decision-making. Through joint research and information sharing, both sectors have been able to identify areas of unmet community needs and develop specific interventions to extend equitable access to nutritional commodities. These partnerships can also enhance health education campaigns through the leveraging of marketing and outreach capabilities from private industry in an effort to change consumer behavior sustainably. As per the suggestions made in the DRA Project Report, stakeholder engagement has to be extensive and active in considering various community forces so as to guarantee that actions not only attack prevalent health inequalities but also encourage future resilience. These collaborations can therefore serve as an example of how the progression in public health not only solves immediate nutritional needs but also builds long-term empowerment and equality in the community (Grindle et al., 2014; Birnbaum et al., 2011).

10.6.3. Community Involvement in Nutritional Initiatives

Community involvement is at the heart of the effectiveness of nutritional interventions aimed at enhancing public health. By developing community involvement, interventions guarantee that the methods employed are culturally appropriate and address the specific needs of the community. By involving members of the community in planning and implementing nutritional programs, they are more likely to embrace such interventions, which will lead to improved diet and health. The Robert Wood Johnson Foundation states that effective actions to promote health, particularly in vulnerable populations, must take into consideration the unique circumstances of the community. This local approach is crucial since it encourages the existence of unhealthy eating barriers and the creation of solutions that appeal to community values, hence empowering people to be in charge of nutritional decisions. Incorporating agricultural practices within community nutritional programs adds another level of participation that can contribute greatly to public health outcomes. By leveraging local agriculture, communities have the opportunity to immediately link food production to nutrition education, whereby residents obtain fresh and healthy food. An illustration is employing smallholder value chain models, whereby the producers' involvement in the local food supply chain, both in terms of income and the consumers' access to nutrients, is increased. This strategy aligns with the findings of existing research, which indicates that improved nutrition can be a byproduct of improved agricultural productivity, particularly for vulnerable groups. These complementary approaches not only make local economies more resilient but also improve community resilience, creating a self-reinforcing feedback loop where food security and nutritional health are both enhanced. Moreover, the creation of community partnerships between health agencies, agricultural units, and local governments is apt to increase the impact of nutritional programs. These types of partnerships have the potential to share resources, capabilities, and infrastructure to enable communities to build comprehensive programs that support a healthy diet. When multiple stakeholders work towards the same goal, as in research, the effectiveness of health interventions is significantly enhanced. With combined resources and expertise, communities can bridge significant gaps in nutrition education, outreach, and access to healthy foods. According to the reports cited above, achieving a balance among the various aspects of nutrition and public health, with active involvement of the community, offers scope for innovative interventions that hold promise to introduce lasting changes in the overall health (Figure 10.16).

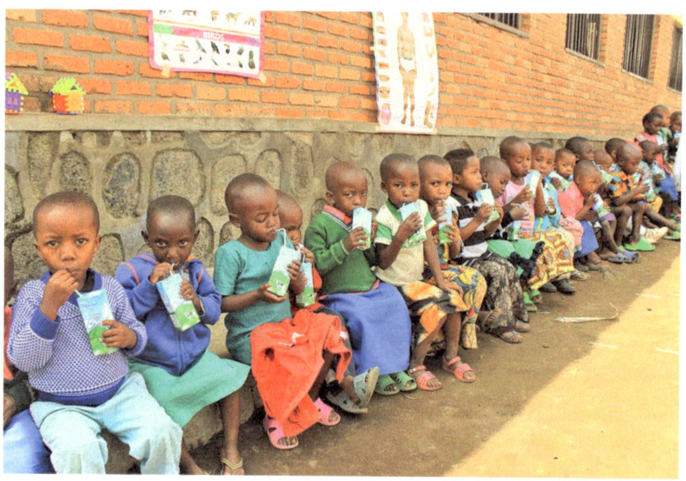

Figure 10.16. Community involvement in nutritional initiatives.

Source: https://e3az4yc7762.exactdn.com/wp-content/uploads/2021/10/hero-nutrition.jpg?strip=all&lossy=1&ssl=1.

CLOSER LOOK

FUTURE DIRECTIONS FOR NUTRITIONAL STRATEGIES

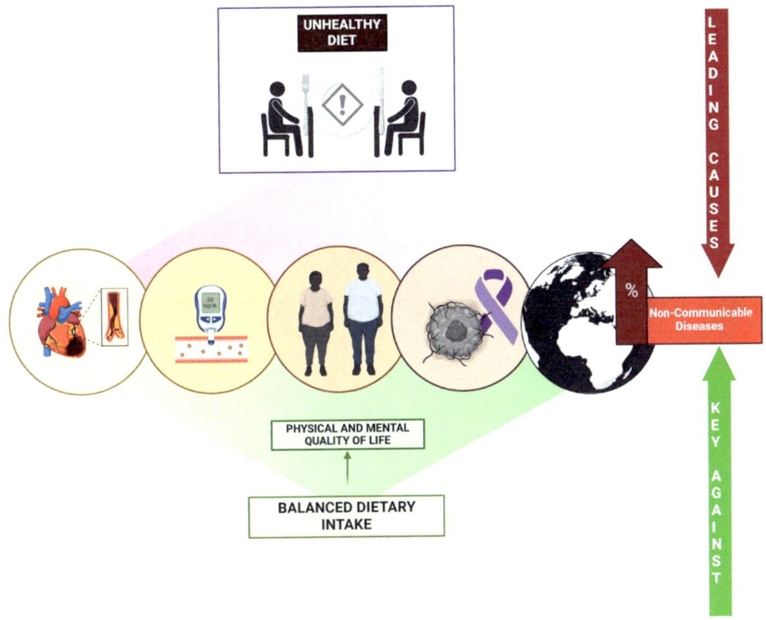

With societies increasingly faced with public health issues, dietary approaches in the future need to highlight integrated mechanisms that can address the complex nature of health and nutrition. A possible way forward lies in the creation of programs that can integrate nutritional education with community involvement, enabling people to make healthier food choices. Such programs can create settings that promote healthy food eating habits, especially among vulnerable groups affected by socioeconomic inequalities. By the use of local stakeholders and resources, communities can create programs that not only educate but also enhance access to healthy options. This approach not only targets individual behavior change but also aims to create an enabling infrastructure supporting long-term dietary enhancement, particularly important in addressing issues such as childhood obesity, reinforced by prevalent socioeconomic risk factors and state initiatives for promoting health in varying contexts. Combined with community-based strategies, sustainable agricultural practices present an important future frontier for nutritional strategy. Emphasizing coordination between agricultural scientists, nutritionists, and policymakers ensures the development of food that meets diverse dietary requirements at lower environmental cost. The SUSVAR Visions workshop is an exemplar of such a collaborative environment, prioritizing where sustainable cereal farming intersects with nutritional needs. Musings in forums like these can lead to innovative breeding strategies and crop management practices that prioritize nutrition outcomes as heavily as traditional agricultural goals. By integrating these perspectives, subsequent nutrition strategies can enhance food security alongside safeguarding biodiversity and resilience within agricultural systems, ultimately enhancing community health more holistically. Moreover, the evolving landscape of technology provides additional opportunities for the improvement of nutrition strategies. Enhanced analytics capabilities, mobile applications, and digital platforms can facilitate personalized nutrition strategies tailored to unique individual health needs, personal tastes, and cultural backgrounds. These technologies hold the promise to bridge knowledge gaps and induce behavior change through real-time feedback and dietary counseling. In addition, social media-based public health campaigns can easily communicate nutritional information, thereby reaching more communities of people and promoting community engagement. Integrating these technological advancements with traditional community customs can have a synergistic effect that promotes healthy living and improves public health. As we progress, nutrition strategies must continue to be adaptive, innovative, and inclusive, setting communities up to prosper in the face of continuous health challenges.

SUMMARY

The endeavor to enhance public and community health by nutrition involves a multi-dimensional approach that operates within the lived experiences and needs of diverse populations. An understanding should be appreciated that food selections are significantly influenced by many variables, including accessibility, affordability, and social dynamics. Research indicates that in college students, the consumption of fast food is generally a convenience and social affair, where a full 67% attributed to social opportunities for food selection, and 60.3% chose quick service and flavor, as reported by Nurrahima et al. (2015). Thus, developing interventions intended to facilitate healthier eating must also consider these social considerations and include measures to offer settings where healthy food consumption is encouraged. In addition, the integration of information and communication management (ICM) systems is likely to enhance food security and public health programs significantly. One systematic method of addressing food availability and accessibility presented in Msuya et al. (2025) outlines primary information that supports community involvement in nutrition strategies. With enhanced capacity among natives in these areas, communities can develop personalized interventions that address their specific dietary needs and neighborhood traditions. These programs enable individuals to make well-informed decisions and hence create a healthier society in general. The successful incorporation of ICM principles into models of public health not only improves food security but also creates an informed society that is respectful of nutritional information and improved ways of life. Lastly, active collaboration between stakeholders—governments, schools, non-governmental organizations, and community leaders—is crucial in creating effective change in public health through nutrition. Programs to strengthen food systems and fund nutritional education have the power to create a ripple effect, promoting healthier lifestyles and diets on the ground. As argued in the context of capacity strengthening requirements articulated in Msuya et al. (2025), emphasis needs to be placed on sustainable approaches that empower people with knowledge and resources to make better choices. Through investment in such programs, communities can move towards not just enhancing public health but ensuring that the coming generation is equipped to continue these gains in nutrition and health.

An appreciation of public and community health requires a keen sense of the pivotal role that nutrition plays in overall health. Nutritional interventions operate not only to maximize personal health outcomes but also to maximize communities' total health. Evidence-based nutrition intervention can be used to address issues such as obesity and malnutrition, both of which affect marginalized populations disproportionately. The HEART initiative is a standout example of this movement, with its emphasis on the worth of Blue-Green spaces in urban planning and the potential that nature access and diet hold in significantly influencing health outcomes. Through participatory engagement and facilitated workshops, stakeholders are positioned to identify together nutritional access obstacles and create specially tailored methods to empower community health, providing a solid foundation for subsequent programs aimed at reducing health disparities and ensuring urban program sustainability (Levi et al., 2024). Not least, the significance of education in evidence-based practices among healthcare professionals cannot be overstated. The incorporation of behavior science in nutrition education is a key moment in building sustainable healthcare. This is underpinned by implementation studies' evidence of translating scientific evidence into practice through increased capacity among health professionals. Instances of such initiatives aimed at enhancing diet care in the healthcare setting have underscored the need for equipping professionals with the knowledge and skills that enable the utilization of nutritional measures effectively. When physicians and other healthcare professionals understand the intricacies of their communities' nutritional demands, they can lead initiatives that drastically reduce access barriers and mobilize public involvement. With health systems focusing on prevention like never before, these experienced professionals can serve as drivers of successful change by integrating nutrition into key areas of concern on public health agendas (Bawab et al., 2020). Finally, community participation is a cornerstone in effective nutritional program planning. Citizens' participation in the identification of the nutritional issues and collective efforts to formulate solutions enhances responsibility and ownership for programs of community health. Effective programs are found to come with benefits from community members in terms of returns through facilitating individualized intervention that is significant to the population's specific tastes and requirements. Moreover, research has indicated that participatory workshops such as the ones organized by the HEART project enable stakeholders to share information and resources, thus creating synergies among public health practitioners, nutritionists, and community members. By providing such a setting in which various voices inform public health policy, communities are able to maximize the effectiveness of nutritional interventions, thus promoting improved health and overall welfare (Levi et al., 2024).

REFERENCES

1. Acheson, D., Barnes, M., Bartley, M., Beresford, P., Blenkinsop, S., Bremner, J., Brewer, M., et al. (2007). *Policy Initiatives to Address Low-Income Households' Nutritional Needs in the UK.* https://core.ac.uk/download/47325.pdf (accessed on 11th June 2025).
2. Amutah, N., King, J., Leverett, C., Mahadevan, M., et al. (2015). Project THANKS: A socio-ecological framework for an intervention involving HIV positive African American women with comorbidities. https://digitalscholarship.unlv.edu/cgi/viewcontent.cgi?article=1239&context=jhdrp (accessed on 11th June 2025).
3. Bawab, N., Moullin, J., Bugnon, O., Perraudin, C., Morrow, A., Chan, P., Hogden, E., et al. (2020). *Proceedings of the Virtual 3rd UK Implementation Science Research Conference. Implementation Science: IS, 15.* https://www.semanticscholar.org/paper/cdeaf6c7db3c2f96b1e137d68626f27318e20648 (accessed on 11th June 2025).
4. Birnbaum, N., Masterson, E., & Schoomaker, H. (2011). *State of Health Equity Movement, 2011 Update Part C: Compendium of Recommendations DRA Project Report No. 11-03.* https://core.ac.uk/download/pdf/18491812.pdf (accessed on 11th June 2025).
5. Bowie, A., & Walker, K. E. (2004). *Linking the Child Care and Health Care Systems: A Consideration of Options.* https://core.ac.uk/download/71341350.pdf (accessed on 11th June 2025).
6. Cabrera, O. A., Gostin, L. O., Magnusson, R., Nygren-Krug, H., et al. (2017). *Advancing the Right to Health: The vital Role of Law.* https://core.ac.uk/download/83109641.pdf (accessed on 11th June 2025).
7. Chen, A., Ayub, M. H., Mishuris, R. G., Rodriguez, J. A., Gwynn, K. B., Lo, M. C., Noronha, C., et al. (2023). Telehealth policy, practice, and education: A position statement of the Society of General Internal Medicine. *Journal of General Internal Medicine, 38*, 2613–2620. https://www.semanticscholar.org/paper/afb0748b3e2fc60054f30ce0bc1346a453446926 (accessed on 11th June 2025).
8. Dorp, M. van, Torgerson, S., & Wiegers, E. S. (2025). *Improving Nutrition Through Agriculture: Viewing Agriculture-Nutrition Linkages Along the Smallholder Value Chain.* https://core.ac.uk/download/pdf/29235287.pdf (accessed on 11th June 2025).
9. Garrett, J., Gelli, A., & Peña, I. de la. (2020). *Nutrition-Sensitive Value Chains from A Smallholder Perspective: A Framework for Project Design.* https://core.ac.uk/download/288633652.pdf (accessed on 11th June 2025).
10. Garson, A., Jr., Engelhard, C. L., & Dorn, S. (2009). *Reducing obesity: Policy Strategies from the Tobacco War.* https://core.ac.uk/download/71348457.pdf (accessed on 11th June 2025).
11. Ghany, M. G., & Morgan, T. R. (2019). Hepatitis C guidance 2019 update: American Association for the Study of Liver Diseases–Infectious Diseases Society of America recommendations for testing, managing, and treating hepatitis C virus infection. *Hepatology, 71*, 686–721. https://doi.org/10.1002/hep.31060 (accessed on 11th June 2025).
12. Gilbert, J., Robert, S. A., & Schindel, A. E. (2018). *Just Transitions in A Public-School Food System: The Case of Buffalo, New York.* https://core.ac.uk/download/219377025.pdf (accessed on 11th June 2025).

13. Grindle, A. K., Smith, D., Longo, M. P., & Murray, M. (2014). *Shared Value in Chile: Increasing Private Sector Competitiveness by Solving Social Problems*. https://core.ac.uk/download/75779234.pdf (accessed on 11th June 2025).

14. Hill, C., Guarner, F., Reid, G., Gibson, G. R., Merenstein, D., Pot, B., Morelli, L., et al. (2014). The International Scientific Association for Probiotics and Prebiotics consensus statement on the scope and appropriate use of the term probiotic. *Nature Reviews Gastroenterology & Hepatology, 11*, 506–514. https://doi.org/10.1038/nrgastro.2014.66 (accessed on 11th June 2025).

15. Hussain, S., Naveed, M., Sharif, M. A., Tahir, A., & Raza, H. M. U. (2025). Impact of the Mamta UNICEF: A fortified food nutrition program on childhood malnutrition during pregnancy in Pakistan. *Cureus, 17*. https://www.semanticscholar.org/paper/983ab216743395a8319d1c64c35335c81e4a8eb8 (accessed on 11th June 2025).

16. Levi, J., & Mathey, L. (2024). Enhancing urban vitality: Insights and strategies for optimizing blue-green spaces. *Proceedings of the International Congress Public Health–Achievements and Challenges–Zbornik Radova*. https://www.semanticscholar.org/paper/ba46075486b521cd407be6039694dec7b30ec154 (accessed on 11th June 2025).

17. Livingston, G., Huntley, J., Sommerlad, A., Ames, D., Ballard, C., Banerjee, S., Brayne, C., et al. (2020). Dementia prevention, intervention, and care: 2020 report of the Lancet Commission. *The Lancet, 396*, 413–446. https://doi.org/10.1016/s0140-6736(20)30367-6 (accessed on 11th June 2025).

18. Lungelo, J. (2024). Potential risks and benefits associated with the genetic modification of crops for improved nutritional content in South Africa. *International Journal of Food Sciences*. https://www.semanticscholar.org/paper/25f1640b616cabbf9cd33a2db33a5a7a85ad0d75 (accessed on 11th June 2025).

19. Mikkelsen, L., & Chehimi, S. (2007). *The Links Between the Neighborhood Food Environment and Childhood Nutrition*. https://core.ac.uk/download/71346749.pdf (accessed on 11th June 2025).

20. Morganstern, A. M., & Putnam-Walkerly, K. (2009). *Making the Case and Getting Underway: A Funder Toolkit to Support Healthy People in Healthy Places*. https://core.ac.uk/download/75778427.pdf (accessed on 11th June 2025).

21. Msuya, E. E., & Temu, A. (2025). *Capacity Building in Information and Communication Management (ICM) Towards Food Security*. https://core.ac.uk/download/pdf/7306199.pdf (accessed on 11th June 2025).

22. Murphy, C. G., Alendy, C., Cooper, J., & Simpson, L. (2008). *Childhood Obesity: The Role of Health Policy*. https://core.ac.uk/download/71342400.pdf (accessed on 11th June 2025).

23. Nagujja, S., & Potts, M. J. (2025). *A Review of Agriculture and Health Policies in Uganda with Implications for The Dissemination of Biofortified Crops*. https://core.ac.uk/download/pdf/6344738.pdf (accessed on 11th June 2025).

24. Nurrahima, A., Rinanta, F., & Anggiesa. (2015). *Factors Affecting Fast Food Consumption Behavior in Students of Nursing Faculty of Medicine Diponegoro University*. https://core.ac.uk/download/76929073.pdf (accessed on 11th June 2025).

25. Østergård, H. (2008). *Discussion Documents–SUSVAR Visions Workshop, Karrebæksminde, Denmark, April 2008*. https://core.ac.uk/download/10928157.pdf (accessed on 11th June 2025).

26. Russo, A. (2024). Urban green spaces and healthy living: A landscape architecture perspective. *Urban Science*. https://www.semanticscholar.org/paper/c5a72c1c452cda8783a64ba803448c57b32d62e5 (accessed on 11th June 2025).

27. Subarno, A., Koesuma, S., & Sukatiman, S. (2025). Integrating environmental health into disaster-resilient villages: Strategies, challenges, and solutions in Surakarta, Indonesia. *Jurnal Kesehatan Lingkungan*. https://www.semanticscholar.org/paper/952edd5ba7ec332a03d70367199817bd91d0d29b (accessed on 11th June 2025).

28. Ugwu, D., Ajayi, A. A., & Kaiser, F. (2025). Strategies to improve health equity through targeted public health initiatives. *International Medical Science Research Journal*. https://www.semanticscholar.org/paper/e1758837bbf1593164aad5d346769e19a664db6b (accessed on 11th June 2025).

29. Wendel, C., Hills, G., & Borgonovi, V. (2012). *Shared Value in Emerging Markets: How Multinational Corporations Are Redefining Business Strategies to Reach Poor or Vulnerable Populations*. https://core.ac.uk/download/71360050.pdf (accessed on 11th June 2025).

30. Winterfeld, A., Shinkle, D., & Morandi, L. (2009). *Promoting Healthy Communities and Reducing Childhood Obesity: Legislative Options*. https://core.ac.uk/download/71354061.pdf (accessed on 11th June 2025).

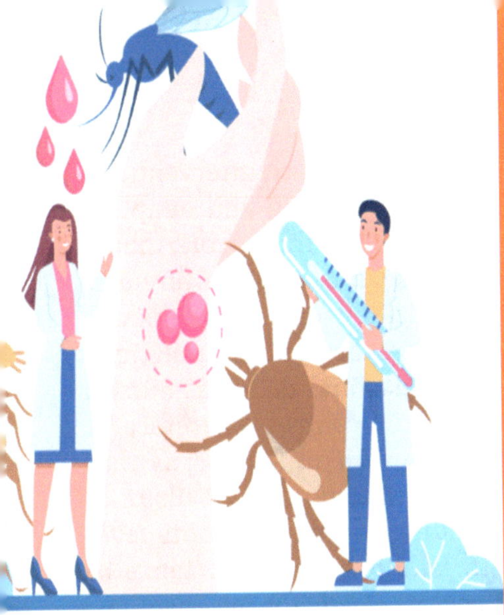

Chapter 11

VECTOR-BORNE DISEASES AND ENVIRONMENTAL FACTORS

Contents

Introduction

Vector-borne diseases (VBDs) constitute a serious global health issue, particularly in low and middle-income nations that exist in tropical environments. Environmental determinants regulate the dynamics of transmission of VBDs to a great extent, including temperature, humidity, and environmental processes that may impact vector populations and behaviors. VBDs such as malaria, dengue, and filariasis are reliant on specific environmental factors that facilitate vector breeding and survival, including mosquitoes. With increasing urbanization and agricultural change, especially in regions like Southeast Asia, human activities and environmental processes increasingly cross paths. Rubber plantations, for instance, have emerged as new disease vector habitats, and thus proper surveillance and control interventions need to be implemented to decrease the chances of outbreaks happening in such an environment (Wilson et al., 2017). Understanding these environmental and ecological interactions is critical in the formulation of effective vector management policies. Effective vector control interventions are crucial in efforts to combat VBDs, and a crucial component of such interventions is the use of integrated vector management (IVM). IVM enhances evidence-based and adaptive implementation of different vector control methods, which provides an inclusive framework that is not only focused on health sector engagement but also with other sectors such as agriculture and urban planning (Tangena et al., 2016). Through the utilization of insecticide-treated nets, indoor residual spraying, and environmental management practices, IVM will decrease vector populations in a sustainable manner. Besides, challenges with resistance to insecticides and deficient human and infrastructural resources hinder capacity building for effective vector control. Therefore, it is important to generate good-quality evidence through systematic reviews and field trials that will contribute to policy decision-making and strengthen vector control interventions (Wilson et al., 2017). IVM requires an effort over the long term in capacity building at the grassroots level to avoid thinly spread diseases and win better health outcomes. In addition, the importance of proper surveillance methods cannot be overstressed in the fight against vector-borne diseases. Surveillance allows health officials to monitor vector densities and the disease epidemiological patterns, knowledge that is crucial in making sound interventions at the appropriate time. New vector breeding grounds occasioned by developments in agriculture demand permanent environmental surveillance to identify breeding grounds and predict possible epidemics. For example, studies conducted in rubber plantations have considered the mosquito biodiversity and its connection with human activities and land use (Tangena et al., 2016). Additionally, active participation of local communities in surveillance enhances better collection of data and involvement in vector control. Hence, an integrated approach of environmental management, community participation, and efficient surveillance systems is required to reduce the load of VBDs and manage the impact on public health effectively. Public Health and Policy (Figure 11.1).

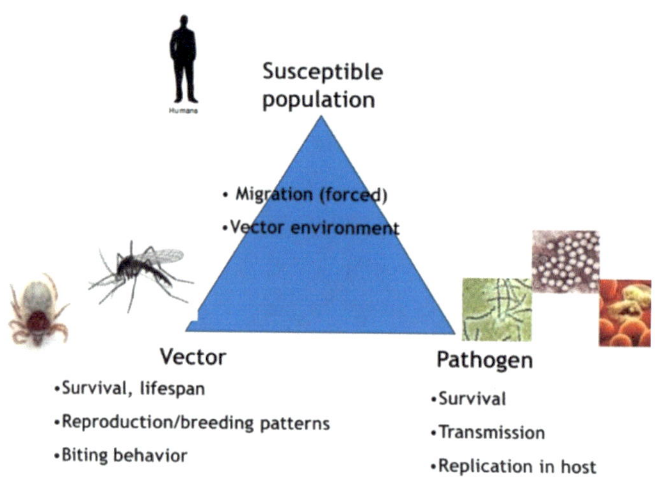

Figure 11.1. Vector-borne-disease-dynamics.

https://image5.slideserve.com/9307096/vector-borne-disease-dynamics-l.jpg.

Definition and Significance of Vector-Borne Diseases

VBDs are illnesses caused predominantly in humans by bites of arthropod vector-borne infected vectors, such as fleas, ticks, and mosquitoes. These illnesses comprise various infections such as malaria, dengue, and filariasis, and represent a significant public health issue globally. Transmission epidemiology of these diseases depends predominantly on environmental determinants such as temperature, humidity, and biodiversity, which affect the vector population as well as their ecosystem. Effective management of such diseases requires a multi-disciplinary approach involving environmental management, public health interventions, and community involvement to counteract the risks from vectors and improve the surveillance systems. As climate change alters the geographical range of the majority of vectors, understanding the definition and meaning of VBDs is necessary in order to combat proactive intervention measures capable of continuously updating themselves in terms of new environmental patterns and vector behavior. The impacts of vector-borne diseases extend beyond health effects, having influences on productivity and social cohesion, particularly in regions disproportionately affected by the diseases. Economic impacts are generally healthcare costs, loss of workforce contribution through illness, and the additional burden to health systems. For instance, regions suffering from malaria experience schooling and agricultural output interludes as infected individuals are kept away from school or labor by the disease. The treatment of VBDs calls for vector control measures and environmental management to reduce the risk of transmission. Interventions such as indoor residual spraying, insecticide-treated bed nets, and community-based programs have helped diminish incidences of dengue fever and malaria. However, these interventions must be tailored to local contexts, as their impact depends on a combination of ecological, sociopolitical, and cultural determinants (Montenegro-Qui et al., 2021). Besides, advancing knowledge in terms of vector-borne disease dynamics is essential for effective public health control measures. The exploration of how the environment and the human population interact with vector behavior can provide valuable insights that inform surveillance and control activities. The significance of the diseases has prompted global health entities to prioritize their elimination to achieve comprehensive data collection and analysis in guiding policy advice. This scientific approach is of critical significance in determining knowledge gaps and designing particular interventions, as suggested in vector control strategy meta-reviews. By integrating scientific evidence and conventional practices at the field level, the health community can build a way to eliminate and control such diseases as leishmaniasis, malaria, and dengue and ensure global health security (Richard, 2020).

Overview of Major Vector-Borne Diseases

In epidemiology, vector-borne diseases such as malaria, dengue, and filariasis are significant threats that have higher impacts on populations in tropical and subtropical regions. Malaria, caused by *Plasmodium* parasites transmitted by *Anopheles* mosquitoes, is a cause of major morbidity and mortality across the world, particularly in Sub-Saharan Africa. Dengue fever, which is induced by the dengue virus and primarily transmitted by Aedes mosquitoes, has seen an explosion of cases over recent years, driven by causative determinants of urbanization and climate change. Filariasis, which is typically caused by parasitic infections transmitted by mosquitoes, continues to be a cause of public health problems in the majority of developing nations. The intricate interaction among such diseases and their environmental and socioeconomic contexts necessitates an ecological appreciation of the environmental determinants influencing their transmission dynamics. Environmental determinants are fundamental to the transmission and dissemination of vector-borne diseases, particularly in the context of breeding habitats conducive to vector multiplication. Urbanization creates water bodies that are stagnant and serve as a breeding ground for mosquitoes, thus increasing their population and, indirectly, risk of transmission. Land use alterations, seasonal climatic variations, and climatic extremes all add to the complexity of vector-borne disease dynamics. For instance, excess rainfall generates new breeding sites, whereas droughts bring vectors and hosts into contact with each other, leading to even higher transmission rates. To effectively control these diseases, it is critical to consider these changes in the environment since they have a direct impact on vector-pathogen interactions, influencing endemic and outbreak patterns. Due to the need for greater vector control, there is a critical need for a systematic review of vector control competence. Countries must perform thorough assessments of their vector control programs to identify vulnerabilities in dimensions like vector surveillance and insecticide resistance, which have been highlighted by studies on the requirements of countries in the Middle East and South Asia.

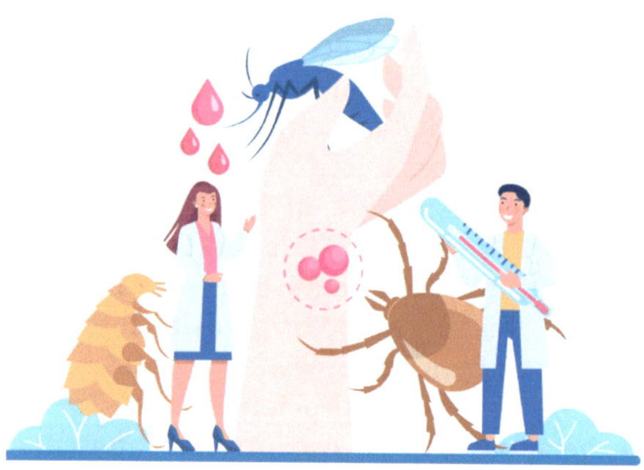

Figure 11.2. Illustration highlighting common vector-borne diseases transmitted by insects such as mosquitoes, ticks, and lice.

Source: https://images.ctfassets.net/uwf0n1j71a7j/6bngZbXA7H0RXPoIRhu7KP/d78c115c59a31a8010a33f8eabcf957b/common-vector-borne-diseases.png?w=1920&q=75.

Effective mechanisms for vector control must not only enhance the surveillance activities but also establish the mobilization of communities and intersectoral coordination to support public health interventions. By giving high priority to comprehensive vector control needs assessments, nations can formulate targeted strategies considering local ecological and social determinants, thereby ensuring the effective control of vector-borne diseases and facilitating the attainment of overall public health goals. This integrated approach harmonizes with sustainable development goals, reaffirming the importance of integrated vector management strategies towards sustainable health (Figure 11.2).

Importance of Studying Environmental Factors

It is important to know the environmental forces that influence vector-borne diseases so that effective, comprehensive measures can be offered to overcome their impact. Temperature, humidity, and availability of water are some of the environmental factors that most importantly influence the life cycles of vectors such as mosquitoes. For instance, certain species of mosquitoes only thrive in warmer temperatures, which enhances their breeding and survival rate. This augmented presence has a direct impact on disease transmission of diseases like malaria and dengue, impacting public health worldwide. Therefore, the research on these environmental factors not only helps in predicting outbreaks but also in making decisions with respect to vector control strategies tailored for the ecological environment. Given that over three thousand million people are exposed to malaria, it is crucial to identify such environmental factors in the development of effective intervention measures that are capable of responding to alterations in climate and habitat, thereby improving the overall public health response (Wolf et al., 2023). Incorporating the study of environmental factors into the management of vector-borne diseases has implications that go beyond biology; it aids in better surveillance activity. Environmental data-integrated surveillance systems have the potential to provide early warning signs of probable outbreaks. For instance, understanding seasonal variations in temperature and rainfall enables health authorities to estimate mosquito population highs and the attendant disease risk. This is facilitated by geographic information systems (GIS) and remote sensing technology, through which high-risk environments can be recognized based on environmental factors. This proactive strategy is most essential in economically vulnerable regions where healthcare and sanitation facilities are few and far between. By giving environmental aspects priority, health authorities can optimize resource allocation within vector control programs so as to reduce transmission rates of filariasis and dengue and allow resilience against impending outbreaks (Wolf et al., 2023). Besides, education on environmental factors is essential to innovation and the practice of sustainable measures in vector control. Traditional vector control methods have declining returns with the advent of resistance in vector populations. For instance, as measures of vector control lose effectiveness, disease risks like dengue rise, and other possibilities must be explored. Integrated vector management (IVM) principles allocate precedence to ecologically sound interventions such as the sterile insect technique (SIT) and genetic approaches for an efficient population reduction of vectors. The efficiency of the new strategies relies on insight into the nuances of environmental controls on vector biology. Thus, interdisciplinarity between ecologists, health professionals, and policymakers is essential to model and promote interventions based on socio-environmental processes, which will further reduce the vector-borne disease burden globally (Dyck et al., 2020).

11.1. Malaria

The complex interaction of environmental factors and malaria transmission is a significant area of research under public health programs to contain the disease burden. The climatic conditions, such as temperature, rainfall, and humidity, play an important role in controlling the survival and the reproductive cycle of the Anopheles mosquito, the primary vector of the transmission of malaria. As evidenced by various research records of climate-associated oscillations, regions with altered precipitation patterns are likely to record concomitant increases in the prevalence of malaria. For instance, studies in Senegal indicated outstanding correlations between climatic factors such as insolation and evaporation and malaria morbidity rates, indicating that environmental modification can alter the epidemiology of malaria transmission and complicate intervention efforts (Keita et al., 2025). This demands an appropriate malaria surveillance strategy that not only tracks disease endemicity but also tracks environmental determinants that may affect transmission patterns. The focus on integrated vector management can be no greater in the control of malaria. Multisector coordination of health, environmental, and meteorological authorities will be required in an efficient strategy to come up with a comprehensive plan. Research has highlighted the need for adopting a multisectoral One Health strategy that harmonizes human, animal, and environmental health while fighting vector-borne diseases. For example, in Senegal, there has been a functioning sentinel surveillance system to assess malaria cases and climatic weather (Keita et al., 2025). There are still challenges with the timeliness, accuracy, and completeness of the systems. These shortcomings must be dealt with in the planning of sensitive responsive interventions attuned to the environmental dynamics of malaria transmission. As affirmed in a number of reviews, the effectiveness of vector control operations will rely on combined measures featuring environmental management alongside behavioral and infrastructural upgrades. Education and community participation also play significant roles in malaria prevention strategies. Evidence underscores the contribution of socio-economic determinants to heightening vulnerability to malaria, so that poverty, low educational levels, and restricted access to health care services significantly enhance susceptibility to malaria. Interventions at the community level that enhance awareness and promote behavioural change are crucial for good vector control and prevention of malaria. Focused interventions aiming to address gender inequities can also enhance health gains. For instance, the participation of women in decision-making makes communities stronger and aids in the implementation of effective malaria control measures. This combined strategy is more and more a recognition that not only biomedical methods propel effective malaria control but also address social determinants of health, strengthening the relationship between conditions in society and susceptibility to disease. To bring these variables into public health policy could seriously diminish the effects of malaria throughout the world (Figure 11.3).

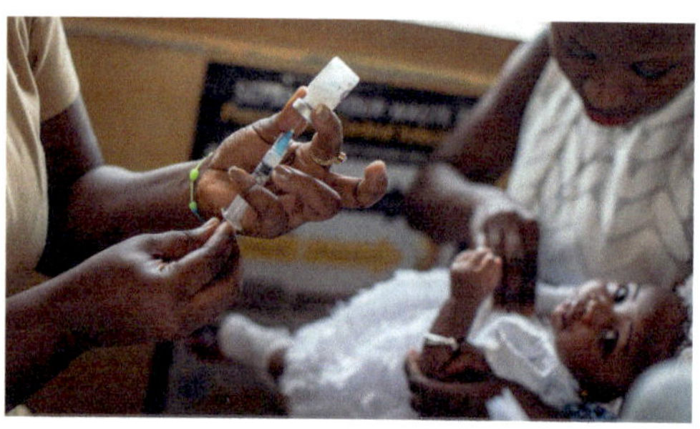

Figure 11.3. Malaria vaccine.

https://external-content.duckduckgo.com/iu/?u=https%3A%2F%2Fstatic01.nyt.com%2Fimages%2F2021%2F10%2F06%2Fscience%2F06malaria-ESP-00%2F06malaria1-videoSixteenByNine3000.jpg%3Fvideo-overlay%3Fvideo-overlay&f=1&nofb=1&ipt=3f2b2ed28869d663063121019cd560e2f56cff358cb8fba014ed128d69929305.

11.1.1. Causative Agent and Transmission

The transmission dynamics of the vector-borne diseases are closely wrapped in with the causative agents themselves and present a complex interaction of pathogens with insect vectors. In the case of malaria, the causative parasites are *Plasmodium falciparum* and *Plasmodium vivax,* which are transmitted to humans through an Anopheles mosquito bite. The life cycle of these pathogens largely depends on environmental conditions, with temperature and humidity playing a crucial role in the lifecycle of the malaria parasite within its vector. Similarly, the dengue virus, transmitted most frequently by Aedes aegypti mosquitoes, is influenced by transmission patterns based on urbanization, climatic variability, and the breeding places of mosquitoes. It is crucial to comprehend such interactions to develop targeted interventions and enhance vector management interventions that are capable of interrupting the transmission cycle and lowering disease incidence. The capacity of a region to control vector-borne diseases hinges not only on effective vector control measures but also on efficient surveillance systems in place to monitor the transmission of pathogens. In Sierra Leone, for instance, malaria, lymphatic filariasis, and onchocerciasis are significant public health issues in the context of limited understanding of the transmission dynamics of the diseases and their causative agents. Notwithstanding all the progress that has been made in improving vector control, overall entomological testing and capacity building within the health systems remain a pressing need. As discussed, inadequate robust surveillance undermines predictive outbreak potential and response capability, creating loopholes that can make populations vulnerable to emergent states like dengue and chikungunya. It is imperative that the disease monitoring infrastructure be reinforced for informing public health policy and ensuring efficient resource allocation. Furthermore, the application of microbial resource management (MRM) methods to vector control initiatives offers new approaches to preventing vector-borne disease transmission. MRM includes the possibility of managing insect microbiota to improve the resistance of vectors to disease, while blocking the life cycle of pathogens like malaria and dengue. For instance, strategic management of microbial communities associated with Anopheles and Aedes mosquitoes may lead to the production of biocontrol techniques that reduce vector populations or inhibit pathogen development. Such biotechnological regulation is a promising path towards enhancing the sustainability of vector control practices. This interdisciplinary approach not only acts as a response to immediate vector-borne disease threats but also becomes consistent with greater environmental management and public health objectives, advocating for an integrated approach to the complex health challenges (Alma et al., 2011; Ansumana et al., 2023).

11.1.2. Symptoms and Health Impacts

The symptoms and health outcomes of vector-borne infections, particularly malaria, dengue, and filariasis, highlight the urgent need for effective intervention measures. Malaria, caused by Plasmodium parasites transmitted through Anopheles mosquitoes, is characterized by fever, chills, and influenza-like illness that may progress to severe complications such as anemia, respiratory arrest, or organ failure if not treated. Dengue fever, on the other hand, could be accompanied by severe headache, joint pain, and high fever, advancing to dengue hemorrhagic fever or dengue shock syndrome, both fatal if not promptly treated. Filariasis, transmitted by Culex and Aedes mosquitoes, leads to lymphatic obstruction and extensive swelling, causing physical disability and extreme psychological impact. These diverse symptoms point towards the huge health burden imposed by such diseases, particularly in low-resource settings where the health infrastructure may be fragile to respond to complications effectively (Danso-Appiah et al., 2009). The interplay between environmental changes and the emergence of vector-borne diseases is evidenced in symptomology and health impacts being accounted for in endemic regions. Agricultural expansion, urbanization, and environmental disruption have created favorable habitats for mosquito vectors, increasing human exposure to pathogens. For instance, the establishment of rubber plantations in Southeast Asia has been linked with enhanced dengue exposure among plantation workers because these anthropogenic ecosystems create breeding habitats for Aedes mosquitoes (Tangena et al., 2016). Land-use changes also affect vector dynamics, minimizing malaria vectors in certain environments and maximizing the occurrence of disease in others. Not only do these impacts affect the incidence and severity of symptoms, but they also increase the geographical area covered by such diseases, as well as facilitate the potential to emerge as outbreaks in places where the diseases do not typically exist. It calls for a multi-faceted response that involves health monitoring and outreach within communities to understand the long-term impacts of vector-borne diseases. Socioeconomic factors are major influencers of escalating symptoms and health impacts of such diseases. Individuals living in poor environments do not have access to early medical interventions, causing delayed diagnosis and treatment. Besides, cultural beliefs about health have the potential to affect detection and response to symptoms, prolonging the suffering of the disease. Thus, there is a need to implement vector control interventions that are part of broader environmental management and health education schemes. Such integration has the potential to raise public awareness, support effective prevention measures, and ultimately lead to the prevention of the undesirable health impacts of vector-borne diseases in ecosystems (Danso-Appiah et al., 2009) (Figure 11.4).

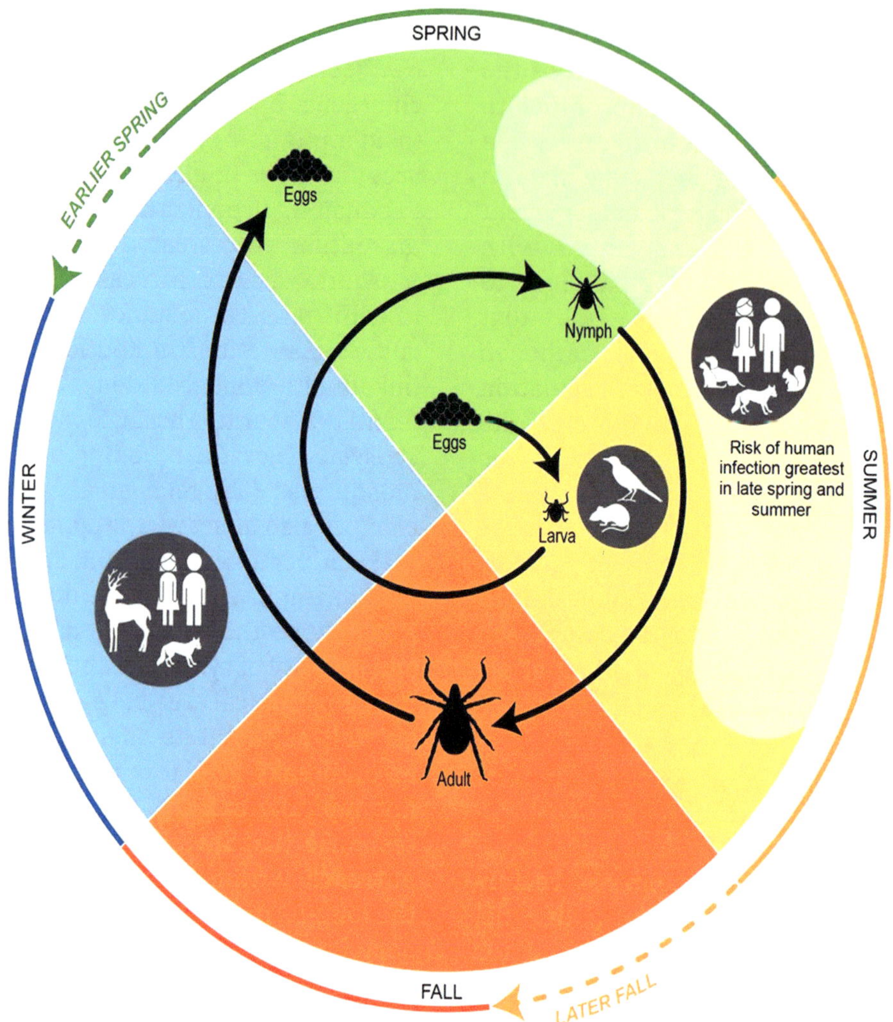

Figure 11.4. Symptoms and health impacts.

https://health2016.globalchange.gov/sites/default/files/styles/large_figure/public/figure/f3-cropped_13.png?itok=QfgiwUqD.

11.1.3. Geographic Distribution and Prevalence

The environmental factors have a very significant impact on shaping the geographic distribution and incidence of vector-borne diseases (VBDs). Environmental factors shape the vector ecology, such as mosquitoes and ticks, by deciding where they live. Climate change has emerged as a significant factor accelerating the process, leading to a disease-friendly habitat for the transmission of diseases such as dengue and malaria. Higher temperatures and altered patterns of rainfall are the causes of the expansion of vector habitats to new regions that were not affected before, primarily in tropical and subtropical areas. This alteration not only increases the risk associated with such diseases but also poses challenges to public health systems that are not normally equipped to deal with sudden spurts in transmission (Zavaleta et al., 2025). In addition, the dynamics of land use and urbanization contribute to the geographic character of VBDs, making them even more complex, thus underscoring the need for coordinated response systems in a bid to effectively respond to these dynamic health threats. Epidemiology of vector-borne illnesses exhibits noteworthy spatial and temporal patterns, which are influenced by numerous ecological determinants. All VBDs have their own unique vector ecology governing its transmission, exhibiting wide-ranging public health implications. For instance, geographic analysis has revealed that disease outbreaks may occur in rural and urban regions, demonstrating the role of environmental variables like bodies of water, irrigation systems, and urban locations in disease dissemination. Accurate knowledge of such factors can assist in pinpointing hotspot locations susceptible to outbreaks (Masimalai, 2024). This information is vital to the development of targeted surveillance and control measures, especially in regions already affected by climatic and environmental alterations, thus demarcating the importance of climates, landscapes, and socio-economic settings in the determination of the geographic range of VBDs. In order to combat the vector-borne disease threats, surveillance and environmental management measures must be optimized to the specificity of affected locations. Geographic information systems (GIS) and remote sensing methods are powerful mapping tools for land cover change patterns and predicting outbreak patterns. Health professionals can recognize timely interventions to mitigate risks through studying the spatiotemporal distribution of vectors and breeding habits. Ecological niche modeling enhances our ability to predict potential VBD transmission in an era of environmental change, allowing us to act proactively (Zavaleta et al., 2025; Masimalai, 2024). Furthermore, supplementing these scientific interventions with community education programs is essential to generate public awareness and encourage preventive practices. An approach that brings together technological advancements and community participation is essential in effectively combating the challenges of vector-borne diseases and ultimately achieving sustainable public health outcomes.

11.2. Dengue

Dengue fever, an infection of viral etiology transmitted by mosquitoes and caused by the dengue virus, is an important public health issue around the world, particularly in tropical and subtropical regions. It is transmitted by the *Aedes* mosquitoes, *Aedes aegypti* and *Aedes albopictus*, which multiply well in urban areas where human habitations and water collections are common. Clinical presentations of dengue range from mild febrile illness to severe cases that may cause hemorrhagic fever and dengue shock syndrome. The process of rapid urbanization through human migration creates conducive breeding habitats for these vectors, amplifying the diseases transmitted. Recognition of the ecological drivers of dengue transmission, including environmental determinants and climate change, lies at the heart of the establishment of effective control strategies aimed at containing outbreaks and preventing related morbidity and mortality. Climate change is a major driver of the epidemiology of dengue transmission, as it alters vector distribution, abundance, and behavior. Higher temperatures favor the geographical spread of Aedes populations, amplifying the risk of dengue transmission in hitherto non-endemic regions. Besides, patterns in precipitation affect the breeding site availability due to water stagnation in urban places because of inadequate drainage systems. According to recent studies, the combination of socioeconomic elements and changing climatic factors exacerbates public health crises, which calls for the adoption of an integrative approach to dengue control. According to Zavaleta et al. (2025), collective efforts in environmental management, technological innovation, and effective surveillance networks must reduce the public health impact of dengue and address climate-induced challenges. Successful vector control remains a cornerstone in controlling dengue outbreaks and demands an integrated strategy with community engagement and education. Chemical insecticide use has been rampant, but resistance in the mosquito populations and environmental concerns have pushed the globe towards searching for alternative and sustainable methods. Measures like larval control, biological control using the use of natural parasites, and genetic alteration of mosquitoes are being increasingly sought after. Besides, robust surveillance systems are essential for prompt diagnosis and outbreak response so that public health authorities can implement timely intervention. As highlighted in Tami et al. (2024), a multicomponent approach bringing together vector control and public health education, environmental management, and community participation is essential for successful long-term prevention of dengue along with other vector-borne diseases (Figure 11.5).

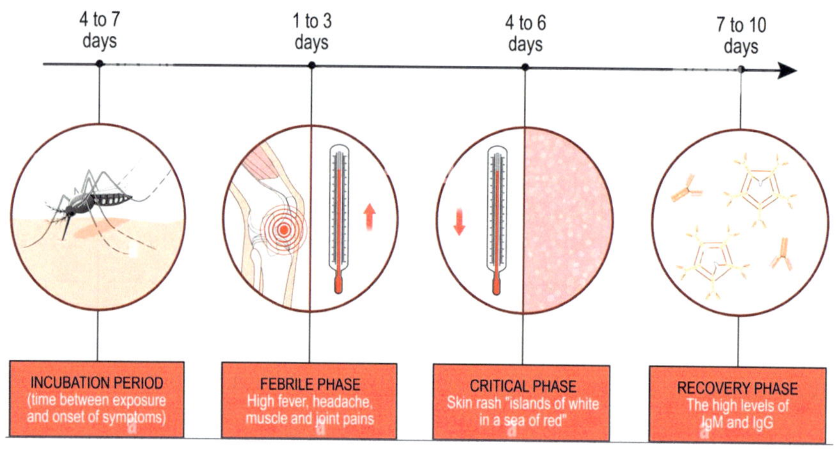

Figure 11.5. Dengue fever.

https://media.istockphoto.com/id/1411455506/vector/dengue-fever-clinical-course-infographics.jpg?s=1024x1024&w=is&k=20&c=qV9ZGeCuAwjSMMxuDQMO-n4fNZIg_ueibH7qjDOubxw=.

11.2.1. Causative Agent and Transmission

The etiologic pathogens of the VBDs are diverse pathogens, predominantly protozoa, viruses, and helminths, which are spread by a variety of vectors such as mosquitoes, ticks, and sandflies. With regard to malaria, the Plasmodium species, particularly *Plasmodium falciparum*, is responsible through the Anopheles mosquito, causing significant morbidity and mortality, mainly in tropical regions of the globe. Similarly, dengue fever is caused by strains of the dengue virus and has Aedes aegypti as its primary vector. Such interaction dynamics reflect on the intricate dynamics of relationships among organisms within ecosystems that define the patterning of such diseases. Recent epidemiological studies focus on the importance of understanding these causative agents because strategic prevention and intervention depend on thorough knowledge of their biology and patterns of transmission (Tami et al., 2024). Further, education in public health regarding such diseases can be an important preventive measure, enabling the community to follow precautions. Environmental factors play a crucial role in the transmission patterns of VBDs, such as climatic trends and anthropogenic factors. For instance, temperature, humidity, and rainfall patterns can favor the populations of vectors, influencing their life cycle and the rate of breeding. Of most crucial significance is the observation that shifts in climate could lead to vectors expanding into new locales, thus increasing the risk of outbreak in the non-endemic region. Dengue fever and malaria both demonstrate clear-cut associations between changing weather patterns and incidence, with socioeconomic factors magnifying the process. For this reason, understanding the interaction between environmental context and vector dynamics becomes critical in predicting impending outbreaks. The transmission dynamics, apart from relying on the biological traits of the vectors and pathogens, also rely on anthropogenic activities that modify their habitats and ecological niches (Masimalai, 2024). Surveillance and control interventions are the main elements to regulate VBD transmission. Environmental management, along with public health interventions through integrated vector management, can reduce the spread of such diseases. GIS surveillance and remote sensing technology facilitate the mapping of vector habitats as well as the detection of areas that have the potential to act as hotspots for disease outbreaks. This is essential in anticipatory health planning and resource distribution. Furthermore, the population control of vectors through ecological means, such as draining flooded areas as well as promoting community-led sanitation, directly destroys breeding sites. Public health interventions targeting vector behavior, personal protective measures, and immunization, where necessary, may supplement these environmental measures. Control of the complex factors involved in VBD transmission is essential in developing an overall strategy for the control or elimination, at least of the occurrence of disease in vulnerable groups (Tami et al., 2024) (Figure 11.6).

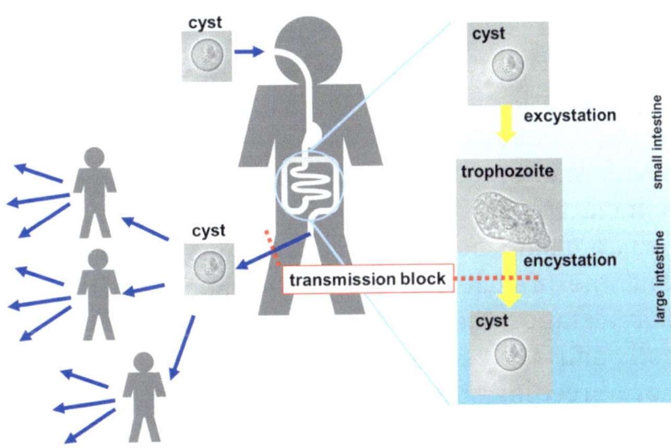

Figure 11.6. Causative agent and transmission.

11.2.2. Symptoms and Health Impacts

Symptom and health impact identification of vector-borne diseases is vital for effective control and surveillance. Malaria, transmitted by the Anopheles mosquito, presents serious symptoms such as fever, chills, and vomiting that may progress to acute complications if not treated. The World Health Organization shows that in 2020, malaria caused an estimated 627,000 fatalities globally, a representation of the health impacts of the disease. Similarly, dengue fever, caused by the Aedes mosquito, features high fever, severe headache, and muscle pain, potentially resulting in dengue hemorrhagic fever, a fatal disease. The increasing incidence of the conditions is inextricably connected to environmental determinants like climate change and urbanization, which increase vector habitats. Such an interaction necessitates a combined public health response in dealing with both environmental determinants and health outcomes. Filariasis, a mosquito-borne illness, also tends to have less serious initial presentations, such as fever and swelling, but can lead to long-term debilitating conditions, such as elephantiasis and lymphedema. The psychosocial and economic implications of such illnesses are extremely high because the afflicted may become unable to work or make any contributions to society. Secondly, emotional suffering arising from visible physical disfiguration may also lead to social stigma, another negative mental health consequence. Such long-term health effects highlight the significance of early diagnosis and successful treatment modalities for vector-borne diseases. Preventive interventions such as vector management and environmental control are crucial not only in reducing the spread of these diseases but also in enhancing the quality of life for victim populations. The information gathered from various research and monitoring programs points to a demanding relationship between environmental aspects and the prevalence of vector-borne diseases. For instance, land use change, increased rainfall, and temperature fluctuations can cause more breeding sites for mosquitoes, leading to higher transmission levels of diseases such as malaria and dengue. In addition, an appreciation of these dynamics from the perspective of One Health that unifies human, animal, and environmental health is essential for the formulation of integrated intervention policies. The convergence of different factors calls for a multidisciplinary approach to disease management that addresses community education on prevention and the deployment of strong surveillance networks to track populations of vectors. Speaking about the symbiotic relationship between environmental management and the outcomes of health impacts will ultimately enhance public health interventions in mitigating the impact of vector-borne diseases on populations worldwide, thus advancing resistance to future epidemics (Vil et al., 2021; Ellwanger et al., 2021).

11.2.3. Geographic Distribution and Prevalence

Geographic distribution and prevalence of vector-borne diseases play a significant role in shaping health outcomes globally, particularly for tropical and subtropical areas. There are places where malaria, dengue, and filariasis are endemic since the environment is favorable to sustain their respective vectors, such as the Anopheles mosquito for malaria and the *Aedes* mosquito for dengue. The transmission of such vectors depends directly on climatic factors like temperature, humidity, and rain, affecting their breeding and mortality. Warm regions with higher rainfall thus tend to see a rise in the prevalence of diseases. For instance, malaria remains endemic in parts of Sub-Saharan Africa, and dengue has extended its range due to urbanization and the associated land-use changes, illustrating the dynamic relationship between vector populations and environmental determinants ultimately affecting disease distribution and prevalence. In addition to climatic determinants, socio-economic determinants and public health infrastructure play a key role in the geographic spread of vector-borne disease. Populations with limited access to medical care, poor sanitation, and a lack of adequate vector control measures have higher rates of incidence. Slums in urban areas, typically characterized by high population density and poor sanitation, are most vulnerable to outbreaks of dengue fever. In contrast, populations with a robust healthcare system may have good surveillance and vector control measures, reducing the risk factor attached to these diseases. The historical reliance on insecticide-based interventions, as evidenced by the development of vector control programs, has been met with varying levels of success globally, with some areas experiencing dramatic disease incidence declines and others struggling with ongoing epidemics due to resistance and environmental factors, emphasizing the need for targeted public health strategies (Anne et al., 2020). The destiny of the battle against vector-borne illnesses relies on a fine understanding of their spatial dispersion in response to adjusting to changing environmental contexts. As global warming and urbanization continue to redefine ecosystems, health systems must employ holistic approaches to environmental management appropriate for local conditions. For example, understanding the distinctive ecology and habits of vector species is crucial in the development of sustainable control methods beyond the employment of chemical pesticides. The war on vector-borne disease will need to involve spending on state-of-the-art surveillance techniques and rallying the community for the purpose of instilling awareness and prevention practices. It is only when geographic prevalence information is matched with effective, evidence-based interventions that public health interventions stand a hope of reducing the disease burden of such conditions as malaria and dengue, ultimately improving the health outcomes of at-risk populations (El G-Batiha et al., 2020).

11.3. Filariasis

Filariasis is a tropical illness that is primarily brought about by parasitic worms spread to humans through the bite of infected mosquitoes. The vector-borne disease manifests itself in the predominant form as lymphatic filariasis, which is responsible for severe disfigurement and disability from limb and genital swellings. The socio-economic impact of filariasis is significant in that the sufferers are most likely afflicted by stigma and unemployment, thus creating more poverty in endemic regions. Understanding the vectors' ecology, here the Culex, Aedes, and Anopheles mosquitoes, is essential for effective control. Environmental factors such as pools of stagnant water, where the larvae of the mosquito stage develop, are key to the filariasis transmission process. Research indicates that intensification of agricultural activity within endemic zones for filariasis may further complicate these dynamics, and this is one example of the fine interface between environmental management and dissemination of disease (Jason et al., 2019). IVM programs have been the most important public health interventions as far as the fight against filariasis is concerned. IVM strategies combine environmental management, biological control, and insecticide use to reduce mosquitoes. Community participation in these activities is important to support sustainability and adherence to the vector control interventions. Community population participation can lead to increased impacts, both on awareness generation regarding filariasis and collective ownership of implementing the preventive measures (Haldane et al., 2019). Such community-based approaches have been shown to boost public health interventions, where communities are well-equipped to make informed decisions regarding their health and environment. Control of filariasis, therefore, requires an integrated approach dealing with the ecological, socio-economic, and cultural determinants of disease transmission. Surveillance is also essential in the control and eventual elimination of filariasis. Through monitoring of disease distribution and vector patterns, public health practitioners can design targeted interventions and target resources to places where they will be most effective. Advances in technology, including GIS, have improved the ability to map disease prevalence as well as identify high-risk groups effectively. Ongoing surveillance also helps to evaluate the effectiveness of interventions, guide future interventions, and keep community participation at the cornerstone of such efforts. Since vector-borne diseases like filariasis continue to be tough due to emerging environmental dynamics, a combination of robust surveillance systems with interventions at the community level emerges as a basis for sustained disease control and further development of public health (Jason et al., 2019) (Figure 11.7).

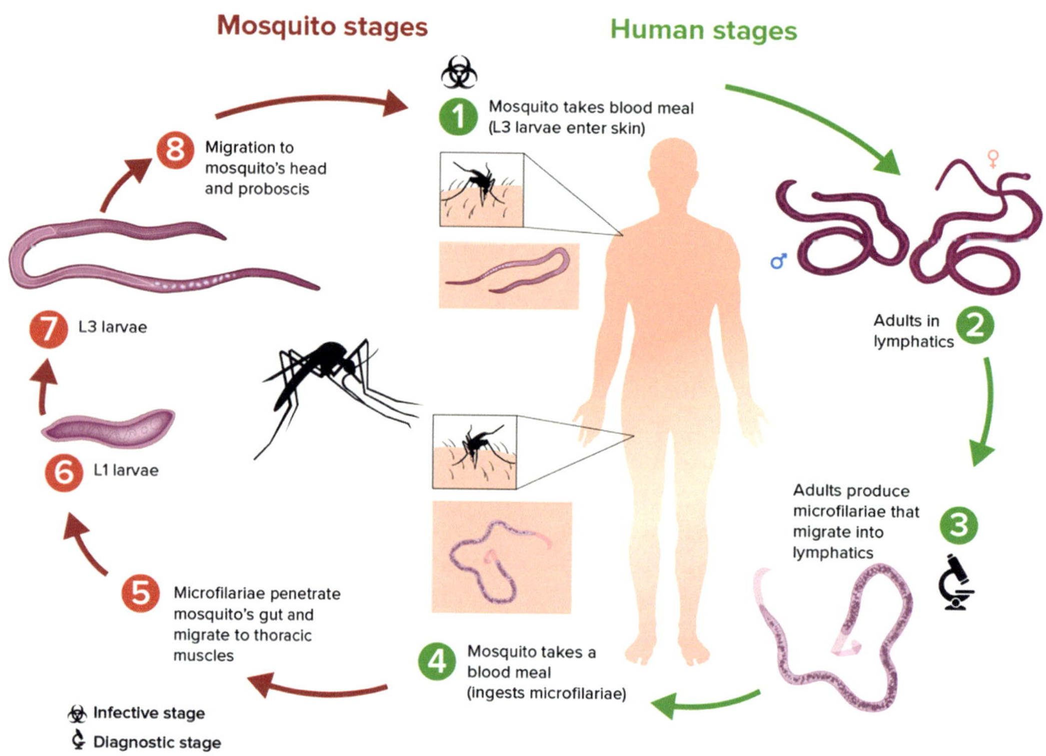

Figure 11.7. Lymphatic filariasis.

Source: https://external-content.duckduckgo.com/iu/?u=https%3A%2F%2Fcdn.lecturio.com%2Fassets%2FFilarial-life-cycle.png&f=1&nofb=1&ipt=2208f0ea0dc13b88efcae2fddb70c06c9f9e1e102b6c637ff695d00341b2028d.

11.3.1. Causative Agent and Transmission

The causative agents of vector-borne infections, such as malaria, dengue, and filariasis, are largely pathogens that rely on specific vectors to complete their life cycles. These vectors, primarily mosquitoes, are the primary transmission modes of these pathogens, which facilitate the transmission of the diseases to human hosts. For example, *Plasmodium* spp., which cause malaria, are transmitted through the bite of infected female Anopheles mosquitoes, whereas. Dengue virus and lymphatic filariasis are transmitted by *Aedes* mosquitoes. In order to create control methods, knowledge about the dynamics of interaction of these pathogens with their vectors is crucial. When environmental conditions fluctuate, so does the behavior and ecology of such mosquitoes, which have significant effects on transmission levels and patterns of infection, hence the necessity for effective vector control and disease surveillance in the avoidance of outbreaks, particularly among regions at risk due to climatic variability (IV Lănescu et al., 2023). Vector-borne disease transmission usually relies on environmental conditions like temperature, humidity, and rainfall patterns. Changes in these climatic variables can affect vector populations through offering more conducive breeding conditions. For instance, higher temperatures will likely extend the breeding season of mosquitoes and enhance the development of pathogens within them. Research foresees a rise in mean temperatures that will result in longer transmission periods for these diseases, such as malaria and dengue, and subsequently result in increased incidence rates in endemic regions (IV Lănescu et al., 2023). This is an indication of the need to build specially tailored vector control programs that counter increased environmental circumstances. Furthermore, these programs should be geared towards integrating environmental management strategies targeting breeding sites and vectors for a holistic disease control and prevention. Sound surveillance systems play a pivotal role in the monitoring of transmission dynamics of vector-borne diseases and in assessing the efficacy of control interventions. These systems provide valuable information on vector abundances, pathogen prevalence, and environmental factors that could be employed to inform interventions in a prompt manner. With climate change, the design of surveillance programs will need to be dynamic to allow the utilization of real-time data for earlier, more effective identification of possible outbreaks. Enhanced surveillance not only aids in the detection of shifts in transmission due to environmental changes but also aids in informing public health responses. With the implementation of stringent monitoring systems with a focus on geographical and seasonal variations, health authorities can predict and mitigate the impact of vector-borne diseases. It further builds disease emergence resilience such that the environment and human beings remain safeguarded.

11.3.2. Symptoms and Health Impacts

Vector-borne diseases like dengue and malaria are leading causes of morbidity all over the globe, manifesting a plethora of symptoms that can significantly reduce the quality of life. Malaria typically presents with fever, chills, and influenza-like manifestations, and if left untreated, can progress to severe conditions like anemia and respiratory failure. On the other hand, dengue fever is characterized by its intense headache, high fever, and widespread muscle and joint pain, commonly referred to as breakbone fever. The severity of these symptoms can intensify into dengue hemorrhagic fever, which is a severe illness that can cause shock and death, particularly among vulnerable individuals, such as children and the elderly. In order to counteract such health impacts, integrated vector control measures are required to help reduce the incidence of such incapacitating diseases (Puerta et al., 2022). Filariasis, another vector-borne infection as severe as Chagas, also illustrates the widespread health impacts associated with such illnesses. Often asymptomatic in its early stages, filariasis may progress into debilitating chronic illnesses like lymphedema and hydrocele that significantly influence daily activity and reduce patients' quality of life. Filariasis has not just long-term physical effects on body health but also social stigma, which equates to psychological issues and economic deficit for the infected. The state of filariasis also leads to complex health requirements like repeated medical therapy and prolonged use of health care, which contribute to healthcare strains. Comprehensive management of the health consequences and symptoms of filariasis involves a multi-component strategy of vector control measures and education at the community level on health (Montenegro-Qui et al., 2021). Environmental interactions with vector-borne diseases increase the symptoms and health implications of the disease. Changes in environmental conditions, such as increasing urbanization and deforestation, fuel vector production, such as mosquitoes, which increases disease transmission. The public health consequences of vector-borne disease are therefore not only the result of biological determinants, but also environmental and socioeconomic inequalities. For instance, residents of slum areas may have additional vulnerabilities because of inadequate access to health care, sanitation, and vector control measures. These are interrelated factors that highlight the need for environmental management and surveillance systems that are integrated to monitor and control the health effects of vector-borne diseases effectively, such that interventions are culturally acceptable and accessible to the target populations (Puerta et al., 2022).

11.3.3. Geographic Distribution and Prevalence

Environmental factors tightly regulate the spatial occurrence and spread of vector-borne diseases such as malaria, dengue, and filariasis. Regions with warm weather and high humidity support breeding conditions for vector populations, particularly mosquitoes. For instance, certain regions in sub-Saharan Africa are more susceptible to malaria due to congenial climatic conditions that support breeding of the Anopheles mosquito. Similarly, rapidly changing urban environments such as those of Southeast Asia are prone to experience an increase in dengue cases since vectors of dengue breed in man-made breeding sites for water, illustrating the linkage between environmental control and disease spread. Understanding this spatial pattern is critical to implement effective vector control and modify public health action to the specific ecological context of affected areas. The impact of human activities on the prevalence of vector-borne diseases cannot be exaggerated. Deforestation, urbanization, and agricultural use of land have severe impacts on habitats, influencing not only abundance but also diversity of vectors. A meta-analysis across mosquito species indicates a general reduction in diversity and prevalence following these activities, with some species, particularly those tolerant of human-altered landscapes, rising. These shifts augment the risk of disease emergence, as such successful species are usually the prime vectors of diseases. Such distribution of mosquito populations geographically emphasizes surveillance complexity and demands for targeted interventions to check vector-borne disease epidemics in modified ecosystems. This underlines the significance of having a One Health response to address the interconnected health of people, animals, and the environment (Pitt et al., 2024). Surveillance systems must evolve to provide accurate estimates of vector populations across varying geographic locales. Effective environmental management relies on timely information and innovative strategies to counter the shifting dynamics brought about by climate change and urbanization. The dynamic relationships between the epidemiology of disease and environmental shifts necessitate a solid structure of vector biology as well as the socio-ecological environment upon which they operate. Improved surveillance allows stakeholders to anticipate outbreaks and come up with anticipatory measures to protect at-risk populations. By promoting collaboration between various stakeholders like public health, environmental authorities, and communities, there is potential to implement practices that not only lower vector populations but also improve sustainable practices in habitat management. By acknowledging the relevance of geographic prevalence and distribution in vector-borne diseases, we are in a good position to prepare and respond to these public health risks (Perrin et al., 2022) (Figure 11.8).

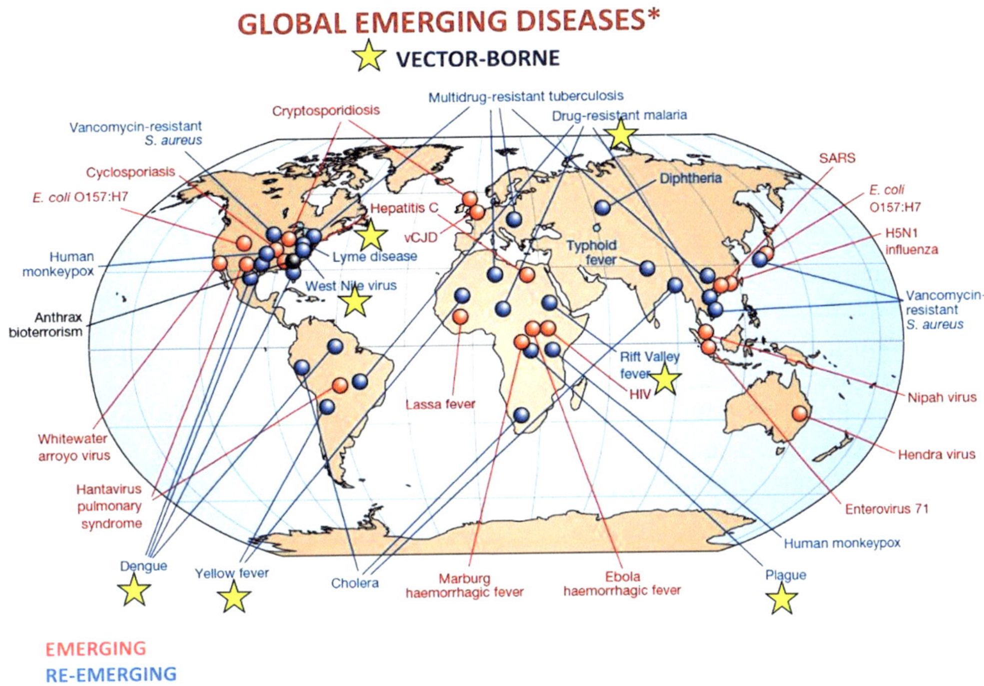

Figure 11.8. Climate change and vector-borne disease.

Source: https://image2.slideserve.com/3920598/slide4-l.jpg.

11.4. Vector Control Methods

The complexity of vector control methods necessitates a multifaceted strategy for managing the mounting vector-borne disease burden of diseases such as malaria, dengue, and filariasis. Conventional strategies have largely relied on insecticides and environmental control methods for population reduction of vectors. However, resistance to these insecticides is increasing, diminishing their potency and prompting a search for alternative intervention methods. IVM synthesizes various strategies that fit local ecological and socio-economic settings. For example, new genetic control techniques, including the sterile insect technique (SIT), offer promising vectors for suppression, especially in urban areas where conventional measures fail to deliver. The natural demand for innovative solutions is underscored by the re-emergence of mosquito-borne diseases owing to increased globalization and urbanization (Dyck et al., 2020). Repairing the transmission dynamics of vector-borne diseases within the urban setting also underscores the importance of having a complete understanding of vectorial capacity and co-infection scenarios. Recent studies outline significant knowledge gaps in the contribution of asymptomatic infection and the environment to disease transmission, particularly in crowded conditions. Surveillance systems play a vital role in monitoring the dynamics of these processes to enable interventions at the appropriate time for the control of outbreaks. Both timely information dissemination of vector-borne disease risk and public involvement in control efforts are also crucial. Public health policy must embrace an integrated stakeholder framework involving governments, communities, and healthcare providers in order to optimize the overall effectiveness of vector control practices. Developing these relationships will become crucial in the development of adaptive strategies tailored to the needs of emerging diseases and changing environmental conditions (Eder et al., 2018). In addition, the quest for environmentally sustainable vector control measures needs a multi-disciplinary approach incorporating environmental, social, and technological considerations. Environmental management through habitat modification and water source control supports chemical control measures and is integral to reducing breeding sites for mosquitoes.

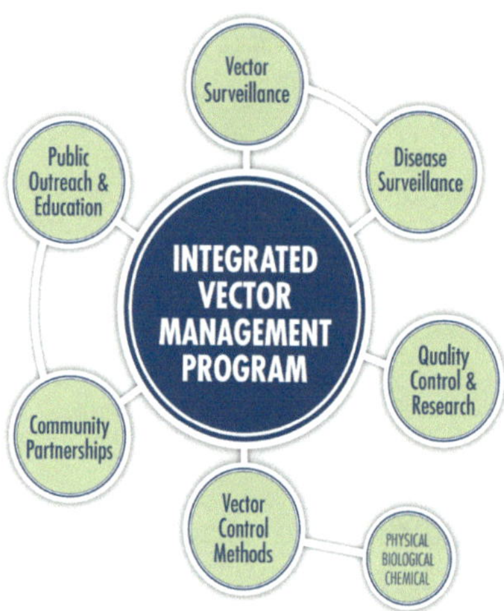

Figure 11.9. Integrated vector management (IVM).

Source: https://streamline.imgix.net/8f98e66a-7f3c-485c-ab3d-2e2789a612a8/d6c633b0-45ca-4200-9cff-8f250f7a40d7/ivm.png?ixlib=rb-1.1.0&w=2000&h=2000&fit=max&or=0&s=f233d280501e06e9f86d91b44ee31bc6.

Application of environmentally friendly measures not only reduces vector populations but also supports concomitance with global international health efforts towards sustainable development. Furthermore, technologies such as biocontrol mechanisms, which utilize natural predators of the mosquito, can be used in conjunction with traditional control methods and reduce reliance on chemical controls. Through this cohesion of various measures, vector control is made more dynamic and robust, ensuring long-term performance in the face of environmental oscillations and shifts in public health concerns (Dyck et al., 2020) (Figure 11.9).

11.4.1. Chemical Control Strategies

Chemical control strategies have a central role to play in the management of vector-borne diseases such as dengue and malaria. The strategies are generally geared towards the application of insecticides, the aim being to reduce directly the number of mosquitoes and hence the spread of the disease. However, the effectiveness of the above chemical controls has been significantly undermined by resistance against such insecticides, as evidenced by ongoing research indicating that trends towards resistance have reversed earlier gains in disease control (Safaa et al., 2022). This necessitates a re-evaluation of chemical control measures at once, in which new agents combined with new methods of delivery may enhance effectiveness against resistant vector populations to make them a fundamental part of any vector control strategy. The failure of chemical control methods brings to the forefront the need to adopt an IVM approach integrating environmental, biological, and chemical means for maximum effectiveness. Current reliance on conventional insecticides must be weighed against their environmental effects and the potential for resistance. Policies supporting environmentally friendly chemical control must be implemented, such as rotating active ingredients and mixing these with other methods of control (Safaa et al., 2022). This coordinated approach is intended to address existing vector control needs as well as maintain long-term effectiveness. Moreover, public engagement in the implementation of these strategies matters in enhancing public health benefits while minimizing environmental impacts, particularly as VBDs continue to be dynamic since their human surroundings are in constant change. Emerging technologies are also shaping the future of chemical control methods against VBDs. Methods such as the Sterile Insect Technique (SIT) and the incompatible insect technique (IIT) can offer a paradigm shift in vector control by reducing density levels using new approaches that are less reliant on chemical insecticides. They apply genetic manipulation to reduce mosquito population levels without maintaining chemical exposures (Dyck et al., 2020). This strategic integration of the genetic methods within chemical control strategies puts front and center the imperative for science-informed surveillance and monitoring systems to enable efficient application and response to such technologies. Overall, the synergy offered through the merging of chemical controls with novel methods and tight environmental regulation will be key to successful long-term vector-borne disease control (Figure 11.10).

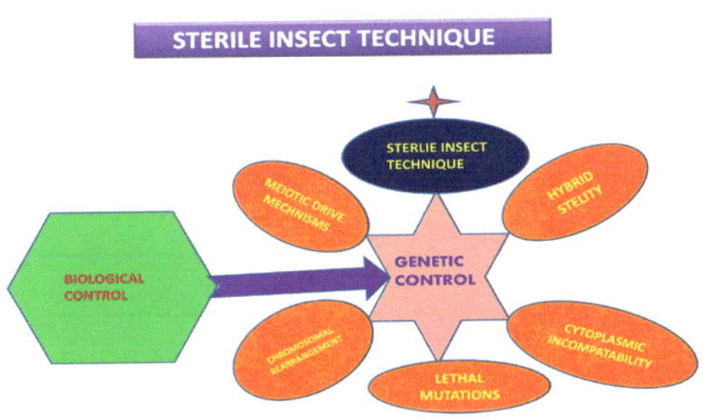

Figure 11.10. Sterile insect technique.

Source: https://external-content.duckduckgo.com/iu/?u=https%3A%2F%2Fimage.slidesharecdn.com%2Fsit-160302080837%2F95%2Fsterile-insect-technique-4-638.jpg%3Fcb%3D1456906271&f=1&nofb=1&ipt=b6b910f851412970dc7785ca7ea0afca36d489e83e7043f209410d7b28b5f085.

11.4.2. Biological Control Strategies

The use of biological control measures offers a promising line in the control of vector-borne diseases such as malaria, dengue, and filariasis. Among the numerous measures that have been proposed, larval source management (LSM) stands out in the sense that it acts against the aquatic phase of mosquito vectors. LSM involves the use of larvicides and environmental sanitation measures focused on reducing mosquito breeding sites. Its effectiveness is borne out by numerous research-based studies that reflect the relationship between LSM implementation and reduced transmission rates. While it shows potential, LSM is frequently underutilized in communities of modest financial resources. The emphasis on insecticidal strategies, even though effective in the short run, fails to offer answers to the ecological forces demanding a long-term response, and that is why more investment and dedication to LSM programs are essential in the battle against stagnation in malaria elimination activity (Okumu et al., 2025). The evolving interface between environmental forces and vector control policy grows increasingly important in the context of climate change. With rising temperatures and altered weather patterns, areas where vector species are flourishing are extending, thereby making measures for control more challenging. The frequency of outbreaks of such diseases as dengue and chikungunya illustrates how climate variability has the ability to amplify public health crises. Biological measures must react to such evolution by incorporating ecological management practices that are adaptive to local ecological and socioeconomic contexts. For example, coordinated endeavors that increase community engagement in sanitation and habitat change assist in consolidating vector control endeavors such that they are better attuned to endure climatic impacts. Such types of alterations must be multifaceted and emphasize the need for public health experts, environmental scientists, and the grassroots to converge to further sustainable and effective disease control interventions (Zavaleta et al., 2025). In addition, successful deployment of biological control interventions calls for stringent surveillance systems that monitor vector populations and determine the effectiveness of applied measures. Surveillance is not deployed as a respondent strategy but as a key element for guiding active public health responses. By being systematic in data gathering on vector behavior, distribution, and population density, health authorities can better forecast outbreaks and refine their approaches accordingly. Integration of biological control mechanisms with surveillance facilitates a complex understanding of the dynamics of transmission, ultimately allowing targeted responses to address the specific challenges that are presented by new environmental contexts. Strong development of surveillance coupled with biological control programs can therefore be the basis for an integrated public health response to mitigating the effects of vector-borne disease in a new world (Okumu et al., 2025) (Figure 11.11).

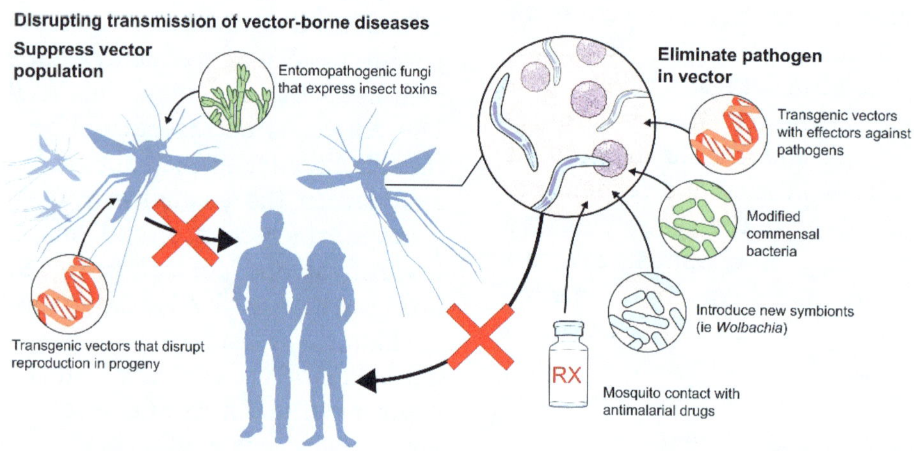

Figure 11.11. Biological control strategies in vector-borne diseases.

Source: https://external-content.duckduckgo.com/iu/?u=https%3A%2F%2Fwww.science.org%2Fcms%2F10.1126%2Fscience.abc2757%2Fasset%2Fc0506249-8ed4-4834-acba-93fdecc04035%2Fassets%2Fimages%2Flarge%2Fscience.abc2757-f3.jpg&f=1&nofb=1&ipt=6b27c26ec03c540344110d3fcb51298b41053c3c9425e059f1f0917a601c38ea.

11.4.3. Integrated Vector Management

IVM is a key strategy for vector-borne disease (VBD) prevention and control, including malaria, dengue, and filariasis. IVM comprises the integration of various vector control tools using an intersectoral approach and offers a forum that ensures the optimization of vector control program effectiveness and sustainability. The WHO promotes IVM as a strategy to address the challenges that are presently faced, such as the limitation of resources and rising insecticide resistance. Significantly, IVM emphasizes adaptive management and evidence-based interventions, thereby allowing programs to evolve in terms of changing epidemiological data and local environmental contexts. Such a dynamic and integrated strategy is not only crucial for the short-term control of vectors but also synchronizes with broader public health objectives, ensuring interventions are tailored to address particular local requirements and environments and therefore enhancing the overall effectiveness of vector control initiatives (Wilson et al., 2017). The implementation of IVM as a strategic strategy necessitates robust surveillance systems comprising both entomological and epidemiological data. Programs, through highly sensitive surveillance, can monitor the transmission of VBD and respond early to any recrudescence of cases. Data-driven decision-making plays an important role in informing the choice of vector control interventions and their deployment where it is most necessary. Furthermore, integration with environmental metrics and decision-support technology holds promise to facilitate the creation of relevant control targets beyond traditional epidemiological indices. With these advanced tools and techniques, IVM highlights a future-oriented process of vector management that facilitates strategic use of resources where most needed. As highlighted by existing studies, such as those from Liverpool School of Tropical Medicine, the adoption of IVM would enhance decision-making ownership in endemic countries, thus resulting in higher responsibility and sustainability for vector control programs (Adams et al., 2015). Moreover, IVM is a call for intersectoral coordination and strategic planning, which are absolutely critical for the successful incorporation of vector control strategies. Engaging stakeholders across various sectors, including environmental, agriculture, and health organizations, is critical to having a coordinated battle against vector-borne diseases. Through collaboration, it improves resource consolidation and the sharing of knowledge, minimizing redundancy in activities while enhancing the impact of interventions. Despite its potential, IVM is undermined by limitations such as poor political will and entrenched organizational silos. To overcome these barriers, there is a requirement for a coordinated effort to foster political will and disburse the necessary financial resources. Human capacity investment and infrastructure investment are essential in shaping an environment of partnership that captures the adaptive nature of IVM, which translates to proper VBD management and eradication (Wilson et al., 2017).

11.5. Environmental Management

Environmental control is crucial in the management of VBDs such as malaria, dengue, and filariasis. Environmental control entails various steps that are designed to minimize vector breeding places to decrease the risk of transmission of these diseases. Conventional vector control measures rely considerably on ecological knowledge and indigenous practices particular to given environments. More obvious has been the tendency, though, to over-sustain on the application of insecticides, as reflected by the issues of resistance to insecticides. In response to these tendencies, it is necessary to restore an integrated environmental management strategy that considers the subtle relationships between vectors and their ecosystems. Sustainable measures, including habitat manipulation and biological control methods, can be optimally synergistic with vector control action and predict more sustainable practices of disease management in the long run, ultimately mitigating public health effects of VBDs (Dyck et al., 2020). Furthermore, vector control effectiveness relies a lot on regular monitoring and evaluation, underlined by the increased complexity of vector ecology due to climate change and urbanization. Being effective in managing the environment requires knowledge of local epidemiology and ecological environments, thereby increasing the intricacies involved in the dynamics of disease transmission. The re-emergence of apparently controlled diseases highlights the application of evidence-based practices that combine local and scientific studies. Encouragement of IVM is a major aspect of environmental management since it encourages the use of various forms of control that are specific to a certain environment, following the ecological dynamics of vector habitat and behavior (Anne et al., 2020). The integrated approach can lead to improved surveillance and response efforts against VBDs, thus generating a more sustainable and effective public health approach. With developments in vector control methods, the incorporation of new technology becomes essential as part of environmental management. Newly emerging innovations, such as the SIT and genetic sexing strains, have exciting potential in the development of vector suppression. When combined with traditional practices in environmental management, such technological innovations can attain synergies that lead to improved vector control methods. By targeting the environmental sources of vector breeding, such as waste and bodies of standing water, interventions are effective in reducing breeding areas to a considerable extent. By incorporating community mobilization and education in environmental management programs, public participation and awareness of the necessity of reducing vector habitats are enhanced. Such an integrated strategy is crucial in ensuring the sustainability of long-term vector control programs and enhancing community resistance to vector-borne diseases, thereby leading to enhanced health outcomes (Dyck et al., 2020) (Figure 11.12).

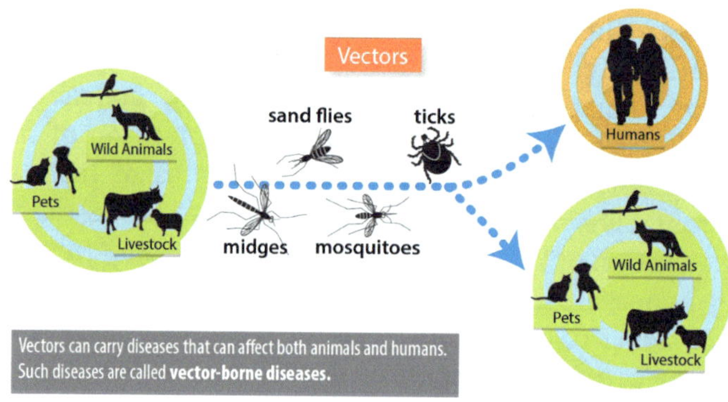

Figure 11.12. Environmental factors in addressing vector-borne diseases (VBDs).

Source: https://www.breakdengue.org/wp-content/uploads/2014/10/dengue12.jpg.

11.5.1. Role of Environmental Factors in Disease Transmission

Understanding how environmental elements play a role in the transmission of vector-borne diseases is crucial in coming up with effective control measures. Various factors such as temperature, land use, and urbanization can influence vector survival and breeding, thus disease spread. Temperature variations, for instance, have the ability to impact the life cycle of mosquitoes, with rising temperatures likely to boost their breeding cycles. Moreover, climate change also causes the patterns of rainfall to shift, which in turn creates optimal breeding sites through water stagnation, enabling more mosquitoes. As a result, regions that are exposed to climate change or urban development activities witness a synchronous rise in vector-borne diseases such as malaria and dengue. Aiming at these environmental determinants is vital for the development of effective vector control interventions that are responsive to the ecological conditions that drive disease dynamics, and it highlights the relevance of comprehensive strategies that honor the interdependence of environment and health (Wilson et al., 2017). Vector management intervention should be informed by an understanding of the ecological contexts that support vectors. IVM has emerged as a key strategy that promotes adaptive application of different vector control interventions in the context of existing environmental conditions. Not only is this more efficient towards increasing the effectiveness of existing measures, such as insecticide-treated bed nets and indoor residual spraying, but it also supports the involvement of sectors other than health towards more sustainable effects. For example, urban landscape planning may significantly influence the breeding behavior of mosquitoes, illustrating the imperative of collaboration between urban planners, environmentalists, and public health professionals to manage vector populations. With the adoption of IVM, health authorities are in a position to mobilize local ecological data to tailor interventions and maximize the overall efficacy of vector control while ensuring that environmental factors are always monitored and regulated (Adams et al., 2015). Competent surveillance activities are most important in comprehending and addressing the challenges arising from environmental factors contributing to disease transmission. Surveillance systems that integrate environmental data can offer important information about vector behavior and risk trends to enable early and adaptive responses to outbreaks. For example, tracking climatic parameters and land use alterations enables public health authorities to anticipate vector population booms and take preemptive control actions. Moreover, the integration of epidemiological information with entomological studies can account for disease occurrence in terms of environmental determinants and alert policymakers to necessary interventions. Appreciation of the role played by environmental factors in disease transmission emphasizes the necessity to foster interdisciplinary collaboration towards enhancing data collection, analysis, and communication. This integrated strategy can ultimately be used to lead to more effective surveillance systems to inform health policy and facilitate the response to vector-borne diseases (Wilson et al., 2017) (Figure 11.13).

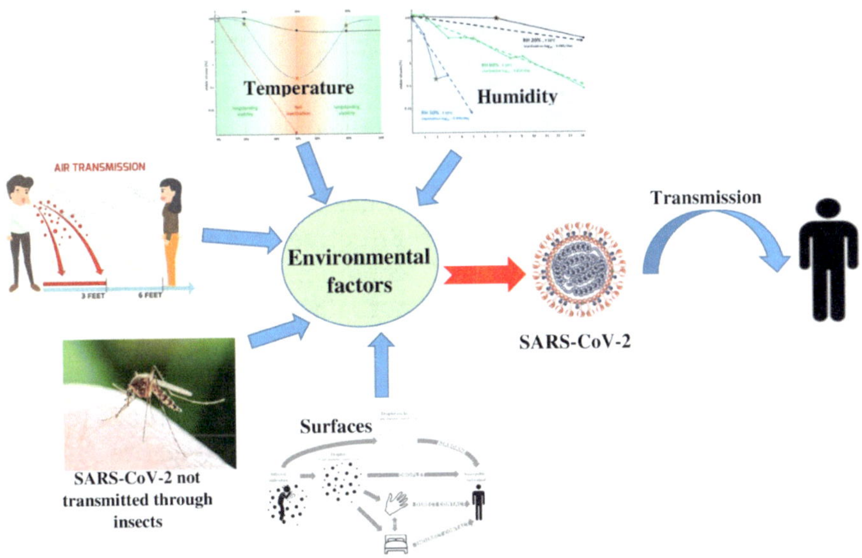

Figure 11.13. The role of environmental factors in the transmission of SARS-CoV-2 (COVID-19).

Source: https://media.springernature.com/lw1200/springer-static/image/art%3A10.1186%2Fs13568-020-01028-0/MediaObjects/13568_2020_1028_Fig1_HTML.png.

11.5.2. Strategies for Environmental Modification

Good environmental modification practices are critical in vector control for the transmission of various diseases like dengue, malaria, and filariasis. Environmental modification reduces the breeding of vectors in places where they can develop and grow. For instance, manipulation of water resources can assist in controlling the incidence of dengue fever because Aedes mosquitoes breed around stagnant water. Drainage system installation in urban and rural settlements can substantially diminish breeding opportunities, and community participation in water management processes instills a feeling of communal responsibility. Coordination with defoliation landscaping plans, minimizing shade, and standing water, is also an effective passive vector control process. These strategies emphasize the necessity of harmonizing environmental management with public health goals to properly tackle vector-borne conditions and community resilience, especially where climatic uncertainty prevails (Raimi et al., 2021). Further, landscape modification entails an integrated strategy, embracing ecological factors into city planning and agricultural production. The use of bioengineering techniques can support siting interventions by allowing natural competitors and predators for vector species to be established. For example, the use of salinity gradients in rice paddies can suppress freshwater-preferential mosquito populations. Similarly, the use of certain native vegetation for planting can help draw in natural enemies of vectors. These ecological interventions not only suppress vectors but also enhance biodiversity and climate change resilience. Public education campaigns coupled with rigorous surveillance and monitoring schemes enable stakeholders to modify such environmental interventions effectively. The existence of human populations alongside disease vectors, therefore, calls for an innovative application of ecological knowledge and community engagement, ensuring a sustainable path towards improving public health outcomes in vulnerable regions (Dahmana et al., 2020). In response to the challenge posed by climate change, it becomes imperative to continually optimize environmental modification measures. The impact of altered climatic conditions is not just on straightforward vector distribution; it reaches the entire ecosystem's dynamics, which could make one more vulnerable to vector-borne disease. Preparations must evolve hand in hand with climate adaptation needs, fortifying infrastructure against the stresses of extreme weather while simultaneously offering ecological intervention. For instance, urban plan design resisting flooding can incorporate vegetation that not only precludes water stagnation but also repels vector habitation. Moreover, the existence of protective policies ensuring responsible land use will curb deforestation and its attendant impacts on vector behavior. Through environmental shifts viewed in terms of climate resilience, actors can create adaptive capacities that protect public health from the increasing repercussions of environmental degradation and global warming (Raimi et al., 2021).

11.5.3. Importance of Sustainable Practices

Sustainable management is a crucial aspect in preventing the risk of vector-borne diseases, which are still a threat to public health globally. Effective management of environmental conditions is vital in significantly reducing the breeding sites of disease vectors like mosquitoes and, consequently, limiting the transmission of pathogens. For instance, plastic waste has been discovered to provide an ideal condition for such vectors because plastics that are discarded may retain still water that harbors Aedes mosquitoes populations, which are responsible for diseases like dengue and Zika virus. To address this issue, integrating effective waste management systems and promoting recycling efforts can alleviate the danger posed by plastic pollution, eventually creating a healthier environment. Without them, danger from vector-borne diseases is sure to grow with growing urbanization and plastic consumption, threatening more communities to outbreaks (Pierre-Maquart et al.,

2022). Besides, the merging of environmental management and sustainability recognizes the urgency to adopt a multi-strategy effort in managing vector-borne diseases. Sustainable agricultural practices, such as integrated pest management, can also lower the use of harmful chemicals that would otherwise lead to further environmental deterioration. The adoption of these practices is beneficial in maintaining the biodiversity necessary for natural pest management. Since resistance to current vector control technologies, especially in mosquitoes, is increasing, reconsidering our methods is crucial. Incorporating environmentally friendly practices in vector control can make current methods more effective while conserving non-target organisms and ecosystems. These synergistic strategies not only aim to counteract health impacts from diseases like malaria but also strive towards worldwide sustainability of public health and environmental conservation (Dyck et al., 2020). Sustainability in health interventions not only decreases the incidence of vector-borne diseases but also enhances resilience in communities against future health threats in a changing environment. Educating communities about the need for waste management, sanitation, and environmental care motivates active participation in public health interventions. Once communities are educated on the relationship between their immediate environment and health conditions, they can better perform acts that promote sustainability. Such a communal effort not only takes away the avenues for the transmission of diseases but also enhances the quality of life. Furthermore, the formulation of sustainable processes and wider awareness among the community can drive novel solutions that address environmental drivers in the fight against vector-borne illnesses, eventually leading to healthier communities and a more sustainable future since the diseases are expected to keep evolving and adjusting alongside human beings (Pierre-Maquart et al., 2022; Dyck et al., 2020).

11.6. Surveillance of Vector-Borne Diseases

Surveillance of VBDs is integral to public health practice, particularly in regions where the diseases are endemic. Effective surveillance allows for early detection of disease outbreaks, monitoring of trends in disease, and evaluation of control measures. The intricacy of VBDs, including malaria, dengue, and filariasis, justifies the value of integrated systems of surveillance. These kinds of systems must integrate entomological, epidemiological, and environmental data to aid immediate response to looming threats. Systematic vector and case surveillance through their continuous monitoring aids public health officials in identifying high-risk groups and locations, thereby allowing effective targeting of interventions. Collection and sharing of data in real time, enhanced through the use of new technologies such as mobile health applications, is also enhanced. It is thus critical that an effective surveillance system be in place to prevent VBD effects and safeguard population health. This involves optimizing control interventions for effectiveness in the detection of VBDs, particularly in cases of resistance to insecticides. Recommendations from the World Health Organization include IVM, which involves adaptive use of pluralistic control methods that are appropriate to specific ecological and epidemiological contexts. An effective understanding of resistance patterns and vector behavior is necessary to control these effectively. Surveys and research have proven that periodic reviews of these interventions, such as the efficacy of insecticide-treated bed nets and indoor residual spraying, are necessary in order to guide informed public health policy decision-making. In addition, effective vector control relies on ongoing monitoring for insecticide resistance, as illustrated by the spatial and temporal patterns in populations of mosquitoes like Anopheles gambiae and others. Such an all-encompassing approach supplements an evidence-based strategy in surveillance as well as control, assuring sustainable outcomes in VBD control. Environmental determinants are paramount in the surveillance and control of vector-borne diseases. Land use changes such as agricultural expansion and urbanization strongly drive the behavior and habitat of mosquitoes and directly influence disease dynamics. For instance, studies in rubber plantations have noted mixed populations of mosquitoes and species richness, which brings to light the ecological role of such locations on the VBD risk of transmission. The interface between vector environments and human activities is complex, combining the behavior of the human population and the ecology of vectors. Such environmental determinants must be considered by good surveillance, employing data from various sources to estimate the risk factors and implement intervention accordingly. For example, identification of hotspots for breeding of vectors in anthropogenic environments enables public health programs and mobilization of the community. Thus, knowledge of environmental influences is central to the holistic surveillance strategies which aim to reduce the incidence of VBDs globally, testifying to the necessity of inter-disciplinary cooperation between health and environmental domains (Figure 11.14).

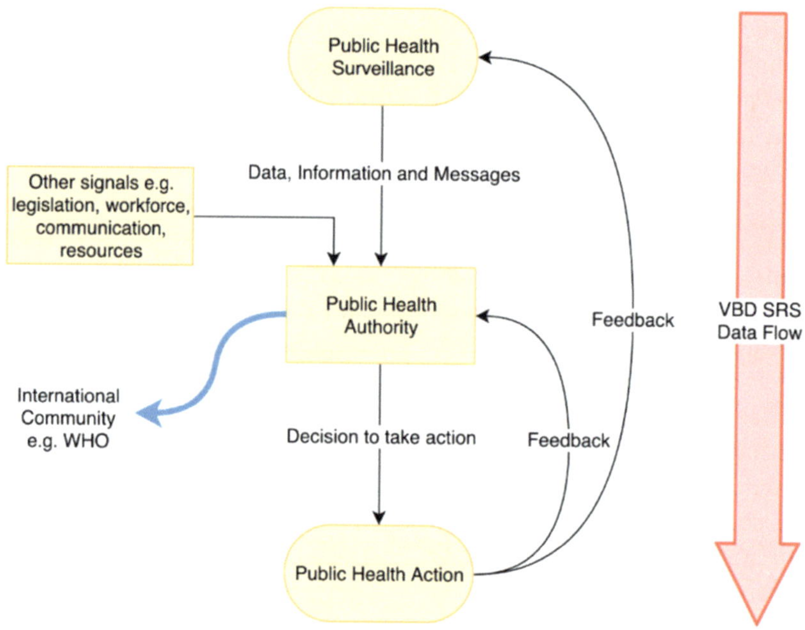

Figure 11.14. Exploring vector-borne disease surveillance and response systems.

Source: https://www.mdpi.com/ijerph/ijerph-17-08512/article_deploy/html/images/ijerph-17-08512-g001.png.

11.6.1. Importance of Surveillance in Disease Control

Surveillance plays a key role in the control of vector-borne diseases through early detection, disease transmission, and prevalence surveillance. With vector-borne diseases still posing a persistent risk to public health, effective surveillance systems are required to identify outbreaks and risk groups. This involves combining data from diverse sources, including clinical notification, laboratory testing, and environmental surveys, to generate an informative picture of the disease epidemiology. Besides, surveillance informs public health interventions, which include interventions such as vector control interventions in specific locations and vaccination. For instance, Egypt conducted a situational analysis, which revealed gaps in preparedness for vector-borne illnesses, necessitating increased surveillance to assist with disease management operations and mitigate risks of impending outbreaks of malaria, dengue, and filariasis (Eassa et al., 2022). The economic costs associated with vector-borne diseases highlight the importance of efficient surveillance systems in controlling disease. Besides the direct health effects, vector-borne diseases may lead to heavy economic losses affecting healthcare costs and productivity. The World Health Organization, for example, has recorded over a billion cases of vector-borne diseases annually, with malaria and dengue leading to heavy economic losses for affected countries (Ortega, 2014).

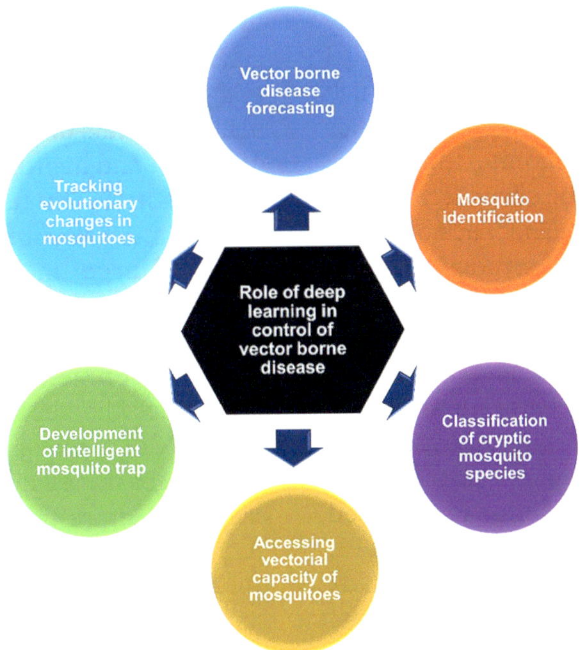

Figure 11.15. Role of deep learning for the control of vector-borne diseases.

Source: https://www.researchgate.net/publication/366273578/figure/fig2/AS:11431281113808926@1674097040185/Role-of-deep-learning-for-the-control-of-vector-borne-diseases.png.

Surveillance not only aids in following trends in disease, but also aids in effective resource allocation, targeting interventions where there is the most exposure to such diseases. Upon the identification of epidemiological trends, surveillance programs are able to aid policymakers in formulating effective strategies in averting transmission and reducing economic impacts, ultimately ensuring community immunity against vector-borne attacks. Moreover, the integration of technology and environmental management into surveillance programs aids in achieving maximum functionality of disease control. Geospatial analysis, remote sensing, and data platforms can provide real-time data on vector habitats and environmental drivers of disease transmission. A case in point would be awareness of the environment in which mosquito breeding occurs to inform the targeted application of insecticides and amplify vector control programs. The synergy between surveillance, environmental management, and community action provides a One Health philosophy, which responds to the convergence of human, animal, and environmental health in disease prevention. In Egypt, effective communication and intersectoral coordination can lead to improved surveillance and response efforts, ultimately leading to vector-borne disease control and associated health and economic consequences (Eassa et al., 2022) (Figure 11.15).

11.6.2. Methods of Surveillance

Effective surveillance methods are inherently enforcement-based in the management of vector-borne diseases, particularly those such as malaria, dengue, and filariasis. Surveillance entails various methods of monitoring as well as regulating populations of such vectors, for instance, mosquitoes that transmit such diseases. Among the most innovative strategies is the use of drone technology, which can yield vast amounts of information on mosquito breeding habitats and environmental parameters favoring vector breeding. With the integration of remote sensing and predictive modeling, scientists can delineate transmission hot spots and sites of ecological interest, and thus allow for focused intervention policies. However, successful drone surveillance depends on aspects such as affordability, regulatory acceptance, and social acceptance, meaning efficient communication and awareness are essential components of any vector control program (Carrasco-Escobar et al., 2022). Moreover, traditional surveillance methods are prone to prioritizing the detection of insecticide resistance among mosquito populations, which is vital to the sustainability of vector control programs. But then there are existing phenotypic tests that quantify this resistance that may not reflect field conditions, and there will be a disconnect between what is seen in the lab and what happens in the field. For instance, environmental parameters such as temperature and humidity can influence the effectiveness of insecticides, and physiological variables related to the mosquitoes themselves—such as age and feeding behaviors—can influence susceptibility to control. This disparity highlights the necessity of constructing standards considering practical resistance, in view of the local settings in which interventions are mounted. Enhanced surveillance practice considering such variations is pivotal towards achieving expected outcomes in vector control and relief of public health burden conferred by transmission of disease (Namias et al., 2021). The employment of advanced surveillance techniques also promises to enhance environmental management in vector control. With the utilization of multi-spectral imaging technologies by means of drones, public health officials are able to assess the ecological condition and habitat suitability of the mosquito population. From such a comprehensive view, it becomes feasible to introduce targeted larval source management activities that provoke more sustainable control practices. Moreover, the ability of drone technology to map environments provides a more robust context for the vector dynamics environmental interaction. With constant advancement in these techniques by researchers, it is increasingly crucial to share findings and best practices to achieve more collective action against vector-borne diseases. Continued advancement in surveillance techniques emphasizes their core role in guiding effective responses to emerging public health issues related to vector-borne pathogens (Carrasco-Escobar et al., 2022).

11.6.3. Challenges in Surveillance Systems

Vector-borne disease surveillance systems are faced with several key challenges that obstruct effective disease monitoring and management. The first is the rapid evolution and adaptation of disease vectors themselves, such as mosquitoes. As a result of climate change, environments have shifted, and vectors like Aedes aegypti, which carry the dengue and Zika viruses, have expanded geographically, resulting in new populations at risk. This shifting scenario makes it more difficult to have sound surveillance procedures in place, which are usually predicated on historical data that no longer applies today. With the mounting burden of vector-borne diseases, with more than half of the world's population now being exposed to dengue alone, the inefficiency of current surveillance methods has to be rectified to prevent the resurgence of diseases that had previously seen a decline (Pierre-Maquart et al., 2022). Furthermore, integrating environmental information into surveillance systems adds an additional level of complexity. Plastic litter, for instance, serves as a breeding ground for several vectors and remains outside the scope of disease surveillance. Proof highlights that plastic litter provides reservoirs of standing water necessary for the larval breeding of mosquitoes, thus increasing disease transmission risks (Pierre-Maquart et al., 2022). However, most surveillance systems do not record such environmental aspects in a proper way due to inadequate aggregated data regarding waste management practices and their direct correlation with rates of disease. Incorporating this inclusion is significant due to the fact that understanding the environmental settings leading to an abundance of vectors can lead to effective public health interventions as well as enhanced community awareness. Finally, the technology gap between the developed and the developing world poses tremendous challenges to effective surveillance systems globally. The majority of middle-income countries, particularly in the tropics, lack the facilities and infrastructure needed to conduct frequent and accurate disease surveillance. This gap leaves populations vulnerable to new vector-borne diseases and hinders coordinated action during outbreaks. Moreover, the dependence on local health systems tends to result in unreliable and heterogeneous data collection across regions. In the absence of a coherent system that utilizes technology and data-exchange facilities, the efficiency of vector control measures will be restricted, reinforcing the current challenges that hinder proper disease surveillance (Dyck et al., 2020). Keeping in view these complexities, the construction of all-around and dynamic surveillance systems becomes essential in order to overcome the challenges of vector-borne diseases effectively (Figure 11.16).

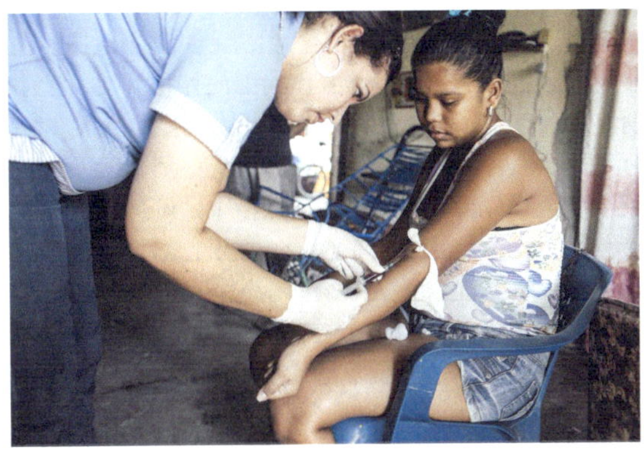

Figure 11.16. Promoting dengue vector surveillance and control.

https://www.who.int/images/default-source/departments/ntd-library/dengue/taking-blood-samples-(c)-paho-je-cogan.tmb-1200v.jpg?Culture=en&sfvrsn=bdd9c5d9_5.

CLOSER LOOK

IMPLICATIONS FOR PUBLIC HEALTH

Public health consequences of VBDs are paramount, particularly where determinants in the environment promote the spread of disease vectors. Mosquito-borne diseases such as malaria and dengue have a stark impact on mortality rates, particularly in low-income countries where health infrastructure can be substandard. Control efforts against vectors, therefore, become imperative. Current intervention strategies encompass chemical, biological, mechanical, and environmental interventions, but there are several of them that require efficiency and application enhancements. Moreover, traditional entomological surveillance methods, despite their imperative role in quantifying mosquito populations, are handicapped by being skill-dependent and labor-intensive, necessitating innovations like computer vision-based image recognition technologies to promote identification processes as well as outbreak responsiveness, as documented in the research of Kittichai et al. (2023). The absence of an effective vector control and surveillance program is a major public health concern, particularly for VBD-risk areas like Qatar. Results of study findings in 2017 and 2019 point to a high prevalence of pathogen-susceptible species of mosquitoes and demonstrate the necessity for more comprehensive management strategies to counteract the threats arising from environmental shifts. For instance, the fact that *Aedes caspius* and *Culex quinquefasciatus* occur in varied habitats points to these species' capacity to sustain virus transmission of the West Nile Virus and Rift Valley fever, which places emphasis on public health resources. Regular surveillance measures are critical to bridging existing knowledge gaps in terms of mosquito ecology and distribution, which is essential for developing impactful interventions, as noted in Farag et al. (2021). Apart from the immediate health impact, the socio-economic consequences of vector-borne diseases are relevant, affecting productivity and healthcare spending in the affected regions. Economic costs of disease control and treatment during outbreaks can strain public health facilities that are already under-resourced. Further, climate variability and urbanization increase the transmission dynamics of VBDs by altering habitats and influencing the breeding activities of mosquitoes. The intersection of these environmental changes with the imperatives of public health requires multilateral resolution through environmental management alternatives. Resolution of the factors of vector multiplication not only allows for the prevention of epidemics but is also an investment in long-term public health readiness against new and emerging infectious diseases, thus pointing to the critical need to integrate ecological understanding in public health planning.

SUMMARY

The increasing threat of vector-borne diseases, including malaria, dengue, and filariasis, requires an immediate re-evaluation of control strategies and environmental management. The pathologies resulting from climate change and urbanization have demonstrated the inefficacy of current vector management strategies, particularly in light of emerging insecticide resistance and the worldwide spread of mosquito species. IVM, which is a composite of strategic elements, offers an attractive model for management. By incorporating advanced surveillance technology, such as using drones for mosquito population surveillance and identification of breeding sites, it is possible for stakeholders to progress in understanding disease dynamics and optimizing intervention strategies. As proposed by emerging surveillance methods, the application of a pluralistic approach is critical in minimizing the effects of these diseases while adapting to their ever-changing nature (Carrasco-Escobar et al., 2022). Moreover, the development and implementation of new suppression technologies, such as the Sterile Insect Technique (SIT) and incompatible insect techniques (IIT), have the capability to complement existing controls. These technologies, particularly in conjunction with environmental management programs, have the potential to suppress mosquitoes substantially, especially in urban environments where high population densities are at greater risk. Technological advancements cannot be overemphasized; they are one of the main factors in combating vector-borne diseases. For instance, SIT has been showing great promise in a number of pilot programs across various nations, which indicates that it can act as a very effective complementary method to the traditional approach (Dyck et al., 2020). With the use of these new technologies, health authorities can considerably enhance the effectiveness of vector control and eventually limit the social and economic consequences of these diseases. To conclude, an integrated approach that integrates environmental management, innovative surveillance, and new control technologies is needed for effective vector-borne disease prevention and control. With continued public health intervention to counteract the challenges posed by these pathogens, constant evaluation and modification will be required. Collaboration among communities, policymakers, and scientists will be vital in implementing sustainable interventions and reducing the incidence of diseases across the world. As such, action on vector-borne diseases presents itself not only as a public health necessity but also as a great challenge that transcends the various aspects of society, environmental management, and technical advancement, requiring collective action to protect vulnerable populations and enable fair global health (Carrasco-Escobar et al., 2022).

A survey of vector-borne diseases such as malaria, dengue, and filariasis reveals the widespread interlinkages between climatic conditions and transmission dynamics of the diseases. Climatic variability, temperature, and precipitation have been shown to affect vector populations and pathogen development significantly. For instance, rising temperatures can enhance mosquito breeding rates and extend transmission seasons of diseases such as malaria and dengue. This relationship underscores the pressing need for intensified surveillance and monitoring to ensure one can predict outbreaks, particularly for climate change-vulnerable zones. According to reports, the projected temperature rise poses tremendous threats, which can potentially enable the prolongation of transmission durations for various pathogens, thereby elevating the risk to such diseases for public health (IV Lănescu et al., 2023). Vector control measures remain key to averting the impacts of these diseases, necessitating integrated pest management measures incorporating environmental management. Proper control of vectors entails not just the use of insecticides but also addressing environmental factors responsible for the proliferation of vectors, such as stagnant water bodies serving as breeding sites. Interventions like environmental alteration, which are favorable to drainage and habitat manipulation, are sustainable interventions capable of significantly reducing vector populations. Furthermore, the incorporation of the involvement of the community is also paramount in such control interventions; when individuals are knowledgeable and, by extension, engage in vector control practices, the effectiveness of these interventions increases manifold. Collaboration between public health authorities and the local community can potentially lead to more sustainable countermeasures against vector-borne diseases. To counter the broader health impacts of climate change, economic investments required for the attainment of Sustainable Development Goals (SDGs) become critical. The attainment of these goals, in particular health-related goals and environmental sustainability, calls for a massive increase in public and private funding. As outlined, an additional estimated 3.8 percent of global GDP will be needed by 2030 to tackle these problems competitively, a significant monetary investment in mitigating the health impacts of climate change. Countries, especially low- and developing nations, can expect to bear higher costs disproportionately on their economic sustainability and public health infrastructure (Aggarwal, 2024). Thus, an environmental management and forward-looking monitoring strategic emphasis can maximize resilience in the face of climate uncertainty against the impending vector-borne disease threats.

REFERENCES

1. Adams, E. R., Bockarie, M. J., Coleman, M., et al. (2015). Fit for purpose: Do we have the right tools to sustain NTD elimination? https://core.ac.uk/download/42615905.pdf (accessed on 11th June 2025).
2. Adams, E. R., Bockarie, M. J., Harrison, R. A., et al. (2015). Mass drug administration and beyond: How can we strengthen health systems to deliver complex interventions to eliminate neglected tropical diseases? https://core.ac.uk/download/77019011.pdf (accessed on 11th June 2025).
3. Aggarwal, R. (2024). Accounting for climate risks in costing the Sustainable Development Goals. IMF Working Paper, 2024, 1–1. https://doi.org/10.5089/9798400264061.001 (accessed on 11th June 2025).
4. Alma, A., Balloi, A., Bandi, C., et al. (2011). Microbial symbionts: A resource for the management of insect-related problems. https://core.ac.uk/download/55756107.pdf (accessed on 11th June 2025).
5. Alqassim, A. Y. (2024). Social, behavioral and environmental determinants of vector-borne diseases: A narrative review of evidence and implications for integrated control approaches. *Journal of Vector Borne Diseases*. https://www.semanticscholar.org/paper/d8f50aed505c259112f5ac356045670a7b89fbfa (accessed on 11th June 2025).
6. Ansumana, R., Hodges, M. H., Jones, R. T., et al. (2023). *The Threat of Vector-Borne Diseases in Sierra Leone*. https://core.ac.uk/download/595481449.pdf (accessed on 11th June 2025).
7. Batiha, G. E. S., Alqahtani, A., Ilesanmi, O. B., Saati, A. A., El-Mleeh, A., Hetta, H. F., & Beshbishy, A. M. (2020). Avermectin derivatives, pharmacokinetics, therapeutic and toxic dosages, mechanism of action, and their biological effects. *Pharmaceuticals, 13*, 196–196. https://doi.org/10.3390/ph13080196 (accessed on 11th June 2025).
8. Belous, M., Amfim, A., & Simion, V. (2023). Food defense, food safety and food industry. *Scientific Papers Journal Veterinary Series, 66*, 44–47. https://doi.org/10.61900/spjvs.2023.03.08 (accessed on 11th June 2025).
9. Bradbury, R. S. (2020). Parasites, Zoonoses and War. MDPI eBooks. https://doi.org/10.3390/books978-3-03936-632-3 (accessed on 11th June 2025).
10. Brown, R., Ferguson, H. M., Fornace, K., Hing, et al. (2018). Evaluation of resting traps to examine the behavior and ecology of mosquito vectors in an area of rapidly changing land use in Sabah, Malaysian Borneo. https://core.ac.uk/download/159067407.pdf (accessed on 11th June 2025).
11. Carrasco-Escobar, G., Moreno, M., Fornace, K., Herrera-Varela, M., Manrique, E., & Conn, J. E. (2022). The use of drones for mosquito surveillance and control. *Parasites & Vectors, 15*. https://doi.org/10.1186/s13071-022-05580-5 (accessed on 11th June 2025).
12. Dahmana, H., & Mediannikov, O. (2020). Mosquito-borne diseases emergence/resurgence and how to effectively control it biologically. *Pathogens, 9*, 310–310. https://doi.org/10.3390/pathogens9040310 (accessed on 11th June 2025).
13. Danso-Appiah, A., Utarini, A., Crampin, A. C., Pond, B., Paul, B. D., Babu, B. V., Braga, C., et al. (2009). *Social Research on Neglected Diseases of Poverty: Continuing and Emerging Themes*. https://core.ac.uk/download/338058.pdf (accessed on 11th June 2025).

14. Dyck, V. A., Hendrichs, J., & Robinson, A. S. (2020). Sterile Insect Technique. CRC Press eBooks. https://doi.org/10.1201/9781003035572 (accessed on 11th June 2025).

15. Eassa, S., & Abd El-Wahab, E. A. (2022). Vector-borne diseases in Egypt: Present status and accelerating toward elimination. Journal of Vector Borne Diseases, 59, 127–138. https://www.semanticscholar.org/paper/9af5e0f38b09c56d420c097f63ad1ec2601a8766 (accessed on 11th June 2025).

16. Eder, M., Cortés, F., de Siqueira Filha, N. T., de França, G. V. A., Degroote, S., Braga, C., Ridde, V., et al. (2018). Scoping review on vector-borne diseases in urban areas: Transmission dynamics, vectorial capacity and co-infection. *Infectious Diseases of Poverty, 7*. https://doi.org/10.1186/s40249-018-0475-7 (accessed on 11th June 2025).

17. Ellwanger, J. H., da Veiga, A. B. G., Kaminski, V. de L., Valverde-Villegas, J. M., de Freitas, A. W. Q., & Chies, J. A. B. (2021). Control and prevention of infectious diseases from a One Health perspective. *Genetics and Molecular Biology, 44*. https://doi.org/10.1590/1678-4685-gmb-2020-0256 (accessed on 11th June 2025).

18. Farag, E., Bansal, D., Mardini, K., Sultan, A., Al-Thani, M., Al-Marri, S., Al-Hajri, M., et al. (2021). Identification and characterization of mosquitoes from different locations in Qatar in 2017–2019. *Parasite, 28*. https://www.semanticscholar.org/paper/9655f276c2f83671231e4884bb79de15043438e0 (accessed on 11th June 2025).

19. Haldane, V., Chuah, F. L. H., Srivastava, A., Singh, S., Koh, G. C. H., Seng, C. K., & Legido-Quigley, H. (2019). Community participation in health services development, implementation, and evaluation: A systematic review of empowerment, health, community, and process outcomes. PLoS ONE, 14, e0216112–e0216112. https://doi.org/10.1371/journal.pone.0216112 (accessed on 11th June 2025).

20. Islam, J., Asif, M., Rahman, S., & Hasan, M. (2024). Exploring mosquito hazards in Bangladesh: Challenges and sustainable solutions. *IUBAT Review, 7*, 1–29. https://doi.org/10.3329/iubatr.v7i2.78792 (accessed on 11th June 2025).

21. Kittichai, V., Kaewthamasorn, M., Samung, Y., Jomtarak, R., Naing, K. M., Tongloy, T., Chuwongin, S., et al. (2023). Automatic identification of medically important mosquitoes using embedded learning approach-based image-retrieval system. Scientific Reports, 13. https://www.semanticscholar.org/paper/a4054c4097a144eb5816e16b90a6ec76c3a70406 (accessed on 11th June 2025).

22. Mabhala, M., Massey, A., Reid, J., et al. (2020). *Mind Your Language: Discursive Practices Produce Unequal Power and Control Over Infectious Disease: A Critical Discourse Analysis*. https://core.ac.uk/download/288345632.pdf (accessed on 11th June 2025).

23. Maquart, P. O., Froehlich, Y., & Boyer, S. (2022). Plastic pollution and infectious diseases. The Lancet Planetary Health, 6, e842–e845. https://doi.org/10.1016/s2542-5196(22)00198-x (accessed on 11th June 2025).

24. Masimalai, P. (2024). Vector borne disease ecology and environment: Remote sensing and GIS for control and management: A systematic review. Journal of Geography, Environment and Earth Science International. https://www.semanticscholar.org/paper/db32a1ad67a67994a47041789c5627c6bf9750f5 (accessed on 11th June 2025).

25. Montenegro-Quiñonez, C. A., Runge-Ranzinger, S., Rahman, K. M., & Horstick, O. (2021). Effectiveness of vector control methods for the control of cutaneous and visceral leishmaniasis:

A meta-review. *PLoS Neglected Tropical Diseases, 15*, e0009309–e0009309. https://doi.org/10.1371/journal.pntd.0009309 (accessed on 11th June 2025).

26. Namias, A., Jobe, N. B., Paaijmans, K. P., & Huijben, S. (2021). The need for practical insecticide-resistance guidelines to effectively inform mosquito-borne disease control programs. *eLife, 10*. https://doi.org/10.7554/elife.65655 (accessed on 11th June 2025).
27. Okumu, F., Moore, S. J., Selvaraj, P., Yafin, A. H., Juma, E. O., Shirima, G. S. G., Majambere, S., et al. (2025). Elevating larval source management as a key strategy for controlling malaria and other vector-borne diseases in Africa. *Parasites & Vectors, 18*. https://www.semanticscholar.org/paper/eb66ab9a57339c3cf7d59a14bd3571797dcc2f4b (accessed on 11th June 2025).
28. Ortega, L. (2014). World Health Day 2014: An opportunity to promote research on vectors & vector-borne diseases. *The Indian Journal of Medical Research, 139*, 481–483. https://www.semanticscholar.org/paper/a9d3b24deccc12d860b1ed32dfcdd385b7b1fac2 (accessed on 11th June 2025).
29. Perrin, A., Glaizot, O., & Christe, P. (2022). Worldwide impacts of landscape enthronization on mosquito abundance and diversity: A meta-analysis. *Global Change Biology, 28*, 6857–6871. https://doi.org/10.1111/gcb.16406 (accessed on 11th June 2025).
30. Pitt, S., & Gunn, A. (2024). The One Health concept. British Journal of Biomedical Science, 81. https://doi.org/10.3389/bjbs.2024.12366 (accessed on 11th June 2025).
31. Puerta-Guardo, H., Manrique-Saide, P., Ayoade, F., Ogunbiyi, T., Baig, A. Z., Aslam, H., Zafar, A., et al. (2022). *Mosquito Research–Recent Advances in Pathogen Interactions, Immunity, and Vector Control Strategies*. IntechOpen eBooks. https://doi.org/10.5772/intechopen.98177 (accessed on 11th June 2025).
32. Raimi, M. O., Odubo, T. V., & Omidiji, A. O. (2021). Creating the healthiest nation: Climate change and environmental health impacts in Nigeria: A narrative review. *Sustainability in Environment, 6*, 61–61. https://doi.org/10.22158/se.v6n1p61 (accessed on 11th June 2025).
33. Rohr, J. R., Barrett, C. B., Civitello, D. J., Craft, M. E., Delius, B. K., De Leo, G. A., Hudson, P. J., et al. (2019). Emerging human infectious diseases and the links to global food production. *Nature Sustainability, 2*, 445–456. https://doi.org/10.1038/s41893-019-0293-3 (accessed on 11th June 2025).
34. Tami, A., Harisi, A., Qadri, M. A., Abdu, A. B., Gaissi, H., Ahmed, K., Salami, E., et al. (2024). Epidemiology in action: Strategies for controlling vector-borne diseases. *Power System Technology*. https://www.semanticscholar.org/paper/7bf69fa43a9b3f18a97f226d9fca96b274630f1d (accessed on 11th June 2025).
35. Tangena, J. A., & Akiko. (2016). The Risk of Vector-Borne Disease Exposure in Rubber Plantations of Northern Lao PDR. https://core.ac.uk/download/76946368.pdf (accessed on 11th June 2025).
36. van den Berg, H., Bashar, K., Chowdhury, R., Bhatt, R. M., Gupta, H. P., Kumar, A., Sabesan, S., et al. (2024). Perceived needs of disease vector control programs: A review and synthesis of (sub)national assessments from South Asia and the Middle East. *PLoS Neglected Tropical Diseases, 18*, e0011451–e0011451. https://doi.org/10.1371/journal.pntd.0011451 (accessed on 11th June 2025).

37. Vilà, M., Dunn, A. M., Essl, F., Gómez-Díaz, E., Hulme, P. E., Jeschke, J. M., Núñez, M. A., et al. (2021). Viewing emerging human infectious epidemics through the lens of invasion biology. *BioScience, 71*, 722–740. https://doi.org/10.1093/biosci/biab047 (accessed on 11th June 2025).

38. Wilson, A. L. (2017). Integrated Vector Management–Generation and Use of Evidence for More Effective Vector Control. https://core.ac.uk/download/82918290.pdf (accessed on 11th June 2025).

39. Wilson, A. L., Courtenay, O., Kelly-Hope, L. A., Scott, T. W., Takken, W., Torr, S. J., & Lindsay, S. W. (2020). The importance of vector control for the control and elimination of vector-borne diseases. *PLoS Neglected Tropical Diseases, 14*, e0007831–e0007831. https://doi.org/10.1371/journal.pntd.0007831 (accessed on 11th June 2025).

40. Wolf, J., Johnston, R. B., Ambelu, A., Arnold, B. F., Bain, R., Bräuer, M., Brown, J., et al. (2023). Burden of disease attributable to unsafe drinking water, sanitation, and hygiene in domestic settings: A global analysis for selected adverse health outcomes. *The Lancet, 401*, 2060–2071. https://doi.org/10.1016/s0140-6736(23)00458-0 (accessed on 11th June 2025).

41. Zavaleta-Monestel, E., Rojas-Chinchilla, C., Molina-Sojo, P., Murillo-Castro, M. F., Rojas-Molina, J. P., & Martínez-Vargas, E. (2025). Impact of climate change on the global dynamics of vector-borne infectious diseases: A narrative review. *Cureus, 17*. https://www.semanticscholar.org/paper/36d78f4c4d2f8bc57e91de3c6bd9ad46413c2841 (accessed on 11th June 2025).

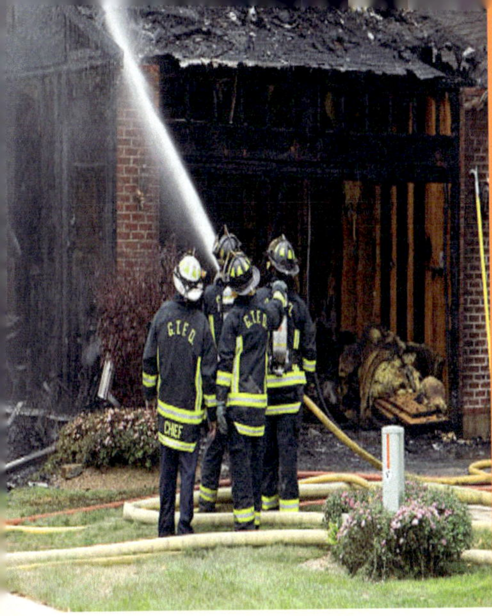

Chapter 12

DISASTER MANAGEMENT AND EMERGENCY RESPONSE

Contents

Introduction

The significance of response to emergencies and disaster management cannot be overemphasized in today's increasingly complicated world, where communities worldwide are threatened by both natural and anthropogenic disasters. Disasters can have the potential to disintegrate the social fabric, leading to loss of lives, economic collapse, and mass devastation of infrastructure. Effective planning and response measures are necessary in mitigating the impacts of such occurrences. The theory of disaster management involves a systematic strategy geared towards tackling the intricacies involved in such occurrences. Through the use of several strategies, such as risk assessment and planning, communities have been able to increase their resilience while boosting recovery. As noted in previous works, an understanding of critical terminologies involved with disasters as well as their management provides the foundation for successful action. The first step towards this endeavor is understanding how disasters happen and thus making it necessary to thoroughly examine both natural and man-made events (Khan et al., 2008). In disaster management, disasters have to be classified into certain categories, where mostly natural and man-made events are of primary concern. Natural disasters, like floods, earthquakes, and hurricanes, are caused by environmental forces and are a direct threat to public safety and health. On the other hand, man-made disasters, like terrorist attacks and industrial accidents, are caused by either single or group human actions leading to disastrous effects. The identification of these types allows for the establishment of precise response systems that cater to the unique nature of each category of disaster. For example, the equipment and training one would need to address a natural disaster would be considerably different from that required to address an artificial crisis. Preparation, response, and recovery systems uniquely adapted to the particularity of such disasters are emphasized in literature, thereby enhancing overall community resilience (Khan et al., 2008). The development of integrated disaster management approaches is imperative not merely for short-term response but also for long-term post-disaster environmental rehabilitation. After the frenzy has passed, recovery must focus on restoring the devastated areas, with attention to public health as well as ecological sustainability. Successful rehabilitation includes an evaluation of the environmental consequences of disasters and actions to restore human well-being along with ecological equilibrium. By integrating public health interventions into disaster management plans, the stakeholders can deploy an integrated response covering the health needs of affected populations and environmental needs in a single intervention. Finally, through such simultaneous consideration, community resilience is promoted through a sustainable recovery system that minimizes future risks and promotes a safer, healthier environment (Khan et al., 2008) (Figure 12.1).

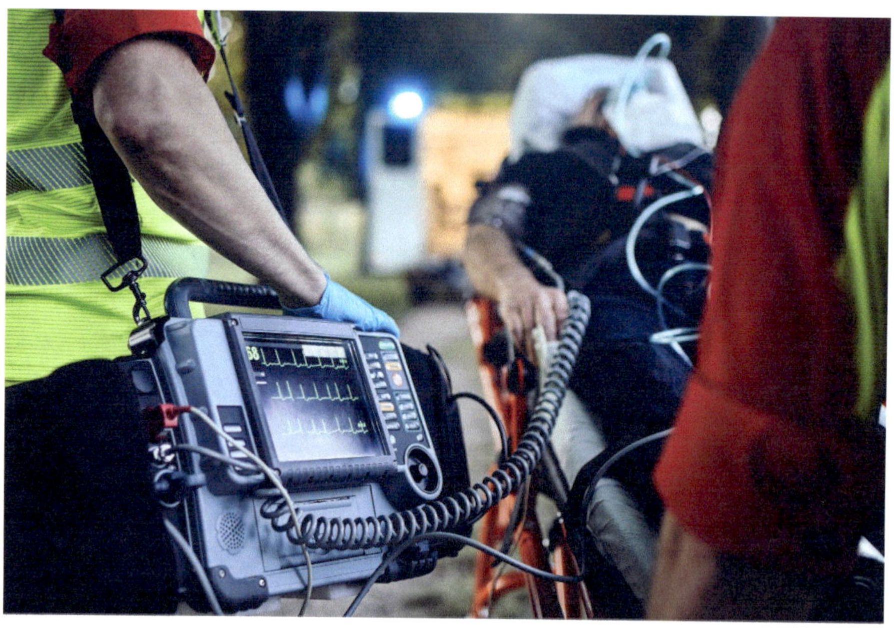

Figure 12.1. Emergency medical responders using a defibrillator on a patient during pre-hospital care.

Source: https://www.facs.org/media/3izlctdp/1177618871.jpg?rnd=132954449329670000.

Definition of Disaster Management

Disaster management is a comprehensive process that includes policies, procedures, and practices to minimize the impacts of disasters and enable a resilient recovery. It is a multi-disciplinary practice across various fields such as emergency response, public health, urban planning, and environmental sciences. Disaster management begins with being prepared, that is, developing plans and preparing individuals in advance so that they can respond well to an unexpected event. Preparation activities also involve public campaigns that inform communities about potential threats and promote self-reliance during emergencies, ultimately developing a culture of resilience. As witnessed in the past, such as the destructive December 2004 tsunami that struck Sri Lanka, effective management steps are centrally responsible for minimizing fatalities and economic loss, which would normally be aggravated by inadequate infrastructure and planning in affected areas (Amaratunga et al., 2006). Phases in disaster management can be divided into four steps: mitigation, preparedness, response, and recovery. Mitigation measures act like they are preventing a disaster or reducing the impact, such as applying building codes to flood-prone areas or restoring ecosystems that can absorb excess water. Preparation is achieved by formulating contingency plans and practice drills to make communities ready to respond. Under the response phase, immediate actions such as search and rescue operations, as well as medical care, are of top priority. Thus, efficient coordination of manpower and resources is essential to response operations. Rehabilitation after disasters focuses on the rebuilding of infrastructure and relief to affected communities in the reconstruction process. Initiatives, such as the Flood Early Warning System launched in Semarang, illustrate the capacity of preventive measures to reduce disaster risk, emphasizing the involvement of community participation in disaster management (Hidayati et al., 2015). One of the most vital aspects of disaster management is interagency cooperation between government, non-governmental organizations, and local communities. Such cooperation optimizes the effectiveness of disaster preparation and response through shared resource pooling, information sharing, and capacity building. Community engagement in disaster management fosters local ownership of risk reduction activities and ensures cultural sensitivity and specificity of the response. Notably, public health is the core of disaster management, in that it ensures the health requirements of the affected population are addressed and outbreaks of diseases are prevented after the occurrence of disasters. Priority given to public health enables communities to safeguard the vulnerable and expedite recovery. Ideally, disaster management must be driven by a unifying understanding of risk, a preparedness culture, and an integrated approach for coping and responding to both man-made and natural disasters.

Importance of Emergency Response

The importance of emergency response cannot be overstated, especially in the context of disaster management. Natural or man-made emergencies can have the ability to cause widespread disruption, impacting health, security, and the availability of essential resources. As witnessed in public health preparedness literature, the magnitude of human distress caused by disasters warrants an effective emergency response system. Such a framework enables communities to act quickly and efficiently, thereby minimizing the adverse effects of emergencies. Public health preparedness enhances societies' ability to resist such adversity more effectively, making them more resilient as well as reducing vulnerabilities. Response measures that emphasize coordination among sectors are crucial in maintaining order and providing quick response, which ultimately enhances the overall capability of a community in handling effectively the effects of a disaster (Gligorov et al., 2008). Along with this, the creation of systematic capacities, such as emergency plans and trained personnel, is also crucial for effective emergency response. The legal institution, coordinating mechanisms, and institutions give a formal structure to addressing emergencies. Public awareness and participation are also very important as they allow communities to recognize threats and take measures for preparedness. According to Gligorov et al. (2008), emergency preparedness demands long-term commitments that allow resilience through training and education programs. This anticipatory approach not only allows for instant restoration but also establishes a safety culture that can anticipate future risks. A good emergency response not only meets urgent demands but also sets the foundation for future resilience and long-term recovery against potential disasters.

Finally, the evaluation and enhancement of emergency response plans following each occurrence are essential in ensuring lessons learned impact future preparation. The preparedness and response continuum stresses constant improvement. Evaluation of community response helps identify gaps in available plans and integration of effective strategies that were successful in past emergencies. This cycle contributes to the development of a culture of safety and resilience because communities learn from past experiences and act on them. Ongoing development of risk assessment methods is of high importance in providing feedback on better emergency response models to enable communities to adapt to ever-changing disaster landscapes. Thus, the integration of serious evaluation in disaster management is in concordance with the overall objective of mitigating the impacts of disasters and strengthening communities for better responding to future emergencies (Gligorov et al., 2008) (Figure 12.2).

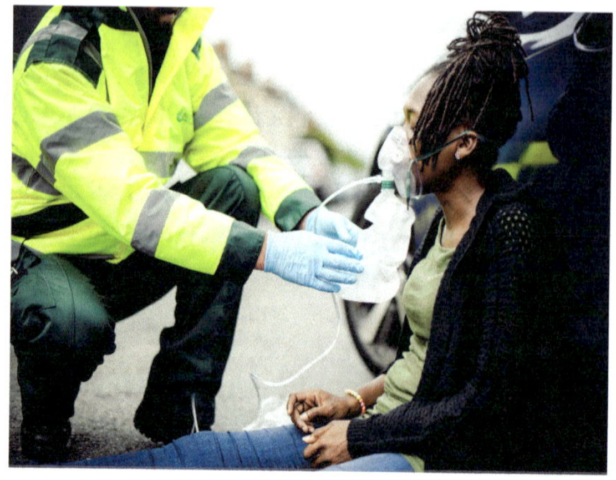

Figure 12.2. First responder administering oxygen to a patient at the scene of an emergency.

Source: https://affinityrescue.co.za/wp-content/uploads/2024/01/repsonse.png.

12.1. Types of Disasters

Disasters can be broadly categorized into natural and man-made disasters, each with different features and consequences. Natural disasters are phenomena such as earthquakes, hurricanes, floods, and forest fires, which are primarily caused by natural processes of the Earth. They have the propensity to produce high levels of loss of life, destruction of infrastructure, and long-term socio-economic disruption. Specific regions may face vulnerabilities due to geographical and climatic factors, thus being susceptible to specific types of natural disasters. Coastal areas, for instance, are susceptible to events like hurricanes and storm surges, requiring special disaster preparedness and mitigation strategies. Understanding the variety of natural disasters, patterns, and occurrences is crucial to effective disaster management, providing readiness measures and population resilience at both local and national levels, as explained in some literature on disaster management (Khan et al., 2008). Conversely, man-made disasters are largely caused by human initiative and may include industrial accidents, chemical spills, and terrorism. Such disasters may occur due to negligence, inadequate regulation, or sudden failure of systems, which frequently result in instantaneous and direct risks to the health of populations. The consequences of man-made disasters go beyond the direct physical impact; they have the potential to trigger environmental degradation, financial disruption, and long-term psychological trauma among those communities affected. Furthermore, uncertainties in human behavior may pose an increased threat of man-made disasters, leading to difficulties in making effective emergency response efforts. It is extremely important to have an intimate understanding of these disasters to enhance risk management systems and implement preventive practices that minimize the frequency and magnitude of such disasters, as emphasized in disaster management literature (Khan et al., 2008). Finally, response to disasters—natural or human-made—needs effective coordination among public health preparedness, emergency response mechanisms, and environmental recovery interventions. Public health interventions remain particularly timely in the event of disaster because they help address immediate health needs, prevent outbreaks of disease, and enhance recovery of populations. Effective disaster management policies incorporate risk analysis, emergency response, and long-term recovery strategies to promote resilience among affected populations. Further, incorporating environmental rehabilitation into such policies is critical for the recovery of ecosystems in rebounding and mitigating future exposures. This multi-faceted strategy not only caters to the immediate needs of the communities but also encourages environmental restoration and sustainable development. Balancing these various sides as a part of national disaster management systems is necessary to effectively implement disaster mitigation measures, as explained in comprehensive research on the subject (Khan et al., 2008) (Figure 12.3).

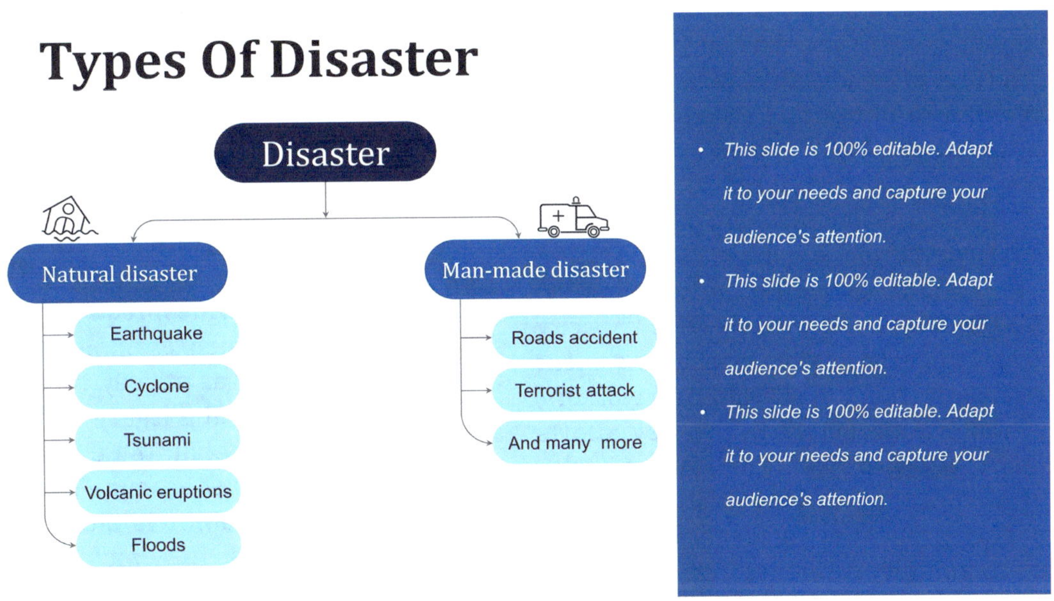

Figure 12.3. Types of disasters.

Source: https://www.slideteam.net/media/catalog/product/cache/1280x720/d/i/disaster_management_powerpoint_presentation_slides_Slide07.jpg.

12.1.1. Natural Disasters

Natural disasters are calamitous events caused by the natural processes of the planet Earth and tend to be devastating in their effect on society and the environment. They include earthquakes, floods, hurricanes, droughts, and volcanic eruptions, all varying in magnitude and effect. Death, property, and livelihood loss are typically the aftermath of such disasters, leading to the necessity for an effective disaster management system. A comprehension of the complex relationships between hazards, vulnerability, and capacity is crucial for the effective response to disasters. The disaster management cycle enables such understanding through preparedness, response, recovery, and mitigation, which are aimed at minimizing overall risk and maximizing resilience in affected communities. Strategies must be appropriate for the most prevalent types of disasters in a specific location, as has been identified by the discussion of several types of disasters and their management systems in Pakistan (Khan et al., 2008). Natural disaster public health response is also critical in preventing secondary effects that may occur later. Health crises usually follow disasters due to disturbances in healthcare services, potential epidemics, and psychological or mental issues for survivors. Preparation needs to include not only initial medical response capacity but also long-term capacity for recovery of the health system. Enhancement of infrastructure, training of healthcare workers, and communication networks are key efforts to be improved. Apart from that, public health campaigns educating communities about risk factors and preventive measures can help enhance community resilience. Effective use of these interventions can significantly minimize the impact on human health and improve overall rehabilitation measures following the disaster (Khan et al, 2008). Rehabilitation of the environment following a disaster is a significant component of sustainable disaster management. The environmental impact of natural disasters, such as soil erosion, deforestation, and water contamination, has lasting effects that need to be met with combined rehabilitation initiatives. The restoration programs normally include reforestation, riverbank protection, and soil purification, which, besides rehabilitating the environment, also enhance community resilience against future occurrences. Engaging local people in rehabilitation interventions strengthens ownership and responsibility, fostering sustainable actions toward the reduction of vulnerability. Moreover, the integration of environmental factors into disaster policy guarantees that recovery will neither contribute to existing vulnerabilities nor create new risks. This holistic approach is essential for strengthening both ecological health and well-being for affected individuals after natural disasters (Khan et al., 2008).

12.1.2. Man-Made Disasters

Man-made disasters are a main type of catastrophes that occur due to human actions or inactions. Some examples of man-made disasters are industrial accidents, oil spills, nuclear meltdowns, and terrorist attacks, among others. The impact of man-made disasters usually goes far beyond the direct physical destruction, causing long-term public health emergencies and widespread environmental destruction. One such example that leaps to mind is the Bhopal gas tragedy, causing not only immediate deaths but a legacy of health issues for survivors. To explain the dynamics behind such events, one must examine underlying risk factors and vulnerabilities along with socio-economic contexts in which they happen. Effective disaster management systems must put these in top priority on their strategies to minimize the impact of future disasters and possess a comprehensive response to human-made crises (Khan et al., 2008). The response to human-made disasters is multifaceted, including coordinated efforts from government agencies, NGOs, and local communities. Initial response has typically been response to search and rescue operations, medical care, and shelter provision for the victims. Yet, the character of these disasters requires a correspondingly complex response strategy that entails consideration of each disaster's singular challenges. Nuclear incidents, for example, require specialized protocols for handling radioactive byproducts and ensuring public health. The crafting of these response plans has largely consisted of strict training as well as simulation to prepare responders for surprise complications. Besides, preparation at the community level is also crucial as it prepares locals to be responsible for their safety and resilience after man-made disasters (Khan et al., 2008). Rehabilitation after a disaster is crucial in rebuilding from man-made disasters and rebuilding damaged communities. Rehabilitation typically involves taking care of the physical and psychological well-being of survivors as well as rebuilding infrastructure, economic balance, and the environment.

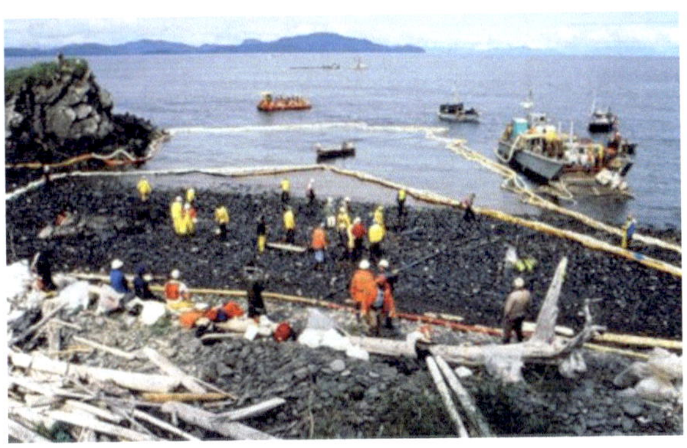

Figure 12.4. Guide helps communities facing man-made disasters.

Source: https://i0.wp.com/alaskaseagrant.org/wp-content/uploads/2019/11/Oil-Spill-image-.jpg?resize=438%2C269&ssl=1.

After incidents like the Deepwater Horizon spill, wide-ranging community engagement is crucial to restore confidence and make recovery programs culturally appropriate and equitable. Rehabilitation is also enhanced by lessons learned for improving future readiness and prevention initiatives. Local stakeholders' participation in planning can lead to more sustainable outcomes, with them holding insights into the setting and community requirements. Lastly, the creation of public health interventions, participation of the people, and ecological restoration form the foundation for effective disaster management for man-made disasters (Khan et al., 2008) (Figure 12.4).

12.1.3. Comparison Between Natural and Man-Made Disasters

The impacts of man-made and natural disasters pose essential challenges to disaster management and emergency response systems globally. Natural disasters, such as hurricanes, earthquakes, and droughts, are the result of geological and environmental factors. Their unpredictability and extensive implications have a tendency to surpass existing preparedness measures, significantly affecting public safety and health. Man-made disasters caused by industrial accidents, terrorism, and pollution are the result of human action or inaction. Such catastrophes often result from system failures such as inadequate regulatory practices and a lack of emergency protocols. Both types require specialized approaches, yet the inherent similarities between vulnerability research and resource allocation mean that the two must be contrasted. Awareness of these contrasts enables policymakers to craft improved responses that take into account each type's unique challenges. Social and health consequences of natural and human-induced disasters call for an empowered and resilient public health infrastructure. Natural disasters have the immediate impact of injuries, displacement, and worsening of underlying medical conditions, which are supplemented by climatic impacts increasing the frequency of the type of disasters due to climate change. For instance, as has been debated in The Climate Change Starter's Guide, climate catastrophes must be tackled immediately through policy change and education to reduce their impact and prepare populations for future events (Deeb et al., 2011). Alternatively, man-made disasters can cause long-term public health crises founded upon pollution and trauma. The public health reaction must not only attend to short-term medical needs but reach further to longer-term recovery and rehabilitation, emphasizing prevention approaches that build on lessons from past events and the unique socio-economic conditions of impacted communities. Lastly, restoration and rehabilitation of the environment following both disasters are contingent upon sound management protocols that address post-disaster complexity. Disaster Management strategies unveil critical knowledge of the recovery process, calling for improved data utilization and information management in a bid to maximize prediction and response activities (N/A, 2021). Integrating risk reduction activities and sustainable practices into the recovery process is crucial, particularly as societies rebuild and redefine their relationship with their environment. This overlap between recovery and management emphasizes the importance of learning from man-made and natural disasters alike in establishing a more resilient structure. In the end, this general understanding is what informs disaster readiness programs that address not just immediate impact but also establish long-term viability and community resilience.

12.2. Causes and Impacts of Natural Disasters

Natural disasters are the outcome of a complex interaction of human and environmental processes, with climate change heightening their frequency and severity. Events such as hurricanes, floods, and wildfires are classic demonstrations of such an interplay, since rising global temperatures induce weather patterns to change and extreme weather conditions to be more prevalent. Further, bad land management and urbanization exacerbate vulnerabilities by placing people in harm's way, especially in developing countries where socio-economic inequalities are pronounced. The effects of such disasters are staggering, covering more than the immediate physical surroundings to social infrastructures and economic stability. Indications reveal that disasters have resulted in over 700,000 fatalities and displaced approximately 23 million individuals; figures such as these put a mark of urgency on anticipatory interventions in disaster risk reduction (N/A, 2018). Furthermore, the impacts of natural disasters extend beyond outright casualties and displacements; they disrupt important systems and services that sustain communities. The financial cost is astronomical, totaling more than $1.3 trillion in recent decades, hindering development progress and exacerbating poverty levels. Marginalized populations such as minorities, children, and women are typically the most affected, at greater risk of such effects as additional complications to health, as well as loss of livelihoods. The disaster risk is further exacerbated by underlying inequalities and drivers such as climate change and urbanization. Various government responses have inadequately managed these intricacies, leading to conditions for the repeat occurrence of disasters rather than preventing them. It is thus required to enhance disaster management steps to resist socio-economic disparities and establish resilience among impacted individuals (N/A, 2018). Adaptation interventions against climate change impacts in urban areas have a tendency to increase inequalities unintentionally. Interventions that prioritize elite groups can lead to the displacement of poor groups by acts of commission, where interventions harm disadvantaged groups. Acts of omission happen when adaptation measures fail to address the requirements of the poor in cities, furthering socio-spatial injustices. Good urban planning must thus prioritize inclusivity, where interventions not only address direct hazards but also enhance the resilience of all members of the community. This calls for a collaborative approach by governments, civil society, and the private sector to create equitable disaster management systems. Finally, equitable policies and practices are crucial to safeguard the interests of the poor and ensure sustainable rehabilitation and recovery following disasters (Figure 12.5).

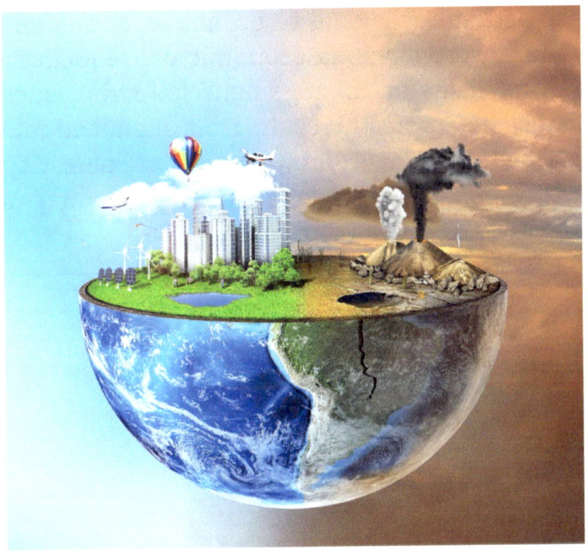

Figure 12.5. A guide to natural disasters: causes, effects & types.

Source: https://images.squarespace-cdn.com/content/v1/64de378da37fe628e3bf97e5/a6aeff48-d23d-4420-9359-c23b68312588/a-guide-to-natural-disasters-causes-effects-type.jpg.

12.2.1. Geological Factors (Earthquakes, Volcanoes)

The geological origins of natural disasters, specifically earthquakes and volcanoes, present special difficulties to disaster management and emergency response planning. Earthquakes, typically resulting from tectonic activity, are catastrophic in high-density urban settlements, resulting in mortality and extensive disruption of physical infrastructure. Urban areas like those in South Asia, with rapid urbanization, are especially vulnerable. This is further aggravated by the complex urban infrastructure and increasing population densities, which make them increasingly vulnerable to the impacts of such geological hazards. For these risks to be managed, they require top-level disaster risk reduction measures, which necessitate that disaster management strategies take cognizance of the multidimensionality of geological hazards and their potential cascading effects (Marta et al., 2022). Volcanic eruptions, although less frequent than earthquakes, are sudden hazards with a greater probability on volcanic islands of multiple hazards compounding the chance of disaster. As indicated in recent research, volcanic islands are particularly susceptible to multi-hazard conditions with simultaneous earthquakes, tsunamis, and ashfall that overwhelm emergency systems with compounded issues. The requirement for multi-hazard management is to deal with the uncertain nature of such geological conditions in an effective way. This strategic perspective not only identifies the requirement of good scientific knowledge in assessing the risk from volcanic activity but also of incorporating community involvement and social considerations in disaster management policy (Marta et al., 2022). A strategy of this kind can assist in guaranteeing well-coordinated emergency responses for the purposes of responding to actual vulnerabilities of the affected. From these geological hazards, incorporating innovative solutions becomes necessary to assist in ensuring that resilience is built in geologically disaster-affected areas. Nature-based solutions, for example, can emerge as necessary in mitigating the impacts of geological disasters. Restorative measures such as reforestation, wetland restoration, and sustainable land use reduce geological risks while also enhancing ecosystem well-being, with spillover benefits to local communities.

Examples of successful case studies of cities in South Asia also demonstrate how proactive measures and effective urban planning can enhance resilience against natural disasters. Through learning from these cases and adopting evidence-based strategies, affected regions can enhance their readiness and response capacities, eventually lending a hand towards their long-term recovery and rehabilitation of the environment (Mukherjee et al., 2022).

12.2.2. Meteorological Factors (Hurricanes, Floods)

Meteorological conditions are responsible for the incidence and intensity of natural disasters, especially hurricanes and floods. The changing climate is enhancing their frequency and intensity, as these events are being fueled by the altering climate. Hurricanes, for example, get their power from warm sea water and atmospheric conditions favorable for their formation. With increasing global warming, sea temperatures also rise, leading to intense storms that can ravage coastal regions. The effects of the disasters are not limited to physical destruction but extend to economic, social, and environmental levels. Higher storm intensity is likely to have enormous economic consequences, affecting the survival of communities and complicating disaster management following such disasters. Flooding, yet another serious meteorological disaster, typically results from sustained rain or out-of-season storms, particularly with hurricane tragedies. The combination of urbanization and inadequately planned drainage systems works to enhance the risk of flooding, leading to calamitous consequences for affected populations.

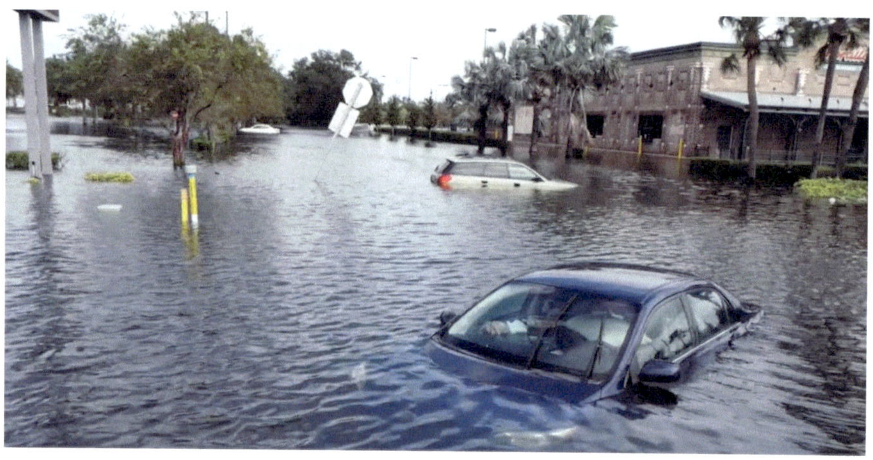

Figure 12.6. Meteorological factors (hurricanes, floods).

Source: https://images.theconversation.com/files/625063/original/file-20241011-15-kehuf3.jpg?ixlib=rb-4.1.0&rect=170%2C0%2C2824%2C1410&q=45&auto=format&w=1356&h=668&fit=crop.

Floodwaters can also be chock-full of debris and harmful chemicals, posing extremely critical public health risks such as waterborne disease, drinking water source contamination, and trauma. Also, ensuing displacement from inundated areas can strain emergency response systems and lead to long-term rehabilitation problems. With populations occupying increasingly more risk-prone areas of flooding, the intersection of urban planning and disaster risk reduction is a critical aspect of managing these risks. Effective disaster management and emergency response must be informed by a comprehensive approach to mitigating the vulnerabilities of meteorological hazards such as hurricanes and floods. The latest trends indicate that concerted efforts are needed to improve disaster preparedness and resilience in society, particularly in high-risk communities where hazard occurrence is associated with socio-economic vulnerabilities. Prevention against the consequences of hurricanes and floods requires that steps such as land use planning, infrastructure investment, and public awareness be given priority. In addition, disaster resilience policy should be taken as an integral part of strategies for poverty reduction and environmental sustainability. As the evidence confirms, investments in management as well as disaster risk reduction are especially crucial where the risk of a hazard is coupled with higher vulnerability, again to ensure a concerted strategy to public health and environmental post-disaster rehabilitation (de Haen et al., 2025; Céline, 2012) (Figure 12.6).

12.2.3. Biological Factors (Pandemics, Infestations)

Pandemics and biological infestations are critical biological factors in emergency planning and disaster management, as their impacts can ripple through societies and economies with devastating consequences. Their emergence in high-density urban environments or in the poorly equipped healthcare infrastructure can result in widespread morbidity and mortality. Historical data show that pandemics are capable of unsettling public health infrastructures, leading to strained facilities and reduced capabilities for emergency response. Public health preparedness involves crafting schemes that support quick identification, containment, and control of infectious disease outbreaks before they have a chance to build into full-scale crises. Responsive systems work when surveillance systems, community engagement, and health infrastructure make emergency response not just timely but equitable and just, as seen in past public health crises when socio-economic disparities aggravated the situation (Ishrat et al., 2024). Biological infestations like pest infestation and crop and animal disease epidemics play a significant role in food security and ecosystems, and therefore need a robust response system in disaster management. Infestations can be brought about by climatic shifts, such as increased temperatures or shifting rainfall patterns, that provide favorable environments to support invasive species. These biological forces can inflict serious economic damage on the agricultural sector, further exacerbating agriculturally dependent communities' vulnerability. In neutralizing such forces, holistic management strategies that combine sustainable agriculture and technological advances must take center stage. By education and building resilience, communities are better placed to withstand the hazards of biological infestations. Promotion of best practices, informed by research and local knowledge, can enhance the capacity to withstand such hazards and thus safeguard food security and environmental health (Li et al., 2024). The dynamic interaction between biological elements and disaster management underscores the importance of an interdisciplinary approach bridging health and environmental issues. The increasing prevalence of zoonotic diseases, which emerge from complex interactions among humans, animals, and environments, determines the necessity for understanding these biological dynamics. Effective disaster management policies must integrate ecological health into public health platforms to tackle biological disasters at a holistic level. Holistic integration can establish community resilience to potential future epidemics by addressing the causes and cross-fertilizing knowledge across effective interventions in one sector to another. Such joint effort on the part of public health officials, environmental agencies, and local communities is thus critical in the face of, and as preparation for, the dual bane of pandemics and infestations. A proactive and inclusive response is therefore critical in maintaining sustainable rehabilitation and recovery after disasters (Li et al., 2024).

12.3. Causes and Impacts of Man-Made Disasters

Disasters brought about by human activities are predominantly the result of human activities, which may range from industrial operations to willful acts of destruction. Industrial accidents, typically due to negligence or lack of safety protocols, also often lead to disasters such as chemical spills, explosions, and fires. In most cases, a lack of adequate regulation and oversight exposes these risks, allowing companies to opt for profitability over safety. Additionally, man-made disasters may result from human warfare in the form of bombings or chemical weapon deployments that indiscriminately destroy infrastructure and human life. Understanding these causes is important in the effective management of disasters since it aids in policy and strategy that not only averts but also minimizes the effects of such disasters, thus promoting public welfare and safety (Khan et al., 2008). The consequences of man-made catastrophes are cross-cutting and affect not just the immediate location where the catastrophe occurs but also broader social, economic, and environmental surroundings. Man-made disasters most often cause extensive loss of life, injury, and mental illness among the affected population. Furthermore, the economic impact can be drastic as businesses may be closed down and community facilities disrupted. This ripple effect tends to require extensive emergency efforts and long-term recovery, putting a burden on public health infrastructure and resources. The psychological impacts upon the community also tend to remain, contributing to long-term societal problems that can complicate recovery (Khan et al., 2008). Proper assessment and planning are therefore integral parts of the effective management of these disasters. Under preparedness and disaster management, an integrated approach would be necessary to address the specific issues of man-made disasters. Principal approaches would be to establish and implement strict measures of safety and training for individuals in risk-prone industries. Public campaigns also play an important role in preparation, educating people about how they must respond in the event of a disaster. In addition, coordination among government and non-government organizations can maximize mobilization of resources and accelerate response, which could entirely preclude the most devastating impacts of such disasters. These must be followed up by an effective disaster management policy that takes into account the intricate interplay between human action, environmental factors, and technological innovation, eventually building resilience in vulnerable communities (Khan et al., 2008) (Figure 12.7).

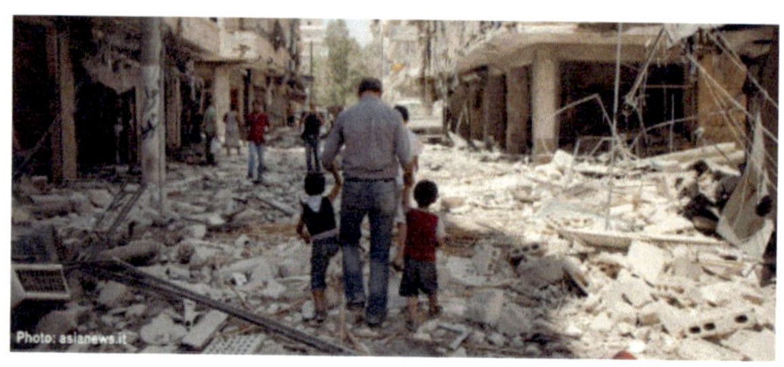

Figure 12.7. The devastating impact of man-made disasters.

Source: https://www.opusa.org/wp-content/uploads/2015/11/Wartorn_Syria_Asianewsit.jpg.

12.3.1. Industrial Accidents (Chemical Spills, Explosions)

Industrial accidents, particularly chemical spillage and explosions, are one of the main categories of man-made disasters with catastrophic consequences for both human health and the environment. They result from many factors, including bad safety management practices, human mistakes, and inadequate emergency preparedness. In the majority of cases, those facilities that handle hazardous substances and are not well-regulated are at greater risk, emphasizing the importance of effective regulatory frameworks and observance of safety standards. For example, analysis of previous incidents shows a consistent trend of correlation between failures in safety management and subsequent major accidents, as depicted in most industries. Identification of such dynamics is beneficial in the design of risk avoidance strategies that are effective in reducing the likelihood of such catastrophes, ultimately preserving community safety and environmental integrity. No effort has been more important to industrial safety than that of discovering human factors concerning industrial accidents. Research has proven that human errors, determined by organizational culture and workstation training, frequently result in incidents such as chemical spillage and explosions. Without effective training programs and a solid safety culture, workers will be unlikely to detect or respond appropriately to hazardous situations. For instance, a study examined a number of high-risk industry accident databases and found machine learning-based forecasting models to be able to predict risky actions and systemic failure in operational practices. Emphasizing the requirement for integrating superior technologies into safety management systems, this preventive measure for accident anticipation underscores the necessity for proper training. By focusing on the human element and leveraging technological advancements, the industries can create more secure environments, lowering the chances of catastrophic events and their effects on public health and safety (Nallathambi et al., 2023). Besides the direct effects, industrial accidents also have long-term effects on environmental rehabilitation and the recovery of public health. Chemical spill disasters have the potential to cause widespread contamination of air, land, and water resources, and thus require a joint response to the clean-up and restoration activities. The response tends to demand intensive responses that require more than a single agent to address immediate health conditions and restore damaged ecosystems. In addition, the growing occurrence of such disasters emphasizes the necessity of creating resilient urban infrastructures that are capable of withstanding future environmental stressors. As observed among areas experiencing climatic and urban stresses, a sustainable development strategy might be necessary in order to reduce risks brought about by industrial accidents and improve efficient recovery measures that can help make communities resilient and the environment sustainable (Emmanuel et al., 2022).

12.3.2. Terrorism and Armed Conflict

The impact of terrorism and war on disaster management is tremendous, pointing to the peculiar problems created by man-made disasters. Unlike natural disasters, which often follow a predictable pattern, terrorism and war present a complex array of challenges related to unpredictability, necessitating a special approach to emergency preparedness and response. Critical elements include the need for systematic risk analysis that quantifies various forms of violence, from conventional warfare to terrorism's asymmetrical violence. Policymakers must also prioritize making vulnerable communities resilient, as social and psychological impacts of violence are as devastating as physical destruction. Local populations must be included in planning responses, as this decreases vulnerability and boosts collective efficacy against similar attacks. Hence, understanding the nuances of man-made disasters is essential for effective disaster management systems. An all-hazards approach needs to be adopted when risk comes with terrorism and armed conflict, as with disaster management systems literature. As N/A (2022) lays down, adopting this comprehensive orientation allows one to look forward not just to deliberate acts but also to accidents and natural disasters, hence creating a resilient emergency management cycle. Each phase—prevention, preparedness, response, and recovery—must be transformed in reaction to the specific connotations of armed violence and terrorism. Preparedness, for instance, can incorporate training first responders to respond to psychological first aid to identify the emotional effects of violent attacks. Furthermore, the recovery phase demands an inclusive effort on reconstruction not only of infrastructure but also of social tissue, which is usually wrecked asunder after such traumas. Such an integrated response ensures that response operations register the whole spectrum of human and environmental resilience. The long-term effects of terrorism and war extend far beyond the immediate devastation and should be duly evaluated in disaster situations. As highlighted in Adebimpe et al. (2008), disasters, whether natural or man-made, place enormous stress on both human and physical environments, which increases vulnerability and affects overall socioeconomic stability. The convergence of public health and armed conflict is particularly dire, as attacks on civilian populations have the tendency to cause public health crises by disrupting essential services. During attempts at recovery from such activities, disaster preparedness interventions in the form of public health preparedness interventions must be part of disaster management plans so that they can prevent disease spread and promote healing within communities. Through proactive collaboration with the different effects of terrorism and conflict, structures of disaster management can promote resilience and a more comprehensive recovery process and eventually contribute to sustainable development and the maintenance of human dignity after disasters (Figure 12.8).

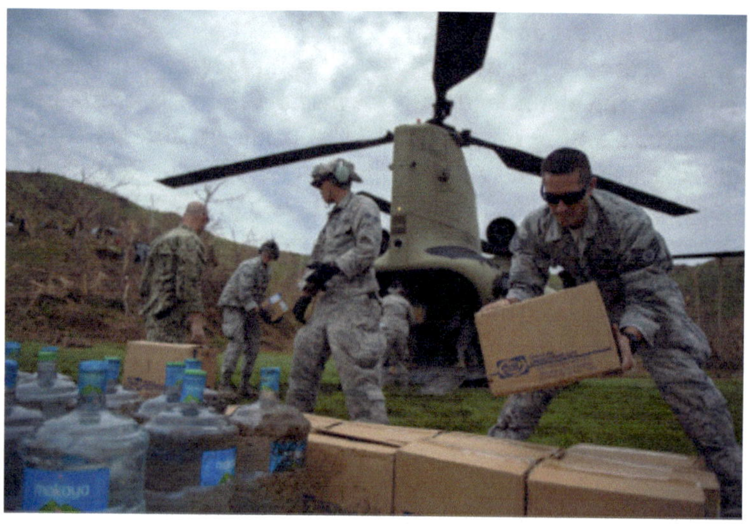

Figure 12.8. Terrorism and armed conflict in disaster management.

Source: https://external-content.duckduckgo.com/iu/?u=http%3A%2F%2Fwww.southcom.mil%2Fportals%2F7%2FImages%2FFocus% 2520Areas% 2520Module%2 FFADR%2520header% 2520pic.jpg%3Fver%3D2016-11-16-114338-427&f=1&nofb= 1&ipt= 9e88dec23eef7f 89bfa6e9fdec 366ea0a0376be096b0d8c1291442f72d655eab.

12.3.3. Environmental Degradation (Pollution, Deforestation)

Environmental degradation in the form of pollution and deforestation is a multifaceted concern intersecting deeply with disaster management and emergency response frameworks. Air and water pollution have the ability to initiate public health crises that are at times inhibiting for emergency agencies. Contaminated surroundings account for respiratory conditions, water-borne ailments, and other diseases, necessitating a structured approach with health education and infrastructural upgrading. Additionally, widespread pollution increases exposure, as poor communities tend to suffer the majority due to a lack of resources for adaptation and compensation. It is not only about short-term reaction but long-term strategies that incorporate environmental health considerations into disaster management policy, echoing ideas outlined in, say, the Climate Change Starters Guide, promoting an integrated process of learning and policy-making for environmental issues (Deeb et al., 2011). Farm expansion, urbanization, and mining result in deforestation that irreversibly alters ecosystems and raises the frequency of natural disasters like floods and landslides. As tree cover is eliminated, the soils' capacity for water retention reduces, resulting in increased runoff that may overwhelm local watersheds and create perilous conditions. The cumulative impact of deforestation makes disaster response a challenge, as governments not only have to deal with short-term emergencies but also have to invest in environmental rehabilitation efforts aimed at balancing the ecosystem. This involves reforestation and public education on sustainable use of land. As emphasized by disaster management policies, deforestation prevention is crucial not only for the environment's sustainability but also for the resilience of the communities facing the increasing occurrence of climate disasters (Khan et al., 2008). The convergence of pollution, deforestation, and disaster management points towards the need to implement an integrated strategy towards environmental recovery after a disaster. Effective policy interventions need to understand the way environmental degradation can have the ability to exacerbate the impact of natural and man-made disasters. By prioritizing learning approaches that equip communities with knowledge on sustainable practices and the importance of taking care of the environment, actors can develop the capacity to withstand impending disasters. Defined in climate change educational materials, integrated disaster preparedness must deal with the root causes of environmental degradation while, at the same time, transferring skills required by communities to restore and prosper after the occurrence of disaster events (Deeb et al., 2011).

12.4. Public Health Response to Disasters

The public health reaction to disasters is a critical component of disaster management with the general goal of mitigating the health effects of natural and man-made disasters. These reactions must be timely and well-coordinated, as they typically delineate the magnitude of morbidity and mortality following a disaster. Effective public health interventions often involve health risk surveillance, the supply of necessary medical equipment, and the mobilization of healthcare professionals into affected areas. Moreover, training programs play a pivotal role in educating communities with knowledge to engage in self-protection and self-mitigation actions. For example, there is a need for effective communication networks in order to issue early warning information regarding impending threats, e.g., disease outbreaks following floods or chemical spills. Ineffective coordination of public health reactions can both intensify exposure and cause massive loss of lives, underlining the importance of having protocols in place and pre-disaster preparedness in disaster situations (Khan et al., 2008). Preparedness is a multi-component aspect of public health reaction to disasters, including training, resource deployment, and community mobilization. Local health officials must take an active role in preparing to have staff and medical supplies on hand when a disaster does happen. This involves not just keeping reserves of appropriate medical supplies on hand, but also ongoing training exercises for health workers to keep them at a moment's notice. Community involvement is also necessary in developing good response plans, as they intimately understand their needs and issues. Community exercises, such as those for community exercises, can foster cooperation between residents and public health authorities, ensuring the efficiency of the health response during the occurrence itself. Effective preparedness ultimately serves to enhance resilience, allowing quicker recovery and minimizing long-term public health impacts that are typically associated with disasters (Khan et al., 2008). Long-term public health impacts greatly rely on what happens in the recovery phase following a disaster. Transformation from relief work to recovery involves thorough consideration of the mental and physical health implications on affected populations. Mental health treatment, indeed, comes to be the need of the hour as individuals cope with trauma resulting from the disaster. Temporary care facilities and integrating mental health treatment with primary care can facilitate complete recovery. Moreover, mitigation of the underlying social determinants of health—e.g., access to food, housing, and sanitation—is also important in building a disaster-resilient health system. Efforts have to be sustained even after the short-term needs are met so that societies may rebuild sustainably and comprehensively. By implementing a holistic recovery strategy, public health interventions can result in improved health outcomes and community resilience in the case of future disasters (Khan et al., 2008) (Figure 12.9).

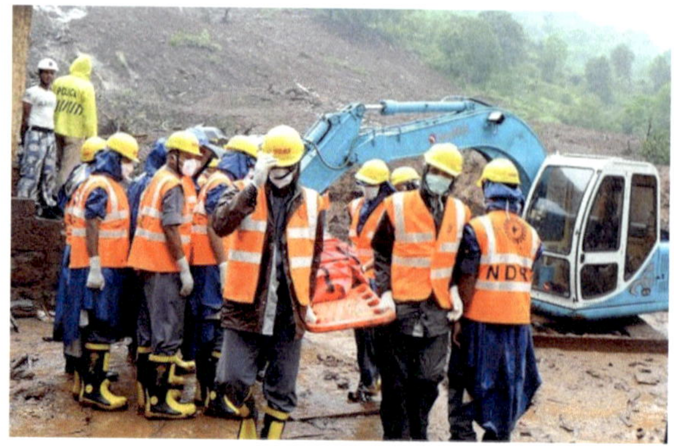

Figure 12.9. Disaster management and public health.

Source: https://aihms.in/blog/wp-content/uploads/2021/06/disaster1.jpg.

12.4.1. Immediate Health Interventions

The concept of immediate health interventions is central in disaster management because it aims to intervene not only against physical trauma but also the psychological impact of natural and man-made disasters. After a disaster, populations in disaster-stricken areas experience acute health emergencies in the form of trauma, epidemics of infectious diseases, and triggering of chronic diseases. Early intervention against these health needs has the potential to reduce both morbidity and mortality. Effective deployment of health resources, such as emergency medical units and mobile clinics, is required to deliver care on a timely basis to the most in-need individuals. And these acute interventions must consider the changing profile of health risks in post-disaster environments, especially with more frequent weather-related events happening and with the need for responsive healthcare strategies, reflecting an all-around response to disaster. Vulnerable groups such as children, the elderly, and those with underlying health issues need special care in the course of immediate health interventions. Identification of the specific health needs of such groups is essential in developing targeted responses that guarantee equal care. Mental health interventions should also be incorporated into the delivery of care in emergencies since trauma can present itself as different psychological disorders that complicate the recovery process. Interventions such as crisis counseling and psychosocial support interventions are key components of an integrated health response. Both the physical and psychological well-being are treated, and disaster management becomes more effective, and ultimately, the outcome of the recovery is better. The emphasis on vulnerability and capacity within disaster management frameworks emphasizes the need to tailor immediate health interventions based on the needs of the individual, further highlighting the importance of holistic health responses during crises (Khan et al., 2008). The guidelines in disaster management and health interventions also depend upon one another because effective health responses have a significant potential to influence the resilience of the affected population as a whole. Quick triage and assessment are necessary in determining priorities in healthcare in order for first responders to distribute resources effectively. An integrated approach to local health systems during the initial response also supports continuity of care, where interventions by health are sustainable and culturally tailored. Moreover, gathering data from health assessments helps in planning for future preparedness and resource distribution. Disaster management policy should reflect a commitment to improving the health outcomes of disaster-affected populations, guided by the evolving relationship between hazard, vulnerability, and health capacity. The presence of rapid health interventions underpins effective disaster management, which ultimately maximizes community resilience and ability to recover (Khan et al., 2008).

12.4.2. Long-Term Health Care Planning

Health care long-term planning is a critical component of emergency response and disaster management, particularly for both natural and man-made disasters. This involves the practice of maintaining health care systems in a position to withstand the impacts of emergencies while continuing to provide basic health services over a period of time. This involves readying healthcare centers not only to deal with immediate health emergencies but also with recovery efforts over the long term. As evidenced by workforce need in disaster response infrastructure, the planning requires a comprehensive evaluation of skill deficits in public health units like law enforcement and emergency services to optimize response capacity and enhance population preparedness (Fichtner et al., 2008). Building the resource base for health care strategically keeps vulnerable groups after a disaster, ultimately defining community resilience and recovery trajectories. In addition, the greatest importance is that lessons obtained from previous disasters are integrated into rational long-term planning for health care. As an illustration, lessons learned from and following such disasters as the Hull flood highlight the requirement for bottom-up public health response informed by the experiences of the affected population (Deeming et al., 2011). With an emphasis on local community involvement in planning, health care systems can more effectively match their response to the specific needs of populations during a crisis. Teamwork with government and community groups produces a more holistic, responsive health care system that adapts to evolving needs, where recovery plans not only react to crises but work proactively to avoid future risks. Lastly, one cannot stress enough the importance of sustainable infrastructure in planning health care after disasters. Investment in facilities, technology, and professional training is necessary for developing long-term capacity for health care systems that will be resilient. Incorporating environmental rehabilitation post-disaster into health care planning allows for the simultaneous development of health and environmental strategy. Since communities are confronted by an increasing incidence of disasters, proper long-term planning for health care is required not just in tackling current health emergencies but also to promote health equity and community flourishing in case of future hardship, positioning these communities for success in the context of change (Fichtner et al., 2008) (Figure 12.10).

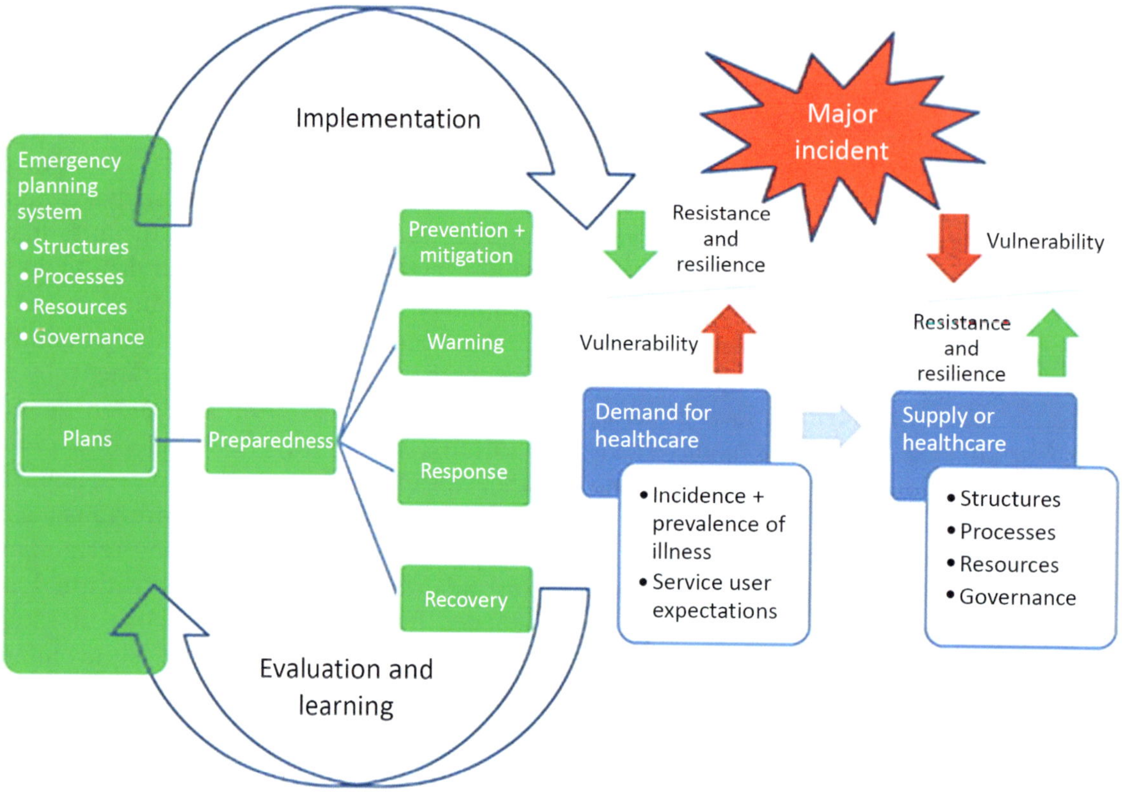

Figure 12.10. Emergency planning and management in health care.

Source: https://www.tandfonline.com/cms/asset/ad47bdca-df9c-452d-8cec-b93da5e8a22a/thss_a_11933249_f0001_ob.jpg.

12.4.3. Role of Public Health Organizations

Public health agencies play a core role in disaster management and emergency response, and they are also key organizations to respond in preparedness, response, and recovery phases. Their work begins far before an actual disaster, as they are part of the process of risk assessment, awareness at the community level, and response plan formulation. Such a forward-thinking effort is essential in mitigating vulnerabilities and enhancing the capacity of the local community to adequately respond when disasters occur. To illustrate, public health agencies participate in educating medical professionals and community volunteers so that they know what to do in the event of an emergency, thus ensuring a concerted response. As Khan et al. (2008) observe, these agencies further assist in drafting disaster management policies at the national level, which guide strategic deployment of resources in emergencies to achieve optimal public health outcomes. In the early response to disasters, public health authorities lead in responding efforts, intervening on behalf of affected populations through interventions. They are legally required to monitor and control epidemic diseases resulting from the disruption of sanitation, water supply, and health services. As evidenced by histories documented during disaster incidents, such as earthquakes or floods, earlier public health interventions can prevent morbidity and mortality rates from shooting up. Additionally, such agencies are very crucial in facilitating access to medical care, mental health care, and preventive health interventions, which allow people to recover more rapidly. Post-disaster role is in harmony with principles as defined in disaster management cycles, as discussed in Khan et al. (2008), and which demands coordinated public health responses that are adaptive to specific disaster settings. The long-term impact of disasters extends beyond medical problems in the immediate aftermath and makes the role of public health organizations central to rehabilitation efforts as well.

They play a central role in environmental rehabilitation through addressing the interdependence of the environment and human health. These include enhancing the health effects of environmental degradation due to disasters, such as contaminated water sources and toxic waste accumulation. Public health organizations usually emphasize collaborative work with government and non-government agencies to embrace sustainable practices that ensure community resilience and long-term recovery. These include expanding public consciousness regarding safe health practices and developing healthcare infrastructure to ensure continuous preparedness for potential future disasters. The prime position of public health agencies in disaster management is thus a reflection of their importance not only in rapid response but also in guaranteeing sustainable health practice for the construction of resilient communities.

12.5. Preparedness Strategies for Disasters

Successful disaster preparedness measures are essential to reduce both human and environmental losses during disasters. These measures include a variety of activities such as risk assessment, capacity building of communities, and resource mobilization. Risk assessment entails the identification of possible hazards and assessment of the vulnerability of communities to enable a prepared response to perceived threats. Community drills and training supplement public information and improve the preparedness capabilities of individuals and households, fostering a culture of preparedness. Moreover, strategic resource allocation in the form of establishing emergency commodity stockpiles and communication systems enables communities to respond rapidly and efficiently in the event of a disaster, thereby reducing the aggregate impact on public health and safety. This integrated approach is essential in building resilience as well as promoting stability in communities during many types of disasters, natural or human-induced (Khan et al., 2008). Another essential disaster readiness component is the availability of an articulated incident command system (ICS), which plays a critical role in facilitating coordinated response activities among varied agencies and organizations. The ICS stipulates roles and responsibilities to facilitate effective communication and coordination during emergencies. Emphasizing training in emergency responders, public health officials, and community leaders is necessary to educate all members of their roles in the system. Regular review and adaptation of readiness plans by simulation exercises and citizen feedback flag weaknesses and emphasize successful actions. Such well-planned systems not only enhance effectiveness at work but also enhance public trust in emergency management processes, ultimately building a resilient disaster-sustaining society (Khan et al., 2008).

Public health response strategies must be integrally woven into detailed disaster preparation plans. One of the key elements is the organization of emergency response teams that are trained to handle medical emergencies resulting from disasters, e.g., infectious disease outbreaks or injury. These are supplemented by public education efforts informing populations of health risks arising from various kinds of disasters, thus making possible anticipatory health interventions. Second, incorporating mental health interventions into disaster readiness ensures that emotional and psychological treatment will be available after the event. Attainment of both physical and psychological health needs is essential for inclusive public health disaster resilience. By prioritizing these at the center of disaster management frameworks, populations are better positioned to safeguard their healthcare systems and enhance efforts at recovery after disaster (Khan et al., 2008) (Figure 12.11).

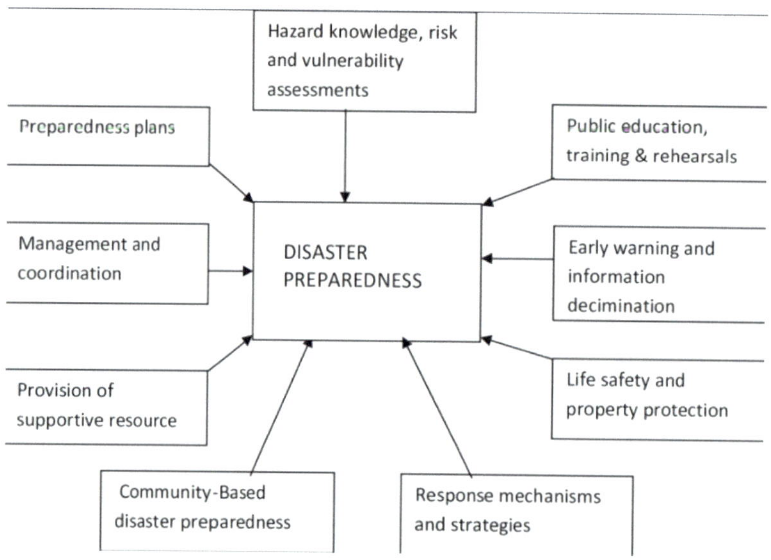

Figure 12.11. Elements and measures for comprehensive disaster preparedness.

Source: https://www.researchgate.net/profile/Md-Sujahangir-Kabir-Sarkar/publication/277934678/figure/fig1/AS:613995346133030@1523399306552/Elements-and-measures-for-comprehensive-disaster-preparedness-Source-Modified-from-IFRC.png.

12.5.1. Community Education and Training

Training and community education form the nucleus for strengthening disaster management frameworks, particularly disaster preparedness for both natural and man-made disasters. Educational schemes increase resilience and response attitude by imparting the required information and skills to the common masses. Local training and workshop schemes can cover an array of topics like disaster preparedness, response systems, and recovery programs. Such projects guarantee that people know their part and role in times of disaster, in the end preventing chaos and inefficiency in times of crises. In regions where certain hazards are common, community education specifically designed with local requirements can prepare residents to respond effectively and quickly. Therefore, community education is aligned with overall disaster management systems, which provide an educated population that can assist in disaster mitigation and recovery efforts. The integration of community training into disaster management is essential for effective public health interventions.

Following a disaster, the educated population can help health professionals deal with health emergencies. With the right knowledge on the public health risks incurred due to disasters, individuals can assume preventive roles such as vaccinations, sanitation, and identification of the health risks. Moreover, as stated in Fichtner et al. (2008), providing the critical workforce training for activities related to disaster management enhances collaboration among various stakeholders in the community, for example, the first responders and health officials.

This collaboration is vital when dealing with health issues that arise during emergencies in order to enable quick identification of needs and distribution of resources. Finally, community training enhances the public health readiness and develops a culture of collective responsibility in the face of disaster-related issues. Community education also establishes a vital connection between local residents and wider disaster management policy, enhancing activities on environmental rehabilitation following disasters and emergencies. Understanding ideas such as hazard, vulnerability, and risk located within local ecosystems allows communities to participate in rehabilitation activities. The incorporation of environmental education within community training can highlight the importance of sustainable practices during rehabilitation phases. The learning from previous disasters, as discussed in Khan et al. (2008), including outcome measures and mitigation measures, can educate communities on the optimal methods of rehabilitation. Having trained community members, there will be a greater chance of utilizing environmentally responsive methods that allow for longer-term recovery. By filling in the gap between action at the level of the individual and policy-level action, community education becomes an essential element of holistic disaster management and recovery planning.

12.5.2. Emergency Response Planning

Emergency response planning is a critical component of effective disaster management, consisting of strategies and procedures to counter natural as well as human-made disasters. A thorough study of the kind of disaster, its nature, and potential consequences is necessary while going through the planning process. For instance, different strategies must be devised for situations involving earthquakes and biological hazards. At the core of this process is the Disaster Management Cycle, consisting of preparedness, response, recovery, and mitigation phases. Through the identification of the hazards and vulnerabilities of different areas, emergency response plans can be made specific to develop resilience and reduce risks. These planning activities allow societies to activate resources promptly so that relief works are properly coordinated and effective during times of emergencies. Understanding these elements is central to developing comprehensive plans that significantly improve performance in the event of disaster, with preparedness listed as vital in minimizing adverse effects (Khan et al., 2008). Coordination of emergency response is important in planning for response. The local government, non-profit organizations, and community members play a major role in developing a strong emergency response mechanism. Each stakeholder brings unique resources and expertise that contribute to resilience. For example, public health agencies can provide critical guidance on health-influenced response measures, while government agencies can give assistance in logistics and infrastructure readiness. Moreover, joint training simulations are crucial to ensuring that every stakeholder understands his/her specific role during a disaster. These exercises can simulate various disaster scenarios in an attempt to test the response capacity of plans and provide suggestions for improvement. Incorporating communities in planning also elevates public awareness and brings about a culture of preparedness and ultimately more effective response measures during crisis situations (Khan et al., 2008). Finally, the role of technology in emergency response planning cannot be overstated. Technological advancements offer new answers that enhance communication, information collection, and resource allocation during a crisis. For instance, geographical information systems (GIS) can provide real-time mapping of disaster-stricken areas, enabling responders to send aid where it will be most beneficial. Social media sites are also essential for delivering information quickly and efficiently to the public, including rapid updates and safety notices. The use of data analytics in pre-disaster planning offers the potential for better forecasting and risk evaluation, and results in better decision-making. As disasters grow more complex and large-scale in character, taking advantage of technology in planning for emergency response becomes increasingly significant in creating responsive and reactive disaster management systems. Not only do these advance quick response operations, but they also improve long-term preparedness planning (Khan et al., 2008) (Figure 12.12).

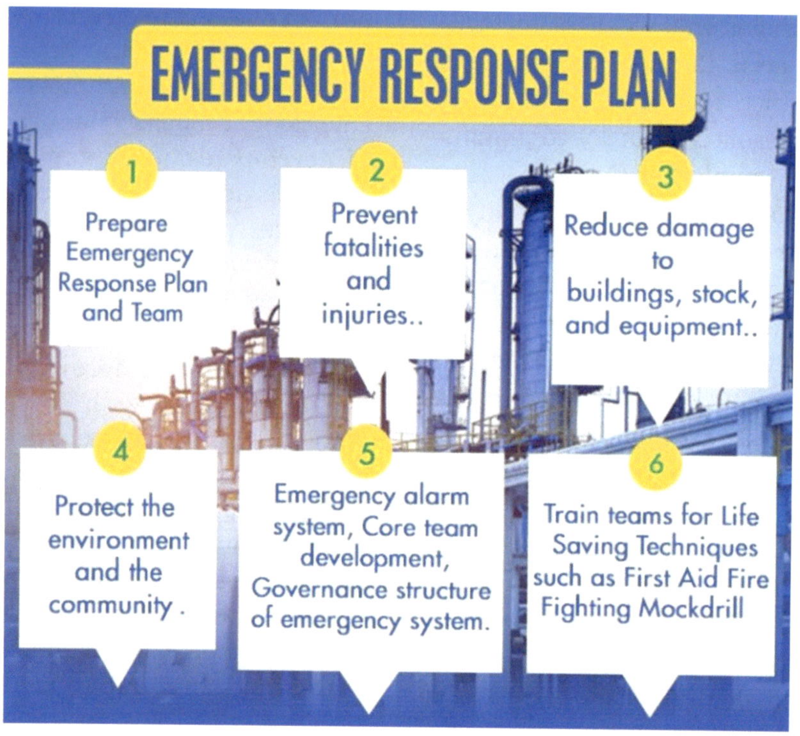

Figure 12.12. The importance of developing an emergency response and disaster management plan.

Source: https://www.thesafetymaster.com/wp-content/uploads/2020/04/WhatsApp-Image-2020-04-06-at-10.36.35-728x675.jpeg.

12.5.3. Resource Allocation and Management

Efficient resource management is central in emergency response planning and disaster management. Efficient deployment of resources during emergencies significantly contributes to the success of relief work, directly influencing communities devastated by natural and man-made disasters. To help in the efficient use of limited resources, there is a requirement to possess organized systems that offer timely access to critical information on risk and resources available. An organized mutual platform for the sharing of knowledge on disaster management interventions, as highlighted in more recent studies, has been central to the enhancement of the effectiveness of ensuing interventions. As demonstrated by the learning experience of the 2004 Asian tsunami, in the case of Sri Lanka, among others, ensuring coordination among stakeholders assists in formulating a thorough understanding of the operating environment, which eventually leads to improved allocation of resources and more effective disaster response programs (Amaratunga et al., 2013). Resource allocation also necessitates a balanced appreciation of the demographic and socio-economic composition of affected populations. Marginalized groups, which are normally disadvantaged in times of crisis, deserve particular attention to ensure equal access to essential services and resources. This involves the identification of specific local ecosystem dependencies of these groups on natural resources and ecosystem services. The intricacy between affected communities and surrounding ecosystems calls for an integrated approach towards resource management that balances recovery with environmental restoration. For instance, as argued in studies that have particularly examined reef ecosystems, poor people's livelihoods are frequently interconnected with the health of settled resources. Through recognizing how changes in these ecosystems affect the poor's livelihoods, resource plans can be realigned so as to foster resilience and sustainability within greater disaster recovery strategies (Whittingham et al., 2010). Finally, strategic resource management in disaster preparedness has to integrate robust planning and coordination processes. Such processes have to consider the shifting nature of disaster risks, along with the potential for sudden-onset emergencies. Effective policies in disaster management have to integrate evidence-based assessments that enable stakeholders to prioritize the allocation of resources based on the highest priority needs of impacted populations. Such a pre-emptive approach not only enhances the capability for immediate response but also facilitates long-term recovery and resilience. Synergy between knowledge sharing, coordination among stakeholders, and resource allocation mechanisms is critical to developing effective disaster management frameworks. By developing a culture in which lessons identified and best practices are exchanged on a large scale, as noted throughout academic research, communities can better prepare for future disasters while enhancing their response efforts (Amaratunga et al., 2013).

12.6. Environmental Rehabilitation Post-Disaster

After a wide-ranging disaster, either natural or man-made, the environmental consequence can be immense and far-reaching, necessitating a rehabilitative process in a formalized format. Effective post-disaster rehabilitation of the environment attempts to restore ecosystems and avoid future deterioration. Rehabilitation involves assessing the extent of damage, which is measuring loss of biodiversity, erosion of land, and pollution of water resources. There is a need to engage local communities in the endeavor since they have indigenous knowledge that can be adapted to enhance the rehabilitation process. Techniques such as reforestation, wetland restoration, and pollution removal are central to revitalizing affected land, eventually resulting in a sustainable environment that can withstand future disasters. Studies have shown that intervention by the community alongside professional intervention will lead to more lasting rehabilitation outcomes (Khan et al., 2008). Knowledge about the diversity of disasters directs the methods employed in environmental rehabilitation. Differing types of disasters, such as earthquakes, floods, and industrial disasters, will have differing ecological impacts and therefore require differing rehabilitation measures. For instance, following flooding events, sediment deposit management and aquatic ecosystems recovery are priorities, but in the case of industrial spills, soil and water decontamination are priorities. The disaster cycle, which involves preparedness, response, recovery, and mitigation stages, emphasizes the need for a coordinated approach where each stage triggers further action (Khan et al., 2008). An iterative learning process allows refining practices and strategies to improve the effectiveness of rehabilitation directly in various contexts.

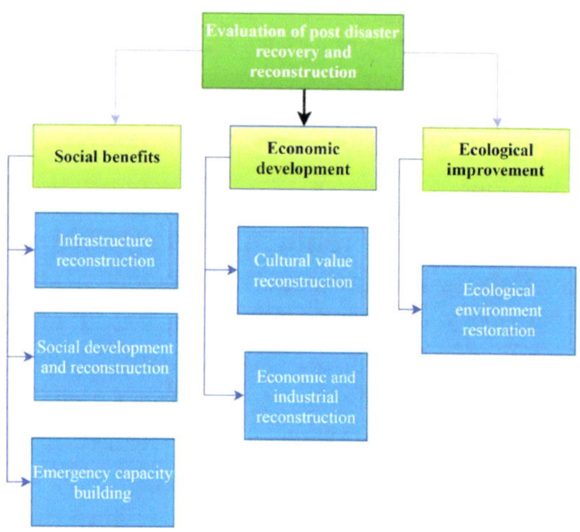

Figure 12.13. Post-disaster recovery and reconstruction effect evaluation.

Source: https://www.researchgate.net/publication/359990661/figure/fig2/AS:11431281095996273@1668067630080/Post-disaster-recovery-and-reconstruction-effect-evaluation-index-system-first-level.png.

Finally, an intersection of environmental rehabilitation and public health cannot be downplayed since the two professions are logically interdependent. Disasters not only harm physical environments but also social networks and the health system of the population. Ecosystem restoration through rehabilitation can lead to improved public health outcomes through the supply of clean air, drinking water, and sustainable food. The integrated effort where ecological integrity is maintained or restored supports the overall health of communities and their ability to recover from disasters. Integration of health monitoring at the environmental rehabilitation planning stage accounts for vulnerabilities and enables pre-emptive measures so that recovery processes are optimized and revolutionary. This focuses on the necessity of ensuring robust policy frameworks that support both public health response measures as well as environmental rehabilitation following disasters (Figure 12.13).

12.6.1. Assessment of Environmental Damage

The assessment of environmental damage following a disaster is an integral part of disaster management and relief operations. This research involves a comprehensive appraisal of the impact not just on physical environments but also on societally ingrained patterns and indigenous economies. Various techniques, such as remote sensing and ground surveys, are employed to quantify damage and assess the severity of resource depletion. Awareness of the level of environmental degradation provides vital information that informs recovery plans so that prioritization and resource utilization can be planned. Also, accurate assessment allows the integration of lessons obtained in future preparedness plans, hence the attainment of a cycle of improvement in disaster response mechanisms, which is paramount in preventing risks in disaster-risk-prone areas (Khan et al., 2008). In environmental destruction management, consideration should also be given to the socio-economic forces of recovery and vulnerability. Disproportionately affected by disasters are marginalized groups, whose resilience is even belittled by other underlying environmental issues. Equitable damage assessments should thus incorporate these socio-economic forces so that remediation strategies consider correcting these inequities. Second, rehabilitation procedures following a disaster do not only require returning the physical environment to how it was, but also building and strengthening community capacity and resilience. Such an effort upholds the concepts of sustainable development and fosters a broader understanding of environmental rehabilitation as both an ecological and a social necessity. Integration of this type brings into focus the importance of integrating environmental assessments within a comprehensive socio-economic context, particularly in regions prone to frequent disasters (Khan et al., 2008). The implications of environmental damage assessment extend far beyond short-term recovery activities. Effective understanding of environmental degradation and consequences allows policymakers to impose stricter regulations and frameworks in an attempt to mitigate disaster risk. Through fostering an active response to environmental health, communities can mitigate vulnerabilities to natural and anthropogenic risks. Effective environmental assessment can also contribute to public health programs, as the degradation of ecosystems has a direct impact on health outcomes among humans. Thus, the interlinkage of environmental assessment and disaster management leads to a key arena of focus in planning for ensuing challenges facing communities to ensure interventions are timely and effective, but catalyze sustainable strategies for long-term resilience (Khan et al., 2008).

12.6.2. Restoration of Ecosystems

Ecological recovery is a key element in disaster response and emergency management, particularly in the wake of natural and human-made disasters. Ecological degradation is most likely to raise the magnitude of disasters and lead to greater vulnerability for affected communities. Post-disaster recovery will have the effect of recovering key ecosystem services, such as flood control, stabilization of soils, and water purification. For instance, appropriate management interventions, including wetland restoration and reforestation initiatives, can help enhance the resistance of a community to subsequent incidents. The role played by the government in facilitating the restoration activities can be immense, especially in terms of funding and policy guidance directions, paying attention with due importance to environmental recovery rather than disaster preparedness activities, like those on research concerning local government initiatives on flood disaster prevention (Chowdhury et al., 2024). Also, integrating local people into restoration activities in ecosystems is necessary to achieve sustainable outcomes. Natural resource-based communities, such as fisheries and forests, should be incorporated into decision-making processes concerning restoration. With this integration, ownership and accountability towards the ecosystem among the inhabitants are created, allowing them to protect their livelihoods and adapt to evolving environmental conditions. Public information campaigns and education programs can also bridge the gap between local traditions and scientific knowledge, facilitating innovative solutions that benefit both the socio-economic organization of these societies and the environment. Restoration of coral reefs, for instance, not only increases biodiversity but also provides economic rewards to impoverished communities that depend on these ecosystems for their subsistence (Whittingham et al., 2010). Thus, public participation is an essential component in the effective implementation of ecosystem restoration measures. In summary, ecosystem restoration needs to be a component of rehabilitation activities in the event of disasters. Effective restoration not only addresses environmental degradation but also contributes to public health impacts through enhanced ecosystem services. Well-functioning ecosystems are capable of minimizing the health risks brought about by disasters, such as waterborne disease and food scarcity. Furthermore, interagency collaboration between governments, non-governmental entities, and the local populace plays a significant role in ensuring the effectiveness of these restorative processes. By establishing policies that put ecosystem health on the same level as disaster risk reduction efforts, societies can become more resilient and avoid the recurrence of future disasters. Ultimately, such concerted action towards ecosystem restoration will not only ensure environmental stability but also facilitate sustainable development in areas subject to disasters (Figure 12.14).

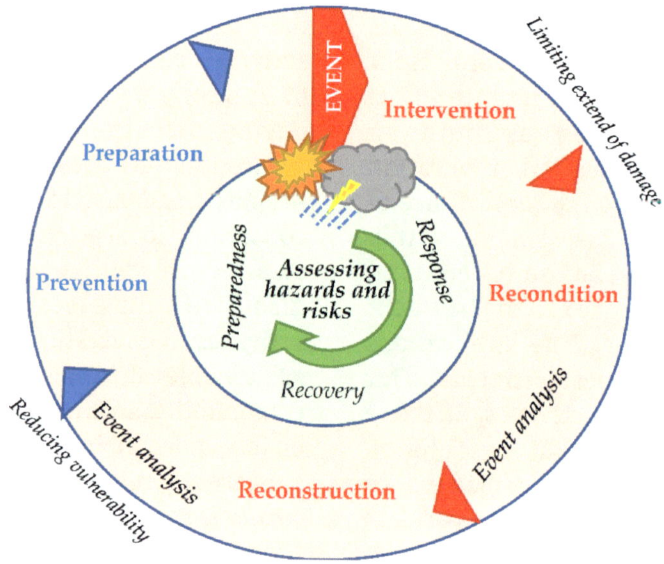

Figure 12.14. Ecosystem-based disaster risk reduction.

Source: https://pub.mdpi-res.com/environsciproc/environsciproc-21-00040/article_deploy/html/images/environsciproc-21-00040-g001.png?1666698333.

12.6.3. Sustainable Practices for Future Resilience

Ecological practices conjoining disaster management are today more than ever becoming a source of strength to build resilience against forthcoming disasters. In a majority of instances, the direct correlation of climate change with the frequency and intensity of natural disasters has directed a shift in the paradigm of preparedness and response. Community-managed disaster risk reduction (CMDRR) is a good example of how resilience can be enhanced because it holds local people accountable for their own preparedness. Involving local resources and knowledge, communities are more likely to understand their vulnerabilities and take preventive measures. As highlighted by the imperative of climate change threats, the building of sustainability at the community level can play a significant role in lessening disaster impacts, facilitating the capacity of communities to adapt and ultimately increase their chances of survival under stress (N/A, 2009). Cultural heritage plays a vital role in shaping the identity of communities and can be a better ally in disaster risk reduction activities. While societies grapple with threats posed by natural and anthropogenic disasters, the understanding and utilization of cultural heritage can enhance collective resilience.

Modern cultural heritage has much more to do with living landscapes and intangible values and traditions than monumental sites; including these elements in disaster management enables disaster strategies to establish solid support systems that are the bedrock of communal solidarity during adversity. Significantly, measures to retain cultural heritage property can further be incorporated into broader disaster resilience policy. Such incorporation maintains historical identity but also enhances public awareness of the imperative to retain cultural histories amidst adversity (Albrito et al., 2013). Sustainable approaches further embrace the multiple-dimensional response required for effective environmental rehabilitation after disasters. When societies bounce back from disasters, green efforts can not only revive devastated ecosystems but also ensure local livelihoods. Employing green infrastructure such as urban parks, reforestation, and environmentally friendly agriculture can greatly improve urban resilience by ensuring biodiversity and natural flood protection. In addition, engaging people in the recovery efforts helps to build ownership and environmental awareness among people. As such practices unfold, they create lasting respect for ecological sustainability, which is crucial in reducing future weaknesses. Ultimately, highlighting sustainable practice is critical not only for existing recovery mechanisms but also in building a culture of resilience that can withstand inevitable assaults of future disasters (N/A, 2009; Albrito et al., 2013) (Figure 12.15).

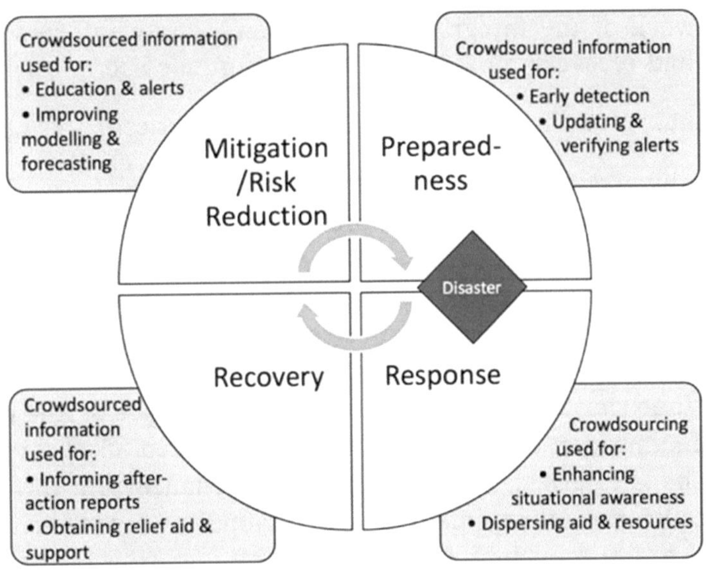

Figure 12.15. Technological innovations for enhancing disaster resilience in smart cities.

Source: https://www.mdpi.com/sustainability/sustainability-15-12036/article_deploy/html/images/sustainability-15-12036-g001.png.

CLOSER LOOK

IMPORTANCE OF INTEGRATED DISASTER MANAGEMENT

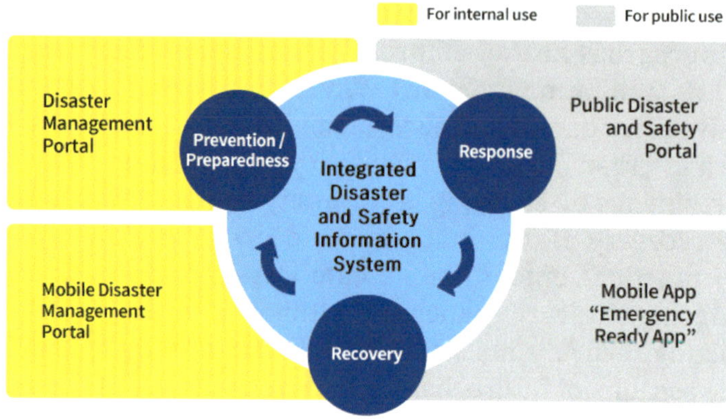

Figure 12.16. Framework of the integrated disaster and safety information system outlining prevention, response, and recovery tools for internal and public use.

Source: https://www.mois.go.kr/images/eng/contents/bestPractices1_img1.png.

IDM is a critical methodology that enhances preparedness and response capability in preparation for natural and man-made disasters. Through the promotion of agency and stakeholder collaboration, IDM enables a comprehensive system of risk assessment, planning, and implementation of disaster management. Such dimensional collaboration is significant as it facilitates the determination of possible dangers and vulnerabilities and the design of effective measures of mitigation. Where stakeholders are synchronized, the resources can be better utilized, ultimately minimizing the effects on communities and shortening recovery time. The pertinence of IDM is also necessitated by the fact that good communication channels need to be established and data needs to be used in a bid to forecast and respond to disaster occurrences. In accordance with various studies, including those that refer to the Disaster Management Cycle, coordination is vital in managing both short-term and long-term needs successfully. Furthermore, the inclusion of disaster management in public health interventions is vital. Most disasters create health emergencies on a large scale, and it is hence crucial for health agencies to be included in planning. Interconnectedness of practice in disaster management with health outcomes suggests that there should be the establishment of inclusive health protocols that can be utilized in times of emergency. Participation of public health authorities in minimizing the risk of disasters as well as in recovery efforts assists communities in preparing and managing ensuing health-related issues after a disaster, for example, epidemic breaks and mental illness. The emphasis on the approach being integrated enables the healthcare systems to succeed in surviving crises, thus ensuring uninterrupted service delivery. This integration of resources and knowledge brings the scenario where public health remains achievable even with devastating disasters taking place, as case studies of successful operations during national disasters prove. Lastly, the use of environmental rehabilitation indicates the contribution made by incorporating an approach into disaster management. The effects of natural and anthropogenic disasters typically result in widespread environmental degradation, posing a risk to ecosystems and human health. It is therefore important to have a management plan for environmental priorities in order to recover sustainably. Addressing environmental issues with public health and socio-economic issues enables communities to attain resilience while preventing probable future disasters. It is a multidisciplinary solution that guarantees the restoration of ecosystems for their capability to buffer future threats. Bridging environmental understanding and technology with disaster recovery planning enhances rejuvenation efforts while enhancing collaboration with long-term sustainability within communities. The importance of all-encompassing disaster management, thus, extends beyond short-term crisis relief, reflecting a conceptually integrated understanding of the complex interdependencies between human activity, health, and the environment.

SUMMARY

The effectiveness of disaster management and emergency response relies on understanding a full range of natural and human-induced disasters. This provides a basis for making proactive responses that reduce impacts and enhance recovery after the disaster has occurred. Interdisciplinary integration of various fields—public health, environmental science, and crisis management—provides a synergistic framework for disaster resiliency. With organizations taking steps to bridge the policy-practice gap, it is then critical to look at the most common challenges to successful implementation seen in many case studies. Also, the methods derived from (Swint et al., 2024) point towards measurable readiness gaps and highlight the significance of adaptive management and systems that can better handle the complexities of current-day disasters. Furthermore, public health readiness is a key component in successful disaster response frameworks. With the availability of high vulnerability in various healthcare facilities, as evidenced in reviews in Khademipour et al. (2022), policy-makers should prioritize capacity-building opportunities as an area of investment. Such schemes must aim at creating reliable infrastructure in the healthcare sector capable of withstanding natural and manmade disasters. By participatory policy formulation, the stakeholders can engage communities so that preparedness mechanisms are guided by local understandings and hence enhance emergency resilience. This collaborative approach demonstrates the potential for significant enhancement in public health interventions in the event of catastrophes. Finally, the rehabilitation phase after a disaster is as critical as the response efforts preceding it. Effective environmental rehabilitation, besides restoring the affected areas, also generates resilience and sustainability within communities in the long term. The integration of disaster risk reduction into urban and rural development planning directs more effective deployment of resources and the prevention of hazards. Such a long-term strategic perspective, supplemented by existing technological advances, offers promising avenues for improving disaster preparedness and response. Lastly, lessons learned should propel relentless enhancement in managing disasters to make communities and systems prepared for the next challenges, as underscored in the findings from the analyses in Swint et al. (2024) and Khademipour et al. (2022).

The impacts of disasters, natural or man-made, are far-reaching, as one can observe from instances such as the 2004 tsunami in Sri Lanka, a central case study in disaster management. In December 2004, a tsunami triggered by an underwater earthquake swept through coastal towns, killing over 35,000 people and leaving millions displaced. Loss of infrastructure in the form of housing, transport, and communication facilities critically impacted recovery and economic stability. It is an example of how huge disasters have the potential to reveal vulnerabilities in public health and civil infrastructure, thereby necessitating effective disaster preparedness efforts. Such traumatic events need to be met not only by short-term relief measures but by sustained recovery programs restoring physical and social capital in affected communities to ensure future shock resistance to potential disasters (Amaratunga et al., 2006). Significant enhancement in disaster management relies on the collective response of stakeholders from government bodies to non-governmental organizations (NGOs) and local society. The recovery process in post-disaster scenarios normally involves not just the restoration of the physical infrastructure but also the strengthening of the socio-economic requirements of the affected groups. Past research has identified that effective disaster management is influenced by a diversity of factors, such as technological and operational factors that span the whole disaster management chain. These factors have critical roles in the mitigation, preparedness, response, and recovery phases. Specifically, social elements of disaster information, including community involvement and dissemination, are critical for resilience and recovery improvement, having communities prepared to deal with future similar crises (Amaratunga et al., 2010). Environmental rehabilitation after a disaster is a critical component of recovery that involves the restoration of natural systems that have been affected. Effective disaster recovery must include environmental concerns to enable sustainable restoration and rebuilding. The relationship between human activity and environmental well-being can exacerbate the effects of disasters, and a comprehensive approach focusing on ecological balance is therefore justified. Inclusion of environmental science in the restoration process not only assists in rebuilding ecologically destroyed ecosystems but also ensures the general well-being and protection of communities. Finally, leveraging disaster intelligence and integrating environmental rehabilitation strategies into the recovery system can foster resilience and preparedness for upcoming disasters and open the door to a more resilient and sustainable emergency management approach (Amaratunga et al., 2006, 2010).

REFERENCES

1. Adebimpe, R. U., & Olorunfemi, F. B. (2008). *Sustainable Disaster Risk Reduction in Nigeria: Lessons for Developing Countries*. https://core.ac.uk/download/478407085.pdf (accessed on 11th June 2025).
2. Albrito, P., Boccardi, G., Dolcemascolo, G., et al. (2013). *Heritage and Resilience: Issues and Opportunities for Reducing Disaster Risks*. https://core.ac.uk/download/20544501.pdf (accessed on 11th June 2025).
3. Amaratunga, D., Baldry, D., Haigh, R., et al. (2025). *Lessons Learned from Asian Tsunami Disaster: Sharing Knowledge*. https://core.ac.uk/download/30730738.pdf (accessed on 11th June 2025).
4. Amaratunga, R. D. G., Haigh, R. P., Pathirage, C. P., et al. (2010). *Identification of Disaster Knowledge Factors: Preliminary Findings*. https://core.ac.uk/download/1661640.pdf (accessed on 11th June 2025).
5. Anguelovski, I., Shi, L. Z., Chu, E., Gallagher, D. B., Goh, K., Lamb, Z., Reeve, K., et al. (2016). Equity impacts of urban land use planning for climate adaptation. *Journal of Planning Education and Research, 36*, 333–348. https://doi.org/10.1177/0739456x16645166 (accessed on 11th June 2025).
6. Charvériat, C. (2012). *Natural Disasters in Latin America and the Caribbean: An Overview of Risk*. https://core.ac.uk/download/pdf/205124388.pdf (accessed on 11th June 2025).
7. Chowdhury, K., & Ishak, B. S. (2024). *The Role of Local Governments in Flood Disaster Mitigation in Makassar City*. https://core.ac.uk/download/617747271.pdf (accessed on 11th June 2025).
8. de Haen, H., & Hemrich, G. (2025). *The Economics of Natural Disasters–Implications and Challenges for Food Security*. https://core.ac.uk/download/pdf/6653435.pdf (accessed on 11th June 2025).
9. Deeb, A., French, A., Heiss, J., et al. (2011). *Responding to Climate Change: The Economy and Economics–Part of the Problem and Solution*. https://core.ac.uk/download/19441204.pdf (accessed on 11th June 2025).
10. Deeming, H., Medd, W., & Whittle, R. (2011). *Recommendations for Changes in UK National Recovery Guidance (NRG) and Associated Guidance from The Perspective of Lancaster University's Hull Flood Studies*. https://core.ac.uk/download/1556070.pdf (accessed on 11th June 2025).
11. Fichtner, A., Cleary, J., & Kauder, R. (2008). *Understanding the Workforce Needs of New Jersey's Public Health and Other Disaster Management Employers*. https://core.ac.uk/download/71341796.pdf (accessed on 11th June 2025).
12. Gligorov, I., Lazarevski, P., & Stikova, E. (2008). *Global Public Health Threats and Disaster Management*. https://core.ac.uk/download/333548437.pdf (accessed on 11th June 2025).
13. Hidayati, I. Y., Rachmawati, Y., Waluyo, M. E., et al. (2015). *The Community-Based Flood Disaster Risk Reduction (CBDRR) in Beringin Watershed in Semarang City*. https://core.ac.uk/download/76939919.pdf (accessed on 11th June 2025).
14. Ishrat, S., & Hameed, N. (2024). The disaster profile of Pakistan and its management strategies. *Research Journal for Societal Issues, 6*, 27–49. https://doi.org/10.56976/rjsi.v6i1.174 (accessed on 11th June 2025).

15. Khademipour, G., & Sheikhbardsiri, H. (2022). Disaster risk assessment of primary healthcare facilities in South East of Iran: A study with approach of disaster risk reduction. *Disaster and Emergency Medicine Journal*. https://www.semanticscholar.org/paper/d7401e828c871a439a010ec5a0046a8b258bece2 (accessed on 11th June 2025).

16. Khan, A., & Khan, H. (2008). *Natural Hazards and Disaster Management in Pakistan*. https://core.ac.uk/download/12017579.pdf (accessed on 11th June 2025).

17. Khan, A., & Khan, H. (2025). *Natural Hazards and Disaster Management in Pakistan*. https://core.ac.uk/download/pdf/7301410.pdf (accessed on 11th June 2025).

18. Li, F., Diop, S., Hirwa, H., Maesho, S., Xu, N., Tian, C., Qiao, Y., et al. (2024). *Dryland Social-Ecological Systems in Africa*. https://doi.org/10.1007/978-981-99-9375-8_9 (accessed on 11th June 2025).

19. López-Saavedra, M., & Martí, J. (2022). Reviewing the multi-hazard concept: Application to volcanic islands. *Earth-Science Reviews, 236*, 104286–104286. https://doi.org/10.1016/j.earscirev.2022.104286 (accessed on 11th June 2025).

20. Mukherjee, M., Wickramasinghe, D., Chowdhooree, I., Chimi, C., Poudel, S., Mishra, B., Faruqui Ali, Z., et al. (2022). Nature-based resilience: Experiences of five cities from South Asia. *International Journal of Environmental Research and Public Health, 19*, 11846–11846. https://doi.org/10.3390/ijerph191911846 (accessed on 11th June 2025).

21. Nallathambi, I., Savaram, P., Sengan, S., Alharbi, M., Alshathri, S., Bajaj, M., Aly, M. H., et al. (2023). Impact of fireworks industry safety measures and prevention management system on human error mitigation using a machine learning approach. *Sensors, 23*, 4365–4365. https://doi.org/10.3390/s23094365 (accessed on 11th June 2025).

22. Ofoezie, E. I., Eludoyin, A. O., Udeh, E. B., Onanuga, M. Y., Salami, O. O., & Adebayo, A. A. (2022). Climate, urbanization and environmental pollution in West Africa. *Sustainability, 14*, 15602–15602. https://doi.org/10.3390/su142315602 (accessed on 11th June 2025).

23. Swint, J., Zhang, W., Marrison, A., & Gabriel, S. (2024). *Syncing Strategy and Execution: A Systematic Review of Public Health Preparedness Policy Implementation*. https://www.semanticscholar.org/paper/bb8fc4f80b5e86f4a496ee3c7015e0dcbb358f8d (accessed on 11th June 2025).

24. Tekeli-Yeşil, S. (2018). *Public Health and Natural Disasters: Disaster Preparedness and Response in Health Systems*. https://core.ac.uk/download/159155913.pdf (accessed on 11th June 2025)

25. Whittingham, E., Campbell, J., & Townsley, P. (2010). *APFIC/FAO Regional Consultative Workshop: Securing Sustainable Small-Scale Fisheries–Bringing Together Responsible Fisheries and Social Development, Windsor Suites Hotel, Bangkok, Thailand, 6–8 October 2010*. https://core.ac.uk/download/75777521.pdf (accessed on 11th June 2025).

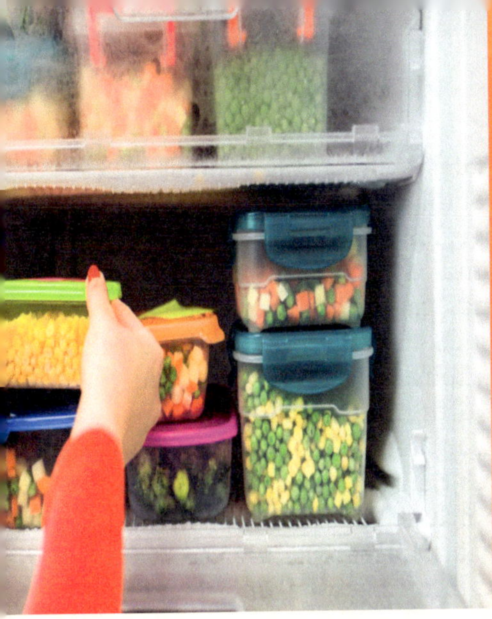

Chapter 13

FOOD SAFETY AND ENVIRONMENTAL HYGIENE

Contents

Introduction

In the current public health situation, environmental sanitation and food safety emerge as the most critical factors in avoiding foodborne illnesses and attaining general welfare. With the ever-growing and urbanizing world population, the complexities of food production, storage, and handling require utmost vigilance. Safe food handling encompasses various practices involving correct storage, cooking, and cooling methods that can potentially minimize the risk of contamination dramatically. The effect of foodborne pathogens is catastrophic, as evidenced in the study on an outbreak of a gastrointestinal illness resulting from a specific catering firm where unsafe hygiene processes facilitated norovirus transmission among the attendees (Chew et al., 2025). This scenario underscores how mishandling of food could result not only in individual health consequences but also in overall economic loss in the form of high productivity losses. The link between environmental cleanliness and food safety cannot be overstressed, especially in vulnerable populations such as children. Research identifies that inadequate access to clean water, sanitation, and hygiene (WASH) facilities has a direct effect on child stunting incidence, which is a public health priority (Dominguez-Salas et al., 2024). It acknowledges this link, which further emphasizes the imperative for combined interventions that incorporate good food safety controls with good environmental hygiene controls. Through the supply of safe food and clean water for drinking, communities can lower the incidence of foodborne illnesses and improve child health status. Further, such interdisciplinary research emphasizes the importance of promoting hygiene practices on a household level and placing a focus on cross-contamination prevention and nutrition protection. Ultimately, building an integral comprehension of environmental hygiene and food safety is necessary for public health advocacy and policy-making. All parties must collaborate to develop measures that will enhance food safety practices in homes and communities, respectively. Measures should include educating food handlers on the importance of personal cleanliness and appropriate food handling procedures to reduce the risk of contamination. In addition, measures towards facilitating improved environmental conditions, such as effective waste disposal and provision of safe water, are essential in creating a safer food environment. With all these concerted efforts, we can combat foodborne illnesses and advance overall nutrition, thereby ensuring community resilience and health for generations to come (Figure 13.1).

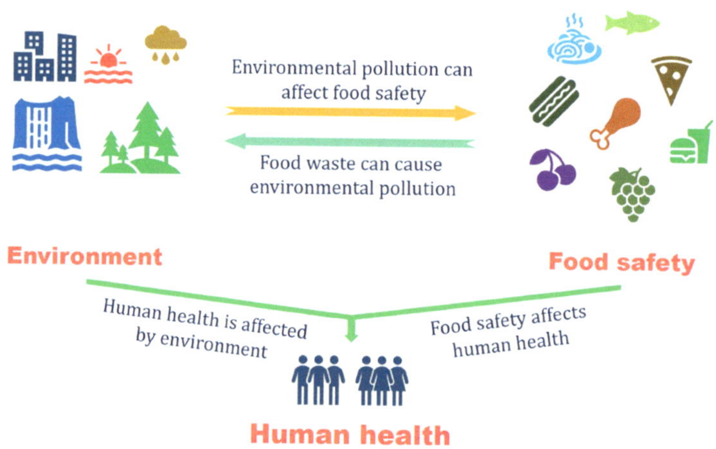

Figure 13.1. Environment and food safety.

Source: https://media.springernature.com/lw1200/springer-static/image/art%3A10.1007%2Fs11356-021-16069-6/MediaObjects/11356_2021_16069_Fig1_HTML.png.

Definition of Food Safety

Understanding the concept of food safety is basic to improving public health and addressing the multifaceted issues of food contamination. Food safety is a wide variety of practices and policy measures intended to ensure that food is safe for consumption throughout its entire lifecycle, from cultivation to processing and ultimately to consumption. Food-safe storage and treatment are of paramount significance, as they discourage the growth of pathogenic microorganisms and toxin formation, which lead to foodborne illness. As outlined in a number of studies, safe food substantially reduces the number of such illnesses, which have long-term serious health consequences on individuals who become afflicted with them and can overburden health systems. These measures are not only essential to individual health but also to the economy, which can experience costly recalls and brand reputation loss as a result of food safety violations. The role of environmental hygiene in food safety cannot be overstated because it plays a crucial part in preventing contamination at various stages of food handling. Environmental factors, including food preparation facilities' cleanliness and sanitization of food contact surfaces, directly influence food product safety. For instance, research indicates that food service workers' knowledge and level of hygiene significantly influence the overall safety of foods presented in facilities like hospitals. Evidence suggests that high levels of training and education correlate with improved food safety behaviors, highlighting the requirement for ongoing education programs in food service environments (Alqurashi et al., 2019). These not only raise awareness but also enable food handlers to implement best hygiene practices that mitigate chances of contamination, fostering a safety culture beneficial to public health. In addition, new food technologies like cell-cultured meat and seafood bring further complexities to traditional definitions of food safety. These novel food production methodologies offer sustainability in satisfying increasing demands for protein, yet require stringent safety evaluations to gain consumer acceptance. Study of the potential risks posed by introducing such goods into production has led to the creation of both chemical and biological risks, further defining the necessity of an elaborate safety evaluation process (Kimberly et al., 2021). This ever-changing world necessitates that classical food safety definitions become more encompassing to incorporate new technology and issues that come with it, so as not to lose sight of consumer health and safety when seeking out new means of food production.

Importance of Environmental Hygiene

Environmental hygiene of food cannot be overstressed because it is the foundation for preventing foodborne illness. Environmental hygiene encompasses a number of practices that guarantee food handling and production environments are hygienic, hence reducing the threats of contamination. A clean environment decreases the chances of microbial growth that can lead to serious health implications. Also, as the topic outlined by the Western Institute for Food Safety and Security reflects, an interdisciplinary approach is important; it stresses the importance of gathering information from environmental science, public health, and food safety to facilitate hygiene practice in food systems (Angelos et al., 2017). Along the way, stakeholders are able to develop effective strategies in accordance with food safety and environmental sustainability, thus ensuring safe consumption without destroying natural resources. Apart from its preventive role, environmental hygiene directly affects consumer confidence in food quality. Whenever individuals believe that food environments are clean and well-regulated, they will be confident that the available food products are safe. This concept affects not only individual purchasing decisions but also broader public health interventions aimed at encouraging healthy consumption practices. The presence of scientists and policymakers, as discussed in the 1995 conference proceedings, underscores the importance of considering the interactions between hygiene control strategies and foodborne pathogen outbreaks throughout the food chain (Anonymous et al., 2025). As in-depth databases, which track hygiene levels and outbreaks of foodborne disease, develop, one can reinforce the invaluable message that environmental hygiene commitments are critical for protecting public health. Environmental hygiene also comes in handy in relation to nutrition, as it leads to the interdependence of food safety and health. Poor environmental hygiene will contribute to food contamination and thus diminish the nutritional quality of the food consumed. For example, the introduction of toxins or pathogens in food due to unhygienic conditions can lead to malnutrition or other illnesses. Thus, a hygienic environment not only ensures food safety but also nutritional purity. With the incorporation of efficient sanitation processes, as suggested under the One Health strategy, policymakers and educators can address such issues collectively, ensuring food safety and nutritional gains with an emphasis on health outcomes (Angelos et al., 2017). Through this, environmental hygiene becomes a fundamental element of combined nutrition and public health, highlighting its integral role in building a healthy community (Figure 13.2).

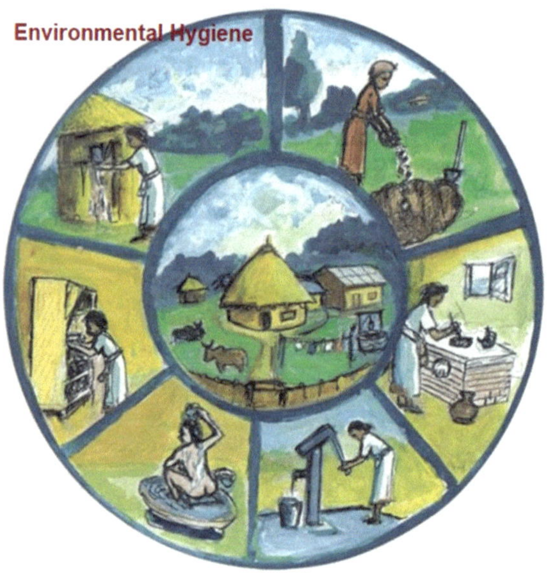

Figure 13.2. Environmental hygiene.

Source: https://hsewatch.com/wp-content/uploads/2022/06/smngoz73iolcdd8k.52f600f6.png.

13.1. Safe Food Handling Practices

In the context of food safety, safe food handling practices are essential in avoiding contamination as well as ensuring the microbiological quality of meals. A survey of a large number of boarding senior high schools in the Volta Region of Ghana discovered that food handlers possess an adequate level of food safety knowledge. But the research also evidenced the prevalence of pathogenic organisms like *Escherichia coli* and *Staphylococcus aureus* in cooked food samples. The findings stress forcefully that there is an imperative need for improved food handling habits that can compensate for the risk of foodborne diseases for school groups. There is a need for good training programs on food storage, preparation, and food hygiene practices. By implementing the appropriate training and resources, food handler microbial contamination incidence can be reduced, thereby contributing to safer school meal environments and national public health. Environmental cleanliness and safe handling procedures must coexist to ensure food safety compliance. Adequate food handling protects food not only from contamination in food preparation but also from ensuring that food storage and serving areas are cleaned and sanitized. The necessity of applying the hazard analysis critical control point (HACCP) protocols shows that there is a requirement for systematic compliance with food safety. Such protocols are directed towards recognizing potential hazards and determining critical control points to reduce hazards along the food production chain. As outlined in the numerous proceedings of food safety policymaker meetings, the lack of integration between pathogen data and food chain operations highlights the need for proper monitoring. Through the application of and enforcement of HACCP, parties can better control food safety hazards, providing increased public confidence in food systems. To fully address the threats posed by foodborne illness, policymakers will need to create and enforce rigorous policies regarding food safety standards. There exists a dramatic incidence of foodborne pathogens that cause direct illness, which necessitates a multifaceted approach to food safety that integrates both policy and education platforms. Training of food handlers, as was evident in the Ghana study, plays a significant role in the reduction of the barriers to proper food safety practice, such as inadequate equipment and poor access to clean water. By investment in food hygiene schemes and the use of proper resources, food safety can be significantly enhanced. As fresh evidence supports the need for improved food safety interventions, sustained collaboration among various stakeholders—from food producers to policymakers—remains essential to preventing foodborne diseases and protecting public health. It thereby contributes to building a healthier food environment (Figure 13.3).

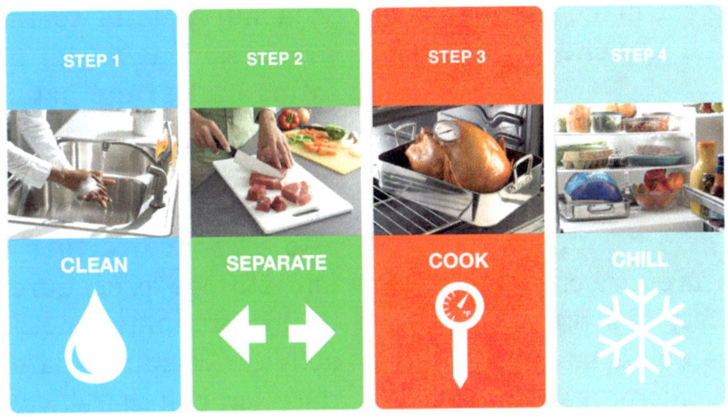
STEP 1
STEP 2
STEP 3
STEP 4
CLEAN
SEPARATE
COOK
CHILL

Figure 13.3. Safe food handling.

Source: https://www.fda.gov/files/SafeFoodHandling_11072023.png.

13.1.1. Personal Hygiene for Food Handlers

Maintaining good personal hygiene levels among food handlers is the most important aspect to ensure food safety and prevent associated health risks of foodborne diseases. Efficient hand washing, the wearing of clean uniforms, and control of cross-contamination by good food handling practices are good personal hygiene practices. A study in Sulaimani Governorate, Iraq, found high levels of food safety knowledge, attitude, and practice among 450 food handlers. The outcome was an indicator of a lack of necessary hygiene practices, such as washing hands and proper handling of raw food, which ultimately contributes to the causation of foodborne illnesses (Nasir et al., 2025). It is thus imperative to increase the level of personal hygiene among food handlers for enhanced public as well as environmental cleanliness, specifically in food service settings. Moreover, personal hygiene beyond minimum needs is something of higher significance that indeed organizes the food preparation and serving setting. Research aimed at food handlers in healthcare institutions has pointed out the risks associated with unsanitary hygiene habits (Surwase et al., 2024). Since patients in such a setup have weakened immune systems, ensuring that food handlers maintain high levels of hygiene can be a major factor in health protection. Proper training on personal hygiene has been found to lead to better outcomes, with handlers who receive such training having better compliance with hygiene standards. Consequently, there is a need for continuous education and reorientation to hygiene procedures to build a food safety culture, thereby enhancing overall food handling effectiveness. Last but not least, adherence to hygiene practices needs to be based on a holistic approach incorporating responsibility at the individual level and institutional support. Organized training sessions and monitoring are required in order for food handlers to have a proper appreciation of hygiene practices, as indicated by the high correlation noted between training and improved knowledge and practices in the said study (Nasir et al., 2025). There is also a need for food outlets to instill a culture that has a focus on hygiene, e.g., provision of necessary resources such as hand-washing stations and adequate personal protective equipment. Through the adoption of these practices as part of the daily food preparation routine, we can significantly reduce the dangers of foodborne illness, drawing attention to personal hygiene in the case of food safety and environmental hygiene in various settings.

13.1.2. Proper Cooking Temperatures

Proper cooking temperatures are crucial to the maintenance of food safety and prevention of foodborne illness, which could be due to the inability to kill harmful microorganisms. The Centers for Disease Control and Prevention (CDC) recommends some internal temperatures that need to be reached in order to kill pathogens such as Salmonella and *E. coli* effectively. For instance, chicken is to be cooked to 165°F (74°C) internal temperature, while ground meat such as beef or pork is to be 160°F (71°C) or higher for it to be safe. Upholding these regulations not only maximizes consumer health protection but also maintains public confidence in food establishments, underlining the significance of the process of operational hygiene in facilitating nutritional safety. The connection between cooking temperatures and the prevention of foodborne illness is also highlighted through existing studies, which revealed that the majority of food handlers possess a basic understanding of these fundamental standards. A study among food handlers in the milk tea industry revealed that people have general knowledge regarding food safety, but certain practices related to cooking and food holding temperatures were poorly understood. Only 44% of the respondents surveyed had received formal training in the proper handling of food, and this was a gap in training that may precipitate cross-contamination and infection. Increased education and awareness of cooking temperatures can help significantly reduce the incidence of foodborne diseases, emphasizing the necessity for increased training programs throughout food service facilities (Joy, 2024). Also, the differing challenges presented in the kitchen environment, such as insufficient staffing and the requirement to cook meals in a hurry, tend to impede correct cooking practices. It is worth noting that while speed forms part of the nature of food service, it is never acceptable to do so at the cost of health and safety. Correct temperature control is not only pertinent to processing raw materials but also extended further to appropriate cooling and storage procedures that have to adhere to predetermined methods to inhibit bacterial activity. An appropriate understanding of both the microbial character of food and the efficient cooking and cooling methods can allow for better, safer food handling within the industry. Its implementation of strict sanitation protocols and temperature controls is indispensable in countering contamination risk between meat and poultry foods, a topic echoed in recent studies on food contamination across various industries (Salama et al., 2024).

13.1.3. Cross-Contamination Prevention

Effective cross-contamination control is critical in maintaining food safety and lowering the rate of foodborne illnesses, particularly in food-serving establishments such as restaurants and open markets. Cross-contamination occurs when harmful bacteria or allergens are transferred from one surface or item of food to another, most of the time through improper handling protocols. For example, a study in open-air markets indicated significant gaps in sanitation protocols, where approximately 89% of the stalls involved had simultaneous handling of money and food by the same personnel, elevating the likelihood of contact between food items and pathogens (Leal et al., 2025). This weakness is further exacerbated by inadequate temperature control and environmental cleanliness conditions that cumulatively offer space for bacterial growth. It is imperative that food handlers are instructed in correct food handling practices, as well as personal hygiene procedures, to minimize these risks and improve the overall safety of food. Foodservice personnel training programs must give top priority to the necessity for food preparation and handling to be conducted in separate zones to prevent cross-contamination. As highlighted by various studies, good Quick-Serve Restaurant (QSR) management practices involve implementing personal hygiene policies as well as workspace separation between cooked and raw foods (Nomzamo et al., 2024). For instance, foodservice managers often make the practice of re-heating the employees' own food using food preparation counters against policy, hence minimizing the opportunity for cross-contaminating surfaces with foreign microorganisms. Correct training and frequent reinforcement of such practices are essential in the construction of a food safety culture in organizations. Lack of proper lead and checks creates opportunities for failures, and ultimately, public health is at risk. Moreover, the application of color-coded equipment and strict processes for raw material handling are essential elements of cross-contamination avoidance. The awareness of foodservice managers regarding temperature control and the quality of ingredients received has to be reflected in concrete measures, such as frequent checks and records of food storage temperatures (Nomzamo et al., 2024). The application of visual markers to ascertain the quality of ingredients and proper disposal of expired or spoiled ingredients goes a long way in minimizing the possibility of contamination. Lastly, it requires an integrated method with training of staff, effective monitoring, and good environmental practices to implement safer food handling. The amalgamation of all these actions not only enhances food safety but also has a positive effect on public health outcomes, delivering a more reliable and hygienic food service environment (Figure 13.4).

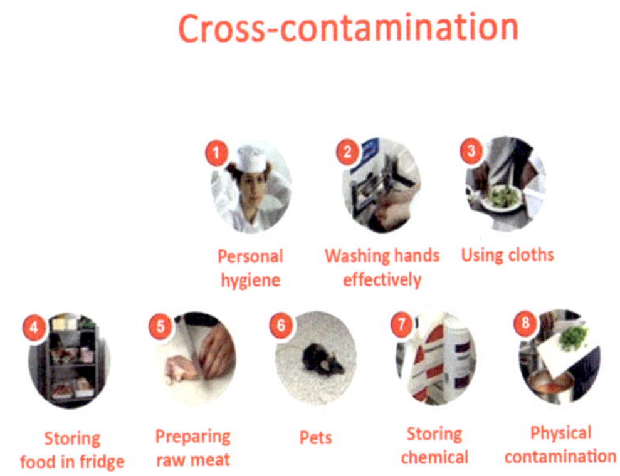
Cross-contamination
1
Personal hygiene
2
Washing hands effectively
3
Using cloths
4
Storing food in fridge
5
Preparing raw meat
6
Pets
7
Storing chemical
8
Physical contamination

Figure 13.4. Cross-contamination prevention.

Source: https://miro.medium.com/v2/resize:fit:1400/1*oNKhRd7WcayNB-y1N8Gucw.jpeg.

13.2. Food Storage Techniques

Correct storage of foods is critical to food safety and preventing contamination. Correct storage significantly slows the growth of harmful microorganisms, which are typically responsible for foodborne illnesses. By way of illustration, foods should be stored at the correct temperatures, with perishable items such as meat, dairy products, and certain vegetables requiring refrigeration at or below 40°F to prevent bacterial growth. Besides, keeping food in sealed containers avoids it from being in contact with air and moisture, the ideal conditions for microbial growth and spoilage. Additionally, one should check storage containers from time to time for functionality and avoid overloading shelves since this will restrict airflow. By using such techniques in food storage, one can avoid foodborne pathogens and achieve a core public health and environmental sanitation objective (Abebe et al., 2020). The increased number of outbreaks associated with fresh produce over the recent years emphasizes the importance of pre-and post-harvest food storage practices. Spoiled fruits and vegetables are potential vehicles for contaminants such as Listeria monocytogenes and Salmonella enterica, which have resulted in multistate outbreaks within the U.S. Storage of food must take into account the entire farm-to-fork process so that fresh fruits and vegetables are protected from contamination during transit or storage. As an example, separating fresh produce from raw meats in refrigerators will deter cross-contamination and consumer illness. Moreover, extensive washing of fruits and vegetables before storage and use can allow for the removal of lingering contaminants. Such efforts are not only essential in averting foodborne disease but also in creating a more sustainable food system (Christina et al., 2019).

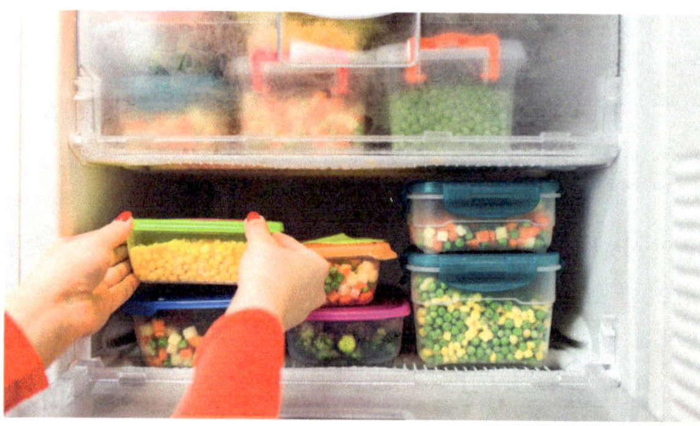

Figure 13.5. Food storage techniques.

Source: https://www.safefood.net/getmedia/945c90e7-11c7-483d-b3f9-ca01aa2e92a4/freezer.jpg?width=2048&height=1152&ext=.jpg.

Finally, routine food storage practices and education continue to be important in home and business environments. Educational sessions about the significance of food handling practices can allow people and food handlers to adopt safer storage practices. Creating a food safety culture entails ongoing education about the hazards of unsafe storage, such as the formation of multidrug-resistant bacteria from contaminated food items. Moreover, knowledge of regional and seasonal differences in food safety can lead to more targeted storage practices. With the creation of a full comprehension of appropriate food storage, society can minimize foodborne disease, which contributes to total public health and raising the contribution of environmental sanitation to nutrition (Abebe et al., 2020) (Figure 13.5).

13.2.1. Temperature Control for Perishable Items

Temperature control is most important for perishable products' safety and integrity, especially for food handling and storage. Suitable temperatures slow the growth of pathogenic microorganisms and ensure the maximum shelf life for food products. The critical temperature range for the majority of perishable products is 40°F to 140°F, which is also called the danger zone that supports bacterial growth. Good refrigeration at a temperature of 40°F and below is necessary for products such as dairy, meat, and fruits and vegetables. Such practice not only helps in avoiding foodborne illnesses but also adheres to standards offered by food safety authorities to ensure consumers are offered safe and quality products. The importance of maintaining such requirements cannot be overstated since slight deviations can lead to severe health implications and financial losses. Food vendor facilities and operations tend to be poor, and this can aggravate temperature control challenges. For instance, Deen et al. (2020) point out that food vendors, particularly those serving university clientele, may lack the basic knowledge required for correct food safety operations. In the majority of cases, limited facility access, such as conventional refrigeration, might lead to incorrect storage methods. Such mismanagement, however, generates an environment conducive to cross-contamination and the dissemination of pathogens. Without the provision of hygienic practice and temperature control, the risk of foodborne illness is extremely high, and there is consequently a public health and safety concern.

Thus, it can make temperature control in food storage more efficient by concentrating on education programs among food handlers. In addition, the role of environmental cleanliness in reinforcing temperature controls cannot be overlooked. Danger from contamination is not only a result of a lack of refrigeration but also a result of environmental factors, such as exposure to open-air elements, such as insects and dust. The facts presented in Deen et al. (2020) show the ways in which food that is prepared in poorly sanitized conditions offers multiple points of contamination. In addition, temperature regulation and overall hygiene procedures are interconnected, indicating a systemic response to food safety. Solving these issues is not merely a matter of complying with temperature control, but also with rigorous hygiene practices that eliminate danger. Training outreach and building facilities are essential to make food handling protocol educated and compliant, and therefore safeguard public health and maximize nutritional benefit in populations.

13.2.2. Proper Packaging Methods

Effective packaging methods are essential in ensuring food safety and preventing environmental pollution. Effective packaging design not only protects food products from environmental conditions outside but also prevents the transfer of pathogens and chemical contaminants that would be harmful to health. For example, packagings that are impermeable to moisture, oxygen, and light can substantially increase the shelf life of perishable foods, thereby preventing foodborne illness. Contamination may occur at any stage of processing and storage, as noted by evidence that attests to the failure to take due care during packaging, leaving the food susceptible to harmful agents like microbes and chemicals from packaging materials themselves (Choudhury et al., 2022). Hence, employing food-safe packaging materials that meet regulatory standards is imperative in minimizing the risk and ensuring the safety of food products throughout their shelf life. In addition to preventing microbial contamination, proper packaging methods are also essential in temperature control and food integrity preservation. Vacuum packaging and modified atmosphere packaging, for instance, have been found to effectively prevent the growth of microorganisms such as Bacillus cereus, which can develop in undeserved conditions and trigger foodborne outbreaks. The recent foodborne outbreak associated with a Malaysian boarding school is a classic example of the possible outcomes of poor food storage and handling operations, highlighting the critical need for environmental control measures such as temperature and humidity in packaging food (Bujang et al., 2019). Through the proper application of suitable processes that are tailored to accommodate the unique requirements of various types of foods, companies can largely improve food product safety and quality, and consequently safeguard consumer health. Also, effective packaging technologies provide environmental cleanliness in the sense that they promote waste reduction and sustainability. Eco-friendly packaging materials not only contribute to a business's reputation but also are driven by increasing consumer pressure for sustainable practices. Food businesses can reduce their environmental footprint while maintaining product safety by utilizing biodegradable and recyclable materials. Secondly, proper packaging contributes to cross-contamination reduction in transportation and storage processes since it creates a barrier that separates products from contaminants from the outer environment (Choudhury et al., 2022). Lastly, the employment of proper packaging processes not only enhances food safety but also the general cleanliness of the environment, thereby improving public health as well as the environment against harmful effects of foodborne disease and contamination (Figure 13.6).

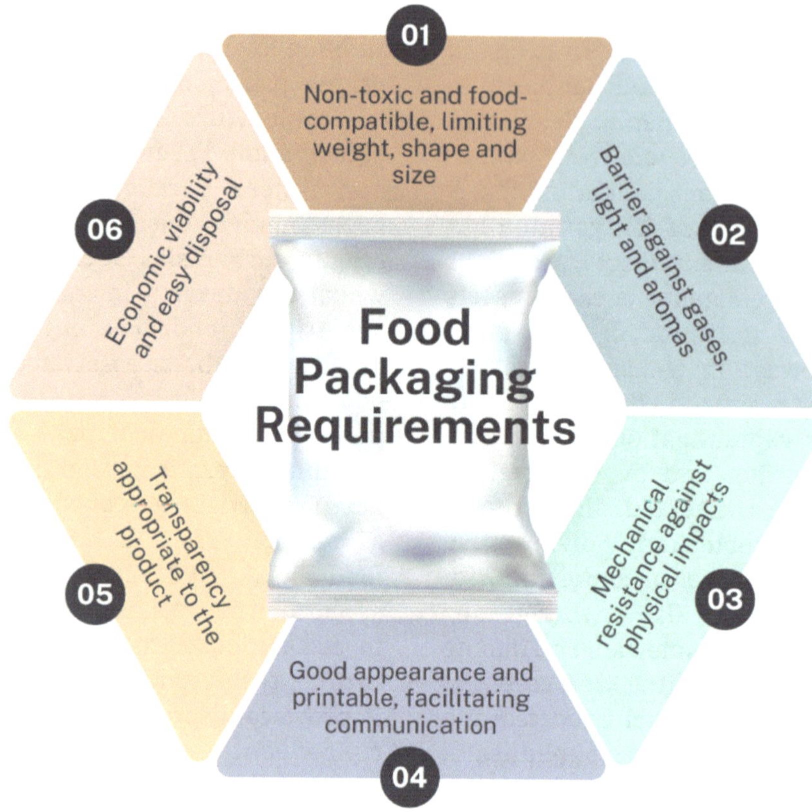
01
Non-toxic and food-compatible, limiting weight, shape and size
02
Barrier against gases, light and aromas
03
Mechanical resistance against physical impacts
04
Good appearance and printable, facilitating communication
05
Transparency appropriate to the product
06
Economic viability and easy disposal
Food Packaging Requirements

Figure 13.6. Packaging methods.

Source: https://www.mdpi.com/foods/foods-13-03327/article_deploy/html/images/foods-13-03327-g001.png.

13.2.3. Shelf Life and Expiration Dates

Shelf life and expiration dates are critical to food safety and the prevention of the risk of foodborne illness. Shelf life is the duration that products can be safely consumed and remain within the desired quality. Shelf life is established by several factors, including storage, packaging, and intrinsic properties of the food. These terms need to be understood by food handlers and consumers alike, as improper handling and storage can lead to contamination and spoilage of food. Education on such parameters, especially for restaurant and other food service unit food handlers, is essential. Most food handlers within the food sector do not possess sufficient knowledge about food safety, which potentially results in increased instances of foodborne disease related to the consumption of spoiled or improperly stored food (Bushu et al., 2022). Consumers utilize the expiration date as a cue to identify the best quality and safety of foods. But uncertainty also exists in the description of these dates, such as best by, sell by, and use by. Any of these terms can indicate a range of food attributes. Based on these, people get the wrong idea about when to discard food. Most consumers, for instance, mistakenly think that food is unsafe to eat just after the expiry date without realizing that some foods can be safe to consume even if stored well. This misunderstanding is the reason for preventable food wastage, aggravating issues in sustainability and food insecurity. Courses of education for food center volunteers have been initiated to induce an increase in knowledge about safe food practices, thus minimizing risks from foods beyond their expiration dates (Anderson et al., 2020). The use of shelf life and expiration dates is not just limited at home but extends to public health at a broader level too. Food distribution channels, particularly those located in lower-income areas, often face challenges due to expiration dates and quality issues. Food bank donations can sometimes be near or even past their expiration dates, which, without proper education and safety precautions, jeopardizes public health. Ensuring that food handlers and volunteers are aware of such considerations for safety can go a long way in minimizing the risk of foodborne disease, thereby ensuring the recipients receive safe and healthy food options. Strengthening food safety education and incorporating an objective perception of shelf life and expiration dates, communities can enhance public health indicators and promote nutritional availability for vulnerable populations (Bushu et al., 2022).

13.3. Understanding Food Contamination

Food contamination is a multifaceted issue underpinning the necessity of proper food handling and storage due to the fact that it literally leads to foodborne illness. Contaminants can, by and large, be categorized as biological, chemical, and physical agents that all represent varying degrees of threat to food safety. Biological contaminants, including bacteria, viruses, and parasites, are of the most concern since they can grow explosively under certain conditions. The global burden of foodborne disease is staggering, with approximately 600 million cases annually, emphasizing the need for adequate food safety procedures. The majority of the countries, particularly in the Middle East and North Africa, have recognized the gravity of this food safety problem and have initiated reformative actions in their systems of food control in order to avoid foodborne diseases as well as protect consumers (Faour et al., 2019). Environmental sanitation plays an essential part in avoiding food contamination. Practices such as regular cleanliness, proper disposal of waste, and the lack of pests are imperative in preventing biological contamination. Cross-contamination, which is typically caused by unsanitary food handling practices, is also a risk factor, and food handlers should practice hygienic methods when they handle and store food.

Training and education in food safety are imperative components in preventing food contamination. In addition, the incorporation of high-tech tools, including next-generation sequencing (NGS), is revolutionizing food microbiology. Through this approach, analysis of microbial communities can be done in great detail, making it easier to identify sources of contamination and improve risk assessment procedures (Jagadeesan et al., 2018). When food contamination is analyzed, it is clear that a systems approach needs to be followed to tackle the intricacies of food safety. The imposition of strict food regulations and enforcement, along with efficient food control management and monitoring systems, can construct a safer food chain. The five essential elements developed by the FAO/WHO provide an essential framework to design effective national food control systems that are important for countries that are grappling with high rates of foodborne illness. But effective implementation relies on mass public participation, continuous learning, and continuous government support to ensure that food safety practices are being done at all levels. Ultimately, building a culture of food safety rooted in cleanliness of the environment is the foundation in preventing foodborne illness and promoting public health (Faour et al., 2019) (Figure 13.7).

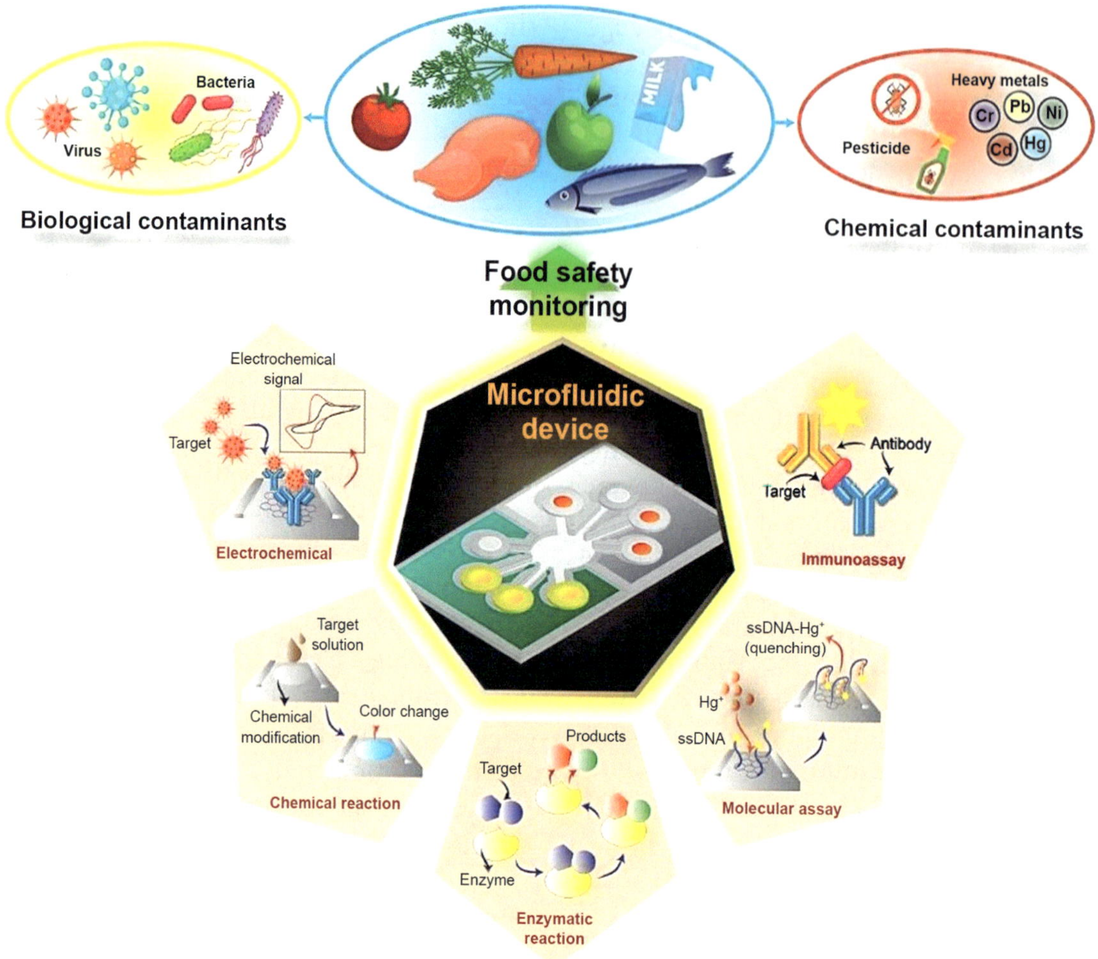

Figure 13.7. Food contamination.

Source: https://ars.els-cdn.com/content/image/1-s2.0-S0963996923013479-gr2.jpg.

13.3.1. Types of Food Contaminants

Food contamination is a critical topic in the area of food safety and environmental sanitation, and it occurs in numerous forms that can be detrimental to human health. Overall, food contaminants are agents that are biological, chemical, and physical. Some of the biologic contaminants include bacteria, viruses, and parasites, and they present the highest potential for the causation of foodborne diseases. The development of such pathogens in food products underscores the need for stringent handling and storage practices to prevent contamination. As expressed in the learning endeavors at the Western Institute for Food Safety and Security, understanding the interaction between environmental factors and food production can enhance efforts directed towards reducing these risks (Angelos et al., 2017). Managing biological contaminants effectively by targeted education is important for the provision of a clean food supply as well as public health. Chemical contaminants, on the other hand, cover a range of chemicals, including pesticides, heavy metals, and food additives, which can enter the food supply inadvertently. The impact of the contaminants is not only immediate health effects, but instead, the contaminants have the potential to cause chronic diseases and disorders in the long run. For example, farming methods using intensive use of chemical pesticides and fertilizers can unknowingly leave toxic residues on crops, necessitating that consumers and producers both have food safety as a top priority. Educational programs, such as those funded by the USDA's Initiative for Future Agriculture and Food Systems, attempt to assist small and medium-sized farms in reducing safety threats related to chemical contaminants in their produce, ultimately contributing to a safer food supply and more sustainable agricultural production (Brady et al., 2005). In addition, physical contaminants such as extraneous materials like glass, metal, and plastic pose a special risk of causing severe injuries when consumed unwittingly by customers. These contaminants are mostly introduced during food handling and processing; thus, food processing environments must have rigorous hygiene practices in place. The use of preventive interventions like staff training and equipment checks can prove greatly effective in combating physical contamination. By developing a culture that makes safety a top priority, stakeholders in the food sector can assist in curbing the occurrence of food contaminants, thereby promoting consumer confidence in food. Recognizing that food contaminants are multifaceted heightens the appeal for a comprehensive food safety approach where environmental sanitation and safe food handling converge (Figure 13.8).

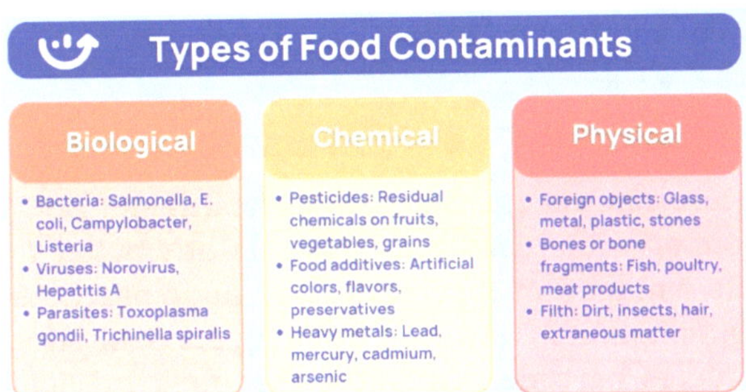

Figure 13.8. Types of food contaminants.

Source: https://cdn.prod.website-files.com/62294553e 9aeea20d15d7bc2/66fc41dd8df66971e19c4e06_649835e783cdc029eee7d924_Xenia%2520for% 2520Trailer%2520Maintenance.webp.

13.3.2. Sources of Contamination

Contamination of food can occur from all sorts of sources, each of which can have serious implications for public health and food safety. Microbial contamination is perhaps one of the most common, usually as a result of poor handling, storage, and preparation procedures. For example, bacteria like *Escherichia coli* and *Staphylococcus aureus* may make their way into food supplies through inadequately equipped food handlers or dirty, unclean kitchen environments. The complexity of the food system calls for multilateral intervention in managing contamination, and understanding the interrelation between food production and environmental practices is central to this. Notification of stakeholders about the correlations can restrict contamination risks and enhance food security, as noted by Angelos et al. (2017). Confronting sources of contamination thus requires cooperation from schools, policymakers, and campaigners on food safety in calling for robust standards of safety. The other significant source of contamination is cross-contamination, where disease-causing agents are transferred from food to food, oftentimes through contaminated equipment or surfaces. This is particularly common in settings like boarding senior high schools, where the food handlers may not have adequate training on safe handling of food. A study that investigated food safety practices and attitudes among the food handlers in the institutions revealed the presence of foodborne pathogens in cooked food, alongside obstacles caused by inadequate equipment and resources. Even though the respondents showed sufficient knowledge regarding food safety principles, application is still ineffective, as reported in Amuquandoh et al. (2020). Understanding these barriers is important in developing successful training and food safety programs that can reduce distinct sources of contamination and promote healthier food environments. Environmental conditions also play a part in contaminating food since they can introduce harmful substances to food supplies. Poor sanitation facilities, poor waste management, and poor water supply all raise the risk of foodborne disease. Where environmental sanitation is weak, as in the case of some developing nations, the likelihood of food contamination is very high. Such interdependence underscores the importance of applying the One Health concept, which encourages a holistic approach to human, animal, and environmental health. By taking environmental concerns into account in the policy-making and education of food safety, the stakeholders aim to create an overall framework that not only ensures food quality but also ensures ecological equilibrium, as noted in Angelos et al. (2017). Holistic intervention in food safety extends beyond immediate handling procedures to include more extensive environmental sanitation facets.

13.3.3. Impact of Contamination on Food Safety

Food contamination has severe consequences for public health and has resulted in increased rates of foodborne diseases. Foodborne diseases are primarily attributed to microbial agents, which can increase through unsafe handling of food and other poor practices like inadequate cooking, poor avoidance of cross-contamination, and lack of adequate sanitation within food preparation environments. Empirical studies have demonstrated that food service workers possess varying levels of food safety knowledge, which affects their ability to undertake safe procedures. For instance, while 50% of food handlers indicated that they washed their hands often during food preparation, high microbial contamination levels continued on food-contact surfaces, particularly in establishments with low food safety consciousness. This inconsistency demonstrates that knowledge is no guarantee of safe food handling practice, thereby implying that it requires a multidimensional intervention to address contamination and achieve food safety effectively (Issa-Zacharia et al., 2025). Environmental sanitation has a key role to play in the prevention of food contamination as well as ensuring the safety of food products. Where sanitary conditions are not good, the risk of contamination is greatly increased. For example, abattoirs in unsanitary areas are discovered, during inspection, not just to be causative of meat contamination but also a source of an extended public health risk. Inadequate waste disposal facilities, inadequate personal hygiene of staff, and overall unhygienic environments may result in mass exposure to pathogens. These findings emphasize the need for high standards of hygiene levels and practices in food production plants. Raising the sanitary levels in food processing plants, for example, abattoirs, is essential to avert the risk from the consumption of contaminated meat and, by default, protect public health (N/A, 2024). Ultimately, the interface between contamination, food safety, and environmental sanitation underscores an important public health problem necessitating concerted action by various stakeholders. Training programs for food service workers, especially, may assist in enhancing their knowledge regarding appropriate food handling practices, but regulatory frameworks with a hard core must be put in place to provide for the discipline of sanitation procedures in food processing facilities. Routine microbial examination and testing should also be included in food safety protocols to detect contamination before the consumers. The long-term goal is to create a holistic system that not only implements measures to address the immediate risks of contamination but also establishes a culture of food safety. This integrative process can significantly lower foodborne diseases, thus safeguarding public health and enhancing nutrition in general (Figure 13.9).

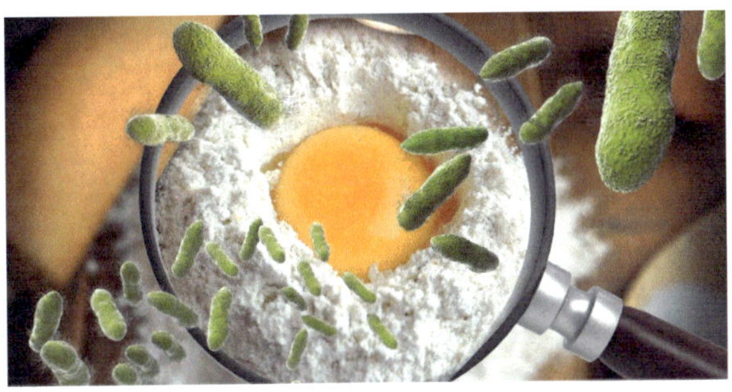

Figure 13.9. Preventing cross-contamination.

Source: https://external-content.duckduckgo.com/iu/?u=https%3A%2F%2Fwww.foodsafe.net.nz%2Fwp-content%2Fuploads%2F2021%2F08%2FPreventing-cross-contamination-risks.jpg&f=1&nofb=1&ipt=a86dcd2b32277f8749d1fe24269a1394d9d370656a8b6b0fc1af6d4265554b23.

13.4. Foodborne Illnesses

Foodborne illness is a serious public health problem caused by the consumption of contaminated food. It can be caused by many factors, including bacteria, viruses, and parasites, which, under improper management and storage of food, thrive to cause infections. The prevalence of foodborne infections calls for acquiring broad knowledge of food preparation and food handling practices. For instance, adhering to safe food handling practices, such as right cooking temperatures and avoiding cross-contamination, is essential in minimizing these risks. An effective education model, such as the One Health model embraced by the Western Institute for Food Safety and Security, defines the relationship between food safety, environmental factors, and public health and emphasizes multidisciplinary efforts towards controlling foodborne pathogens (Angelos et al., 2017). Furthermore, the microbiological quality of institutional food in institutions such as schools underscores the importance of strict measures for food safety. Research aimed at boarding senior high schools indicates that there are disconcerting findings regarding the microbiological safety of food in schools, in that it carries risky bacteria such as *Escherichia coli* and *Staphylococcus aureus*. These microbes can cause severe consequences to health if not controlled, and it is therefore important that food handlers possess well-acquired knowledge in food safety practice. In the case observed in the Volta Region in Ghana, though food handlers demonstrated adequate knowledge in food safety, limitations in the form of a lack of equipment supply and irregularity in water supply are obstacles to effective practice application. Hence, such challenges demand strategic intervention in order to improve food safety in such environments (Amuquandoh et al., 2020). Hygiene in the environment cannot be overstated in the prevention of foodborne illnesses. Proper environmental hygiene allows for safe food handling by creating sanitary conditions needed for food preparation and storage. Without maximum hygiene levels in food preparation rooms, the risk of contamination increases, thus leading to an increase in foodborne illnesses. Implementing strict cleaning protocols and regular health checks enhances compliance with food safety legislation, maintaining food environments safe for consumption. Furthermore, promoting environmental sanitation not only protects public health but also reinforces the broader role of food safety within nutrition. This strict action creates a safety culture and accountability that are essential for preventing future incidents and maintaining the people's well-being (Figure 13.10).

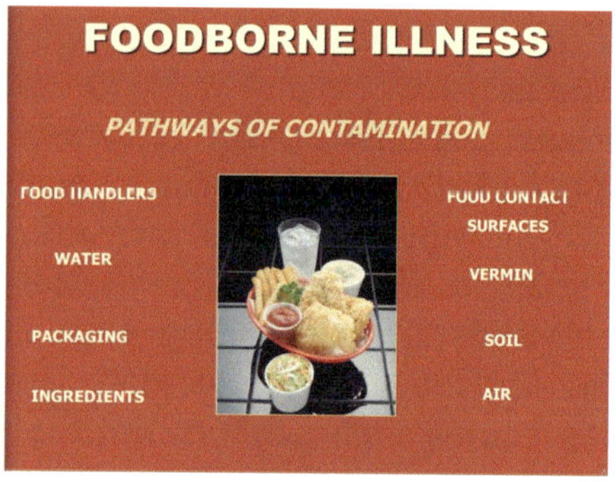

Figure 13.10. Foodborne illness.

Source: https://image.slideserve.com/328925/foodborne-illness6-l.jpg.

13.4.1. Common Pathogens Causing Foodborne Illnesses

Foodborne illness remains a significant public health concern, with a vast array of widespread pathogens that may contaminate food supplies. The most frequently implicated bacteria are Salmonella, *Escherichia coli* (*E. coli*), and *Listeria monocytogenes*. *Salmonella* is particularly known for its association with undercooked eggs and chicken and is highly risky in environments where food handling protocols are substandard. *E coli*, which includes the O157:H7 strain, leads to acute gastroenteritis and is traditionally linked with leafy greens as a contamination vehicle and undercooked ground beef. The ability of Listeria to proliferate at refrigeration temperatures underscores the imperative to have rigorous food safety measures in place. Monitoring and education regarding these pathogens need to be continuous to reduce foodborne illness rates and guarantee public health, particularly among vulnerable populations. Besides bacterial pathogens, viruses such as norovirus and Hepatitis A are also prevalent agents responsible for acute foodborne outbreaks. Norovirus is very contagious and may be frequently spread by contaminated food or contact with contaminated surfaces; therefore, it is a frequent cause of outbreaks in communal settings like restaurants and schools. Hepatitis A, on the other hand, presents a significant hazard via food handlers who have not followed norms of hygiene, repeating the connection between environmental habits of hygiene and food safety. The stark reality of these endemic viruses increases the demand for public health measures that will improve food safety awareness. As noted, it is crucial that food safety and environmental sanitation converge in an effort to reduce risks posed by these viral pathogens and guarantee food preparation and consumption safety, especially within institutions like hospices where patients are immunocompromised (Nkhebenyane et al., 2018). Because foodborne pathogens are of such nature, correct methods of handling, storage, and preparation can significantly minimize risks from contamination. Safe heat treatment temperatures are crucial because the majority of these pathogens are destroyed by proper heat treatment. Clean refrigeration practices also come into play in the prevention of the growth of such pathogens as Salmonella and Listeria. Where susceptible populations are involved in an environment, for example, in hospices, rigorous hygiene practices must be implemented. A holistic approach that combines awareness with in-situ practice for food handlers can significantly reduce the threat of foodborne infection. Emerging evidence regarding antimicrobial resistance among pathogens affirms the need for highly informed food safety experts who can be in a position to modify practices in response to current health trends and studies (Angelos et al., 2017). Consequently, a culture of food safety training is imperative in the avoidance of foodborne illness and instilling a culture of health in food-related industries.

13.4.2. Symptoms and Health Effects

The symptoms of foodborne illness could vary considerably based on the etiological agent and the susceptibility of the individual, e.g., age and overall health. A few of the typical symptoms are gastrointestinal disturbance, which can be nausea, vomiting, diarrhea, and abdominal cramps, and generally occur 24 to 48 hours after consuming contaminated food. In severe situations, symptoms may advance to dehydration, kidney failure, or even death, particularly in most vulnerable groups, such as the elderly and immunocompromised. Furthermore, certain pathogens lead to long-term impacts on health, like persistent gastrointestinal disease or Guillain-Barré syndrome, a rare nervous system disorder. Recognizing these symptoms is important for early detection of foodborne illness so that the individuals may get medical attention promptly and minimize overall morbidity related to such diseases (Monarez et al., 2025). Foodborne illnesses not only carry direct risks for health but also have a wide-ranging effect on public health. According to recent data, approximately 800 foodborne outbreak cases and 15,000 associated cases occur annually in the United States, indicating a significant healthcare system burden (Monarez et al., 2025). The economic cost due to such outbreaks includes medical expenses, lost productivity, and regulatory agency costs in addressing outbreaks. For instance, food poisoning outbreaks from unhygienic handling of food in street markets underscore the significance of environmental hygiene. In Brazil's Colatina, the unhygienic conditions of meat stalls created enormous cross-contamination risks. Hence, control of signs and medical consequences of food poisoning becomes a reminder of the urgency of having more effective food safety steps and public health awareness campaigns. The role environmental hygiene plays in reducing the effects of foodborne disease cannot be overestimated. Food contamination by microbes often results from poor handling practices, including improper hand washing. For example, research indicates that inadequate temperature control and simultaneous food handling and cash handling significantly increase contamination potential in open markets. These breaks in hygiene regimes account for the spread of pathogens as well as bacterial persistence between food storage. As evident from the changing outbreak rates, effective environmental hygiene regimes—like constant monitoring and scrupulous adherence to food safety procedures—are required to alleviate the incidence of foodborne illness (Monarez et al., 2025). By establishing a culture of hygiene in food handling and storage units, the health impact of foodborne disease can be significantly avoided and a safer food supply chain facilitated (Figure 13.11).

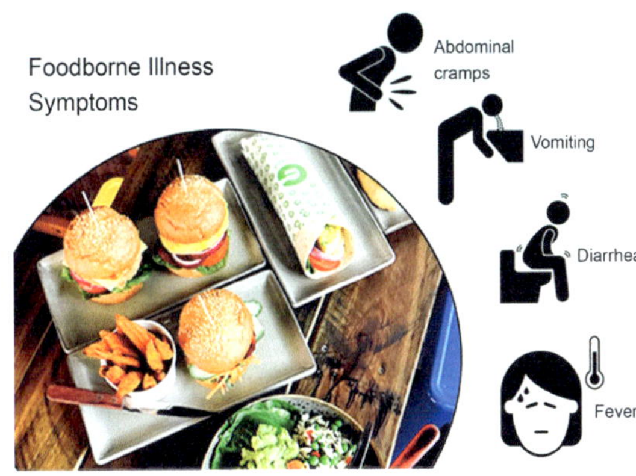

Figure 13.11. Cause of foodborne illness.

Source: https://www.healthcheckup.com/wp-content/uploads/2018/03/foodborne-illness-symptoms-500x292.jpg.

13.4.3. Statistics on Foodborne Illness Outbreaks

Foodborne disease outbreaks represent a major public health concern worldwide, characterized by the transmission of pathogens primarily through contaminated food products. Approximately 600 million foodborne illness cases are estimated to be reported annually, with an alarming figure of 420,000 deaths yearly due to poor food handling. The largest number of outbreaks is traced to animal-derived products, where zoonotic pathogens such as Salmonella and *E. coli* are of special significance. The burden of these diseases precipitates unevenly in developing countries, whose lack of conducive food safety standards and infrastructure can lead to heightened exposure. The understanding of the outbreak trends is thus paramount to the development of successful interventions and public health interventions towards the reduction of the incidences of foodborne diseases, thereby the need for setting up conducive, safe food handling and storage practices in risk reduction. The major foodborne pathogens highlight the complex nature of such outbreaks, particularly aimed at animal foods. Foodborne microbes, particularly pathogenic bacteria like S. aureus and L. monocytogenes, pose serious threats to public health because they grow in conditions that support their multiplication and are commonly associated with meat, milk, and egg foods.

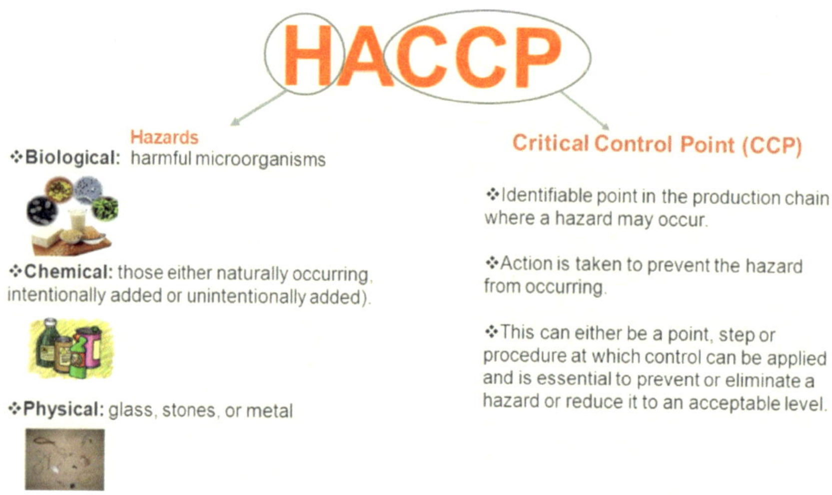

Figure 13.12. Hazard analysis critical control point (HACCP) systems for foodborne illness.

Source: http://isoaudit.or.kr/wp-content/uploads/2020/11/HACCPHazardsCriticalControlPointCCP.jpg?ckattempt=1.

Prevalence of such pathogens necessitates strict monitoring and enforcement of hygiene levels at all levels of the food chain. Hence, good manufacturing practices (GMP), rigorous sanitation protocols, and Hazard Analysis Critical Control Point (HACCP) are essential to reduce the hazards caused by such pathogens. By targeting efforts towards improving these practices, foodborne illness rates caused by contaminated animal products can be significantly reduced, which in turn will enhance public health gains overall. Foodborne illness outbreak data also underscore the significance of education and behavior change among food handlers and consumers. Research shows that the large number of meat handlers with poor knowledge and awareness of maintaining safe food procedures contributes to the possibility of outbreaks. For example, a survey showed that despite 66.4% of meat handlers demonstrating a good standard of hygiene, there remains a disturbing lack of concern for hand washing after various operations like sneezing and coughing. This shortage not only highlights the necessity for more training programs regarding proper food handling but also raises the requirements of county health departments to exert control and direction to ensure compliance. Intervention of such behavior determinants is important since amplifying food handlers' attitudes and behaviors can lead to a food service environment that is safer, eventually protecting consumers against foodborne illness risks (Abebe et al., 2020; Yenealem et al., 2020) (Figure 13.12).

13.5. Environmental Hygiene in Food Preparation Areas

Environmental hygiene integration into food preparation sites is crucial to ensure food safety and prevent contamination that can lead to foodborne illnesses. This intricate practice requires a mix of practices, such as the use of clean surfaces, proper waste disposal, and the provision of proper ventilation. Cleanliness is not only a necessity for bodily appearance but also for microbial control; a dirty area can act as a reservoir for pathogens that have the potential to create severe health risks to consumers. Hygiene is defined by an understanding of the interlinks between food production and environmental impact, as indicated by the subject covered by the Western Institute for Food Safety and Security as requiring a complex understanding of food safety through a One Health perspective (Angelos et al., 2017). Through intensified training and regular practice, food handlers can reduce the risk of contamination and foster a culture of safety in food preparation settings. Cross-contamination is a significant risk in food preparation settings. The risk arises when harmful microorganisms from raw foods, particularly meats and fish, are conveyed to ready-to-eat foods. Preventive measures, such as the use of separate equipment and utensils for each food, are required to minimize such a risk. In addition, the application of systems like Hazard Analysis Critical Control Point (HACCP) is fundamental in scientifically identifying and controlling points of danger in food preparation activities. As policymakers on food safety have stated in their discussions, such gaps require multi-disciplinary measures that combine data from all supply chain levels (Anonymous et al., 2025). By focusing on policies of hygiene and analytical tools, food outlets are capable of providing enhanced protection for public health as well as for consumer confidence in food safety measures. Environmental sanitation should not be overlooked regarding nutrition, as the quality of food can be affected even by dirty preparation environments.

The microbiologic laws underscore that environmental cleanliness is crucial to maintaining food quality and nutritional value. Unless food preparation surfaces are kept in perfect sanitary conditions, not only is the risk of foodborne illness elevated, but the nutritional content of food is decreased by spoilage and by microbial action. Moreover, teaching the importance of cleanliness to food handlers can be extended to community education about safe handling, storage, and food preparation practices. Thus, environmental hygiene is an essential component of the armor against foodborne illness and is a critical component in supporting nutrition and food security in general in society (Angelos et al., 2017; Anonymous et al., 2025) (Figure 13.13).

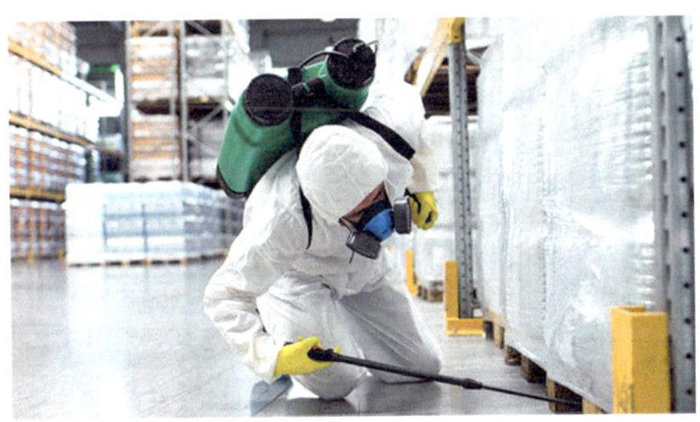

Figure 13.13. Environmental hygiene services.

Source: https://vergo.uk/wp-content/uploads/2022/07/shutterstock-711673786-resized.jpg.

13.5.1. Importance of Cleanliness in Kitchens

Kitchen' cleanliness is an important area of food safety and overall environmental hygiene, and it serves as a first line of defense against foodborne illnesses. As a means of minimizing the risk of foodborne illnesses from poor handling and storage of food, a clean kitchen is the future. It has been demonstrated by research that poor hygiene can be a cause of high production of harmful microorganisms, with pathogens like Salmonella and *E. coli* leading to severe outbreaks of food poisoning. The immediate connection between kitchen cleanliness and contamination rate emphasizes the importance of meticulous sanitation practices, a concern underscored by health department efforts (Waters et al., 2011). Such practices, aside from providing a safer eat-out experience, also provide long-term sustainability of food centers through the guarantee of consumer confidence and repeat patronage. Also, the enforcement of rigorous cleanliness protocols complements the ongoing training and education of food handlers. By inducing a hygiene culture in the kitchen, employees are encouraged to maintain safe food handling practices every day. An aggressive strategy like this is necessary for the prevention of foodborne illness relating to contamination caused by unsafe food handling or cooking. The success of regular audits and subsequent appraisal, demonstrated in various studies, depicts how notified inspections can suppress major violations such as equipment sanitation and hygiene protocols by an enormous extent (Waters et al., 2011). These processes are the solution to having a workplace where compliance and the health and well-being of all guests are priorities, revealing the manifold benefits of enjoying a clean kitchen. In regions where foodborne illnesses are prevalent, cleanliness becomes even more important. For instance, warm and humid climates in certain regions may enhance the growth of bacteria, and it is therefore important that food establishments maintain high cleanliness standards. Governments usually respond by implementing stringent levels of sanitation controls as well as food handlers' education programs emphasizing the importance of their role in preventing contamination threats. Through observing the relationship between food consumption-related health benefits and sanitation, food service managers have an educated basis for altering procedures. Only through a sustained commitment to cleanliness can kitchens be successful in preserving public health while optimizing nutritional advantages for the consumer. Environmental cleanliness has an unavoidable function to safeguard both the food supply and population health.

13.5.2. Sanitization of Surfaces and Equipment

Surface and equipment cleaning is an important component of food safety and environmental sanitation in foodservice operations. Surfaces that come into contact with food, such as counters, cutting boards, and utensils, become breeding grounds for pathogens if they are not sanitized. Routine sanitation not only protects against the hazard of cross-contamination but also significantly lessens the likelihood of foodborne illness from microbial contamination. Furthermore, compliance with standardized sanitation protocols is crucial to ensuring health regulations and industry best practices. A food safety audit's evidence shows that inadequately executed sanitation protocols were associated with high levels of microbes on food preparation surfaces, suggesting a need to enhance such protocols further in order to improve overall food safety outcomes in various food service settings (Asim et al., 2017). Microbiological safety of raw foods, particularly of ready-to-eat foods such as salads, relies on the cleanliness of cutting boards and equipment on which they are handled. Recent evidence indicates that despite visual inspection scores not always correlating with microbial counts, issues like cross-contamination do have concrete implications on pathogen levels, such as Listeria spp., on cutting boards and utensils. It is evident that regular checking and improving sanitization procedures are needed in order to reduce threats regarding foodborne pathogens (Faour-Klingbeil et al., 2016). Facilities should implement thorough training procedures on the effective sanitization technique and give high priority to maintaining clean environments to safeguard public health. Moreover, successful sanitization not only guarantees reducing contamination risk but also promotes growing customer satisfaction and trust. As food service organizations demonstrate consistently respect for hygiene and food safety standards, they not only ensure regulatory requirements but also have a positive image in the eyes of consumers. Consumer trust is vital, particularly with the growing demand for healthy and safe food. Units that implement rigorous sanitation are likely to find that their adherence to hygiene protocol effectively reduces the number of foodborne illness outbreaks, ultimately enhancing public health programs and maintaining a safer food environment for society (Asim et al., 2017). Thus, ongoing investment in sanitation facilities and staff training is essential to food safety success (Figure 13.14).

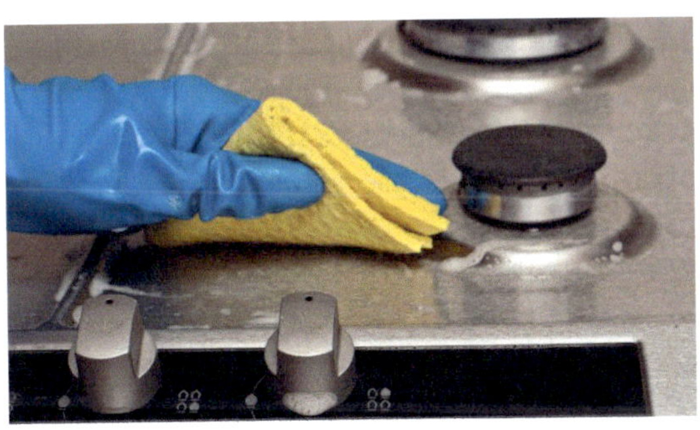

Figure 13.14. Sanitization of surfaces and equipment.

Source: https://blog.foodsafety.ca/hubfs/Imported_Blog_Media/Understanding_the_difference_between_cleaning_sanitizing.jpg.

13.5.3. Pest Control Measures

Effective pest control measures are crucial in ensuring food safety and environmental sanitation. Infestation of rodents, insects, and other pests in food storage units and food preparation environments can result in high levels of contamination. Such pests carry pathogens, which could result in foodborne illness, posing a direct risk to public health. An efficient pest control program is comprised of both preventive and remedial measures, including thorough facility inspections, sealing every possible entry point, and following strict sanitation procedures. It is essential that food operations adopt an integrated pest management (IPM) system, which combines several means of monitoring and controlling pests without having a negative impact on food safety. By prioritizing these steps as the most important, institutions can minimize the likelihood of contamination and establish a sanitary environment for safe food handling practices. Education cannot be overemphasized in implementing measures of pest control, particularly in agricultural environments. Farmers, educators, and policymakers need coordination to establish a multi-pronged strategy that counteracts food safety concerns. Educational courses, such as those developed by the Western Institute for Food Safety and Security, aim to inform stakeholders of the intersections of food production, pest management, and environmental health. The learning system in these courses emphasizes understanding of pest behavior and the ecological ramifications of agricultural practices, therefore informing pest management decisions. Research indicates that capacity building and training small- and medium-scale farms with resources can significantly enhance their ability to mitigate pest-related risks and promote sustainable practices (Brady et al., 2005). Ultimately, cultivating a pest control culture of awareness and sensitivity is crucial to ensuring safe food systems. Bringing pest management into food safety protocols not only guards individual health but also has broader environmental sustainability implications. Effective pest management can reduce the application of chemical pesticides, which may be dangerous to the environment and result in resource depletion. In taking environmentally friendly approaches to pest control, such as through biological controls or habitat modification, food producers can maintain ecological balance without compromising food safety. Moreover, enhancing pest control strategies enhances food security initiatives that stabilize food availability without compromising environmental integrity. As per the guidelines released by various agricultural programs, implementation of this knowledge into practice will have significant benefits for the consumers as well as the producers (Angelos et al., 2017). In summary, pest management is an essential element in a comprehensive food safety plan that links public health, environmental sanitation, and nutrition.

13.6. The Role of Environmental Hygiene in Nutrition

Good environmental hygiene is a cornerstone of nutrition since it minimizes the risks of foodborne illness, which otherwise can significantly detract from dietary health. Food can be contaminated with a range of pathogens of illness and therefore can interfere with nutrient absorption and general health. Poor hygiene in food preparation, handling, and storage not only heightens the risk of food contamination but also presents major obstacles to sustaining good dietary health. For instance, food handling techniques such as washing and cooking ensure fruits and meat are free from pathogenic and disease-causing bacteria. By ensuring clean surroundings, whether at home or in manufacturing facilities, people can significantly reduce the risk of foodborne diseases, thus improving nutritional outcomes. This principle focuses on adding rigorous hygiene processes as an integral part in a comprehensive strategy for enhanced food safety and nutritional health. The active interface between agronomic practices and the sanitation of the environment is a key function to ensure food safety. Filthiness usually originates from the farm surroundings, and hence, soil and irrigation water are a priority area of concern. Research indicates that there are significant health risks from bacteria such as Salmonella and *E. coli* that could be transported in contaminated irrigation water and farm soil (Iwu et al., 2019). Besides posing a danger to human health, such pathogens risk developing antimicrobial resistance, complicating treatment and setting higher standards for food safety. Recognizing that the path to nutritious food begins well before it reaches the consumer's plate emphasizes the importance of the implementation of hygiene measures on the preharvest stage. Public health and the integrity of our food supply are safeguarded by interventions in minimizing contamination during agricultural operations, demonstrating the inextricable link between environmental sanitation and nutrition. Moreover, advancements in food technology, such as cell-cultured meat and seafood cultivation, offer new opportunities for enhancing food hygiene and safety. Such technologies require an efficient system for measuring safety to ensure the nutritional benefit of such products is attained without imposing new hazards (Kimberly et al., 2021). Comprehensive safety assessments for both potential biological and chemical hazards in the production process are critical. Not only do these assessments ensure consumer health safety, but they also foster consumer confidence in novel food technologies. As more attention is called for regarding food's safe and environmentally friendly sources, integrating environmental sanitation into these technologies becomes essential. Lastly, the meeting of food technology and hygiene procedures will become crucial for the future of nutrition, such that innovations become magnified for public health benefits (Figure 13.15).

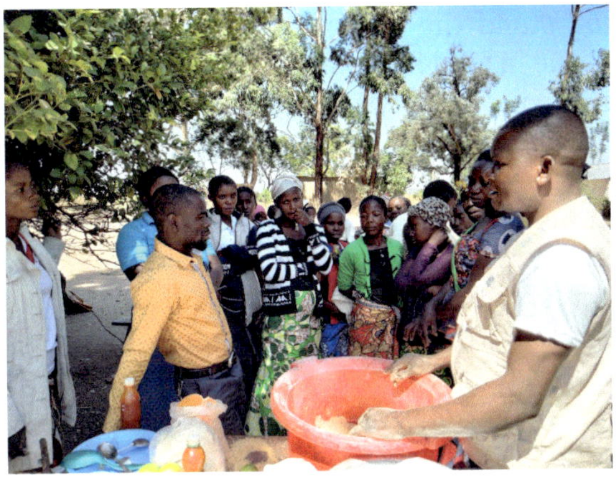

Figure 13.15. Nutrition, hygiene, and environmental protection.

Source: https://www.coopi.org/admin/assets/js/ckeditor/kcfinder/upload/files/images/IMG20220604124140%281%29.jpg.

13.6.1. Connection Between Hygiene and Nutrient Preservation

The relationship between hygiene practices and nutrient preservation plays a significant role in ensuring food safety and nutrition. Following due respect in terms of hygiene protocols in food handling and storage significantly reduces the chances of food contamination by harmful pathogens that lead to food spoilage. Foodborne illnesses often originate from poor food environments characterized by unhygienic conditions conducive to the proliferation of harmful bacteria, as manifested by outbreaks of Salmonella in contaminated foods. When food is contaminated, not only does it pose health risks, but the nutritional value can also be forfeited through spoilage and the destruction of essential vitamins and minerals. Hence, adopting good hygiene habits is paramount for maintaining consumer health as well as food product purity of nutrients, which underscores the significance of raising awareness and compliance with standard food safety standards. Furthermore, having sound environmental hygiene practices is crucial in the maintenance of nutrients. Contamination can be brought about by a number of factors, including improper storage of foods, inadequate cleaning of preparation plates, and raw material handling. For instance, cross-contamination between raw and cooked food can introduce pathogens that not only undermine human health but also undermine food quality and nutrient preservation. Techniques such as correct refrigeration and effective cleaning procedures play a central part in minimizing such risks by maintaining foods under the best conditions for intake. As mentioned under food safety systems, enhancing environmental sanitation is also a move towards safeguarding the nutrients for effective human nutrition, thus also enhancing not just health but also well-being in populations. Besides the direct impact on food safety and nutrient preservation, there is an even broader implication for sustainable food systems. Maintaining clean food environments extends beyond individual health, as it enhances overall food security and nutritional quality within communities. The significance of safe food systems, according to food security rhetoric in Africa, encompasses the worth of good nutrition, productive agriculture, and equitable access to safe food. Practices that promote hygienic habits not only improve the safety of food items but also strengthen consumer confidence in their nutritional adequacy. Lastly, it is crucial to discuss hygiene and how it impacts the maintenance of nutrients to make sound strategies that underpin public health and maximize equity in food systems, such that food becomes accessible to everyone in a safe and nutritious form (Onyeaka et al., 2024; Oluteru et al., 2024).

13.6.2. Impact of Environmental Factors on Food Quality

The influence of the environment on food quality is significant, with varying factors such as soil condition, water quality, and atmospheric conditions directly affecting agricultural output. For instance, soil nutrient level determines the level of crop development and health, which, in effect, determines the nutritional quality of the output food. Sustainable agriculture, which involves natural resource preservation, is an important factor in reversing the adverse impact of pollution and climate change on food quality. Practicing techniques like crop rotation and organic farming can improve soil fertility and its biodiversity, consequently making the crops healthier. As reiterated in recent research, incorporating a One Health perspective in food safety education can promote awareness of the environmental implications of food production (Angelos et al., 2017). This interdisciplinary approach is able to instill a greater appreciation of the fact that environmental stewardship is essentially intertwined with food quality and safety. Water quality, which is otherwise an overlooked environmental factor, plays an important role in food safety and nutrient retention. Contaminated sources of water could bring pathogens and chemical residues into food, which could contribute to foodborne illnesses. Research determining individual cases, such as those conducted in boarding senior high schools in Ghana, shows that poor supply and sanitation facilities directly hinder food safety practices among food handlers (Amuquandoh et al., 2020). Lack of access to clean water not only limits the ability to perform proper hygienic practices when preparing food but also taints the overall safety and microbiological quality of the food being served. It is thus crucial that the food handlers are provided with clean water and good sanitation facilities so as to promote food safety and public health outcomes. Environmental hygiene extends beyond the food manufacturing process and into food storage and handling, where temperature, contamination, and airborne pathogens can have a profound impact on food quality. Storage conditions, such as temperature control, humidity, and sanitation, directly influence the shelf life and sensory attributes of food products. Uncontrolled storage conditions may lead to spoilage, loss of nutrients, and increased risks of contamination by pathogenic organisms. It is important to understand the role played by environmental hygiene in food handling operations in managing foodborne disease. As indicated in the literature available, training programs that help raise awareness about food safety among food handlers can assist in upgrading operational procedures to ensure food quality is preserved from farm to table (Angelos et al., 2017). With these environmental components addressed, stakeholders are able to increase the production of safe and quality food (Figure 13.16).

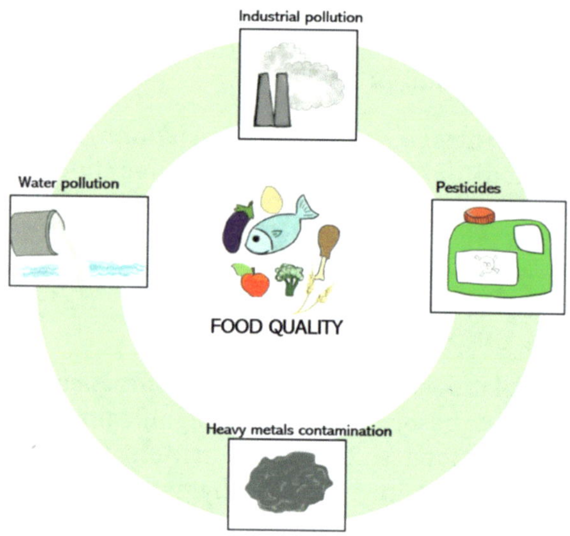

Figure 13.16. Impact of environmental pollutants on food quality.

Source: https://www.researchgate.net/publication/359657684/figure/fig1/AS:11431281211791371@1702493822308/Impact-of-environmental-pollutants-on-food-quality.tif.

13.6.3. Strategies for Improving Environmental Hygiene

Good environmental hygiene is essential in foodborne disease prevention and general food safety. Good manufacturing practices (GMPs) play a critical role in the provision of high levels of hygiene in factories where foods are produced. GMPs entail several preventive actions, including regular cleaning and sanitizing of surfaces, equipment, and storage areas to minimize the risk of contamination. In addition, education programs for procedures related to hygiene can do much to enhance awareness and compliance among food handlers. When staff understand possible hazards, such as zoonotic disease pathogens commonly linked with animal food items, cross-contamination risk is significantly minimized. According to research, some zoonotic bacteria, such as S. aureus and Salmonella species, are the principal causes of a high percentage of foodborne outbreaks, hence emphasizing the importance of strong hygiene practices in reducing exposure to such pathogens (Abebe et al., 2020). Besides the inclusion of strong hygiene practices, the development and use of standardized hazard analysis critical control points (HACCP) systems in food companies are key practices for enhancing environmental hygiene. HACCP provides a methodical system for identifying potential food safety hazards and introducing preventive controls at the food chain's critical points. Targeting risk management and instituting control measures, companies can systematically deal with potential sources of contamination, ultimately providing assurance of public health. Coordination of all these efforts among various stakeholders, such as farmers, distributors, regulators, and consumers, is necessary. This multi-faceted approach recognizes that food safety is not only for food producers but for all those who have an interest in the food chain. Policies and investments that enhance stakeholders' awareness and capacity-building can help further enhance food safety outcomes (Jaffee et al., 2018). In addition, continuous surveillance and monitoring of environmental sanitation practices are essential for addressing emerging issues in food safety. With the rise of multidrug-resistant zoonotic bacteria, robust monitoring programs become essential. Coordinated efforts in the collection and analysis of data on foodborne pathogens can be utilized to inform public health programs and interventions in reducing foodborne disease prevalence. The integration of technological innovations, such as rapid tests and real-time tracking systems, can enhance these monitoring programs. By actively identifying points of contamination, food supply chain actors can intervene in a timely manner to lower risks. Success in such measures relies ultimately on an organic understanding of food safety risks and its commitment to continuous improvement in environmental sanitation practices (Jaffee et al., 2018).

CLOSER LOOK

FOOD HANDLING AND HYGIENE PRACTICES

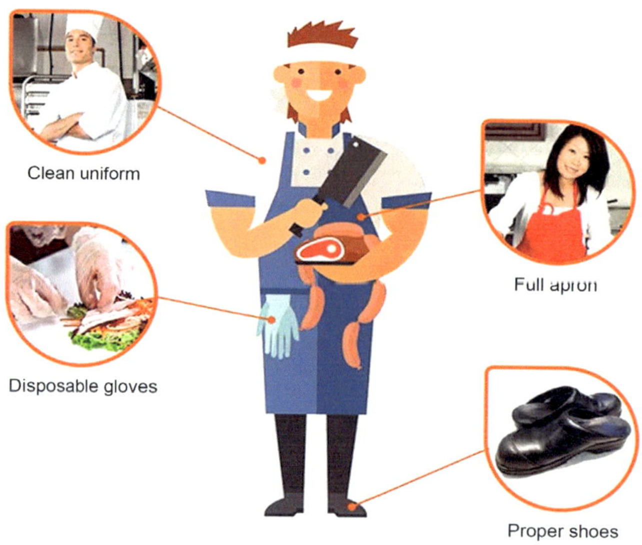

Figure 13.17. Essential personal hygiene and safety practices for kitchen staff, including clean uniforms, aprons, gloves, and proper footwear.

Source: https://www.unileverfoodsolutions.com.my/en/chef-inspiration/food-safety/personal-hygiene-kitchen-safety-tips/jcr:content/parsys/content-aside-footer/textimage_1885460863/image.transform/jpeg-optimized/image.chef_en.jpg.

Food safety requires the call to action to improve food handling and hygiene measures to be central to averting risks associated with foodborne illnesses. The presence of foodborne pathogens justifies extensive education of food handlers, particularly in vulnerable settings such as hospices. Research indicates that a majority of food handlers are not given adequate training, which results in unsafe food preparation practices. For example, it was found that only 32% of food handlers in some studies had formal training on food hygiene standards, highlighting the urgent need for systematic education programs to fill knowledge gaps. By emphasizing good food handling habits, such as avoiding cross-contamination and adequate cooking temperatures, we can really help to minimize outbreaks of foodborne disease, thereby safeguarding the health of high-risk groups, such as those with weakened immune systems due to diseases like HIV/AIDS. Furthermore, the integration of a successful hygiene strategy should be given top priority within total health programs that seek to improve food safety. It is not merely an individual responsibility but a part of public health that requires collective effort from the healthcare professionals, legislators, and society. A unified message regarding the importance of food safety through hygiene practices can bring about behavior change among people of all sections. This appeal is beyond the passing of information regarding proper food handling, but establishing a system where hygiene habits become part of everyday life. By addressing existing obstacles, such as the availability of limited resources and inadequate management support in various food service settings, we are in a position to optimize safety regulation adherence, thus protecting community health. Finally, the role of environmental hygiene in providing safe handling of food cannot be overlooked. Maintaining a clean state for food preparation areas, kitchens, and food storage rooms at all times is crucial in preventing the transmission of pathogens. This entails developing routine cleaning schedules, employing effective cleaning agents, and training workers on the importance of having a clean environment. Research suggests that inadequate infrastructure and poor kitchen conditions usually hinder food safety efforts, requiring investments in food service infrastructure in line with health needs. Joint working between scientists, health authorities, and the public sector can facilitate innovative solutions and dialogue. By paying heed to these critical elements of food safety and environmental hygiene, we can lobby for a healthier future for all, reducing the risk of foodborne illness and enhancing nutritional outcomes.

SUMMARY

The intricate relationship between food safety and environmental sanitation is crucial for the avoidance of foodborne illnesses and public health. The findings presented in this essay clarify that safe storage and handling processes of foods are crucial to protect the integrity of food consumed by vulnerable populations, such as senior high school students in boarding schools. For instance, a study from Ghana revealed pathogens in school food, highlighting the importance of well-planned food hygiene programs as well as adequate training of food handlers to ensure that they are not contaminated and decontaminate themselves to protect the consumers. Barriers, like adequate equipment and erratic water supply, must be removed in order to introduce a culture of safety and hygiene in schools (Amuquandoh et al., 2020). Moreover, understanding how the environment impacts food safety enables stakeholders to integrate effective interventions. Analysis of food safety practices in Louisiana feeding locations was indicative of typical issues such as temperature control and lack of proper personal hygiene, these being the factors that have a significant impact on foodborne illness. These violations help indicate the necessity of the creation of targeted educational materials and hands-on tools for food providers to ensure greater compliance with food safety procedures. With greater focus on food safety as a result of dangers such as the COVID-19 pandemic, the stakeholders have no choice but to make use of advanced communication channels to promulgate accurate information and best practices to effectively (Haynes et al., 2021). Ultimately, constant education and awareness for consumers and handlers alike is still the ticket to improved food safety and nutrition. Through the establishment of a culture that emphasizes hygiene and safe handling of food, public health can be significantly enhanced. The collaboration between stakeholders—e.g., policymakers, teachers, and food service operators—will not only enhance the food safety measures but also provide a sustainable platform for future food security. As this essay suggests, the convergence of food safety within a broad context of environmental hygiene can confer enormous benefits on community health, dietary practices, and the overall well-being of society. As it is apparent, there is a need for ongoing investment in food safety initiatives to ensure that generations yet to come will enjoy access to safe and healthy food (Amuquandoh et al., 2020; Haynes et al., 2021).

Among food safety and environmental sanitation, the most important are the complexities of safe handling and storage of foods. Perhaps one of the essential issues is the risk level of contamination at many stages of food production and consumption. As argued in more recent published works, the issue of linking pathogen data throughout the food supply chain is a pervasive limitation to effective prevention strategies. Inability to trace foodborne pathogens from farm to table undermines efforts to know and manage health risks (Anonymous et al., 2025). There should be more public health interventions and controls directed not just at specific pathogens but also at the general environment of food handling practices in an effort to make consumers safe and decrease the incidence of foodborne illness. Contamination is harmful to health, evidenced by frequent outbreaks of foodborne disease that lay bare systemic flaws in the food safety regulatory system. To design effective preventive strategies, it is crucial to establish the primary drivers of the diseases. A compromised system of regulation has been cited to be at the core of the majority of the contemporary food safety issues, and a redrawing of practices and policies (Levi et al., 2008) is required. The implementation of concerted actions that address the causes of contamination can significantly reduce public health threats. Highlighting the significance of enhancing consumer awareness and education on correct safe food handling procedures can further support such efforts, thereby leading to a drastic reduction in food-related health threats. The role of environmental hygiene in nutrition cannot be overstated, as it dictates the quality of food being supplied to the consumers. Sustaining a sanitary environment during food preparation and food storage significantly lowers risks associated with foodborne pathogens. The connection between environmental hygiene and nutrition indicates that there is an imperative for comprehensive hygiene practices in the food service industry. By undertaking a multidisciplinary approach focused on improving environmental hygiene practices, stakeholders are in a position to successfully control the incidence of foodborne disease and encourage overall public health. Further, successful discoveries and imposition of safer food handling are critical in enhancing a safety culture that focuses on consumer health and nutritional adequacy in food systems (Anonymous et al., 2025; Levi et al., 2008).

REFERENCES

1. Abdul Mutalib, N. A., Nordin, S., Sakai, K., et al. (2015). *An Overview of Foodborne Illness and Food Safety in Malaysia*. https://core.ac.uk/download/153816888.pdf (accessed on 11th June 2025).
2. Abebe, E., Gugsa, G., & Ahmed, M. (2020). Review on major food-borne zoonotic bacterial pathogens. *Journal of Tropical Medicine, 2020*, 1–19. https://doi.org/10.1155/2020/4674235 (accessed on 11th June 2025).
3. Ackerley, L., Bloomfield, S. F., Bockmühl, D., et al. (2018). Containing the burden of infectious diseases is everyone's responsibility: A call for an integrated strategy for developing and promoting hygiene behavior change in home and everyday life. https://core.ac.uk/download/226614717.pdf (accessed on 11th June 2025).
4. Alqurashi, N. A., Priyadarshini, A., & Jaiswal, A. K. (2019). Evaluating food safety knowledge and practices among foodservice staff in Al Madinah hospitals, Saudi Arabia. *Safety, 5*, 9–9. https://doi.org/10.3390/safety5010009 (accessed on 11th June 2025).
5. Amuquandoh, E. F., & Appietu, M. E. (2020). Examining food safety knowledge and the microbiological quality of school meals in Ghana. https://core.ac.uk/download/489417615.pdf (accessed on 11th June 2025).
6. Anderson, S. (2020). *Food Safety and Risk of Foodborne Illness at A Food Center Extension: Toolkit for Front-Line Volunteers*. https://core.ac.uk/download/334981578.pdf (accessed on 11th June 2025).
7. Angelos, J. A., Arens, A. L., Cadriel, J. L., Johnson, et al. (2017). One Health in food safety and security education: Subject matter outline for a curricular framework. https://core.ac.uk/download/323068605.pdf (accessed on 11th June 2025).
8. Anonymous, Jensen, H. H., & Unnevehr, L. J. (2025). *Tracking Foodborne Pathogens from Farm to Table: Data Needs to Evaluate Control Options*. https://core.ac.uk/download/pdf/6551081.pdf (accessed on 11th June 2025).
9. Aramouni, F. M., & Blakeslee, K. (2006). *MF2269*. https://core.ac.uk/download/33360363.pdf (accessed on 11th June 2025).
10. Asim, S. H. (2017). Initial Assessment of Environmental Microbial Hazards in Doha Restaurants. https://core.ac.uk/download/84995789.pdf (accessed on 11th June 2025).
11. Brady, P. L., & Morris, J. R. (2005). *Production and Handling Practices for Safe Produce*. https://core.ac.uk/download/215463406.pdf (accessed on 11th June 2025).
12. Bujang, N., Abd Wahil, M. S., Abas, S. A., Alkhair Khairul Amin, K. H., Zulkifli, N. I., Mohd Shah, S., Aziz, N. F., et al. (2019). Outbreak of foodborne disease in a boarding school, Negeri Sembilan State, Malaysia, 2021. *Western Pacific Surveillance and Response Journal, 14*, 1–7. https://www.semanticscholar.org/paper/cddae9f87efd201f6dc14134465edbb7c5e6687a (accessed on 11th June 2025).
13. Bushu, E. G. (2022). Food safety knowledge, attitude, and practice of food handlers in kitchens of foodservice establishments in Lideta Sub-city, Addis Ababa, Ethiopia. https://core.ac.uk/download/534424777.pdf (accessed on 11th June 2025).
14. Carstens, C. K., Salazar, J. K., & Darkoh, C. (2019). Multistate outbreaks of foodborne illness in the United States associated with fresh produce from 2010 to 2017. *Frontiers in Microbiology, 10*. https://doi.org/10.3389/fmicb.2019.02667 (accessed on 11th June 2025).

15. Chew, A., Greenville, F., Pingault, N. M., Barrett, S., Waters, N., Hudson, L., & Post, J. (2025). A foodborne norovirus outbreak associated with six events and a single caterer, Canberra, November 2022. *Communicable Diseases Intelligence, 49.* https://www.semanticscholar.org/paper/39e7d2c2707ca96d5e679bb416c7424b9df12325 (accessed on 11th June 2025).

16. Choudhury, S., Medina-Lara, A., Smith, R., & Daniel, N. (2022). Research on health impacts of chemical contaminants in food. Bulletin of the World Health Organization, 100, 180–180A. https://www.semanticscholar.org/paper/0c58b946d80de6d8ce8ae843288344379dfe1152 (accessed on 11th June 2025).

17. Deen, A., & Khuluse, D. S. (2020). *Hygiene and Safety Practices of Food Vendors.* https://core.ac.uk/download/334754644.pdf (accessed on 11th June 2025).

18. Dominguez-Salas, P., Waddington, H., Grace, D., Bosire, C., Moodley, A., Kulkarni, B., Dasi, T., et al. (2024). Understanding the role of household hygiene practices and foodborne disease risks in child stunting: A UKRI GCRF Action Against Stunting Hub protocol paper. BMJ Pediatrics Open, 8. https://www.semanticscholar.org/paper/cbe56a6d09da0f10a7dd542240e7b213ead837fb (accessed on 11th June 2025).

19. Ellwanger, J. H., da Veiga, A. B. G., Kaminski, V. de L., Valverde-Villegas, J. M., de Freitas, A. W. Q., & Chies, J. A. B. (2021). Control and prevention of infectious diseases from a One Health perspective. *Genetics and Molecular Biology, 44.* https://doi.org/10.1590/1678-4685-gmb-2020-0256 (accessed on 11th June 2025).

20. Faour-Klingbeil, D., Kuri, V., & Todd, E. C. D. (2016). Microbiological quality of ready-to-eat fresh vegetables and their link to food safety environment and handling practices in restaurants. https://core.ac.uk/download/74390081.pdf (accessed on 11th June 2025).

21. Faour-Klingbeil, D., & Todd, E. C. D. (2019). Prevention and control of foodborne diseases in Middle-East North African countries: Review of national control systems. *International Journal of Environmental Research and Public Health, 17,* 70–70. https://doi.org/10.3390/ijerph17010070 (accessed on 11th June 2025).

22. Haynes, P. E. (2021). *Evaluation of Food Safety Practices at Louisiana Summer Feeding Sites and Food Safety Communication Via Social Media During Crises.* https://core.ac.uk/download/478717093.pdf (accessed on 11th June 2025).

23. Issa-Zacharia, A., Lubanji, R., & Matondo, J. (2025). Evaluation of food safety knowledge among food service workers and microbial contamination of food contact surfaces in university restaurants in Morogoro, Tanzania. *International Journal of Nutrition and Food Sciences.* https://www.semanticscholar.org/paper/1577406f1fe2287d7ad2151672e1d1c1207afca3 (accessed on 11th June 2025).

24. Iwu, C. D., & Okoh, A. I. (2019). Preharvest transmission routes of fresh produce associated bacterial pathogens with outbreak potentials: A review. *International Journal of Environmental Research and Public Health, 16,* 4407–4407. https://doi.org/10.3390/ijerph16224407 (accessed on 11th June 2025).

25. Jaffee, S., Henson, S., Unnevehr, L. J., Grace, D., & Cassou, E. (2018). The Safe Food Imperative: Accelerating Progress in Low- And Middle-Income Countries. Washington, DC: World Bank eBooks. https://doi.org/10.1596/978-1-4648-1345-0 (accessed on 11th June 2025).

26. Jagadeesan, B., Gerner-Smidt, P., Allard, M. W., Leuillet, S., Winkler, A., Xiao, Y., Chaffron, S., et al. (2018). The use of next generation sequencing for improving food safety: Translation into practice. *Food Microbiology, 79*, 96–115. https://doi.org/10.1016/j.fm.2018.11.005 (accessed on 11th June 2025).

27. Leal, S. D. M. L., Pieper, A. O., de Oliveira, M. A., Cardozo, R. D., & Carvalhai, J. F. (2025). Condições higiênico-sanitárias no comércio de carnes e derivados em feiras livres em Colatina, Espírito Santo. Pubvet. https://www.semanticscholar.org/paper/aa0c612482253b2e8405e69840b8f7f58f8db03f (accessed on 11th June 2025).

28. Levi, J., Segal, L. M., & Vinter, S. (2008). *Fixing Food Safety: Protecting America's Food Supply from Farm-To-Fork*. https://core.ac.uk/download/71351319.pdf (accessed on 11th June 2025).

29. Martinez, M. J. J. (2024). Critical analysis of the practices of shop food handlers regarding safety and hygiene: Case study in Paranaque City. *African Journal of Biological Sciences*. https://www.semanticscholar.org/paper/372d6ecf379e6a8eaae045c0ebcf84785d5be48f (accessed on 11th June 2025).

30. Marule, N. L., du, G., & Marx-Pienaar, N. (2024). Gauteng's managers' implementation of food safety protocols and practices in their QSR environments. Journal of Consumer Sciences. https://www.semanticscholar.org/paper/506df82b5101cd300059e28908a5d233ff44c5d6 (accessed on 11th June 2025).

31. Nasir, K. A., & Ezzaddin, S. A. (2025). Food handlers' knowledge, attitudes, and practices regarding food safety in Sulaimani Governorate, Iraq: A cross-sectional study. *Journal of Contemporary Medical Sciences*. https://www.semanticscholar.org/paper/c5cc69025dc65cd2e2256cc9b5dd89faa12c19b6 (accessed on 11th June 2025).

32. Nkhebenyane, J. S. (2018). Food Hygiene Risks and Related Practices in Central South African HIV/AIDS Hospices: A Qualitative Assessment. https://core.ac.uk/download/222968072.pdf (accessed on 11th June 2025).

33. Ong, K. J., Johnston, J., Datar, I., Sewalt, V., Holmes, D., & Shatkin, J. A. (2021). Food safety considerations and research priorities for the cultured meat and seafood industry. *Comprehensive Reviews in Food Science and Food Safety, 20*, 5421–5448. https://doi.org/10.1111/1541-4337.12853 (accessed on 11th June 2025).

34. Onyeaka, H., Siyanbola, K. F., Akinsemolu, A. A., Tamasiga, P., Mbaeyi-Nwaoha, I. E., Okonkwo, C. E., Odeyemi, O. A., et al. (2024). Promoting equity and justice: Harnessing the right to food for Africa's food security. *Agriculture & Food Security, 13*. https://doi.org/10.1186/s40066-024-00505-0 (accessed on 11th June 2025).

35. Orimaye, O. E., Ekunseitan, D. A., Omaliko, P. C., & Fasina, Y. O. (2024). Mitigation potential of herbal extracts and constituent bioactive compounds on Salmonella in meat-type poultry. Animals, 14, 1087–1087. https://doi.org/10.3390/ani14071087 (accessed on 11th June 2025).

36. Poole, N., Donovan, J., & Erenstein, O. (2020). Viewpoint: Agri-nutrition research: Revisiting the contribution of maize and wheat to human nutrition and health. *Food Policy, 100*, 101976–101976. https://doi.org/10.1016/j.foodpol.2020.101976 (accessed on 11th June 2025).

37. Salama, Y., & Chennaoui, M. (2024). Understanding microbial contamination in meat and poultry production. Journal of Research in Agriculture and Food Sciences. https://www.semanticscholar.org/paper/0b74241a08d879d5e1413af6b4ea3395d4840634 (accessed on 11th June 2025).

38. Surwase, K. K., Doibale, M., & Lakhmawar, N. (2024). IJCM_291A: Hygiene practices among food handlers in a hospital setting: A case study from District Hospital Parbhani. *Indian Journal of Community Medicine, 49*, S84–S84. https://www.semanticscholar.org/paper/ecf84a8459cd89fec275eece62ddad2cc27af1d4 (accessed on 11th June 2025).

39. Waters, A. B. (2011). Doctor of Philosophy. https://core.ac.uk/download/276264220.pdf (accessed on 11th June 2025).

40. Yenealem, D. G., Worku, A., & Abdulmajid, S. (2020). Food safety practice and associated factors among meat handlers in Gondar Town: A cross-sectional study. *Journal of Environmental and Public Health, 2020*, 1–7. https://doi.org/10.1155/2020/7421745 (accessed on 11th June 2025).

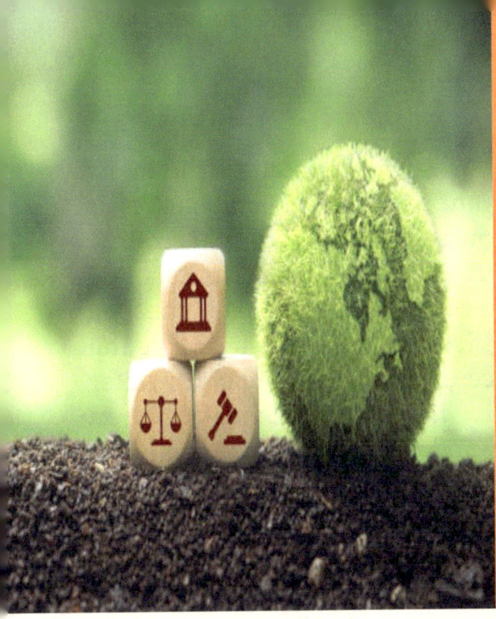

Chapter 14

LEGISLATION RELATED TO ENVIRONMENTAL AND PUBLIC HEALTH

Contents

Introduction

The increasing emphasis on environmental and public health legislation constitutes a major reaction to growing concerns about pollution and natural resource depletion. Conventionally, the Environmental Protection Act (EPA), Water Act, and Air Act are pillars of environmental regulation infrastructure in most nations, outlining the government's roles and supplying the legal stipulations necessary for natural resource preservation and public health. These pieces of legislation aim to curtail the adverse effects of industrialization and urbanization, which went uncontrolled for decades. The enactment of these fundamental laws is reflective of a paradigm shift towards the realization of environmental sustainability as part of public health, rather than approaching the debate on how legislation can induce positive change in society. Due to interconnections between environmental determinants and public health, robust regulatory mechanisms have become essential in offering unpolluted water and air, and protecting ecosystems that support human existence. Institutional inefficiencies, poor resources, and a lack of political will have posed difficulties for the implementation of environmental laws in many places. As in the debate over environmental regulation, it is important to examine the dynamics of governmental directives and judicial intervention. Judicial intervention, and by extension courts, has come to serve as a necessary check on the limitations of executive enforcement in issues of environmental conservation. For instance, judicial activism has been considered as an extra check in a federal system, particularly where executive branches are not sufficiently holding environmental standards to account. Interestingly, the judiciary's perception of access to clean air and clean water as rights has evoked significant decisions that have impacted policy implementation approaches, showing the judiciary's responsiveness to urgent environmental and public health issues (Rao et al., 2025). The function of non-governmental organizations (NGOs) is also crucial in assisting government agencies in enforcing environmental law. NGOs are watchdogs over manufacturers and public agencies, being a voice for marginalized communities victimized by the degradation of their environment. Further, the push from NGOs has the capacity to bring about policy change through raising awareness among the public and mobilizing the grassroots. In general, NGOs collaborate with institutions of government to develop comprehensive policies that aim to reduce the harmful effects of pollution and promote environmentally friendly patterns of behavior. The collaborative approach is increasingly appreciated as essential for comprehending and addressing complex environmental issues that transcend geographical and political boundaries. As witnessed in Indonesia, a convergence of internal drivers and external pressures, including civil society influence, has propelled environmental regulation to a policy priority in discourse, pinpointing the dynamic interdependence among legislation, governance, and activism at the grassroots level (Elston et al., 1994) (Figure 14.1).

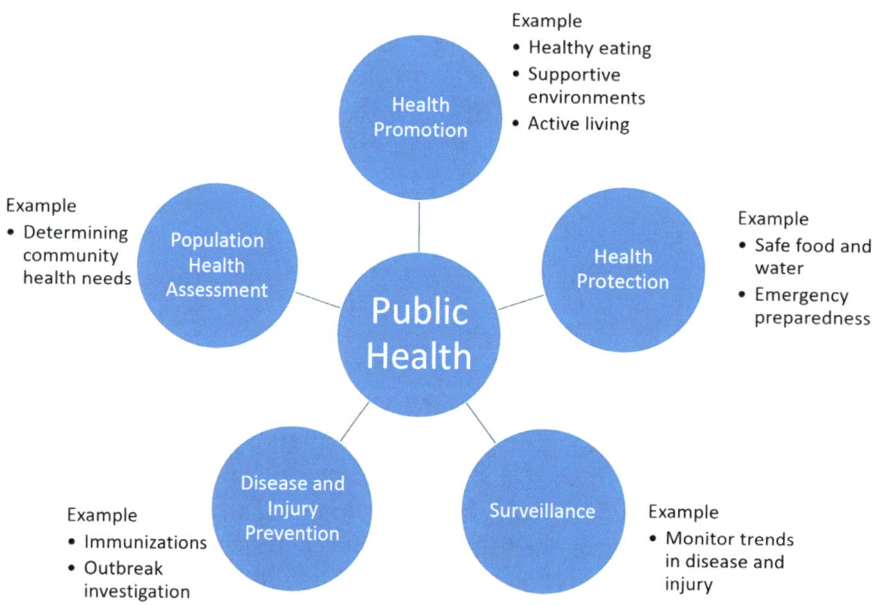

Figure 14.1. Public health legislation.

Source: https://www.engagenlarchive.ca/sites/default/files/5_functions_of_ph.jpg.

Definition of Environmental and Public Health Legislation

Public and environmental health law is a system that has been established to protect the health of individuals and the environment against the operations and activities that are likely to create harm or danger. It consists of a broad range of legislation and regulations aimed at decreasing pollution, providing clean drinking water, and strengthening public health programs. They encompass such paradigmatic examples as the Environmental Protection Act, Water Act, and Air Act, each addressing specific domains of environment and health concerns through structured enforcement procedures. By establishing norms and protocols for industrial and community operations, these legislative instruments play a crucial role in maintaining ecological harmony while safeguarding population well-being. Lastly, robust environmental and public health law is needed for ensuring sustainable development as well as the protection of human rights, which are inherently linked to health and environmental security (Dias, 2025). Environmental and public health law in most countries also needs intervention by government agencies and NGOs in ensuring enforcement and publicity. The government institutions are mandated with monitoring environmental factors and public health indicators, whereas the NGOs can engage communities by means of education and awareness campaigns. Such a participatory mechanism enables one to grasp public health issues arising from the environment in an integrated manner. Effective implementation is as dependent upon the legal provisions spelled out in these acts as it is upon the willing effort of all parties to ensure that communities are provided with the support needed for sustainable health gains. This coordination among public institutions and NGOs can be helpful in building creative solutions that address immediate environmental health requirements, as highlighted by studies that focus on the effectiveness of such coordination in varying settings (Lungu et al., 2010). Owing to the complexity of environmental and public health laws, their impact needs to be recognized outside the direct context of legal compliance. It informs policy-making regarding public health issues, guides socialization on health and environmental conservation, and enables inter-sectoral dialogue required to tackle pressing and complicated health challenges. Through a convergence of principles from multiple fields such as environmental science, public health, and justice, law forms a holistic framework for understanding the manner in which environmental factors directly determine human health outcomes. Forward-looking establishment of research agendas and action plans, as advocated in research gap assessments of environmental health, ensures policies are made relevant and responsive to the emerging concerns. Ultimately, the success of environmental and public health law hinges on its ongoing evaluation of implementation and collective action of various stakeholders towards the protection of human rights and attainment of full community health (Dias, 2025).

Importance of Legislation in Protecting Health and the Environment

Law plays a significant role in the safeguarding of public health and environmental integrity by providing the framework for society to minimize detrimental effects from industrial activity. The Environmental Protection Act, for instance, consolidates authority for federal and state authorities to set standards controlling the sources of air and water quality degradation. These are essential to prevent pollution-related health issues, such as respiratory illness and waterborne disease. Regulating emissions of sulfur dioxide and nitrogen oxides can reduce major environmental issues, such as acid rain, which has been shown to decrease soil fertility and impact crop yields in regions such as Punjab, as illustrated in the results of (N/A, 2025). This connection between environmental regulation and health identifies the necessity for stringent legislative intervention to sustain the well-being of populations and ecosystems. Furthermore, the enforcement of public health legislation in the environmental law paradigm identifies an engaged reaction towards the management of health hazards. Policy and legislation need to be constantly overseen and implemented with parameters of water and air quality, with direct influence on the health outcomes of communities. This type of monitoring enables the reversal of any deteriorating trend caused by elements in the environment, thus decreasing the incidence of disease caused by environmental degradation. Research has demonstrated that populations that are greatly affected by pollution experience significant public health challenges, including the increase in respiratory ailments among vulnerable groups, particularly children and the elderly, as highlighted in N/A (2025).

Consequently, law not only protects the environment but also enhances public health by bringing a required link between regulatory mandates and public well-being. The combined efforts of government agencies and NGOs enhance the efficiency of these legislative controls, making public enlightenment and mobilization easier. NGOs play an important role in campaigns promoting environmental health awareness as well as ensuring compliance with environmental law. They can also act as crucial intermediaries between regulatory institutions and communities, making sure that affected groups have a voice in policy-making. Collaborative work among sectors initiates the sustainable use of agricultural practices and anticipatory regulation of pollutants. It leads to coherent strategies addressing short-term health matters and long-term environmental sustainability. Therefore, the multisectoral strategy with effective legislation, government regulation, and community participation is crucial in the conservation of public health as well as the environment (Figure 14.2).

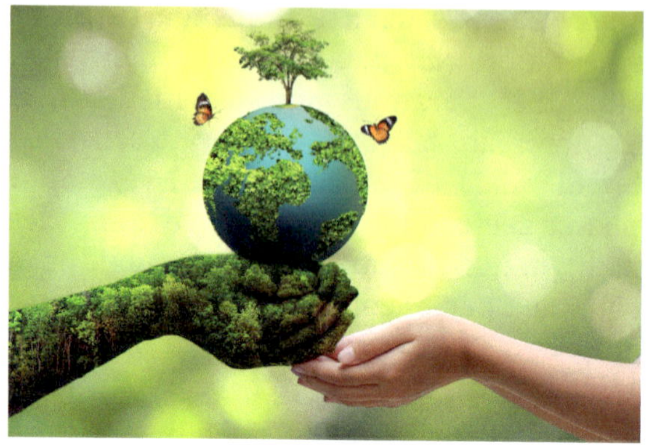

Figure 14.2. Symbolic representation of environmental conservation and the responsibility of protecting Earth's ecosystems.

Source: https://external-content.duckduckgo.com/iu/?u= https%3A%2F%2Fwww.aimsindia.com%2Fwp-content%2Fuploads%2F2022%2F06%2Fworld- environment.png&f= 1&nofb= 1&ipt=926221109c76b0cad5610ee94fb9987b9dcf75 ddc937044cd1e9e55e61700ba9.

14.1. The Environmental Protection Act

The Environmental Protection Act (EPA) assists in the compilation of an integrated framework with the intention of safeguarding the environment and enhancing public health. Enacted in response to growing environmental issues, the Act consolidates scattered legislation, paving the way for the uniform application of rules governing air quality, water supply, and hazardous waste disposal. By encouraging cooperation among federal, state, and local governments, the EPA facilitates uniform implementation of environmental standards, minimizing the chances of jurisdictional variations. The Act also provides citizens with a voice in environmental regulation, with an emphasis on transparency and accountability. This legal structure, therefore, not only addresses necessary immediate environmental concerns but also works to impart a broad appreciation of human development and human rights and places environmental health at the forefront of overall public welfare initiatives (Muntarbhorn, 2025). Enforcement of the EPA is paramount to its effectiveness and demonstrates an interest in compliance with regulation. The agencies tasked with implementing its provisions must operate within an interdisciplinary environment that integrates environmental science, policy, and public health factors. In this regard, the EPA has a twofold purpose—serving as both a guardian of environmental integrity and a police force that imposes penalties for infractions. This policing mechanism is essential to deterring violations that detract from air quality and water purity, thereby safeguarding communities from potentially hazardous conditions. While doing so, it also builds a supportive regulatory framework that is able to respond to the evolving character of environmental hazards. Strict enforcement of the EPA is also making the most out of the pivotal role played by non-governmental organizations (NGOs), whose on-the-ground work and public campaigns complement government efforts, to prioritize public health in environmental policy (Choudhry et al., 2025). The convergence of the Environmental Protection Act with other acts, such as the Water Act and Air Act, necessitates an integrated approach to environmental management. The interconnectedness enhances a whole-of-system perspective in addressing issues of water scarcity, air pollution, and ecosystem degradation. Each of the pieces of legislation complements the others to constitute a total method of resource management and public health protection. As is demonstrated in water-scarce countries, effective governance must consider all stakeholders, from the government and consumers to industries. The EPA framework for cooperation facilitates the development of policies around water that prioritize environmental protection and equity in access. Therefore, government policies, complemented by the facilitating role of NGOs, are instrumental to ensuring the law not only reacts to emerging threats but also prevents new environmental issues (Choudhry et al., 2025) (Figure 14.3).

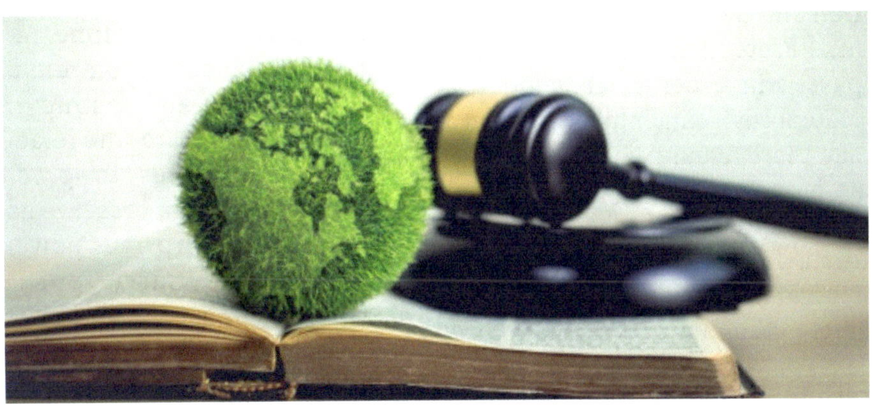

Figure 14.3. Environmental Protection Act.

Source: https://external-content.duckduckgo.com/iu/?u=https%3A%2F%2Fwww.scclegal.com%2Fwp-content%2Fuploads%2F2023%2F10%2FNavigating-Environmental-Law-and-Regulation-Expert-Insights.jpg&f=1&nofb=1&ipt=9815f3a98af4d5c5f25a059f533e8fd1aeda81020ad8d1a4b4eaf324e0a7afdd.

14.1.1. Historical Context and Purpose of the Act

The historical context of environmental legislation portrays a complex interplay between rapid industrialization and increasing public awareness of environmental issues. For the majority of nations, the latter half of the twentieth century represented a decisive turning point when citizens began to recognize the adverse effects of pollution and other forms of environmental degradation on public health and natural resources. This growing awareness was further fueled by landmark events, such as the publication of Rachel Carson's Silent Spring, which identified the dangers of pesticides and sparked a larger environmental movement. As pressure for change grew, governments were pushed increasingly to enact legislation that would protect natural habitats and public health, preparing the ground for comprehensive legislation such as the Environmental Protection Act and other milestone legislation regarding air and water quality. The purpose of such environmental measures was finally motivated by the necessity of protecting both public health and the environment against the degrading effects of pollution and depletion of resources. The Environmental Protection Act, to take one instance, was passed in order to consolidate and harmonize federal environmental protection programs so that there would be an orderly way of managing hazards. Similarly, the Water Act and Air Act attempted to manage specific sources of pollution, prescribing standards that the municipalities and industries have to follow. By setting concrete guidelines and regulations, this legislation sets out to create a platform for sustainable development and resource utilization, for the sake of a healthier environment and, ultimately, maintaining citizens' rights to clean water and air. Attempts at such legally mandated protection of the environment against ecological harm went beyond not causing ecological damage and also addressed the social and economic effects caused by environmental degradation to humans. To this end, as well as enforcing the laws, enforcement of environmental regulations has also largely relied on collaboration between various stakeholders, including governments and non-governmental organizations (NGOs). Success in enforcing the laws had relied on judicial control to ensure responsibility and compliance, particularly where local governments did not approach environmental issues resolutely. The judiciary has played a necessary part, defining environmental rights as fundamental rights and stepping in to fill the gaps generated by government inertia, as evident from the increasing number of cases of judicial activism in environmental protection. Under this comprehension, the legal system's success is not just based on legislation but also on the collective action of all those participating in the governance process—executive bodies, the judicial system, and NGOs—acting in unison to facilitate positive change for the benefit of environmental and public health welfare (Rao et al., 2025; Elston et al., 1994).

14.1.2. Key Provisions and Regulations Established

The EPA is a cornerstone in the legislative framework focused on ensuring levels of environmental and public health. Its key provisions mandate the elaboration of far-reaching guidelines to preclude pollution, regulate wastes, and preserve natural resources. The Act further provides powers to regulatory authorities to carry out environmental monitoring and assessment. This regulatory authority not only attempts to limit harmful discharges and emissions but also promotes sustainability through practices that encourage renewable energy sources and ecological restoration. Furthermore, the EPA emphasizes cooperative action among government agencies, NGOs, and society, thereby developing an inclusive mode of environmental governance. This multi-dimensional strategy ensures proactive action in conserving ecosystems as well as making provisions for public health concerns based on environmental determinants. In addition to the EPA, the Water Act has a crucial role to play in managing water quality and quantity, which are the pillars of public health. The Act outlines rigorous standards for the surface and groundwater, in consideration of avoiding pollution by means of industrial effluent, run-off from agriculture, and other poisonous sources. Through the establishment of stringent enforcement measures, the Act ensures that water bodies are protected against degradation and therefore contribute significantly to the health and well-being of communities dependent upon such natural resources. Some of the most important provisions in the law include regular water quality checks and installation of pollution control mechanisms, as well as public education campaigns to inform communities of the importance of having access to clean water. The law not only protects aquatic life but also ensures the basic rights of citizens to safe and clean drinking water, ultimately proving the link between environmental integrity and public health. Secondly, the Air Act reinforces this legislation by specifically focusing on air quality management, which is crucial in the protection of the public's health from the adverse effects of air pollution. Measures under the Air Act include provisions for National Ambient Air Quality Standards (NAAQS) to regulate and control atmospheric pollutants. The act provides powers to authorities to impose control measures on industries and automobiles, causing deterioration of air quality. Furthermore, the Act invites the public into action through compulsory open publication of air quality data, enabling communities to lobby for cleaner air. Through the enforcement of these essential provisions, the Air Act plays a pivotal role in reducing respiratory diseases and enhancing the general standard of living. The joint efforts of government agencies and NGOs also draw attention to the importance of working together in rendering guarantees for air quality standard compliance, again reinforcing the public's devotion to health and environmental safety.

14.1.3. Impact on Environmental Conservation Efforts

The enforcement of such acts as the Environmental Protection Act has had a significant impact on the climate of environmental conservation activities in the United States. The act established a solid platform for the protection of environmental health through managing pollutants and encouraging sustainable development in various industries. By giving a legal platform on which pollution control is enforced, the act has spurred the incorporation of new technology and methods with the aim of reducing environmental degradation. In addition, the oversight responsibility played by government agencies, in collaboration with NGOs, has been instrumental in promoting awareness and compliance, increasing the effectiveness of conservation initiatives. In analyzing the complex interrelations in this regulatory environment, one can see a trend towards more holistic measures that emphasize environmental sustainability, highlighting the importance of balanced legislative efforts in bringing effective conservation results (Gladys, 2005). The Water Act is another significant component of the environmental conservationist legislation cache, particularly where conserving water resources is concerned. The Water Act not only controls the quality of water but also focuses on sustainable management practices that do not pollute and ensure safe drinking water. Therefore, strides have been made in water conservation measures that promote the aims of environmental conservation. The coordination between government institutions and social agencies has also enhanced the impact of this act, as a collective effort allows for increased public awareness and involvement in the conservation of water. The combined approaches promoted by this legislation have translated into innovative solutions to specific local water problems while maintaining ecological harmony concurrently. The Water Act thus constitutes the catalyst that triggers desirable change in water resource management (Hersh et al., 2025). In addition, the Air Act plays a central role in environmental protection activities, particularly where air quality and public health are concerned. Through its implementation, it provides for the imposition of stringent air quality standards for the purpose of avoiding the detrimental effects of pollution on the environment and on human health. The act encourages the utilization of cleaner technology and practices and emphasizes the reduction of emissions from industry and motor vehicles. Government responses, together with NGOs' support, in disseminating information and best practices, are significant in public awareness and compliance with air standards. Furthermore, international discussion of air contamination and global warming is increasingly influenced by the experience of the Air Act, indicating its global significance to environmental policy-making. By doing this, the law not only addresses spontaneous issues of air quality but also establishes a conservation culture whose lasting impacts on the environment are profound (Gladys, 2005) (Figure 14.4).

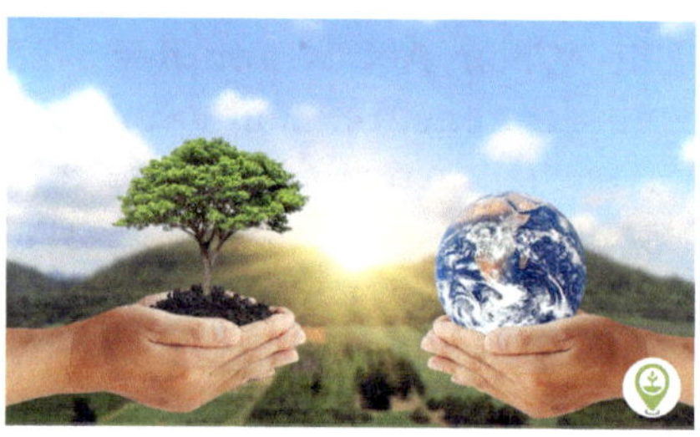

Figure 14.4. Environmental conservation efforts.

Source: https://external-content.duckduckgo.com/iu/?u=http%3A%2F%2Fwww.ecomatcher.com%2Fwp-content%2Fuploads%2F2022%2F09%2Frestore.jpg&f=1&nofb=1&ipt=3c50cccf77 2b6c4d82ad7343cb3f46f3ca7b5334ded334e134295cfe02e1d3df.

14.2. The Water Act

The Water Act serves as a critical component of legislative frameworks aimed at safeguarding water quality and ensuring the sustainability of freshwater resources. This legislation addresses various dimensions of water management, including the allocation of rights, regulatory standards for pollution control, and the frameworks for public health protection. By establishing guidelines for water usage and waste management, the Act attempts to balance competing interests among agricultural, industrial, and municipal water consumers. Moreover, it emphasizes the necessity for an integrated approach to water management, recognizing that water resource issues are often intertwined with broader ecological and socio-economic factors. Such an inclusive strategy is essential, particularly in regions characterized by vulnerable ecosystems and communities reliant on aquatic resources for their livelihoods, as described in detailed case studies within various environmental research literature (Bryceson et al., 2001). Furthermore, the enforcement mechanisms embedded within the Water Act underscore the importance of governance in achieving the legislation's objectives. Effective enforcement not only relies on regulatory bodies but also requires the collaboration of NGOs and community stakeholders who play a crucial role in monitoring compliance. The ongoing dialogue between these entities facilitates the exchange of knowledge and resources, thereby enhancing the efficacy of water management practices. Importantly, the role of NGOs extends beyond mere compliance monitoring; they often engage in public education initiatives aimed at raising awareness about water conservation and pollution prevention. Thus, the multifaceted approach to enforcement outlined in the Water Act reflects a broader perspective on public health, recognizing that clean water access is foundational to community well-being and environmental integrity (Behrman et al., 2025). Lastly, the interaction between the Water Act and public health laws illustrates the legislation's dual purpose in safeguarding both the environment and human health. Contaminated water sources can lead to a multitude of health issues, and thus, the Water Act integrates public health considerations into its framework. It enshrines the principle that water integrity is paramount to disease prevention and promotes the establishment of water quality standards to protect vulnerable populations, especially in underserved regions. This interconnection is vital in recognizing the lessons learned from various case studies related to sustainable water resource management, which point to the necessity of adopting comprehensive strategies that address both environmental sustainability and public health imperatives. Through collaborative efforts among government bodies, NGOs, and local communities, the Water Act embodies a holistic approach to addressing these critical issues, solidifying its position as a cornerstone of environmental and public health legislation (Bryceson et al., 2001) (Figure 14.5).

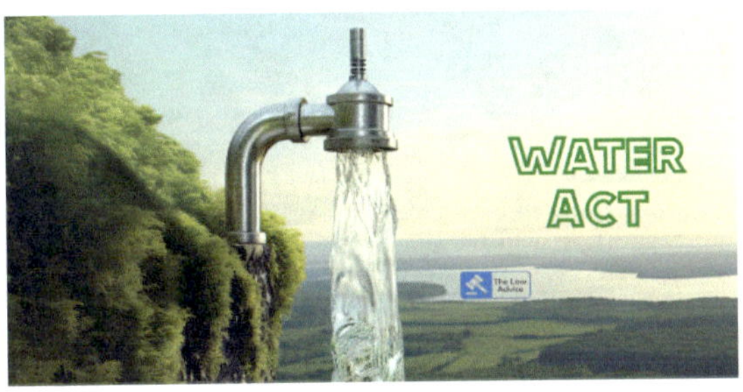

Figure 14.5. The Water Act.

Source: https://external-content.duckduckgo.com/iu/?u=https%3A%2F%2Fcdn.thelawadvice.com%2Fwebsite%2Farticles%2Fe9294dc1-d388-4e5b-b274-8066e0b5cfb3.webp&f=1&nofb=1&ipt=0a703fc3b333189ac14df8f8f4cbc8e59cc92cf5fbbc30732121d8f05707e9a7.

14.2.1. Objectives of the Water Act and Its Significance

The objectives of the Water Act are predominantly centered on sustainable management and protection of water resources in order to ensure a secure and adequate water supply to the public. The act offers a framework for the regulation of water use and quality, acknowledging the role of water in human health as well as environmental sustainability. Besides, the Act strives to address water scarcity, water pollution, and equitable distribution, emphasizing the necessity of conserving water resources for future generations. Through its facilitation of integrated management of water resources, the Water Act is looking to establish an arrangement in which the stakeholders are actively engaged in decision-making. This regulatory structure is significant in the sense that it lays the groundwork for a coordinated response by various government organs, civil society, and communities to ensure unity in addressing severe issues of water access and sustainability. Notably, the Water Act also emphasizes good governance and multi-stakeholder involvement in water management. The Act posits that sustainable water management is not a sole government mandate but requires engagement by non-governmental organizations (NGOs), the community, and the private sector. Through the inclusion of governance in water management, the Act provides for partnerships that enhance service and accountability. These collaborations are crucial, especially in more exposure-prone regions, as they are able to seize the dynamic character of vulnerability along with the intricacies of the problems of climate change. This is in line with the mandate that effective adaptation needs to be context-specific and consider social, economic, and cultural factors (Thomas et al., 2018). The inclusion of various stakeholders ensures that the regulatory system is holistic and able to address particular water concerns of various communities. Additionally, the Water Act is pivotal to achieving broader environmental goals and aligning with international systems, such as the United Nations Sustainable Development Goals (SDGs). Focusing on access to water and water quality, the Act contributes towards the accomplishment of various SDGs, including sanitation and clean water, as well as sustainable cities and communities. The significance of the Act also emerges in the case of managing solid waste, where good governance facilitates the regulation of pollution arising from the disposal of waste into water bodies (Rodi et al., 2017). This symbiotic relationship between waste administration and water management is a classic example of the transdisciplinary role of environmental law. Generally, the Water Act is central to the protection of water resources, highlighting the vital balance between public health and environmental protection underpinning good governance in modern society.

14.2.2. Regulations on Water Quality and Pollution Control

Management of water quality and pollution control is a crucial aspect of environmental law that provides protection for public health and the' conservation of ecosystems. Under this, a range of legal instruments, such as the Environmental Protection Act and the Water Act, have been passed to address the challenges posed by water body pollutants. Specifically, such a law imposes strict controls over the discharge of pollutants, ensuring that water quality is maintained at standards acceptable for use by humans and aquatic life. For instance, regulations in the Environmental Protection Act mandate the monitoring and reporting of water quality parameters, which serve as compliance standards. These steps reiterate the importance of proactive regulatory policies in curbing pollution and promoting sustainable water management practices, which benefit the well-being and safety of individuals as a whole (N/A, 2025). Furthermore, monitoring water quality regulation is periodically supported by local and national authorities in collaboration with each other. These agencies are responsible for conducting regular inspections, testing water bodies for pollutants, and taking remedial measures wherever standards are lacking. Such regulations must be enforced not just for the protection of natural water resources but also for the protection of public health, especially of the vulnerable sections. For instance, water quality decline due to industrial effluents could lead to severe health complications such as gastrointestinal illness and long-term exposure risks. Therefore, policy implementation is crucial, and strategic action must be taken to create awareness among people regarding water quality decline and compliance with established rules (Yew, 2019). Aside from the function of government, the role of NGOs cannot be underscored in the case of water quality and management of pollution. NGOs tend to plug gaps within regulatory policy and enhance community engagement and greater transparency in environmental policy formulation.

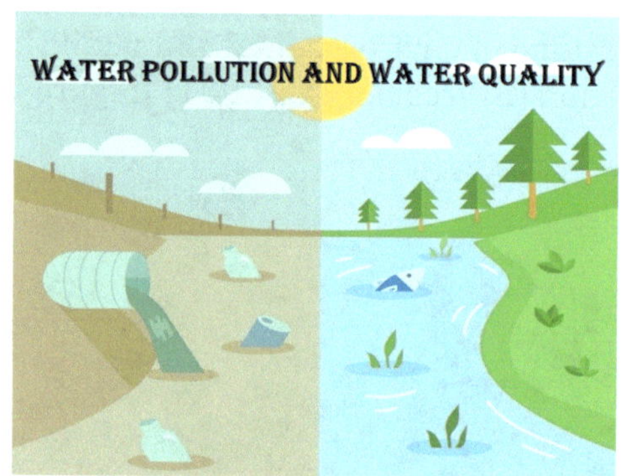

Figure 14.6. Regulations on water quality and pollution control.

Source: https://external-content.duckduckgo.com/iu/?u=https%3A%2F%2Fequest.co.in%2Fimages%2FCourses%2FWP.png&f=1&nofb=1&ipt= d85211d52f5833ca6e70 b828043389db0d07 1c0b9e48fbd81a2eb36a61d97ed2.

Through the medium of awareness campaigns, NGOs remind citizens of the necessity of clean water and the effects of pollution on society. They also play a significant part in holding private as well as public entities accountable for their green activities. Processes such as community monitoring programs make the local stakeholders active stakeholders in the protection of water quality. By promoting collaboration between governments, society, and NGOs, more efficient strategies can be devised to address water pollution and not only guarantee compliance with regulations but promote a culture of environmental responsibility among the populace (N/A, 2025) (Figure 14.6).

14.2.3. Case Studies of Successful Water Management Initiatives

Effective water management initiatives highlight the turning point of law and how it is applied practically, particularly in environmental sustainability. Across various countries, case studies pinpoint robust water quality and availability gains triggered by rigorous legislative tools such as the Water Act. For instance, the Murray-Darling Basin Plan in Australia is a model of successful water management, where the government has taken steps to allocate water resources equitably between agricultural, industrial, and ecological needs. This initiative not only succeeded in ending overdraft but also restored ecosystems, showing how widespread government and community cooperation can lead to sustainable water management practices. Impacts noted in such cases emphasize the necessity of robust regulatory frameworks enforcing compliance and stakeholder engagement across various sectors (Rodrigues, 2022). A second exemplary case is that of the implementation of integrated water resource management (IWRM) in the Netherlands. This highlights government institutions' collaborative strategy with NGOs and local communities in tackling the problem of water caused by climate change, as well as urbanization. Through facilitation of cooperation in surface water management, groundwater management, and water quality management, the Netherlands has developed an international model for resilience planning. It is backed by legislation, offering a comprehensive system that balances water issues with urbanization and agriculture, thus safeguarding the health of the public and the environment. The success of the Dutch water management shows the strength of policies that foster multi-stakeholder cooperation and adaptive frameworks capable of responding to changing environmental trends (Yaya et al., 2018). Through the successful water management outcomes , legislation becomes more critical since it not only guides environmental conservation activities but also promotes public involvement. Interventions influenced by the Environmental Protection Act and other legislation seek to induce awareness and responsibility among industries and citizens of their water consumption and its implications on health and ecology. These interventions prioritize a change from punitive governance to cooperative governance, where diverse stakeholders collaborate to evaluate and control water resources in a sustainable manner. These instances highlight the importance of continued legislative aid and civil society mobilization to ensure water management practices adapt according to new challenges of the time, finally guaranteeing water quality for generations to come (Rodrigues, 2022).

14.3. The Air Act

The Air Act is an important environmental law that aims to safeguard public health through the regulation of the air. Enacted largely to control air pollution, the Act empowers government agencies to set standards for allowable concentrations of pollutants and subsequently regulate them. This all-embracing approach not only addresses the proximate environmental problem but also collaborates with general public health initiatives. Research indicates a direct link between air quality and various health outcomes; therefore, adequate regulation under the Air Act is required to avoid causing health hazards due to air pollution. Regulators also play the role of ensuring compliance by the industry, thereby preventing the release of harmful emissions that aggravate respiratory diseases, cardiovascular issues, and other ailments prevalent in places with poor air quality (Dudek et al., 2025). In addition to the Air Act regulation, the performance of government and nongovernment organizations (NGOs) also plays an important role in promoting compliance and public awareness. The government agencies are responsible for overseeing the monitoring of air pollution levels, policymaking, and emission reduction programs from activities such as vehicles and factories. But NGOs also play a vital role by advocating for increased controls and engaging communities in air quality issues. NGOs typically serve as a bridge between the government and citizens, highlighting the significance of pure air on general health and happiness. Their outreach activities tend to include educational campaigns emphasizing the connection between air pollution, human health, and rights, in constructing a more informed citizenry that can demand accountability from public and private sector actors (Dias, 2025). Enforcing the Air Act to the fullest will need to be the joint effort of a multitude of stakeholders spanning from regulators to industry and civil society. The success of the Act is contingent on how willing such bodies are to accept regulation and give priority to sustainable practices. Regular review and revision of air quality standards, based on scientific research, keep the Air Act current in the face of emerging environmental concerns. Building synergy between governmental institutions and NGOs might further enhance accountability, data collection, and public involvement in tracking air quality. Last but not least, the Air Act's vision is more than regulation; it hopes to construct a healthier and more equitable environment where the right to air is recognized as a basic human right and part of human development (Dias, 2025) (Figure 14.7).

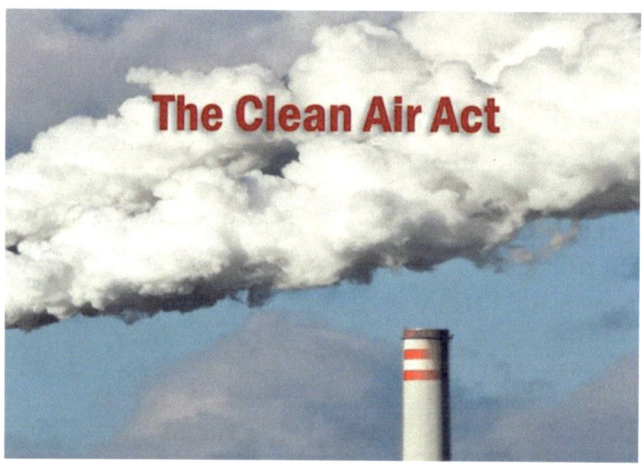

Figure 14.7. Clean Air Act.

Source: https://external-content.duckduckgo.com/iu/?u=https%3A%2F%2Fcleanwaterpartners.org%2Fwp-content%2Fuploads%2F2017%2F07%2Fclean-air-act.jpg&f=1&nofb=1&ipt=dfe1b01bfabf862c2e76e4506eee89db5f6f38a77d01722ad56cece395c870d4.

14.3.1. Overview of the Air Act and Its Legislative Framework

The Air Act, or officially known as the Air (Prevention and Control of Pollution) Act of 1981, is an important law that deals with air quality in India. Initiated as a response to growing levels of air pollution due to industrialization, urbanization, and car emissions, the Act is intended to avoid, control, and disperse air pollution within various regions. The legislative framework consists of measures for regulation and penalties for contravention, including a structural model for the establishment of State Pollution Control Boards, the purpose of which is to bring into effect the Act's provisions. These boards play a key role in the monitoring of air quality, the issuing of permits to establishments that give rise to pollutants, and ensuring public health safety, thus fitting into the general thrust of environmental and public health law. The legislative framework under the Air Acts is intertwined with other environmental legislation, such as the Environmental Protection Act and the Water Act, which gives a comprehensive environmental governance system. This convergence draws attention to a general natural resource management approach, which is required due to the interdependent nature of air, water, and land pollution. Moreover, the Air Act not only enforces responsibilities on governmental agencies but also empowers local communities and civil society entities to oversee compliance as well as advocate for stricter air quality standards. Since air pollution continues to be a pervasive health risk, the collaborative effort of these stakeholders becomes increasingly essential to promote public health and sustainable growth in accordance with global environmental standards. Besides, the effectiveness of the Air Act is always being challenged by political, economic, and social pressures. Industries that rely on oil and gas are usually the cause of a challenging implementation of stringent air quality standards, such as in regions where coal mining still remains dominant, an instance of a sensitive balancing of economic pressures and environmental urgency (Brauers et al., 2020). Besides, public health issues have also gained increased prominence in recent times, with studies highlighting the dangers posed by deteriorating air quality. Studies done by organizations focusing on health disparities accentuate the urgent imperative of systems change to improve air quality, particularly in urban areas (N/A, 2020). The Air Act must, thus, keep in step with empirical realities and public perceptions to remain effective and relevant in addressing air pollution challenges.

14.3.2. Standards for Air Quality and Emissions Control

A comprehensive mechanism for air quality and emission management is essential under the framework of environmental law, most significantly articulated in the Clean Air Act. The Act provides the foundation for federal air quality standards that agencies are required to implement in an attempt to protect public health and the environment. Appreciation for the value of these standards is evident by knowing their effects on air pollutants like particulate matter and ozone that directly put human health at risk. Also, the regulation encourages improved practices in industries, enforcing compliance by forcing reductions in emissions. The implementation of National Ambient Air Quality Standards (NAAQS) establishes the necessary yardstick to encourage states to develop implementation plans tailored to local circumstances, yet in accordance with overarching federal standards. It is only through such regulation that populations are able to benefit from better air quality and the prevention of environmentally induced ailments, illustrating the importance of the regulatory mechanisms in public health. Moreover, the use of pollution controls with legislative tools such as the Environmental Protection Act provides a robust base to address air quality management complexities. Interestingly, improvements in regulatory methods tend to involve the use of integrated pollution control (IPC), which has seen extensive application in countries like the United Kingdom, as seen in many studies. The UK's Environmental Protection Act of 1990 is a good example of progress toward full pollution controls by establishing a unified inspectorate focused on the Best Practicable Environmental Option (BPEO) for varied pollutants. One strategy has the benefit of facilitating cross-media considerations, where air quality improvements do not have a tendency to create a pollution shift in other environmental media unintentionally. By embracing IPC measures, the Act is a shining example of legislative systems' resilience to new environmental concerns, ultimately advocating for an integrated approach to public health and environmental protection (Hersh et al., 2025). Lastly, collaboration between the government and non-state agencies (NGOs) in regulating air quality standards cannot be overstressed. Collective efforts make legal systems become effective on the ground as pragmatic interventions, promoting stakeholder engagement and awareness. NGOs usually mobilize the public, getting individuals aware of air pollution and pushing for stronger regulation. They can also bridge the gap between science and policy-making because they provide thought-provoking insights towards improved air quality policies. Through collaboration with government agencies, the organizations encourage compliance with established air quality standards, assist in monitoring levels of pollution, and assist in public campaigns to reduce exposure to harmful pollutants. In the long term, the collaboration enables effective environmental policy, prioritizing consideration of public health in air quality management (Dudek et al., 2025) (Figure 14.8).

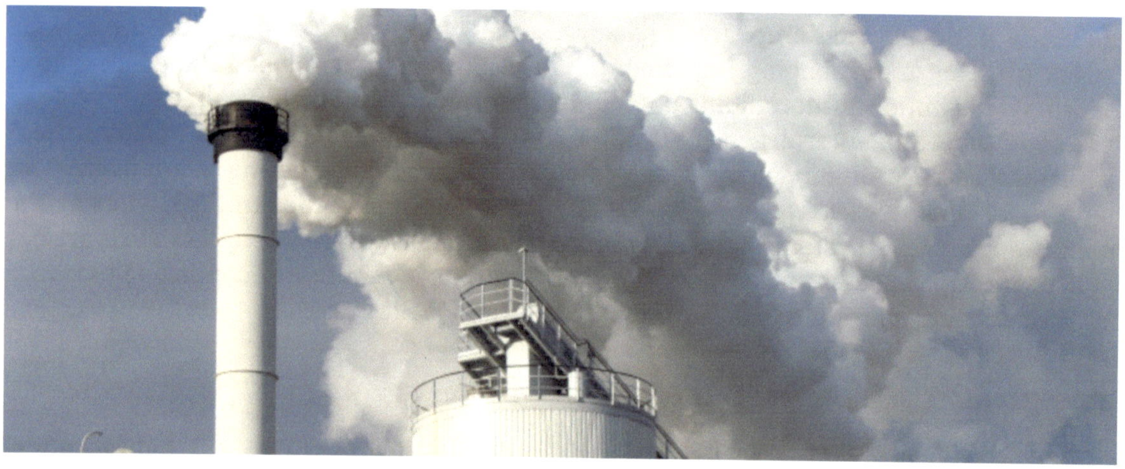

Figure 14.8. Air pollution control.

Source: https://external-content.duckduckgo.com/iu/?u=https%3A%2F%2Fwww.britannica.com%2Fexplore%2Fsavingearth%2Fwp-content%2Fuploads%2Fsites%2F4%2F2019%2F03%2Fair-pollution-control-hero.jpg&f=1&nofb=1&ipt=83ba22092ff87453671205e6fa0b40c8817d124c2d5d58d184e19d7a212b71fb.

14.3.3. Challenges in Enforcement and Compliance

The enforcement of environmental and public health laws is confronted by a plethora of issues that significantly hamper their effect. One key problem is that political polarization has intensified, coupled with the lack of comprehensive legislative efforts. Congress failed to approve crucial environmental bills since the 1990s, rendering a large part of regulatory policy obsolete and lacking impact in many individuals' perceptions. The stagnation is like a reliance on executive actions that, although promising, are not properly authorized and mandated to bring about significant change. As elaborated in van de Biezenbos et al. (2017), the failure to find broad congressional support for environmental change can be regarded as a symptom of a greater issue of political procrastination hindering the creation of sustainable solutions. The absence of the use of effective and robust standards dilutes compliance and enforcement mechanisms, leaving communities vulnerable to the related health risks of environmental contamination. Compounding these issues, local authorities typically face legal obstacles in enforcing their own laws that aim to mitigate environmental damage. Many states have established preemption legislation that bars municipalities from banning practices like hydraulic fracturing, leaving local governments deprived of the ability to properly address environmental concerns at hand. This regulatory climate is one of the greatest challenges to cities and towns, which would want to prioritize environmental security and public health, but have their capacity limited by state controls. As van de Biezenbos et al. (2017) note, even if municipalities attempt to enforce existing state environmental laws, they are limited by conflicting jurisdictions. These intricacies complicate the enforcement of local as well as state regulations and challenge the ability of communities to safeguard public health in their own jurisdictions. In addition, enforcement is frequently impaired by the lack of resources and poor institutional capacity. The regulatory agencies, for example, the Environmental Protection Agency (EPA), are commonly underfunded and short-staffed, and thus limit their ability to track compliance. The combination of limited funds and an increased number of bodies to regulate creates daunting control challenges. These imbalances can lead to selective enforcement where crimes are not enforced due to prioritization of urgent matters or an insufficiency in manpower. With this reality, the critical necessity for renewed congressional backing, as mentioned in Case et al. (2014), becomes apparent by the day. It is only through renewed commitment to effective and adequately funded enforcement mechanisms that the goals of environmental law can be met and compliance and public health objectives fulfilled.

14.4. Public Health Laws and Their Enforcement

Use of public health law is a key factor in safeguarding community well-being and ensuring equitable access to health facilities. Public health law consists of several types of regulation intended to combat public health threats, e.g., epidemics and environmental hazards. Effective use requires coordination among governments, as well as partnership with NGOs and civil society organizations. However, bureaucratic inefficiency and lack of resources usually hinder it. The recent review found that even when there is a clearly defined regulatory system, the potential of public health policies remains disempowered by weak capacity and the power of influential actors who can direct health priorities toward their agenda (Rao et al., 2025). Therefore, the responsibility of maintaining public health often descends to the judiciary, which intervenes when regulatory roles cannot protect vulnerable segments of society, representing an aggravating gap in public health regulation. Judicial activism is a compound influencing factor in enforcing public health legislation, inclined to function as a necessary brake on government inertia. In the majority of instances, courts have been requested to interpret public health rights, and they have emphasized the inherent right to clean air and water as a component of health itself. This intervention is particularly applicable in countries where public health crises resulting from pollution and environmental degradation are not being addressed by government agencies, either because they are unwilling or incapable. Judicial action not only compels the government to comply with codes of public health but also draws attention to better management of resources and policy reform (Rao et al., 2025). But this reliance on the judiciary for action also poses problems related to the sustainability and efficacy of such action, as courts are ill-equipped to implement complex public health measures on a systemic level. The broader implications of compulsory public health legislation extend to social equity and the advancement of sustainable development goals. The enforcement process should ensure that there is careful consideration and transparency so that minority communities are not disproportionately affected by environmental policy. Furthermore, the role of NGOs in advocating for public health reforms cannot be overstated, considering that they primarily play the role of intermediaries who offer a megaphone for silenced voices. Through advocating for more robust public health laws and their implementation, NGOs shape a healthier world in alignment with national and international public health agendas. Thus, the interplay among government, judiciary, and civil society organizations is important for a complete strategy towards public health laws, ultimately leading to more robust communities to tackle contemporary health challenges (Figure 14.9).

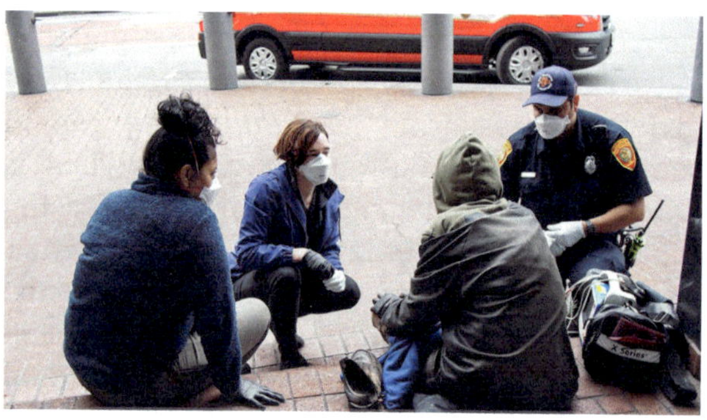

Figure 14.9. Law enforcement and public health.

Source: https://mspgh.unimelb.edu.au/_data/assets/image/0008/4142951/varieties/Banner.jpg.

14.4.1. Overview of Public Health Laws and Their Objectives

Public health law has the crucial role of defending populations' health by establishing the principles that inform the interplay among persons, the state, and health organizations. Public health law attempts to avoid disease, promote health, and protect populations' health through the regulation of sanitation, the prevention of disease, and the control of environmental risks. With the passing of regulations and policies to address public health concerns, such as non-communicable and communicable diseases, these laws impose essential measures of protection on vulnerable populations. Aside from that, the objectives of public health laws are inclined to coincide with those of environmental laws because they understand that a healthy environment is the very core of public health. For instance, water quality law, air quality law, and pollution control law have a direct bearing on population health outcomes, calling for an integrated strategy to health legislation. In the current public health matters, the interdependence of public health law with environmental law has become clear. Legislations that aim at protecting the environment, such as the Environmental Protection Act, the Water Act, and the Air Act, all help significantly in curbing exposures to harmful substances and health inequalities across different groups. For instance, in imposing air and water standards through public health legislation, controls are created that are essential in preventing pollution and environmentally caused diseases. The enforcement of these policies, with powerful enforcement mechanisms and community outreach programs, is vital to their realization. The blend of public health policy and environmental policy enables the possibility of comprehensive public health interventions, not merely treating short-term health hazards but also working towards ensuring long-term sustainability of communities in relation to environmental perspectives. The role played by the government and NGOs in the passage and implementation of public health law is pivotal in achieving their objectives. Governments at all levels have the responsibility to formulate sound legislation, appropriate funds, and create awareness among the citizens about public health schemes. NGOs can, in return, be key allies, advocating for policy changes, orienting citizens on issues of public health, and upholding compliance with existing laws. This partnership increases the possibility of addressing public health problems effectively and directs community resources towards a common goal. Public health laws, therefore, are not merely legal instruments but also a part of the social fabric that works towards health equity and access to secure settings. Combined intervention of government and NGOs is important in realizing the full potential of the laws to reinforce public health results and strengthen community resilience against environmental shifts.

14.4.2. Mechanisms for Enforcement and Public Health Monitoring

Effective enforcement mechanisms and public health surveillance mechanisms are also essential to ensure compliance with public health and environmental legislation. Of key relevance to this enforcement is the establishment of regulatory systems defining the roles of stakeholders like government agencies and NGOs. These frameworks not only describe the legal limits of pollution control and public health measures but also specify the enforcement mechanisms available to authorities in order to encourage compliance.

For example, the Environmental Protection Act gives agencies the authority to inspect, monitor, and enforce sanctions for non-compliance, thus reiterating the necessity to comply with established environmental standards and public health measures. By providing a clear avenue for accountability, the law facilitates a proactive response for safeguarding public health and the quality of the environment. A monitoring system for public health can effectively be enhanced by large-scale data collection and coordinated efforts among governmental and nongovernmental actors. Partnership is crucial since it brings in different capacities and resources, allowing it to have an improved response to issues of environmental health. Routine monitoring of air and water quality, mandated by the Air Act and Water Act, is the focus of surveillance in detecting potential hazards and preventing public health risks.

The incorporation of people's feedback levels and NGO monitoring activities further reinforces this system, with local issues addressed and with public health policy responsive to changing environmental factors. Further, the use of technology and the analysis of data facilitates ongoing checking and reporting, thereby enhancing transparency and trust with stakeholders. The interplay among law, enforcement capacity, and public health surveillance is critical to the effective functioning of the public health and environmental system.

As noted in Elston et al. (1994), global pressures, including foreign donors and international obligations, have successively influenced Indonesia's environmental policies, providing a setting in which enforcement mechanisms are driven by both internal and external pressures. Increasing realization of environmental deterioration and its socio-economic consequences has also emphasized the importance of successful coordination among NGOs and government institutions. This participatory approach not only ensures closer public health law enforcement but also enables ecological activities that are commensurate with higher causes of social justice and environmental preservation. Through the integration of such systems within a comprehensive legislative framework, the state becomes better equipped to safeguard public health as well as build a more resilient environment (Figure 14.10).

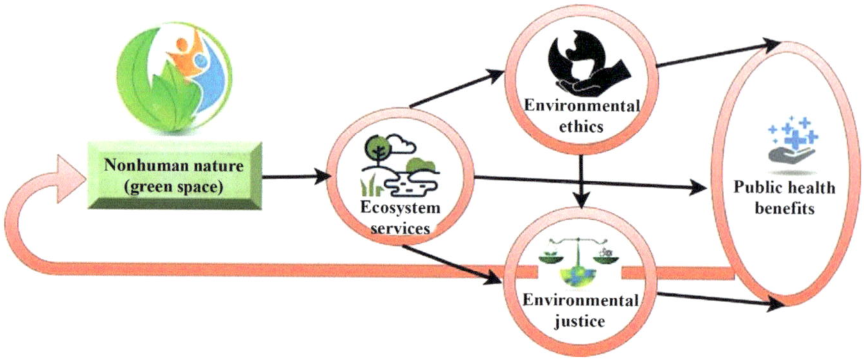

Figure 14.10. Mechanisms for enforcement and public health monitoring.

Source: https://www.researchgate.net/publication/373885906/figure/fig3/AS:11431281188435040@1694612604231/Process-of-Environmental-Law.jpg.

14.4.3. Role of Public Health Agencies in Implementation

Public health agencies are centrally responsible for the implementation of public health and environmental legislation. By interpreting provisions made under enactments such as the Environmental Protection Act, Water Act, and Air Act into actionable programs, public health agencies ensure legal mandates are met to the letter. Public health authorities, in general, are involved in assessing environmental risks, ensuring compliance, and sensitizing society towards the relevance of public health law. Their involvement is essential in averting adverse health effects as a result of environmental pollutants since they facilitate the implementation of science in policy-making. Science and policy coordination help in putting in place holistic public health interventions for both acute and future health problems, which ultimately lead to a healthier environment (Jeevanandam et al., 2018). Moreover, the active participation of public health organizations in the enforcement of public health laws significantly ensures their enforcement. These organizations not only ensure compliance with environmental law but also develop guidelines and resources that help local communities comply with laws. By engaging themselves directly in the enforcement process, public health officers can swiftly and efficiently address cases of non-compliance and thus forestall public health emergencies from spiraling out of control. Their role includes conducting inspections, managing health surveys, and collaborating with other stakeholders like government departments and non-governmental organizations (NGOs). This collaborative system maximizes the capability of public health systems to answer complex environmental issues and encourages sustainable ways of living among the communities (Robert, 2016). In addition to their policing function, public health agencies also play a critical facilitation role for public participation and education on issues concerning environmental health. Through conducting outreach programs, the agencies educate the public about potential risks in the form of environmental hazards such as water pollution and air pollution. Through awareness and provision of the information, they empower the communities with information that enables them to act proactively to defend their health and well-being. The outreach programs also facilitate public involvement in environmental decision-making, creating an informed citizenry that can push for better policies. Therefore, public health institutions not only implement policy but also contribute to enhancing the capability of populations to counteract environmental risk, thus bridging the gap between policy and public health outcomes (Jeevanandam et al., 2018).

14.5. The Role of Government in Environmental and Public Health

The government plays a key function in ensuring public and environmental well-being through an apparatus of law that aims to minimize risks and promote the health of its citizens. The Environmental Protection Act is a classic example of such devotion, for it serves as the foundation of regulatory policies that regulate and limit pollution, ensure the conservation of natural resources, and promote sustainable development. Through the creation of the Environmental Protection Agency (EPA), the government created an independent agency tasked with enforcing the laws and generating regulations that must be followed by individuals and industry. In addition to direct participation in environmental matters, such legislation acknowledges the interconnection between public health and the environment. For instance, air and water pollution can lead to severe health implications, referring to the need for collective action that lays down the causes of such risks (Sandra et al., 2019). Additionally, the Water Act and the Air Act are integral components of this extensive regulatory framework, focusing on the prevention and limitation of the release of pollutants into watercourses and into the air.

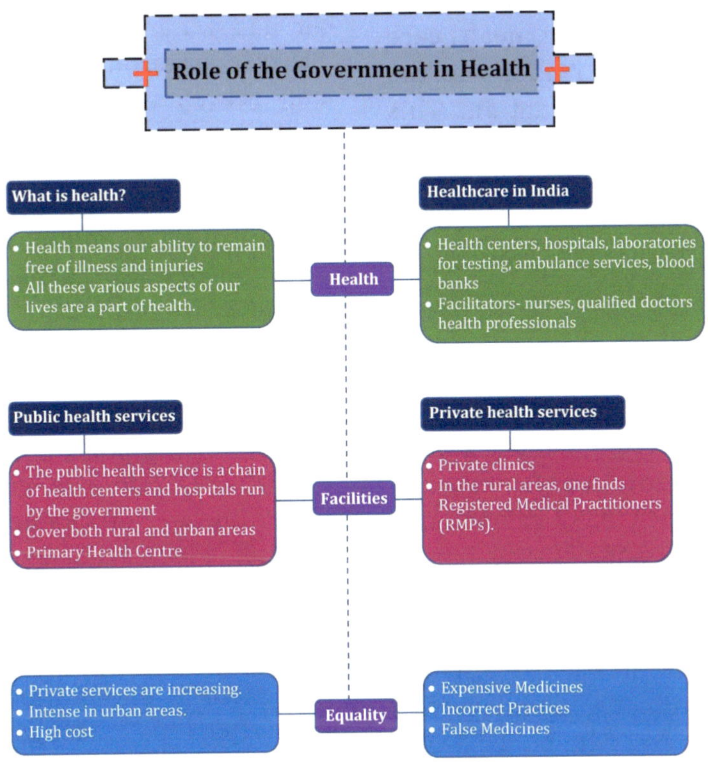

Figure 14.11. The role of government in healthcare.

Source: https://res.cloudinary.com/dpzpn3dkw/image/upload/w_1200,f_auto,q_auto/v1738143664/l0zf0whuwadz2gscv8eg.jpg?_upload_ref=ic_img_tool&__ar__=0.97.

These acts define clear standards for emissions in the air and water, enabling the government to impose fines for noncompliance and facilitate enforcement by various agencies. The effectiveness of these acts does not solely rely on legislative patronage but also on continuous monitoring and public involvement. Government agencies most often collaborate with non-government organizations (NGOs) to educate the public on environmental health risks and complement participatory methods that enable citizens to enhance their health and the environment. By the promotion of government-NGO partnership, a holistic solution to the issues of public health is achieved, which is fundamental to creating long-term change and immunity to environmental risks (Robert, 2016). Its enforcement complements the role of governance in ensuring that healthcare systems are in a position to respond to the effects of environmental degradation. This encompasses the regulation of healthcare providers, the establishment of public health standards, and the monitoring of health-related information to monitor trends and potential crises. With their extensive public health legislation that could comprise mobile health campaigns and community interventions, the government can respond efficiently to endemic and epidemic threats that are usually worsened by environmental conditions. The involvement of NGOs is usually a complement to these legislations that adds greater impact through local knowledge and resources used to enhance the health outcome. As such, the role of government now transcends mere legislation to an active one that promotes the integration of environmental protection with public health policy in order to safeguard society and preserve nature for future generations (Sandra et al., 2019) (Figure 14.11).

14.5.1. Government Agencies Involved in Health and Environmental Protection

The development and implementation of health and environmental protection laws in the United States significantly rely on federal agencies such as the Environmental Protection Agency (EPA) and the Centers for Disease Control and Prevention (CDC). The EPA, which was created in 1970, develops and implements regulations under primary environmental laws, such as the Clean Air Act and the Clean Water Act, that are central to safeguarding public health and the environment. These agencies work together to monitor pollutants as well as regulate public health risks that have been caused by environmental pollution. In exchange, they handle issues ranging from air and water quality to the management of hazardous waste. Adherence to these laws not only prevents environmental dangers but also promotes healthier communities as it reduces exposure to toxins and promotes sustainable methods that conserve natural resources for generations to come. State and territorial governments also have an important function to fulfill in enforcing environmental and public health legislation. Each state possesses an environmental protection agency that is tasked with implementing federal regulations and modifying policies to accommodate local conditions. The agencies control air and water quality, impose health regulations, and monitor waste management, acting rapidly to react to environmental emergencies posing a threat to health. With collaborations with local governments and NGOs, these state agencies guarantee public education and community participation, increasing awareness of environmental health concerns. As can be seen, successful public awareness campaigns have the ability to encourage individual engagement in environmental stewardship, thereby leading to healthier, more resilient communities. The dynamic inter-activity of federal and state institutions guarantees a multi-faceted approach to health and environmental protection and enables differential reactions to different challenges for varying jurisdictions. Apart from the government role, there is also a significant role of non-governmental actors in advocating for the protection of the environment and health. NGOs serve as a middleman between the public and the regulator and speak on behalf of impacted local communities whose livelihoods are at risk due to environmental degradation. They directly participate in policy-making practices, presenting studies and evidence-based policy recommendations to inform decision-makers on issues of concern, such as water contamination and air quality degradation. NGOs also often conduct outreach programs, raising awareness among the general public on environmental health risks and promoting sustainable living. This collaborative framework enhances accountability by government officials, as public pressure can lead to more effective enforcement efforts and more effective legislative measures. Lastly, government institution-NGO cooperation plays a central role in addressing complex environmental challenges, calling for collective solutions, and safeguarding the welfare of the general populace, as seen in efforts to combat such issues as acid rain and air pollution in the context of comprehensive environmental policies (N/A, 2025; Hamilton, 2017).

14.5.2. Policy-Making Processes and Stakeholder Engagement

Effective policy-making processes play a critical role in the making and enforcement of environmental and public health legislation, for example, the Environmental Protection Act and the Water Act. These processes typically begin with the identification of issues that must be regulated, following which there is intensive engagement with stakeholders. Stakeholders like government, NGOs, community members, and industry players play a significant role in conveying the needs and values of affected populations. This is not only essential to receive wide, diverse opinions but also to create consensus around desired policies. Open communication promotes trust and enables stakeholders to collaborate to address intricate problems, especially when environmental issues have implications for public health. The engagement between the interests that participate in stakeholder dialogue can optimize policy decisions' adaptability to the pressing concerns of environmental sustainability and public health administration. Moreover, stakeholder engagement in the policy development process facilitates legislative systems to become efficient. The Air Act and other environmental policies are supported by a foundation of scientific information and public involvement. Stakeholder involvement allows policymakers to incorporate local knowledge and community practice within the decision-making system, so the laws that are passed become meaningful and relevant. Proper participation is also characterized by two-way feedback loops, where stakeholders can review and comment on working policy documents and proposals. This participatory process has the ability to increase the legitimacy of policies as well as raise compliance levels among the population subject to regulations. In addition, examination of major policy decisions indicates that inclusion can alleviate possible conflicts through balanced consideration of environmental, social, and economic priorities in environmental and public health legislation. To reinforce stakeholder involvement in policy-making, the implementation of procedures that emphasize equity and transparency is of critical importance. The efficiency of public and environmental health laws relies on the direct participation of marginalized communities that are often disproportionately affected by public health crises and environmental deterioration. Research has established that the integration of participatory practices within governance can significantly improve policy benefits through addressing social justice and equity concerns. This is particularly important in developing environments where there may be power disequilibrium benefiting all other parties while undermining quality governance. Policymakers need to then engage in an effort to create forums for dialogue that allow the marginalized and invite them to be involved in the legislative process so that policy choice is reflective of varied voices and experiences. Good stakeholder participation will, in the long term, contribute to improved governance and drive the larger goals of environmental and public health legislation, and thus towards sustainable and just outcomes in community wellbeing and environmental management.

14.5.3. Funding and Resources Allocated for Health and Environmental Initiatives

Effective funding and resource allocation are key to effective health and environmental programs as outlined in legislation like the Environmental Protection Act, Water Act, and Air Act. The enactments necessitate a coordinating financial plan to ensure that resources offered can be effectively utilized to facilitate public health and environmental sustainability. Finance is not only about government budgets but also partnerships with NGOs and private institutions. Such partnerships may expand the reach and impact of health and environmental programs, particularly among marginalized groups. Second, fair and transparent use of resources is necessary in order to trust and engage people and enable stakeholders to take active roles in enhancing their health and environment. The urgent need for collective efforts in the conservation of freshwater ecosystems highlights the failure of current financial measures. While freshwater ecosystems offer a home to most of the world's biodiversity, the ecosystems are undergoing catastrophic losses with wetlands disappearing at breathtaking rates. The pursuit of concentrated environmental activities—such as improving water quality and natural resource management—requires firm financial support. Governments should prioritize spending on extensive recovery plans to discourage biodiversity loss effectively. Furthermore, increased access to resources via international collaborations or grants can help preserve such significant ecosystems. By emphasizing sustainable practices and rehabilitation efforts, funding approaches can bring about dramatic health changes, showing the interconnection between public and environmental health improvements (Tickner et al., 2020). Laws regarding environmental protection and public health also rely on effective monitoring and evaluation of funded activities. Unless well regulated, financial resources can lose their intended effects, which is important in maintaining public trust and raising funds in the future.

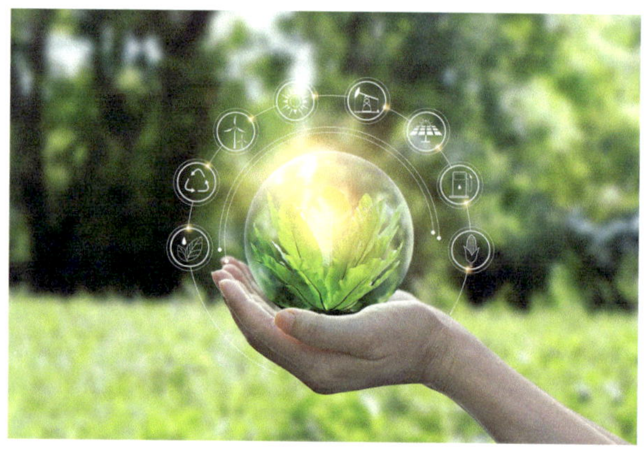

Figure 14.12. Visual representation of sustainable development and environmental protection through renewable energy and conservation practices.

Source: https://getlegalindia.com/wp-content/uploads/2021/11/environment-protection-act.jpg.

For instance, engaging communities in the process of evaluation can provide critical information on the effect of health interventions and policies on the environment.

Also, enhancing coordination between the government institutions and NGOs can create higher awareness and induce advocacy action, mobilizing environmental and health project resources even more. Periodic review paves the way to strategy realignment and the improvement of fund allocations to properly address new issues. Ultimately, the success of environmental and health programs relies on strategic resource allocation and sustained commitment to environmental management and public health improvement (Hilty et al., 2020) (Figure 14.12).

14.6. The Role of NGOs in Environmental and Public Health

The contribution of NGOs in environmental and public health campaigning cannot be overemphasized, particularly in the context of different legislative initiatives. These bodies at times perform crucial middleman roles between the government and the general public, pushing for adherence to the laws in place and pointing out loopholes within policies that can compromise environmental integrity and public health. By mobilizing individuals and creating awareness, NGOs are able to elevate the rate of debate on environmental issues, compelling government bodies to enforce legislation effectively. Such positive involvement brings about a culture of accountability, ensuring that provisions in legislation not only exist but are enforced and also regularly updated to address emerging issues in public health and environmental protection (Kelly et al., 2004). In addition, NGOs are also critical to public health surveillance and data collection alongside the efforts of the state to enforce laws. They will carry out research and dispatch resources to get key data on pollution levels and public health status so as to facilitate informed intervention and advocacy initiatives. As environmental health becomes increasingly complicated, experts hold that there must be a functional partnership to be able to make significant strides. For example, if NGOs are operating in cooperation with grassroots communities, they can identify the environmental hazards prevailing at present and demand mitigation by resorting to legal action. The autonomy of NGOs from state bureaucracy enables them to respond promptly to emerging public health crises, improving the efficiency of existing legislation (Kelly et al., 2004). Finally, the incorporation of NGOs in the ecological governance framework reinforces the values of transparency and democratic accountability.

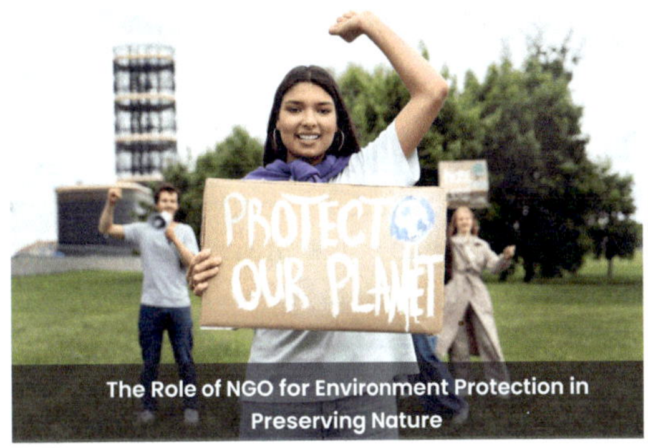
PROTECT OUR PLANET
The Role of NGO for Environment Protection in Preserving Nature

Figure 14.13. The role of NGO in environmental protection.

Source: https://www.socialforaction.com/blog/wp-content/uploads/2024/12/ngo-for-environment-protection.png.

By engaging in active policy debate, such groups ensure that peripheral voices are heard, particularly those most heavily impacted by environmental degradation and health disparities. Their participation tends to produce more nuanced policies that merge local customs and community demands with environmental policy. As enacted by models like the IPPEP Model, good governance of the environment requires the joint engagement of plural groups of stakeholders, including NGOs. Without them, "Third Parties," as established in the IPPEP

Models findings, environmental laws might be toothless, highlighting the imperative role NGOs play in buttressing legislative measures that safeguard environmental and public health (Butzel et al., 2014) (Figure 14.13).

14.6.1. Contributions of NGOs to Advocacy and Awareness

The position of NGOs in promoting environmental and public health law is central to policy formation and raising public consciousness. NGOs typically provide a voice for disadvantaged groups suffering from environmental breakdown and pollution, since they strive persistently to bring attention to injustices and drive legislative change. Their grass-roots campaigns galvanize public opinion, resulting in critical pressure on governments and companies to embrace stronger environmental regulations. Over the past few years, the fate of communities affected by the oil sector has come under public scrutiny, with NGOs bringing to light violations of human rights and degradation of the environment. Rising pollution of local ecosystems puts the livelihoods of marginalized groups at stake, who depend on healthy habitats for their survival. Hence, NGOs play a central role in framing these narratives, demanding accountability and justice under the provisions of current environmental law, as noted by Certomà et al. (2013). Apart from raising awareness, NGOs promote advocacy using legal structures that enable private enforcement mechanisms. In the US, the Environmental Citizen Suit provision empowers individuals and entities to bring suits against environmental law offenses, marking a significant point in environmental management. This provision emerged from intensive environmental activism during the 1960s and 1970s, proving that environmental non-governmental organizations (ENGOs) can appeal to legal safeguards to further public health and environmental protection. By facilitating engagement by civil society organizations, such legal avenues establish a participatory process for citizens in order to hold polluters accountable and seek redress. These mechanisms emphasize the need for implementing good policies through civil action, which is the central component in promoting compliance with Acts such as the Environmental Protection Act and the Water Act, as seen through the comparative study of legal practice from Wang et al. (2021). The cooperation of NGOs around the world also broadens the scope and horizon of advocacy work everywhere. Environmental issues are by their nature transnational, even surpassing state legislation and regulation; thus, NGOs have come together to tackle intricate environmental issues as a group. Such alliances compound their impact through collaboration, sharing of resources, tactics, and accomplishments on the international level, thus establishing a collective global strategy to issues like global warming and biodiversity loss. The combined efforts also drive collective campaigns to identify legislative loopholes and push for broad legal reforms that can directly affect the environmental and public health systems. While NGOs campaign for the creation of international legal systems, their advocacy and awareness drive the legitimate requirement for organizations to adapt to changing challenges to environmental governance, ultimately contributing to increased accountability and pushing for sustained public interest.

14.6.2. Collaboration Between NGOs and Government Agencies

The collaboration of government agencies and NGOs takes a principal position in effectively enforcing public and environmental policy. NGOs, in most cases, function as intermediaries, bridging the gap between government policy and the needs of the community. Their presence at the grassroots level enables them to gather important information and opinions from the public, which is effective in shaping policy change. This partnership is particularly imperative in view of the complexity of certain environmental issues that require a similar collaborative approach to address legislation such as the Environmental Protection Act. By working together, NGOs can leverage their expertise and practical experience to enhance government efforts, and in so doing, ensure maximization of the coverage and effectiveness of environmental protection legislation and public health regulations. Secondly, the collaboration between NGOs and governments typically involves shared resources, expertise, and best practices. For e-waste management, NGOs can play a critical role in educating individuals regarding the harmful consequences of improper disposal and encouraging sustainable practices. As emphasized in current research, active involvement of NGOs allows for the application of extended producer responsibility (EPR) and schemes of producer responsibility, key ingredients in sound management of e-waste. Not only do these partnerships ensure joint action, but also openness and accountability in waste management systems, hence creating a firmer legal framework that is essential for environmental sustainability. The synergy between government agencies and NGOs transcends compliance; it enables innovative solutions to complex environmental challenges. Through the sharing of resources and expertise from both parties, collaborative action can address emergent issues such as water and air quality standards. The IUCN-WCPAs Best Practice Protected Area Guidelines are an example in themselves through prioritizing collaboration among specialist practitioners, enabling improved protected area management through shared expertise. These partnerships are needed to transform bills into on-the-ground outcomes that benefit public health as well as conservation. In this, the dynamic relationship between governments and NGOs is a key factor in granting the resistance needed for future environmental health challenges, where both are well-matched in intent (Figure 14.14).

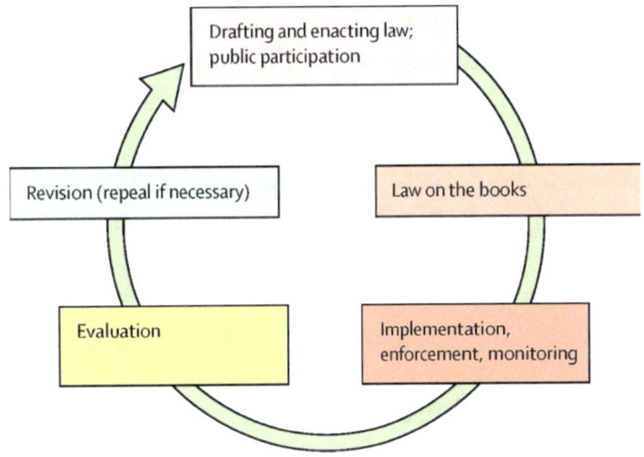

Figure 14.14. The legal determinants of health.

Source: https://www.thelancet.com/cms/10.1016/S0140-6736(19)30233-8/asset/fc6f85a1-1832-4fdd-b108-159024d8f713/main.assets/gr6_lrg.jpg.

14.6.3. Case Studies of Successful NGO-Led Initiatives

In assessing the role of NGOs toward environmental and public health initiatives, case studies highlight their ability to implement effective grassroots interventions that complement measures imposed by legislation such as the Environmental Protection Act. One such explicit example is the intervention activities offered by organizations that lobby for enhanced protection of freshwater habitats. NGOs engaging in such activities usually develop elaborate plans that not only raise awareness but also initiate legislative change. Through cooperation with local communities in documenting declining freshwater biodiversity, these NGOs can effectively mobilize public and government support for policies that are aligned with sustainable development agendas. These efforts show the capacity for NGOs to operate as central stakeholders facilitating legislative objectives while advancing community involvement in ecological conservation and the overall improvement of public health outcomes concerning access to clean water and biodiversity protection (N/A, 2022). The case of a pioneering environmental NGO presents the large-scale influence of focused interventions within the purview of public health legislation. The organization initiated a campaign for wetland revival, which is instrumental to water quality and biodiversity conservation. The program took evidence-based steps towards pollution control and sustainable natural resource management that resulted in wetland revival in large areas. Through partnership with government agencies and local community members, the organization gained funding and volunteered for grassroots projects. In addition to the environmental metrics, the worth of this program extends further, encouraging better health in the community through protection of the drinking water supply and reducing the occurrence of waterborne illness. This illustrates the degree to which NGOs can ensure effective operationalization of public legislation concerning health, thus showing the crossover between environmental protection and public health (Tickner et al., 2020). NGOs also have a critical function in agendas for legislative proposals on air quality and pollution abatement. Successful projects have already shown how NGOs can use scientific evidence to campaign for improved air quality standards. For instance, an NGO conducted a series of community-based monitoring programs to assess levels of air pollution in cities. The findings were strong enough to influence local government policy to incorporate new regulations implemented to reduce emissions from industrial units and vehicles. Through the role of a bridge between residents, scientists, and policymakers, these NGOs facilitate a concerted response towards environmental health concerns to ensure that legislative policy works in defense of public health. Through the power of having localized information, advocacy becomes more solidly grounded, ultimately leading to better environmental law intended to secure the health of exposed people (N/A, 2022).

CLOSER LOOK

FUTURE OF ENVIRONMENTAL AND PUBLIC HEALTH LEGISLATION

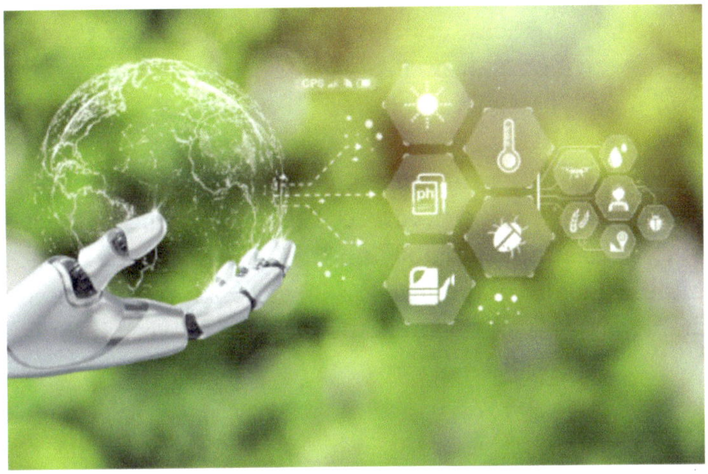

Figure 14.15. Application of artificial intelligence in environmental monitoring and sustainable development.

Source: https://external-content.duckduckgo.com/iu/?u=https%3A%2F%2Fwww.einfochips.com%2Fwp-content%2Fuploads%2F2023%2F06%2FUsing-Artificial-Intelligence-for-Environmental-Protection-and-Sustainable-Development-Blog-Featured-Image-2-scaled-1.jpg&f=1&nofb=1&ipt=dec9008215ee8ae2d4252c2044fcbc62e16d47d481f3f9d9a00bd3c662218d45.

Amidst the shifting landscape of environmental and public health legislation, guidance for the future must center around cross-cutting policymaking to address the interconnectedness of various ecological and health issues. Legislative frameworks such as the Environmental Protection Act and the Water Act will need to evolve to include more fluid threats like climate change and loss of biodiversity. The role of multi-actor systems emphasizes the necessity of interaction between various actors, including governmental agencies, NGOs, and civil society, to introduce legislation that is responsive and adaptive to emerging challenges. Increased focus on sustainable management that honors the multiple socio-environmental interactions is required, and by doing so, enhances resilience in the face of increasing ecological change. This strategy will not just manage current threats but also provide avenues for innovative solutions that can fortify public health systems against environmental degradation. Public health legislation must also adapt to incorporate a more preventive rather than responsive strategy, particularly in the context of the increasing number of health crises linked to environmental factors. As air and water pollution are still huge threats to human health, legislative efforts must be followed by strict enforcement. The integration of the findings on mangrove ecosystems is crucial as these ecosystems provide essential services that have a direct association with public health. Mangrove conservation and recovery not only address natural disasters but also serve to improve air and water quality. Therefore, the future legislative agendas must include biodiversity conservation as a health priority for the public. This shift in strategy will be through concerted action to align environmental and public health legislation so that defense procedures are founded on scientific consciousness and participation at the community level to legitimize their validity and effectiveness. Lastly, the future of environmental and public health policy must be one of equity, particularly for the most underserved populations that contribute to most of the ecological costs. Having an understanding that inequities in health are typically exacerbated by environmental injustices, policies in the future should be geared towards tackling inclusive models that give voice to marginalized groups. Bringing those people along into the policymaking process not only creates trust but also brings local forms of knowledge into solving problems effectively. The role of NGOs becomes increasingly vital in representing the interests of marginalized communities and in ensuring inclusive stakeholders' engagement in policy-making. As the equity considerations are included in future legislation, policymakers shall be able to create a more robust framework that addresses not only the environmental concerns but also ensures social justice and equitable health outcomes for all. A comprehensive strategy shall result in comprehensive, sustainable, and effective public health and environmental legislation.

SUMMARY

The climax of this examination of public and environmental health law presents the imperative interplay between regimes of law, state enforcement, and public pressure. The success of such legislative measures as the Environmental Protection Act, the Water Act, and the Air Act is evident in their ability to prescribe standards that protect public health and natural environments. But the anarchic process of implementation demonstrates that legislation alone is not always sufficient. Working with the combined efforts of government agencies and NGOs requires a synergetic attempt to ensure these legislations are translated into actions that count. The synergy yields innovative solutions and enhances accountability, albeit with continued challenges in implementing regulatory mechanisms with bureaucratic complexities. Furthermore, the integrated pollution control (IPC) strategy is an illustration of harmonizing environmental regulations in different sectors, as reflected through the experiences of countries such as the United Kingdom and the Netherlands. Through a holistic strategy towards pollution management, IPC promotes beyond-compliance collaboration, which generates improved environmental outcomes for air, water, and land. Policy implementation based on the principles of sound science and public participation is thus crucial in managing the intricacies of modern environmental governance. As recognized in ongoing arguments, the imperatives of adaptive measures and emerging technologies only go to further emphasize the necessity for concerted action towards such chronic issues as pollution and declining public health (Hersh et al., 2025). Finally, judicial activism has been a blessing and a curse in the regulatory sphere. While it is a necessary ingredient for filling gaps where governmental enforcement falls through, judicial intervention can only be a temporary solution. The courts have come a long way in upholding environmental rights, but without profound changes in the executive branch's incentive structures, real reform will remain elusive. Ultimately, the sustainability of environmental and public health programs depends on building capacities for governance and nurturing a culture of accountability that balances forward action with rear-guard reactions. Sync of the government's and civil society organizations' roles can thus force the paradigm shift towards good environmental stewardship as encapsulated in the experiences chronicled in this analysis (Rao et al., 2025).

Key Points

In examining the framework of environmental and public health law, cross-references illustrate the intricate interrelationship between regulation, enforcement, and public impact. The Environmental Protection Act provides general principles intended to safeguard natural resources and minimize the impact of pollution on human health. Together with the Water Act and the Air Act, the legislation collectively constitutes a comprehensive regulatory scheme addressing the quality of essential resources that affect population health. Robust enforcement provisions are critical to the degree that violations are addressed promptly and transparently, thereby ensuring public health protection. The legislative convergence illustrates the meaning of uniform policy implementation in health protection, with the reality that law in itself is insufficient without active surveillance and public accountability. The concord between legislation and implementation not only claims to enhance environmental quality but also aims to remedy health disparities caused by environmental factors. Furthermore, public health legislation is the foundation and guarantor of community well-being and health. The controversy surrounding this legislation surrounds the requirement to address issues comprehensively, enlisting the participation of both the private and public sectors towards advancing society's health. Governments and NGOs are both institutions that are vested with the responsibility of implementing health legislation, and this therefore suggests the need for a collaborative rather than siloed public health strategy. The multi-actor approach is all-important since it involves multiple actors in the governance of health, thereby making interventions in health policy more effective. The relationship between government intervention and NGO work manifests itself in the form of community resilience and health security, especially among marginalized populations. Thus, strong public health law enforcement and effective multi-sector coalitions are crucial in addressing health disparities and supporting sustainable well-being across populations. Lastly, emphasis on the importance of evidence-informed policy is necessary to fully value environmental impacts on public health outcomes. The necessity of robust data accumulation and analysis, as outlined for the multi-actor systems discussion, puts evidence-informed decision-making into the spotlight. Effective policy not only requires a clear understanding of the issues in question but also the capability to win over diverse stakeholders. The multi-disciplinary style ensures that a variety of perspectives are considered, and consequently, more targeted and effective health interventions are formed. By taking advantage of the intricacies of socio-technical systems, under direction from frameworks such as those in Enserink et al. (2022), policymakers can forecast problems and switch strategies accordingly. Lastly, the marriage of policy, stakeholder participation, and empirical evidence accentuates the complexity in establishing an equitable and sustainable public health climate, necessitating ongoing commitment to legislative innovation and public health expenditure.

REFERENCES

1. Abubakar, I., Dalglish, S. L., Angell, B., Sanuade, O. A., Abímbọ́lá, Ṣ., Adamu, A. L., Adetifa, I., et al. (2022). The Lancet Nigeria Commission: Investing in health and the future of the nation. *The Lancet, 399*, 1155–1200. https://doi.org/10.1016/s0140-6736(21)02488-0 (accessed on 11th June 2025).
2. Akram, H., Hussain, S., Mazumdar, P., Chua, K. O., Butt, T. E., & Harikrishna, J. A. (2023). Mangrove health: A review of functions, threats, and challenges associated with mangrove management practices. *Forests, 14*, 1698–1698. https://doi.org/10.3390/f14091698 (accessed on 11th June 2025).
3. Barroso, G., Custódio, I. G., Borges, C. E., dos Santos, E. A., Pinto, T. A. A., Soares, M. A., Duque, T. S., et al. (2025). Pesticide residues in Brazil: Analysis of environmental legislation and regulation and the challenge of sustainable production. *Sustainability*. https://www.semanticscholar.org/paper/3501eb2a44a5fdbb685edc0051d34bbc94108433 (accessed on 11th June 2025).
4. Behrman, J., Meinzen-Dick, R., & Quisumbing, A. (2025). *The Gender Implications of Large-Scale Land Deals*. https://core.ac.uk/download/pdf/6237661.pdf (accessed on 11th June 2025).
5. Brauers, H., & Oei, P.-Y. (2020). The political economy of coal in Poland: Drivers and barriers for a shift away from fossil fuels. *Energy Policy, 144*, 111621–111621. https://doi.org/10.1016/j.enpol.2020.111621 (accessed on 11th June 2025).
6. Bryceson, I., & Francis, J. (2001). *Tanzanian Coastal and Marine Resources: Some Examples Illustrating Questions of Sustainable Use*. https://core.ac.uk/download/75777471.pdf (accessed on 11th June 2025).
7. Butzel, A. K., Ottinger, R. L., Parker, J. L., et al. (2014). *Assessing Environmental Governance of the Hudson River Valley: Application of an IPPEP Model*. https://core.ac.uk/download/46712887.pdf (accessed on 11th June 2025).
8. Case, D. W. (2014). *The Lost Generation: Environmental Regulatory Reform in the Era of Congressional Abdication*. https://core.ac.uk/download/62567150.pdf (accessed on 11th June 2025).
9. Certomà, C., Greco, L., Greyl, L., et al. (2013). *Digging Deep the Oil World: Corporate Liability and Environmental Justice Strategies*. https://core.ac.uk/download/55815053.pdf (accessed on 11th June 2025).
10. Chan, G. K. Y. (2019). Environmental pollution control in Singapore: The intersection of torts, statutes, regulations and community norms. *Vietnamese Journal of Legal Sciences, 1*, 77–88. https://www.semanticscholar.org/paper/66180bac9de546fa354af5aec2cf1b45a5f3f271 (accessed on 11th June 2025).
11. Choudhry, Y. A., & Faruqee, R. (2025). *Improving Water Resource Management in Bangladesh*. https://core.ac.uk/download/pdf/6373479.pdf (accessed on 11th June 2025).
12. Dias, A. (2025). *Human Rights, Environment and Development: Special Emphasis on Corporate Accountability*. https://core.ac.uk/download/pdf/6248783.pdf (accessed on 11th June 2025).
13. Díaz, S., Settele, J., Brondízio, E. S., Ngo, H. T., Agard, J., Arneth, A., Balvanera, P., et al. (2019). Pervasive human-driven decline of life on Earth points to the need for transformative change. *Science, 366*. https://doi.org/10.1126/science.aax3100 (accessed on 11th June 2025).

14. Dudek, D. J., Simonis, U. E., & Xue, L. (2025). *Environmental Governance in China*. https://core.ac.uk/download/pdf/6628229.pdf (accessed on 11th June 2025).
15. Elston, K., & Warren, C. (1994). *Environmental Regulation in Indonesia*. https://core.ac.uk/download/11242754.pdf (accessed on 11th June 2025).
16. Enserink, B., Bots, P. W. G., van Daalen, E., Hermans, L., Koppenjan, J., Kortmann, R., Kwakkel, J., et al. (2022). *Policy Analysis of Multi-Actor Systems*. TU Delft Open eBooks. https://doi.org/10.5074/t.2022.004 (accessed on 11th June 2025).
17. Hamilton, L. (2017). *Public Support for Environmental Protection*. https://www.semanticscholar.org/paper/374dc044b773abd8190f4c57f92208bd0a63430d (accessed on 11th June 2025).
18. Hersh, R. (2025). *A Review of Integrated Pollution Control Efforts in Selected Countries*. https://core.ac.uk/download/pdf/9307942.pdf (accessed on 11th June 2025).
19. Hilty, J., Worboys, G. L., Keeley, A. T. H., Woodley, S., Lausche, B. J., Locke, H., Carr, M. H., et al. (2020). *Guidelines for Conserving Connectivity Through Ecological Networks and Corridors*. https://doi.org/10.2305/iucn.ch.2020.pag.30.en (accessed on 11th June 2025).
20. Jeevanandam, J., Barhoum, A., Chan, Y. S., Dufresne, A., & Danquah, M. K. (2018). Review on nanoparticles and nanostructured materials: History, sources, toxicity and regulations. *Beilstein Journal of Nanotechnology, 9*, 1050–1074. https://doi.org/10.3762/bjnano.9.98 (accessed on 11th June 2025).
21. John, E. I., & Bello, I. E. (2025). Assessing the role of good governance and policy making in land use abuse monitoring and management in Nigeria. *International Journal of Research and Innovation in Social Science*. https://www.semanticscholar.org/paper/3f602965bce0a2c802b6263e9748ba123c47a13a (accessed on 11th June 2025).
22. Kelly, W. P. (2004). *Citizens Cannot Stand for It Anymore: How the United States' Environmental Actions in Afghanistan and Iraq Go Unchecked by Individuals and Non-Governmental Organizations*. https://core.ac.uk/download/144226335.pdf (accessed on 11th June 2025).
23. Lungu, K., Morse, T., & Taulo, S. (2010). *Gap Analysis of Environmental Health Research in Malawi: Report to the National Commission of Science and Technology*. https://core.ac.uk/download/19610167.pdf (accessed on 11th June 2025).
24. Muntarbhorn, V. (2025). *Human Rights and Human Development: Thailand Country Study*. https://core.ac.uk/download/pdf/6248764.pdf (accessed on 11th June 2025).
25. Murthy, V., & Ramakrishna, S. (2022). A review on global e-waste management: Urban mining towards a sustainable future and circular economy. *Sustainability, 14*, 647–647. https://doi.org/10.3390/su14020647 (accessed on 11th June 2025).
26. Mutangadura, G. B. (2005). *Sustainable Development in Southern Africa: Progress in Addressing the Challenges*. https://core.ac.uk/download/75779752.pdf (accessed on 11th June 2025).
27. Peel, J., & Lin, J. (2019). Transnational climate litigation: The contribution of the Global South. *American Journal of International Law, 113*, 679–726. https://doi.org/10.1017/ajil.2019.48 (accessed on 11th June 2025).
28. Permono, B., & Kurniati, A. (2024). Decision-making processes in resource management: Lessons from the agriculture sector. *Journal of Resource Management and Decision Engineering*. https://www.semanticscholar.org/paper/03ead763741fb3d4ce0023c1026765d06a032226 (accessed on 11th June 2025).

29. Rao, M. G., & Mandal, S. (2025). *Overlapping Fiscal Domains and Effectiveness of Environmental Policy in India*. https://core.ac.uk/download/pdf/6604651.pdf (accessed on 11th June 2025).

30. Rejikumar, J., & Vishnu, M. (2025). Legal aspects of environmental protection in India. *Juni Khyat*. https://www.semanticscholar.org/paper/5d16b135dfa410542151cc4bdd3e61377a4d12fe (accessed on 11th June 2025).

31. Rodić, L., & Wilson, D. C. (2017). Resolving governance issues to achieve priority Sustainable Development Goals related to solid waste management in developing countries. *Sustainability, 9*, 404–404. https://doi.org/10.3390/su9030404 (accessed on 11th June 2025).

32. Rodrigues de Lima, A. C. (2022). *Soil Quality Assessment in Rice Production Systems*. https://www.semanticscholar.org/paper/1ff2e0338843618761dac766054b362253103082 (accessed on 11th June 2025).

33. Sikes, R. S. (2016). 2016 Guidelines of the American Society of Mammalogists for the use of wild mammals in research and education. *Journal of Mammalogy, 97*, 663–688. https://doi.org/10.1093/jmammal/gyw078 (accessed on 11th June 2025).

34. Thomas, K. A., Hardy, D., Lazrus, H., Méndez, M., Orlove, B., Rivera-Collazo, I., Roberts, J. T., et al. (2018). Explaining differential vulnerability to climate change: A social science review. *Wiley Interdisciplinary Reviews: Climate Change, 10*. https://doi.org/10.1002/wcc.565 (accessed on 11th June 2025).

35. Tickner, D., Opperman, J. J., Abell, R., Acreman, M., Arthington, A. H., Bunn, S. E., Cooke, S. J., et al. (2020). Bending the curve of global freshwater biodiversity loss: An emergency recovery plan. *BioScience, 70*, 330–342. https://doi.org/10.1093/biosci/biaa002 (accessed on 11th June 2025).

36. van de Biezenbos, K. (2017). *Where Oil Is King*. https://core.ac.uk/download/144231844.pdf (accessed on 11th June 2025).

37. Wang, H. (2021). *Assessing China's Environmental NGO Public Interest Litigation Against the U.S. Citizen Suit Model*. https://core.ac.uk/download/480448110.pdf (accessed on 11th June 2025).

38. Yaya, R., Wibowo, S., Ulfaturrahmah, & Jalaludin, D. (2018). Environmental disclosure practices after mandatory disclosure policy in Indonesia. *Journal of Business & Retail Management Research*. https://www.semanticscholar.org/paper/d6d057d87908defe2214dd147eda471ff6aeffcd (accessed on 11th June 2025).

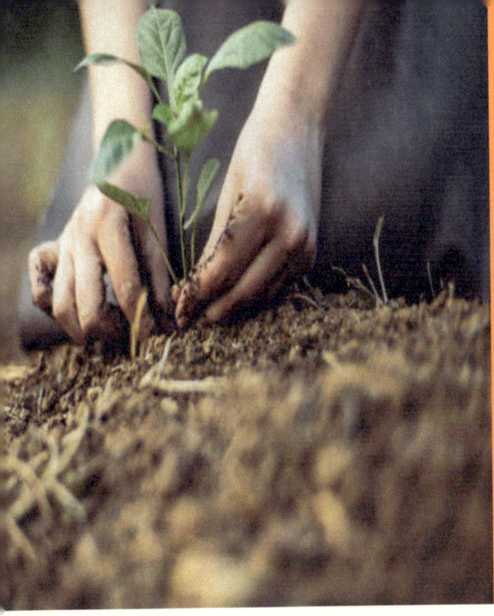

Chapter 15

SUSTAINABLE DEVELOPMENT AND ENVIRONMENTAL HEALTH

Contents

Introduction

The overlap between sustainable development and environmental health is gaining common acceptance as a paradigm to address current global challenges. As urbanization continues, the intricacy of balancing the resources of the environment and public health has been a concern in urban and rural environments. Sustainable development describes an all-embracing strategy for balancing economic growth, social justice, and environmental protection, thereby ensuring health and well-being for everyone. This coordination is critical, as ecosystem destruction tends to worsen health inequities, particularly in marginalized groups. Approaches that incorporate sustainability into health planning can provide long-term dividends, not only enhancing health outcomes but also promoting ecological stability. Addressing gender equity concerns, utilization of resources, and community building is the way forward for creating environments that enhance human health and make ecosystems more sustainable in the end, leading to better overall quality of life for varied populations of individuals

(Herklotz et al., 2012). The applicability of environmental health in the broader sustainability debate cannot be overemphasized. Effective urban and rural planning, which takes into account the distinctive needs and situations of communities, creates systems that are health-promoting and environmentally appropriate. For instance, sanitation and hygiene programs for improved sanitation and hygiene can efficiently reduce the spread of disease and improve general well-being in communities. Effective application of sanitation and hygiene behavioral change techniques and methods is essential to creating healthier environments. This involves not only the installation of physical infrastructure but also engaging communities to make them understand the importance of sustainable conduct (Evans et al., 2010). The interventions that incorporate community inputs and locally derived knowledge are most effective, supporting cooperation as the foundation for sustainability. In the long term, environmental wellness must be incorporated into all else that is contemplated, again supporting human and ecological systems' interconnectedness. Involvement of citizens and communities in working towards sustainability is a key component of the entire platform. Educating and incorporating local communities into the decision-making process is integral to guaranteeing ongoing efforts in environmental welfare. Where decisions are made by the people, they tend to embrace sustainable practices, which in turn means improved health outcomes and conservation of the environment. Programs aimed at teaching people how to conserve resources, manage waste, and mitigate climate change can create a sustainability culture that knows no borders. By affirming the interdependency between human behavior and environmental well-being, people can develop a sense of accountability for their environment. This collective effort not only reinforces local environments but also abets the global agenda for sustainable development, ensuring current and future generations a capacity for survival within a healthy and balanced environment (Herklotz et al., 2012; Evans et al., 2010) (Figure 15.1).

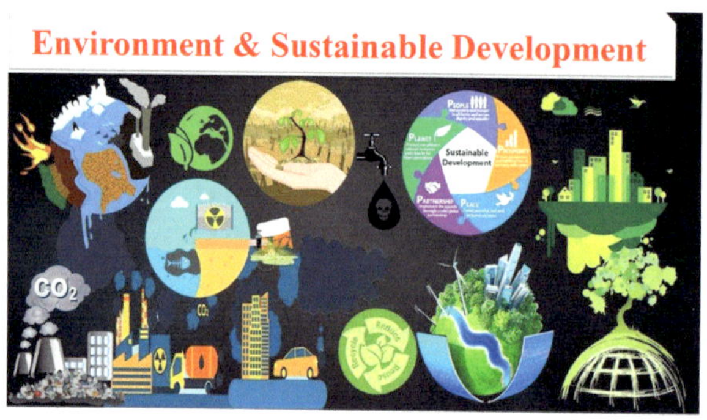

Figure 15.1. Environmental sustainability development.

Source: https://external-content.duckduckgo.com/iu/?u=https%3A%2F%2Ftse3.mm.bing.net%2Fth%3Fid%3DOIP.0km6kNhacFfsycVh4R8OogHaEK%26pid%3DApi&f=1&ipt=08bfb95dbe81d214a3eec7c9ff01f76c94c1f2a4a93cb5c4a9638298705cfae2.

Definition of Sustainable Development

Sustainable development is a three-dimensional concept that entails a whole-brained approach to fostering well-being in society in a way that maintains the integrity of the environment. Anchored in its essence is the triple bottom line, which integrates social, economic, and environmental dimensions of decision-making. This policy focuses on taking into account not only economic viability but also the social impact and ecological consequences of development initiatives. It recognizes that sustainable development is not achievable through individual actions, but through interdependencies between various sectors. As envisioned under the theme of urban wastewater management, a heterogeneous structure based on sustainability principles can guide strategic asset investments as a reaction to community needs and environmental responsibilities (Ashley et al., 2008). This broader vision for development emphasizes that long-term sustainable development is an equilibrium among many aims so that the world is a better place to live for current and future generations. The phrase sustainable development is more than the efficient use of resources. It invites an understanding of how these resources are interconnected within larger systems, especially in urban and rural development. Natural resource management is critical to preserve farm yield and maintaining ecological balance. For instance, agricultural and food system policy must not only aim for short-term economic yield but also for their environmental impacts and health contributions to society (Bellon et al., 2025). Urban planning, in particular, is aided by principles of sustainable development through practices encouraging green spaces, sustainable transport, and the use of renewable energy. Such planning facilitates not only environmental health but also national resilience in the face of climate change, highlighting how holistic strategies can result in a better quality of life. Individuals and communities are critical drivers of the principles of sustainable development. They are both agents of change and beneficiaries of sustainable approaches, underlining the realization of grassroots participation in decision-making. Involving the citizens also creates a sense of ownership of development projects, investing in local sustainability initiatives such as neighborhood gardens or home retrofits for energy efficiency. Education is also a powerful tool, as it allows communities to make informed decisions around sustainable value. Through the highlighted urban planning initiatives, the dynamic interaction between residents, planners, and policymakers can unlock innovative strategies that augment local resources while addressing environmental and health challenges. Ultimately, individuals' and communities' work provides the groundwork for a sustainable future, reflecting the basic premises of sustainable development in diverse social contexts.

Importance of Environmental Health

Environmental health becomes more important in sustainable development with reference to urbanization and accelerating ecological degradation due to increasing population and urbanization. Healthy ecosystems are of prime importance to human health because they provide basic services such as clean air, water, and fertile soil. These factors are not only crucial for personal well-being but for public health as well. Environmental health is irrevocably entwined with the sustainability paradigm since it involves the interdependence of integrity within ecosystems and human health. All environmental health concerns must be resolved through an integrated means of both scientific knowledge and community involvement. By pursuing approaches like ecological restoration, contested by the Society for Ecological Restoration, communities can play active roles in restoring impaired ecosystems, which, in turn, encourages sustainable livelihood and health impacts (George et al., 2019). The appreciation and response to environmental health are thus not necessarily a preference but an imperative for the generation of resilient, sustainable communities. Further, the role of environmental health in planning urban and rural spaces cannot be overstated. Urban environments come with some challenges, such as air pollution and limited green space, that adversely affect the health of citizens. Thus, making environmental health considerations a part of urban planning can significantly enhance living standards and public health. Besides, rural regions, even though conventionally regarded as being healthier due to their location close to natural environments, are plagued by the adverse effects of industrial activities, agricultural runoff, and global warming. Effective planning policies must incorporate sustainability values so that the development activities do not damage the health of the ecosystem but enhance it (N/A, 2018). That means creating policies that safeguard natural resources while encouraging citizens to adopt behaviors that promote environmental stewardship. Ultimately, environmental health is an essential perspective through which urban and rural planners can design spaces focusing on people and ecological health. Community and personal involvement are crucial in advancing the importance of environmental health. Getting communities involved in local sustainability projects fosters a sense of responsibility and ownership for their surroundings.

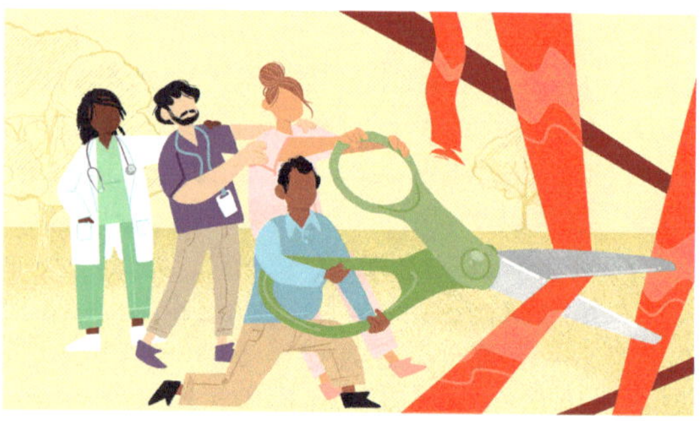

Figure 15.2. Importance of environmental health.

Source: https://rwjf.scene7.com/is/image/rwjf/Public-Health-blog-Illustration?ts=1740613604061&dpr=off.

For instance, community clean-up days or tree planting activities not only make the local area look more aesthetically pleasing, but they also enhance air quality and biodiversity. In addition, education regarding the impacts of pollution and loss of habitat can equip individuals with the skills to advocate for cleaner ways of practice in communities and homes (George et al., 2019). With collaboration from stakeholders—like NGOs, government institutions, and the private sector—communities can formulate end-to-end approaches that address environmental health concerns as well as promote social equity. As soon as individuals realize their part in environmental health, they become agents for change, belonging to a larger movement toward sustainability. Grassroots action not only enhances public health conditions within communities but eventually enhances public health conditions across regions (Figure 15.2).

15.1. Principles of Sustainability

Principles of sustainability actually depend on the interdependence between the environmental, social, and economic dimensions, which are popularly referred to as the triple bottom line. This holistic system recognizes that the health of our planet is inseparably tied to the well-being of its people and society. For instance, sustainable development policies promoting gender equality can advance improved environmental outcomes; women's involvement in managing natural resources contributes to higher resource sustainability, thus in developing healthier communities. Evidence shows that when women have equal access to resources as men, communities are more stable against environmental disturbances and consequently experience sustainable development in their respective fields, for instance, health, education, and energy management (Herklotz et al., 2012). This integrated perspective emphasizes the integration of social equity in environmental actions to ensure end-to-end sustainability. In urban planning and rural planning, the principles of sustainability demand integrated design that harmonizes human activity with nature. Effective urban planning takes aim at creating spaces that maximize minimal environmental footprints and promote social equity. For instance, green transportation systems can reduce greenhouse gas emissions while enhancing access to necessary services for the underprivileged. Through the use of technologies and practices guided by the most current scientific knowledge, planners can guarantee that the two communities are economically prosperous and continue to remain environmentally sound. US Agency for International Development assigns the highest priority to this approach in its international Water and Development Strategy that emphasizes sustainability by engaging partnerships in host countries and the application of emerging technologies to increase water management (N/A, 2013). Sustainable planning must thus address contexts at the local level, seeking to balance ecological integrity and economic and social needs of all members in the community. Moreover, the participation of people and communities towards obtaining sustainability cannot be overemphasized. Community participation is crucial for the implementation of sustainable practices for improving environmental health. When individuals participate directly in efforts towards sustainability, whether it is neighborhood clean-ups, community gardens, or learning programs, they establish a culture of environmental stewardship. Not only does this enrich local ecosystems, but it also instills a sense of ownership and responsibility among people. Studies have determined that dedicated individuals are likely to support policies and practices that allow sustainability on higher levels, a ripple impact that spreads to action and policy beyond the local scale. Since communities exchange information and resources with each other, they are able to utilize their collective strengths for higher environmental and societal contributions, supporting the contention that sustainability is everybody's business and will have to be addressed by everybody (Figure 15.3).

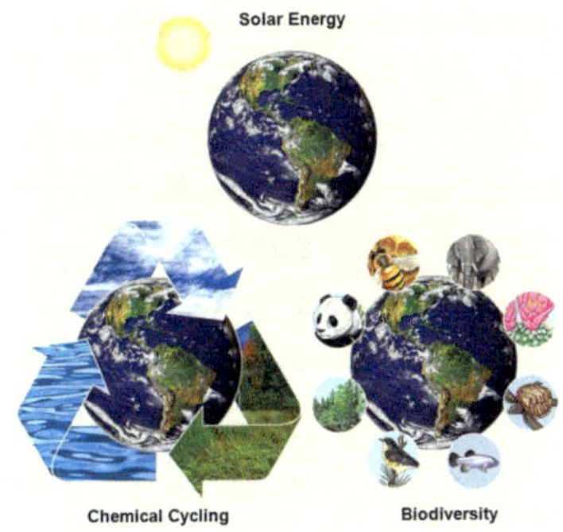

Figure 15.3. Principles of sustainability.

Source: https://venhoevencs.nl/wp-content/uploads/2020/05/the-basic-principles-of-sustainability-2-800x600.jpg.

15.1.1. Economic Sustainability

Economic sustainability remains a core component in the broader framework of sustainable development, uniting ecological sustainability with fiscal sustainability to ensure the availability of resources for future generations. The concept is one of frugal management of economic resources to enhance long-term environmental well-being and social justice. Sustainable economic activity is oriented to profitability as well as its impact on the quality of life of the community and the environment. For example, integrating the circular economy can reduce waste and maximize resource utilization, eventually resulting in cost-effective and sustainable solutions. As indicated by George et al. (2019), these measures can play a very important role in helping to conserve biodiversity and improve ecosystem services, which are very crucial for ensuring the balance required for communities to sustain themselves. Moreover, economic sustainability encourages innovation in such a way that businesses are able to adapt to changing environmental regulations alongside emerging technologies that fuel sustainability goals. Urban and rural planning also contributes a lot towards economic sustainability through well-informed decisions that help in the balanced development of the economy without harming the environment. Effective planning policies integrate economic development with ecological wellness in a way that makes land use strategies conform to sustainable practice. For example, green infrastructure integration, e.g., urban parks and forests, not only adds to urban beauty but also increases local diversity and air quality. According to the analysis of sustainable community development, government agencies and local businesses must coordinate efforts to build a coordinated response to economic, social, and environmental challenges. Furthermore, initiatives like neighborhood food systems can enhance rural economies without compromising food security and reducing the environmental impacts of long-distance transportation, thereby aligning with sustainability principles at the community level. Double focus on both of them is essential to foster resilience against ever-changing global change. Private individuals and communities play a vital part in enhancing economic sustainability through practices that represent collective values of stewardship of the natural world and social responsibility. Community involvement is also crucial in embracing sustainable economic practices because the people living in these areas best understand their economies and environments. Participatory systems, such as community-led renewable energy projects, make communities responsible for their resources while reducing fossil fuel consumption. Similarly, educational programs also raise awareness of the economic benefits of maintaining practices, which increases environmentally friendly practice participation. Promotion of local businesses through sustainable consumerism supports economic sustainability through creating a virtuous cycle—whereby local economies grow and ecosystems are preserved. The link between economic sustainability and community health eventually results in an integrated framework towards sustainable development, ensuring that future generations can enjoy advancements. Sustainable economic practices have the potential to yield significant environmental and economic returns through active engagement by people and communities (Yoshikawa et al., 2020).

15.1.2. Social Sustainability

Social sustainability depicts the concept that the well-being of society is the pillar of sustainable growth. Social sustainability is the significance of developing inclusive access to resources, opportunity, and rights among individuals, primarily among the marginalized classes. With social priorities, communities wish to design environments where individuals can thrive, connect, and excel. For instance, the promotion of gender equality is a critical element of social sustainability because it grants women equitable access to education, health, and economic prospects. Hence, the enhancement of women's roles in all areas not only enriches individual life but also yields general societal advancement, creating a positive cycle that sustains environmental sustainability as outlined in Herklotz et al. (2012). As such, social sustainability must be thought of as an integral part of overall development plans. The planning spaces in rural and urban areas are enhanced by the concepts of social sustainability in the formulation of interventions that address the unique needs of diverse communities. Planning must prioritize both social and environmental needs of a community to facilitate integration towards accessibility and inclusion. For instance, rural sanitation service development is an urgent social problem that overlaps with environmental health and affects the quality of life for the people living in rural communities. There are reports that, although rural sanitation in Latin America has progressed, achieving the Millennium Development Goals is still a challenge, highlighting the necessity of using sustainable, long-term approaches that incorporate local communities and governments in planning, as noted in Pearce-Oroz (2011). Resolving these issues as a whole is capable of harmonizing social development and environmental well-being. The efforts of individuals and communities in progressing social sustainability cannot be overstated. Individuals are often the agents of change in their societies, advocating for policies conducive to equitable access to resources and environmental conservation. Grassroots participation and local organizations offer avenues for empowerment of residents' engagement in sustainable activities, where diversity is incorporated in decision-making to ensure that various voices are heard. Through collaboration and engagement, communities can address key social issues while making themselves resilient to environmental stressors. Through active engagement in activities that strive towards social equity, individuals not only contribute to individual and community well-being but also construct the entire system for sustainability. Last but not least, social sustainability relies on individuals uniting, as the integration of the social, economic, and environmental factors creates a more balanced and fair society that upholds sustainable development's values (Figure 15.4).

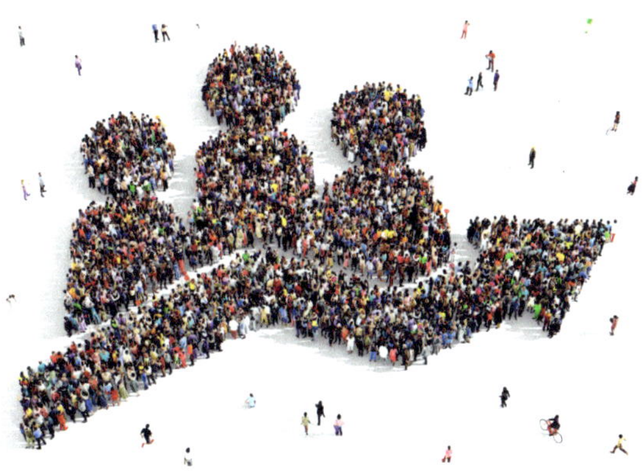

Figure 15.4. Social sustainability.

Source: https://cdn.prod.website-files.com/63638f240463b63a577b5bf9/63e624912ff628ec665d313e_624d63166587e41cff74efce_shutterstock_604150523.jpg.

15.1.3. Environmental Sustainability

Because the implication of environmental sustainability is continually increasing, gender equity's contribution towards promoting such endeavors comes up as a relevant consideration. Research confirms that ensuring the provision of resources in equal proportions to women has the potential to impact sustainability for any sector under consideration, for example, energy, health, and climate change. By enabling women and raising their level of access to resources, societies can leverage their experience and involvement in sustainable efforts to improve not only their individual status but also the general environmental health. The intersectionality of gender and sustainability calls for policies that are inclusive and encourage women's active participation in environmental activities and bring evidence to the forefront that gender equality is not only a social issue but an integral aspect of sustainable development (Herklotz et al., 2012). In urban planning and rural development, sustainability concepts are employed as a benchmarking principle to prevent environmental issues as well as enhance public health. Planning that is effective must accommodate land use, resource management, and community involvement to enhance resilience against environmental degradation. Joining sustainable practices within such settings demands collaboration on the part of all who have an interest in them, including government agencies, community-based organizations, and residents. For instance, the United Nations Development Assistance Framework (UNDAF) prioritizes national priorities that match these goals toward an integrated means of ensuring environmental sustainability. Through constant monitoring and evaluation, the performance of urban and rural planning systems can be quantified so that they can be responsive to environmental and human health needs (N/A, 2014). However, governments and organizations are not solely tasked with encouraging environmental sustainability, but even communities and individuals themselves. Local actions can create huge changes when communities adopt sustainable practices, such as recycling, water efficiency, and advocating for green policies. Public education and mobilization on sustainability can help establish a culture of stewardship whereby citizens see themselves as responsible for protecting the environment. Community activities, such as community gardens and clean-up days, enable one to be actively engaged in sustainability while fostering social integration within communities. As individuals are increasingly made conscious of their ecological footprint, they contribute to a broader movement in the direction of achieving sustainability objectives, thereby reflecting the crucial interdependence of individual and collective action in achieving environmental health.

15.2. Environmental Health in Urban Planning

The environmental health idea remains at the heart of urban planning, especially with cities increasingly grappling with the demands of sustainable development. Urban dwellings present some unique challenges that can have negative effects on public health in terms of air and water pollution, noise, and substandard green spaces. To construct healthier communities, urban planners must place serious emphasis on environmental health as part of their planning. Research has indicated that higher urban densities can enhance public transport and infrastructure, but, in addition, can have significant negative impacts on health and well-being, which are undervalued when planning (Berg et al., 2021). This reality induces a need for a balanced assessment considering both the pros and cons of densification in towns, such that the formed town designs not only enhance sustainability but also the health of the entire population. A key aspect of the debate on environmental health within urban planning is the interface between evidence-based practice and actual planning policy. In some instances, urban planning projects engage core environmental issues superficially while being far too preoccupied with specifics like budgetary and travel benefits of increased density (Alst\ue4de et al., 2021). This alignment is detrimental in that it ignores the social implications of densification, such as putting a strain on recreational facilities and biodiversity conservation.

As city planners become more aware of these imbalances, they can actively work to implement more equitable planning measures that directly target such complex issues. This may encompass the use of green infrastructure and increased public space accessibility, leading to improved urban environments and a healthier quality of life for city dwellers. The role of communities and individuals in furthering environmental health in the city cannot be underestimated. People's participation in planning can yield a high degree of diversity of opinions that enrich decision-making and foster community ownership. Public participation is crucial in the determination of specific health problems associated with urban environments, such as lead poisoning from old infrastructure or heat island diffusion in densely populated areas. Community actions can also be presented as policy influencing to make green areas and eco-friendly transport modes a priority, which can mitigate the negative health consequences associated with urban settlements (Alst\ue4de et al., 2021). Lastly, facilitating communities to contribute to urban planning processes not only benefits environmental health but also enriches social relationships, leading to more sustainable and resilient cityscapes (Figure 15.5).

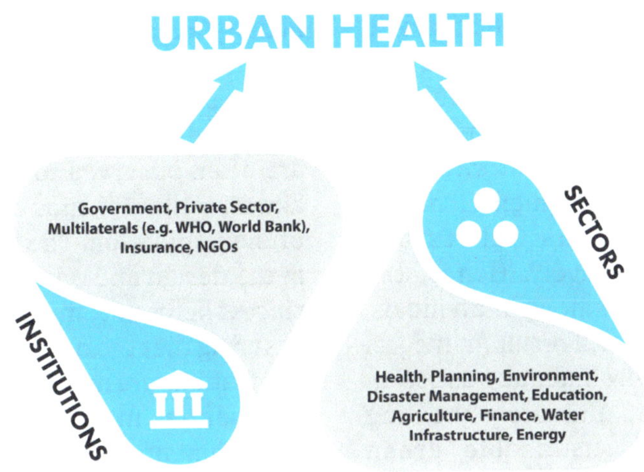

Figure 15.5. Urban health.

Source: https://static.cambridge.org/binary/version/id/urn:cambridge.org:id:binary:20180411085702906-0475:9781316563878:60333fig10_3.png?pub-status=live.

15.2.1. Air Quality Management

Air quality management is a critical part of environmental health and sustainable development, particularly in light of the growing urban population. Deterioration of air quality poses severe health consequences in the form of respiratory diseases, cardiovascular ailments, and premature mortality. Keeping these issues in mind, effective air quality management needs to be incorporated into urban and rural development plans. Such integration not only addresses the timeliness of healthcare issues but also aids in greater sustainability measures in bringing about healthier living environments. Because cities all over the world are grappling with the effects of urbanization, there is a desperate need for innovative policies that deal with air quality, ultimately dictating the well-being of entire communities. Stakeholders like local governments and the private sector must unite to create policies that reduce emissions and enhance air quality monitoring systems. On top of that, community engagement in air management systems will create a sense of shared responsibility towards the health of the environment. Communities play an important role in shaping cleaner air and more environmentally friendly practices and policies. Grassroots activism has the power to pressure local government into undertaking measures that decrease pollution sources such as industrial effluent and automobile traffic. Through sensitization of the public concerning the damaging effects of air pollution and offering the same public the tools with which they can battle for their rights, grassroots activism has the capacity to influence environmentally friendly urban planning. In today's networked world, the integration of air quality issues into broader sustainability efforts can create cities with the potential to design places that support well-being and health. The potential of communities to become active participants in air quality management is the strength that is available within collective action towards achieving sustainability objectives. Socioeconomic issues that are an inherent part of air quality management only act to highlight the need for equity-based policies in policy formulation. Vulnerable groups disproportionately experience poor air quality, which worsens pre-existing disparities in health. Sustainable development is not possible without reducing these inequalities, necessitating targeted measures that ensure everyone in the community has improved air quality. This applies even more so to gender equality, where empowering women through equal access to resources results in better health outcomes for the community. By integrating air quality management strategies with the principles of environmental health and sustainability, policymakers will respond to these inequalities effectively. Hence, the promotion of cooperation among individuals, societies, and governments will result in integral solutions addressing environmental justice in air quality management, ultimately yielding healthier societies and sustainable urban environments (Herklotz et al., 2012; Scott et al., 2016) (Figure 15.6).

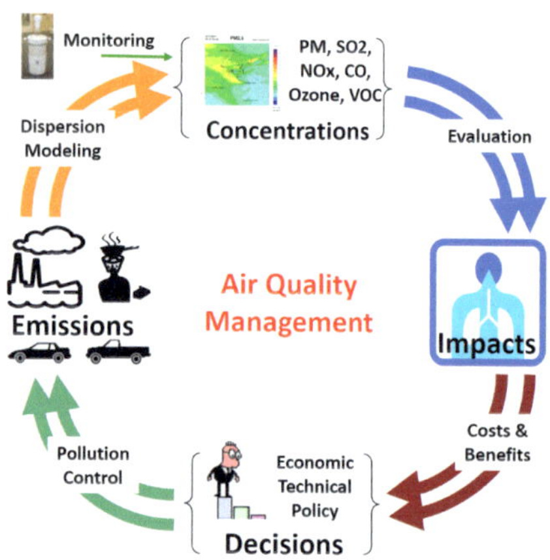

Figure 15.6. Air quality management.

Source: https://urbanemissions.info/wp-content/uploads/images/schematics_air_quality_management.png.

15.2.2. Green Spaces and Public Health

The interaction of green spaces and public health is increasing in prominence as an important discipline among the concepts of sustainable development and environmental health. Green spaces such as parks, gardens, and green roofs offer different ecological services that directly contribute to public health benefits. Groniness around has been discovered to trigger physical activity, counteract stress, and increase social encounters, all of which have positive impacts on physical as well as mental health. Moreover, cities endowed with a lot of green infrastructure are often observed to have reduced urban heat and air pollution, thus overall greater well-being of the population. The stakeholder engagement in the design and operation of such areas is vital since it helps in community ownership as well as ensuring that the needs and interests of different populations are met. Such a participatory process is essential in facilitating sustainable urban environments that give prominence to health and well-being in planning approaches (Gupta et al., 2024). Under the auspices of sustainable development principles, the integration of green spaces in urban and rural planning is a strategic response to addressing health inequalities and enhancing resilience. Green infrastructure not only assists in responding to the environmental degradation exacerbated by urbanization but also in enhancing the socio-economic cohesion of populations. Benefits such as increased property value, new employment opportunities, and augmented biodiversity in the urban setting can be quantitatively and qualitatively assessed. For instance, there has been evidence to suggest that urban areas that have larger green space allocations tend to register higher mental health status due to lower anxiety and depression levels among citizens. Green spaces can also act as natural shields against climate-related health hazards like heat strokes and respiratory illnesses. Hence, green space planning can be regarded as a significant part of public health policy that merges ecological sustainability with health objectives in communities (Adesina et al., 2024). The actions of citizens and communities in undertaking and maintaining green spaces are critical aspects in promoting public health in the sustainability context. Participation from the community does not just inform planning decisions but also fosters collective ownership of the environment. Green-space enhancement projects at a local level, such as neighborhood clean-up days or community gardens, can greatly improve the health of residents and create a sense of belonging. Besides, education will help individuals acquire the knowledge of the health benefits associated with green spaces and push them to actively engage in planning and managing green spaces. Coordination between municipal governments, urban planners, and local people could lead to integrated strategies that place a strong emphasis on health and sustainability, also guaranteeing the inclusion of green spaces in the public's health and well-being. Such partnerships enable communities to be agents of change while seeking a more sustainable, healthier urban future (Gupta et al., 2024) (Figure 15.7).

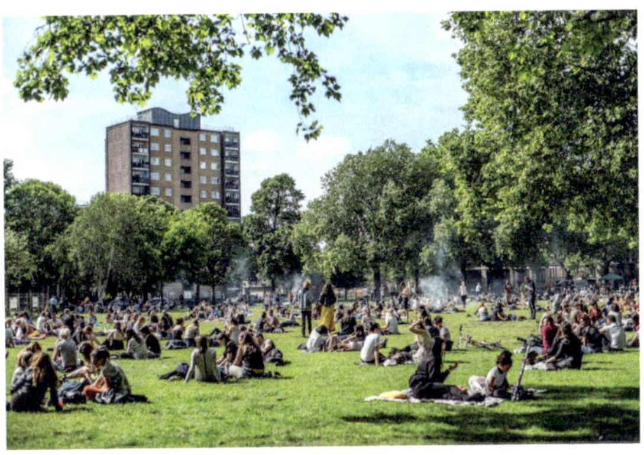

Figure 15.7. Green spaces and public health.

Source: https://s.abcnews.com/images/US/park-01-as-gty-191101_hpMain.jpg.

15.2.3. Infrastructure and Waste Management

The connection between infrastructure and waste management is at the center of the argument of sustainable development versus environmental health. Effective systems for waste management are critical to urban and rural planning since they directly affect public health and environmental health. With ongoing urbanization, waste management becomes increasingly complex. There is a necessity for the application of an integrated framework that considers the waste management interface with other urban systems. Sustainability today is often unattainable, demanding an integrated framework for social, economic, and environmental considerations. The implementation of a "triple bottom line" approach can guide decision-makers on how to make waste management policy effectiveness decisions, thereby fostering a more sustainable urban environment (Ashley et al., 2008). The use of such an all-encompassing perspective enables cities to effectively manage their waste creation and enhance the quality of life of their residents. Just as vital is taking into account the gender dimension in managing waste and infrastructure planning. There is evidence that the achievement of gender equality largely contributes to sustainable development, particularly in urbanization and resource use. Women are likely to assume a crucial role in managing family garbage and the sustenance of environmental sustainability at the community level. In ensuring women's fair portion in resources and choice, not only do we increase individual and family well-being, but also enhance world environmental sustainability (Herklotz et al., 2012). Thus, integrating gender perspectives in waste management and infrastructure planning has the ability to deliver more effective and fair outcomes. The focus not only recognizes women's input but also energizes communities and subsequently reinforces sustainable practice. Ultimately, responsibility for achieving sustainable waste management and infrastructure solutions is transferred beyond governments at the individual and community levels. Involving residents in sustainability activities is essential in establishing a sense of responsibility and care for the environment. Local recycling programs and clean-up initiatives are excellent examples of how groundswell can initiate bigger sustainability agendas. Additionally, education and campaigns can assist in helping individuals make more sustainable lifestyle choices, developing a sense of collective responsibility for waste management. Because urban areas are experiencing increasing waste generation, integration of citizens' opinions and activities in waste management can enhance adaptability and resilience. The hybrid approach to infrastructure and waste management, including gender equality and local involvement, is thus critical in integrating the principles of sustainability (Ashley et al., 2008; Herklotz et al., 2012).

15.3. Environmental Health in Rural Planning

In rural planning, environmental health must be the core element since rural communities seek sustainable development. Rural areas typically experience a high incidence of issues like poor clean water access, poor sanitation, and exposure to contaminants as a result of agricultural production. Successful environmental planning has the power to promote public health by limiting these risks and guaranteeing rural communities the resources necessary to support a healthy living environment. In addition, acknowledging the fact that women's equal access to resources has a major role in ensuring sustainable environmental practice provides an additional dimension to rural planning efforts. As emphasized by the results, integrating gender equity into sustainable actions improves global health outcomes at the local level, thus leading to the welfare of rural communities and promoting sustainable development objectives (Herklotz et al., 2012). Rural planning and environmental health not only address pressing health needs but also broader ecological concerns. The mutual dependency of community health and environmental quality demands the establishment of integrated management practices with respect to the sustainability of the environment. For instance, implementing ecosystem-based approaches to resource management ensures that communities can adapt to climate change impacts while sustaining their local ecosystems. The Solomon Islands model demonstrates how the transfer and replication of community-managed practices, particularly in fisheries, can be achieved to support sustainable operations that preserve vital resources and build community resilience. The process underscores participatory planning and stakeholder engagement due to the significance of local knowledge in formulating good environmental policy (Boso et al., 2011). Communities can play an instrumental part in guaranteeing that environmental health strategies are effectively put into place within rural planning.

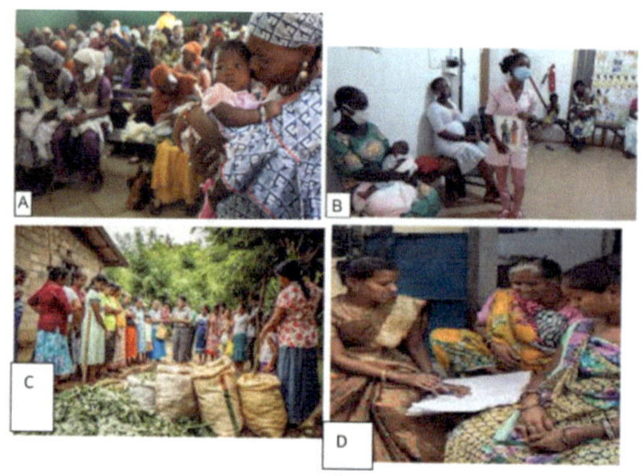

Figure 15.8. Environmental health in rural planning.

Source: https://ars.els-cdn.com/content/image/3-s2.0-B9780323904476000060-f02-02-9780323904476.jpg.

By encouraging a culture of cooperation, individuals are able to work together in lobbying for sustainable practices that address their own health as well as that of the environment around them. Public campaigns and school programs can activate residents to participate in grassroots-level environmental action, thereby giving them a sense of ownership and responsibility for their surroundings. Encouraging local participation not only enhances community relations but also guarantees policies reflect the unique needs and capacities of rural communities.

Ultimately, when communities and individuals are actively engaged in sustainable endeavors, they become active participants in sustaining healthy environments and creating a more sustainable future for rural areas (Figure 15.8).

15.3.1. Agricultural Practices and Soil Health

The connection between farming practice and soil health is a critical factor in achieving sustainable development, particularly under environmental health and urban planning paradigms. Sustainable agriculture promotes practices that not only ensure high yields from crops but also maintain and enhance the quality of the soil. Practices such as crop rotation, cover cropping, and minimum tillage are some of the ways that contribute extensively to soil aeration, nutrient holding, and diversity, and thus foster healthier environments. These practices, if adopted, can decrease the degradation caused by conventional farming, whereby excessive reliance on chemical fertilizers and monoculture cultivation degrades soil fertility in the long term. Additionally, integrating farming with urban planning can trigger synergies that increase food safety and ecosystem health, particularly in peri-urban areas where urbanization is likely to progress at the cost of productive land (Scott et al., 2016). Lastly, conscientious soil management through sustainable agriculture reflects broader sustainability and community resilience values. Additionally, soil health has direct implications for the broader environmental landscape, particularly in the urban and rural development contexts. Urbanization poses unique challenges because it can derange local agricultural systems and contribute to soil degradation as a result of land use changes. But effective city planning with the inclusion of sustainable agriculture can lead to healthier soils and, consequently, improved food systems. For example, promoting food production policies at a city level can minimize the food miles and increase community activity, hence having a positive impact on public health and the local economy. These efforts require collaboration between stakeholders like policymakers, farmers, and citizens who live in local communities to develop plans that prioritize environmental sustainability alongside the reduction of socioeconomic disparities in food access (Allen et al., 1999). By considering soil health in conjunction with farming practices in urban policy, cities are able to support increased resilience levels and drive the sustainability of critical natural resources. Moreover, the contribution of individuals and communities towards supporting sustainable land management cannot be downplayed. Grassroots action will influence innovative approaches to soil management that are in concert with the objectives of international sustainability. Grass-roots activities such as promoting learning and strengthening individuals with the skills needed for sustainable agriculture practices, such as composting, organic agriculture, and permaculture, result in good soil and environmental conservation. Public participation in such processes cannot be overemphasized, as the local populace is usually the first to notice any changes in soil quality and farm yields. Such collaboration between local authorities and community organizations can then amplify such endeavors, facilitating information and resource sharing necessary for sustainable agricultural development. In doing this, soil rejuvenation and integrity are societal responsibilities that can ensure overall environmental welfare and underscore the concepts of sustainability across all levels of society (Scott et al., 2016).

15.3.2. Water Resource Management

Effective management of water resources is crucial in order to achieve sustainable development and environmental well-being in urban and rural settings. As populations grow and climate change takes its toll, water resource demands have heightened, triggering conflicts as well as over-drawal of water systems.

Conservation of water by having sustainable management practices, making provision for equitable access, and guaranteeing the sustainable use of water resources. This encompasses not only policy and regulatory frameworks but also community engagement so that local inhabitants play an active role in the management of water. Such engagement induces a feeling of ownership and stewardship towards local waters and ultimately serves ecosystems and human societies. Applications of scientific research integrating with local knowledge are important in developing effective plans for water management to deal with variation based on site-specific conditions and environmental demands. For dealing with problems arising due to climate change in managing water resources, adaptation and resilience measures also need to be incorporated. Flooding, droughts, and water pollution incidents have intensified with variations in climatic factors. Therefore, building effective disaster risk reduction mechanisms is of paramount importance, particularly in the most disaster-prone areas. Equitable water resource allocation is the foundation of social equity since ecologically responsive societies are affected most by a lack of water or by water pollution. Through the adoption of multi-hazard and multi-sectoral approaches, communities can establish effective water management policies that affect overall disaster risk reduction and sustainability.

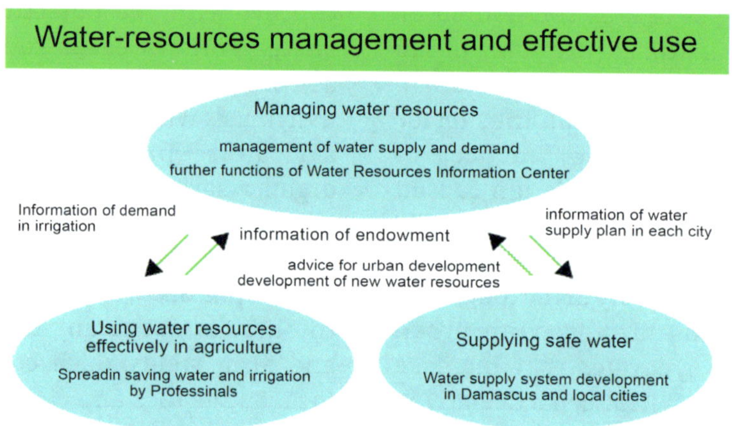

Figure 15.9. Water resource management.

Source: https://fotisedu.com/wp-content/uploads/2024/01/image-58.png.

This interconnectedness is consistent with global efforts, where it is emphasized that governments, civil society, and local actors need to collaborate in addressing the underlying drivers of water insecurity and providing a sustainable future for water, as highlighted by the imperative to plan and reduce disaster risk (N/A, 2018). Finally, but not least, the participation of people and communities in water resource management cannot be overstressed. Grassroots action offers opportunities for innovative solutions to water issues, as local stakeholders possess information about their environment that is usually priceless. Education and awareness raising allow communities to conserve water and engage in watershed restoration efforts. Furthermore, through participatory monitoring and feedback mechanisms, stakeholders are actively engaged in ongoing water quality and availability determinations, thus ensuring that accountability in water management is enhanced. Aligning local efforts with comprehensive policy actions, such as those indicated by the International Principles and Standards for the Practice of Ecological Restoration, provides the foundation for green ecosystems. Conjoining this type of effort affirms the notion that water management is more than a function of the government but also a collective responsibility to ensure environmental integrity and climate change adaptability (George et al., 2019) (Figure 15.9).

15.3.3. Biodiversity Conservation

Conservation of biodiversity is the focus of sustainable development, interweaving ecological health and human health. Biodiversity refers to the variety of living organisms in an ecosystem, such as species diversity, genetic diversity, and ecosystem diversity. Conservation of this biodiversity is not only an environmental concern; it has far-reaching implications for food security, health, and climate resilience. With increasing urbanization and rural landscape transformation, loss of biodiversity could lead to diminished ecosystem services such as pollination and nutrient cycling, which are important for sustainable agriculture. This dependency emphasizes the greatest necessity for concerted action to preserve biodiversity because it has a direct impact on environmental health and community wellbeing dependent on natural resources.

Thus, sustainable development must put biodiversity at the center of planning and implementing policies. The comprehension of the place of biodiversity in the realm of sustainable urban and rural planning is crucial for the enhancement of resilient communities. Urbanization, characterized by population growth and industrialization, tends to lead to habitat loss and fragmentation, thus putting many species and ecologically connected networks at risk. Conversely, integrating conservation of biodiversity in urban development is able to enhance environmental health through the creation of green spaces that offer various benefits, including better air quality and recreation. Rural communities can also benefit from biodiversity conservation activities, particularly through the promotion of agroecological approaches that maintain local ecosystems. For instance, local indigenous biodiversity is relied on by sub-Saharan West African small-scale farmers to support local agriculture and ensure food security. By knowing these interconnections among biodiversity and public health, planning action can become more cohesive, maintaining a sustainable balance between human advancement and environmental wholeness, as with most localized interventions. The role of individuals and communities in spearheading biodiversity conservation cannot be overstated. Grassroots organizations are now major forces for encouraging sustainable behavior and stewardship of the environment. Human society has the potential to assist with conservation through community projects such as restoring habitats, planting forests, and creating biodiversity corridors.

These grassroots efforts enhance ecological resilience by not only contributing to it but also engaging people in active involvement and making them feel stakeholders in their natural resources. Education and awareness are also important contributors to public action mobilization for the conservation of biodiversity. By improving the understanding of the intrinsic value of biodiversity and its direct impact on health and well-being, communities can mobilize their efforts towards sustainable activities. According to several studies, successful interventions in terms of conservation rely on the incorporation of local knowledge and scientific counsel to ensure that the conservation of biodiversity becomes a by-product of the general principles of sustainable development (Herklotz et al., 2012; Fliessbach et al., 2012) (Figure 15.10).

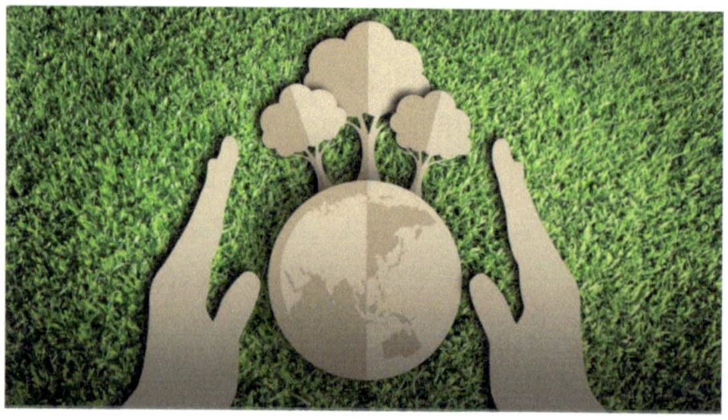

Figure 15.10. Biodiversity conservation.

Source: https://d12aarmt01l54a.cloudfront.net/cms/images/Media-20220330171836/808-440.png.

15.4. The Role of Individuals in Sustainability

Understanding the role of individuals in sustainability calls for respect that each person has the potential to contribute substantially to the well-being of the environment and environmental sustainability measures in urban and rural settings. People can make decisions and actions that collectively result in greater environmental goals. For instance, using environmentally friendly transportation methods such as cycling, carpooling, or public transport, one can reduce carbon emissions and encourage the same amongst their populations. One can observe that individual actions, when multiplied over a number of people, can result in remarkable rises in the levels of environmental well-being, reducing pollution and improving the quality of life.

This coming together of personal action and public mobilization gives a lower layer to achieving sustainable development, highlighting the critical connection between personal responsibility and system change in sustainability initiatives. Under community involvement, people's mobilization into action on sustainability issues enhances awareness and fosters collective mobilization. Grass-root mobilizations that empower people at the grassroots level to get involved in environmental conservation activities are likely to bridge the gap between knowing and doing. For example, clean-up initiatives by communities or waste management through education workshops can be a catalyst for participation in broader sustainability activities. Unmediated people's participation is likely to build a common feeling that focuses on the long-term health of the environment at the cost of short-term ease. Also, meeting in accordance with the special needs of peri-urban zones is pertinent, for it is stated in Allen et al. (1999).

Here, individuals have a main role in achieving environmental sustainability, yet simultaneously, encounter the effects of poverty and scarcity. Also, the ways in which individual choices shape sanitation and hygiene practices are a key factor in achieving sustainability. An understanding of the sociocultural and psychological factors that influence behavior towards optimal sanitation practice is imperative. Behavior change strategies are likely to rely on individuals making informed decisions, leading to improved environmental health. Sustaining solutions may incorporate individuals being enlightened about the necessity for sanitation and hygiene, a requirement highlighted in Evans et al. (2010).

Such learning not only illuminates practice but also instills a sense of responsibility within individuals to contribute positively to their way of living. Individuals, therefore, become integral in shaping the trajectory of sustainable development, influencing environmental health policy and community practices through conscious, discerning action (Figure 15.11).

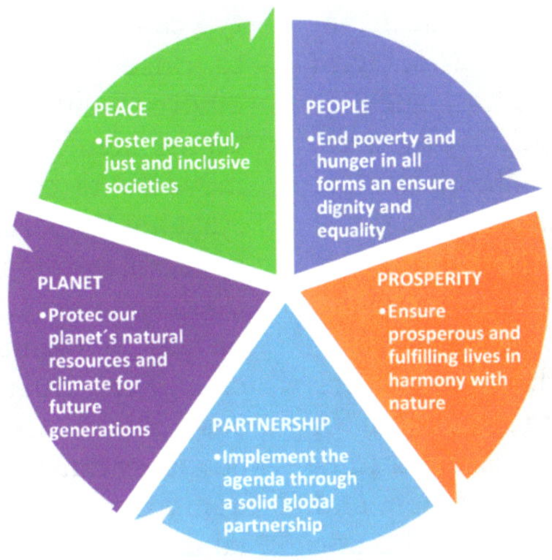

Figure 15.11. Participation and sustainable development.

Source: https://media.springernature.com/lw685/springer-static/image/prt%3A978-3-030-11352-0%2F15/MediaObjects/978-3-030-11352-0_15_Part_Fig2-57_HTML.png.

15.4.1. Sustainable Consumption Practices

Sustainable consumption practices are growing in prominence as societies battle to respond to the environmental degradation brought about by unsustainable resource consumption. These practices have a wide range of behaviors, such as ethical buying, waste reduction, and choosing products that are sustainably produced and ethically sourced. The assumption of sustainable consumption is that individual action has aggregate impacts on larger systems and therefore it promotes a culture of sustainability. By conscious product selection, diminishing environmental impact, consumers are able to influence patterns of demand towards more sustainable choices, and, in a very general sense, influence company behavior and state policy. This coalescence illustrates how informed consumers contribute toward a sustainable economy and environment, and that individual actions are not in isolation but part of an integrated web of social action aimed at inducing conformity with the principles of sustainability. Moreover, consumption behaviors for sustainability extend beyond individual actions to embrace societal responsibilities. Societies play a significant part in encouraging sustainable consumption by supporting local programs and educational campaigns. These can ensure increased awareness of the effects of consumption patterns on the environment and provide information and assistance in adopting more sustainable patterns of consumption. For example, community-supported agriculture (CSA) schemes involve people in food production in local communities, promoting peer networks to prioritize sustainable choices in their diets. Additionally, collective work among people in the community tends to solve problems in innovative ways that bring about common challenges like food deserts or managing refuse, thus improving environmental health. Emphasizing the manner in which collective action can magnify the effectiveness of solo efforts, such social movements initiated by communities reflect a holistic approach to sustainable development in which social and environmental health are interlinked. The two-way intersection of gender and sustainable consumption patterns creates additional levels of debate for the sustainability agenda. Evidence indicates that where women have equal access to resources and to decision-making, there is a positive correlation with improved environmental outcomes, such as greater sustainable consumption practices. Empowering women not only makes home life better but also encourages more thoughtful stewardship of resources at the community level, as evidenced in a variety of sectors ranging from energy to agriculture. For instance, sub-Saharan West African smallholder farmers demonstrate the impact of gender inclusion in sustainable agriculture practice, demonstrating how resource management principles and local knowledge can lead to enhanced climatic resilience and food security (Fliessbach et al., 2012). These findings underpin the recognition that sustainability is multifaceted, necessitating solutions that recognize the vital role of all and every community in enabling fair and sustainable consumption (Herklotz et al., 2012).

15.4.2. Community Engagement and Advocacy

Community involvement and activism play key roles in environmental health and sustainable development, with effective engagement shaping successful programs. Community involvement generates an inclusive setting in which neighbors, local leaders, and organizations join together to address crucial environmental problems. Sustainability principles address not just strategic planning but also community involvement in decision-making. By taking a participatory approach, people are in a position to leverage local knowledge and skills, and thus come up with context-sensitive and culture-sensitive solutions. Grassroots participation ensures that development projects are in tune with the actual needs and aspirations of those affected, and thus enhances the possibility of long-term sustainability and environmental justice. Furthermore, advocacy is a fundamental vehicle through which people can influence policies affecting their health and the environment. These campaign drives typically start as mass movements that try to raise awareness on matters concerning environmental threats at the local level or unjust methods in dispensing resources. Such movements can get the attention of various stakeholders, from local governmentsand non-governmental organizations to even corporate bodies. Such attempts at raising awareness on environmental health concerns and policy change can create a conducive environment for sustainable behavior. The importance of such advocacy campaigns is brought home by models demonstrating the interdependence between land and water resources, illuminating the need for management at both urban and rural levels (Goldman, 2011).

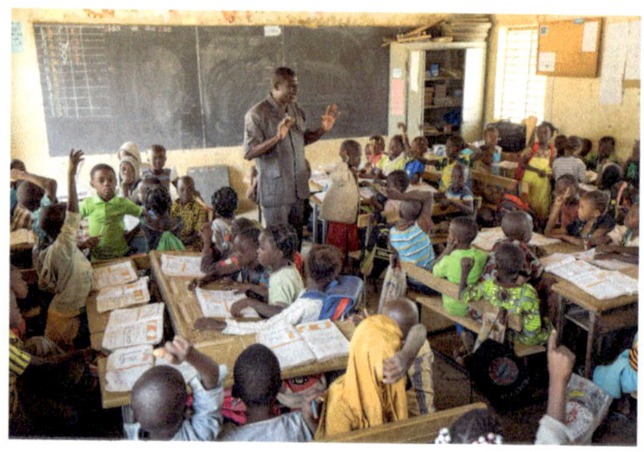

Figure 15.12. Community engagement and advocacy.

Source: https://assets.globalpartnership.org/s3fs-public/styles/standard_blog_banner/public/40710900201_f054c0a526_o.jpg?VersionId=3pqukES6Ce5ewcU8QW1SlvIEKFVsLynI&itok=saa4-pB4.

Furthermore, effective outreach and advocacy initiatives must be complemented by strategic partnerships across sectors. Partnerships between government institutions, non-profit sector organizations, and community organizations can find greater strength in the advocacy of sustainability. These collaborations can open doors to resources, funding, and expertise necessary for the application of sustainable practices. Formal entities, for instance, foundations focused on community welfare, usually dominate this environment through assistance and advice (N/A, 2012). In settings with social and economic inequalities, these collaborative efforts can make sustainability initiatives inclusive. Lastly, through generating a united front, societies can address environmental health matters more effectively, making it possible to implement an integrated sustainable development approach that empowers individuals and promotes overall well-being (Figure 15.12).

15.4.3. Education and Awareness

Education and awareness are the essential premises in the evolution of sustainable development and environmental health within urban and rural planning contexts. Better-informed communities are better able to counteract the sustainability challenges and embrace practices that balance out the adverse impacts on the environment. The sharing of knowledge through education initiatives fosters a community valuing ecological wholesomeness and facilitating sustainable activity. By integrating education for sustainability into school curricula, individuals learn about the interdependencies of social, economic, and environmental conditions early in life, which is vital for making prudent decisions. Such an integrated approach can prepare future generations to gain the awareness needed to place a high priority on sustainability in their work and personal life and to contribute positively towards community-based green programs, thus amplifying the collective effect of such initiatives. Furthermore, public awareness campaigns have the potential to shape the behavior of individuals and communities towards sustainability. Public awareness campaigns are capable of making known the importance of local environmental issues, so that people realize their duty towards being the protectors of their environment. Using different media forms, including social media and community workshops, stakeholders can reach out to different groups of audiences and shape discussions about sustainable behavior. For example, water conservation projects can be helpful in making the communities understand the implications of their water usage patterns and encouraging the proper handling of resources. The importance of joint education and outreach is underscored by initiatives that pay particular attention to illustrating how sustainability analysis can strengthen resource management decision-making, affirming that collective knowledge is important for effective environmental health interventions (Ashley et al., 2008). Besides, addressing the interface between gender equity and sustainable development is of crucial importance in awareness campaigns and education. The empowerment of women through concentrated educational packages enhances their access to resources and decision-making avenues that contribute to preserving the environment. Evidence indicates that with equal opportunities in education and resource access, families are not only benefited but also the environment is bound to thrive (Herklotz et al., 2012). This simultaneity highlights the need for inclusive education that considers the specific challenges of women and marginal communities, thereby allowing for a general appreciation of sustainability by all members of society. Lastly, integrating gender analysis into education on sustainability can lead to concrete gains in environmental well-being and social justice, reinforcing further the argument that awareness and education are integral elements in the realization of sustainable development.

15.5. The Role of Communities in Sustainability

The role of communities in sustainability is at the core, in that they are the foundation for achieving sustainable practices that address local and global challenges. The communities possess unique knowledge and cultural understanding that informs sustainable development strategies, particularly in urban and rural settings. For instance, rural societies often suffer from depopulation and cultural heritage loss that can be counteracted by people-driven initiatives such as the SunCare Hub in Sweden and Spain. The initiative is an exemplary demonstration of how grassroots efforts can be employed to increase access to health care and align with SDGs by strengthening a sense of belonging and shared responsibility. By participating in sustainable projects, communities not only improve their environmental health but also strengthen social bonds, leading to a more robust infrastructure that can survive economic and ecological change. Communities are also an important component in reducing gaps prevalent in urban and peri-urban settings. As urbanization continues to prove difficult, peri-urban interface (PUI) zones are faced with unique environmental sustainability issues as well as poverty-related concerns. Local community initiatives to identify and define such issues can lead to community-wide solutions that promote social justice and environmental preservation.

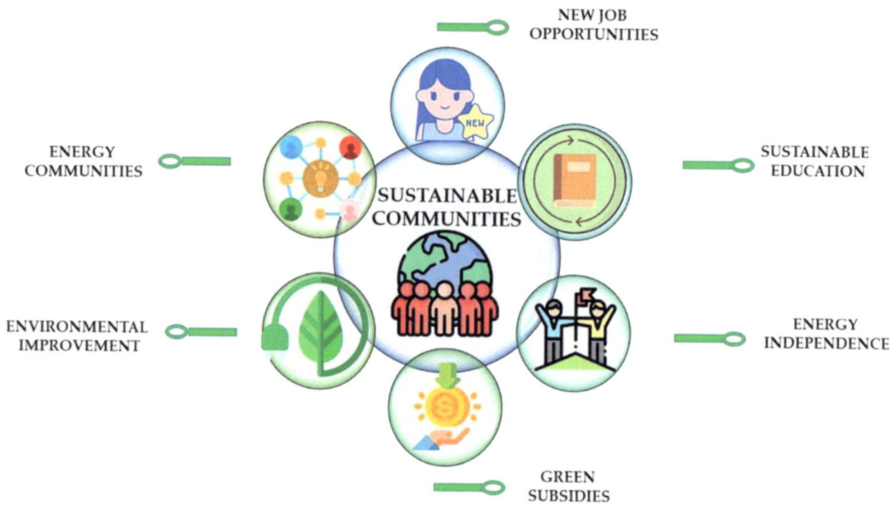

Figure 15.13. Strategies for developing sustainable communities.

Source: https://media.springernature.com/lw1200/springer-static/image/art%3A10.1038%2Fs41598-023-48021-8/MediaObjects/41598_2023_48021_Fig13_HTML.png.

For example, with participatory planning and local government, members of the community can advocate for policies that place priority on sustainable land use, waste management, and environmental health programs. This empowerment of community voices is paramount to generating a comprehensive approach to sustainability because it enables local needs and concerns to be integrated into larger environmental causes. Therefore, resolving these differences is not only consonant with the precepts of sustainability but also improves the overall quality of life for all members of the community. Lastly, the relationship between sustainable economic growth and community action exists in several projects working to advance local economies and increase sustainability. Successful and efficient projects are usually built on partnerships between governmental organizations, non-profit organizations, and community organizations with like-minded goals. The case study of SunCare Hub illustrates how sustainable health infrastructure can be utilized in order to stimulate local economies through the creation of jobs and improved overall health among community members. Here, sustainability is greater than a matter of environmentalism, and it has a sense of interrelation with economics and society. Sustainability-conscious communities not only contribute locally toward global targets such as Reduced Inequalities (SDG 10) but also achieve local resilience against the global economic cycles. Integrated research and planning emphasize the necessity of a model in which the unique requirements of every community are guiding sustainability interventions with a diversified impact geared toward the general objective of sustainable development in society (Figure 15.13).

15.5.1. Local Initiatives and Programs

Local initiatives and programs play a crucial role in the leadership of sustainable development and environmental wellness in cities as well as in rural contexts. Localized programs are specific to suit the needs of the people, promoting innovative approaches that avoid environmental harm while correcting social injustices. For instance, programs can be centered around waste reduction through recycling schemes within the community or city gardens that enhance local food security. These bottom-up strategies engage the people as well and lead to a feeling of ownership and accountability of the populace towards the environment, thus incorporating sustainability principles into the social life of the community. Through decentralization of sustainability initiatives, the communities are able to effectively address their particular issues, ultimately creating environments that are ecologically sustainable and socially equitable. Moreover, stakeholder collaborations involving local governments, non-profit organizations, and citizens also complement the success of local efforts through gaining alternative resources and abilities. Such collaborations are vital for constructing inclusive measures that integrate sustainable planning practices for urban and rural areas. For instance, a community may engage in collaborative ventures for the beautification of green spaces or public transportation systems, thereby promoting sustainable mobility and reducing reliance on fossil fuels. These initiatives reflect a broader vision of sustainability where various perspectives come together to create resilient communities. In particular, community programs can be further incorporated into higher systems, such as in policy reforms that foster healthy agriculture and local well-being (Fisher et al., 2001).

This incorporation enables local initiatives to contribute meaningfully to international targets for sustainability. In addition to promoting environmental health, local initiatives also empower communities and individuals, developing local leaders in sustainability. Education and awareness are usually conducted to familiarize residents with sustainable practices such as composting, conservation of energy, and water management. Not only do such educational processes equip individuals with the knowledge needed to make environmentally friendly choices, but they also mobilize community action. For example, grassroots environmental stewardship can be initiated through community workshops or school programs that will have a multiplier effect and cause collective participation in sustainable activities. Through the promotion of a culture of sustainability at the grassroots level, these programs enhance social cohesion and resilience and therefore emphasize the belief that individuals and communities are principal agents of the achievement of sustainable development (N/A, 2012). Lastly, local action is a powerful instrument through which communities can forge a lasting future in accordance with their particular needs and aspirations.

15.5.2. Collaboration with Government and NGOs

Effective collaboration among governments and NGOs is crucial in the quest for sustainable development goals and the mitigation of environmental health challenges. Collaboration facilitates the concentration of resources, division of labor, and indigenous knowledge to stage successful interventions likely to bring long-term impacts both in urban and rural settings. Governments are likely to provide a regulatory framework, funding, and financial assistance, while NGOs provide field experience and tailor-made approaches to engage local communities. This is particularly true in work towards improving WASH services, where the two can collaborate in identifying the most pressing needs and designing responsive interventions that improve public health levels. Through collaborative action, the organizations can also facilitate a more inclusive environment, enabling the engagement of marginalized groups in decision-making processes affecting their livelihood. Research initiatives made for enhancing universal urban sanitation demonstrate how the collaboration between the government and NGOs is vital. For example, the Urban Sanitation Research Initiative is intended to bridge the gap between policy and research by establishing strong linkages between city and country governments and key stakeholders, such as international donors and financial institutions. This collaborative approach not only derives actionable conclusions but also builds capacity in local institutions for effective management of WASH services. Emphasis is placed on building an enabling environment through supplemented government investment, which is central to the sustainable development of WASH services targeting low-income communities. Such partnerships provide a platform whereby evidence-based approaches can be exchanged so that sanitation innovation is aligned with broader sustainability goals, thereby ensuring healthier urban environments and improved quality of life for the inhabitants. The GLAAS report highlights the continued imperative for governments and NGOs to cooperate well to deal with finance and supporting environments for WASH projects. The data collected from 75 countries and 25 international assistance agencies indicate the diversification of the challenges involved in addressing vulnerable populations. Joint implementation can mobilize resources at a larger scale and improve innovative finance arrangements tied to sustainable development goals. Moreover, through knowledge and resource sharing, government institutions and NGOs are able to share best practices and deploy project templates with social equity and environmental protection underpinnings. As highlighted in recent research, encouraging cooperation has the potential to enable the design of targeted interventions that ensure access to safe water and sanitation since these are essential determinants of environmental health and sustainability in both urban and rural planning contexts (N/A, 2017) (Figure 15.14).

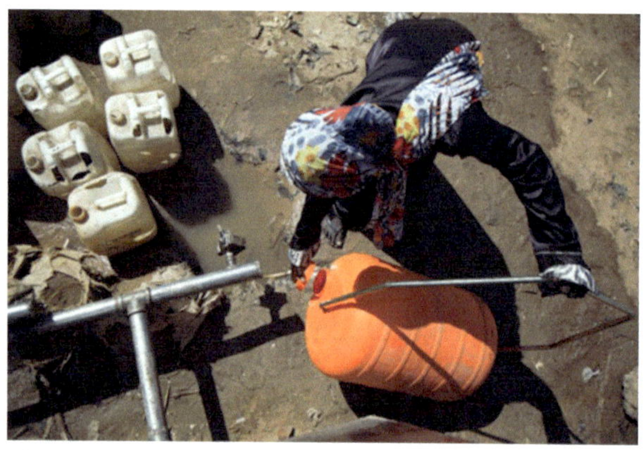

Figure 15.14. Global analysis and assessment of sanitation and drinking-water (GLAAS).

Source: https://glaas.who.int/images/librariesprovider2/default-album/how-we-work/howwework.tmb-479v.jpg?Culture=en&sfvrsn=da71f25_1.

15.5.3. Community Resilience and Adaptation

In sustainable development, the resilience of the community is crucial in minimizing the impact of environmental hazards. Resilience refers to the capacity of a community to cope with altered conditions, either altered climate, natural disasters, or socio-economic transformation. Sustainability principles encompass human health dependence on environmental well-being, with a need to mobilize community resources in a bid to build adaptive capacities. Resilience-focused communities will likely recover from disruptions and maintain essential services. Collective action through local stakeholders can enhance such capacities by managing knowledge and resources, leading to improved environmental health outcomes. Promoting green infrastructure and community practices is one of the best examples of how sustainable approaches can enhance resilience and facilitate successful ecosystems in urban and rural settings, supporting objectives set out in sustainable development frameworks (N/A, 2012). Community resilience is not only a matter of infrastructure but also concerns social factors, including inclusiveness and equity. Participation of diverse groups in the adaptation process is central to building resilience, as it enables trust and cooperation. Overcoming disparities offers a chance for everybody in the community to provide and gain, especially in marginalized groups that are usually worst hit by environmental degradation. Successful adaptation measures need to take account of local knowledge and insights, so that communities can create imaginative solutions adapted to their specific situations. In addition, diminishing vulnerability through available resources like healthcare and education makes societies cohesive and robust. Through the integration of equity-oriented practices in planning and community development, the efforts to build resilience can be made holistic and sustainable and contribute to overall environmental wellness (Herklotz et al., 2012). With the shift to more sustainable urban and rural planning models, the role of people and communities in building resilience becomes more central. Empowering local communities allows them to take ownership of sustainability programs, thereby boosting their capacity to adapt and thrive amidst change. Self-organized initiatives—such as disaster preparedness training, collaborative environmental management, and grassroots mobilization—serve as key components in resilience building. These initiatives not only enhance short-term adaptive initiatives but also foster long-term sustainable initiatives. Active engagement of individuals fosters a resilience culture, where proactive measures are the order of the day rather than a reaction. By prioritizing community-centered approaches, we can leverage the strengths of local populations in tackling environmental problems and fostering sustainable health gain, therefore directing towards overall sustainability objectives of sustainable development (N/A, 2012).

15.6. Challenges to Sustainable Development

The pursuit of sustainable development is beset by numerous challenges that originate from the complex interdependence of social, economic, and environmental factors. Among the major challenges is overdependence on local resources and indigenous knowledge, particularly in agriculture. Smallholder farmers such as those in the sub-Saharan area of West Africa are predominantly reliant on local knowledge systems that have been cultivated over the years. While science-based information can enhance decision-making in such complex scenarios, transition to more sustainable practice commonly encounters resistance from communities that are not willing to relinquish proven methods of operations. This clash between outdated and new approaches demonstrates the thin line required in advancing sustainable agricultural systems that deliver food security and reduce the impact of climate change, exemplifying the intricacies entailed in advancing sustainable development (Fliessbach et al., 2012). Another pressing issue related to sustainable development includes accessibility and sustainability of water and sanitation services, particularly in rural areas. While major steps have been made in the improvement of rural sanitation in Latin America, many areas lag in the achievement of the Millennium Development Goals. The growing population increases the demand for well-functioning sanitation systems, and as such, it is important to ensure their long-term sustainability. One of the main issues is enhancing the capacities of city governments, which must be directly involved in creating and maintaining such services. Furthermore, establishing the right legal and financial frameworks must be achieved in order to support sustainable activities. Lacking these pillars, global access to clean and proper sanitation is just a fantasy that cannot be achieved, showing the complicated interaction of variables that render sustainable development challenging (Pearce-Oroz, 2011). People's and communities' roles in addressing challenges to sustainable development cannot be devalued. Grassroots movements are most likely to become agents of change, suggesting sustainable solutions that are in harmony with needs and cultural conditions in the local context. Empowered local people working on sustainability have a sense of ownership and stewardship of the environment's well-being. Projects that are locally initiated can best address problems at the local level, such as deforestation, pollution, and resource management. By leveraging local knowledge and culture, communities have been able to imagine and institute solutions that are grounded in their unique circumstances. However, these projects have to be coordinated and supported by the various stakeholders like governments, non-profit organizations, and businesses. The interface of community and individual efforts with broader institutional assistance is thus crucial in demolishing the barriers that prevent sustainable development and constructing a more robust and inclusive world for all (Figure 15.15).

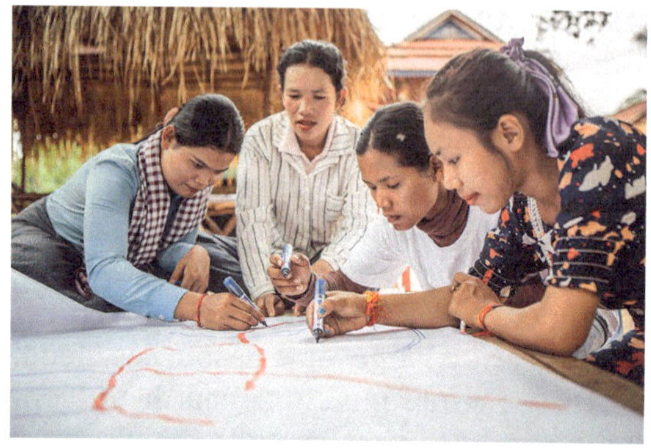

Figure 15.15. Community-led development.

Source: https://outreach-international.org/wp-content/uploads/2023/03/CLD-2.jpg.

15.6.1. Economic Barriers

Economic barriers extensively hinder the realization of sustainable development, particularly in urban and rural areas. The imbalanced distribution of resources typically denies poorer communities access to the funds required to implement sustainable practices or improve the environment in their locality. Economic barriers in most cities restrict access to green technology, such as renewable sources of energy and eco-friendly means of public transport that promote carbon footprint reduction. Moreover, the employment of traditional, resource-based economic models exacerbates environmental degradation through the difficulty involved for communities to finance the costs of adaptation and remediation efforts. This inequality highlights the importance of integrating participatory planning approaches dedicated to equity, where investing in the economy is directed toward solutions that are equitable and can eliminate poverty among underserved populations while establishing sustainable practices in line with sustainability principles (Davis et al., 2025). Breaking through economic hurdles entails new means that utilize the strength of technology and the participation of people to create balanced opportunities. The key to such an initiative is the use of Geographic Information Systems (GIS), through which planners can chart and examine economic disparities and identify locations to tap support for sustainable development from. With GIS-driven terrain analysis, cities are able to rationalize land utilization in a socially just and ecologically sustainable manner. Moreover, the GIS analytical capabilities can pinpoint particular locations where most investment is required, thereby resulting in an evidence-based urban development policy. Despite this, several crucial challenges still exist, ranging from access to quality data to the development of technical skills among the planners. Overcoming such barriers is imperative in using GIS methodology for fostering sustainable urban development with due consideration of economic, social, and environmental interdependencies (Ayomide et al., 2025). The ability of individuals and communities to overcome economic barriers cannot be overstated in attaining sustainable development. Grassroots initiatives and community programs tend to be drivers of change, calling for policies favoring economic equality and environmental conservation. When people realize the economic benefits of sustainability, they tend to adopt practices that decrease environmental degradation while promoting their own well-being and health. Local government, business, and citizen cooperation are the keys to economic incentive creation that leads to sustainable development, which makes possible the realization of a common vision for a better environment. Hence, overcoming economic obstacles makes it possible to advance toward environmental wellness while simultaneously empowering communities to manage their own destiny, thus sustaining the salient connection between the assumptions of sustainable development and the economic well-being of people and families (Davis et al., 2025).

15.6.2. Political and Regulatory Challenges

Political and regulatory concerns have a determinative role in sustainable development, particularly environmental health in urban and rural areas. Disproportionate regulatory systems can establish uneven sustainability procedures, generally obstructing collective actions toward long-term environmental goals. Policymakers are placed most frequently in the situation of balancing economic development and environmental responsibility, an adversarial conflict exacerbated by shifting political circumstances and conflicting interests. Attempts to institutionalize sustainability principles are often hampered by ineffective enforcement tools and a lack of coherence in local, state, and federal policies. This patchwork framework can have loopholes in regulations that oppose effective environmental management, which in turn makes it harder to drive sustainable communities. Resolving these regulatory and political problems requires a harmonized framework that brings together various policies across all levels with a clear roadmap for sustainable development. Where political concerns and environmental health intersect is the issue of community engagement and local participation in sustainability initiatives. Not only do regulatory frameworks need to command compliance, but they also need to compel local communities to become engaged in decision-making forums. This is particularly necessary where local knowledge and resources are central to successful sustainability initiatives. In West Africa, for instance, local knowledge and resources are used heavily by small-scale farmers to control complex farming systems (Fliessbach et al., 2012). Strong governance systems should be cognizant of and incorporate these local perceptions so that local community members can become engaged actors in sustainable environmental management rather than passive actors in state-driven policies. This participatory approach not only empowers individuals but also fosters ownership, guaranteeing a more sustainable and responsive response to environmental pressures. Moreover, the regulatory landscape of water management in a sustainable manner is progressively being shaped by the effects of climate change. Whereas climate variability and climatic extremes challenge conventional water resource management regimes, regulatory frameworks that are flexible and visionary are immediately necessary. The low-impact development principles and the importance of the relationship between water and land must be integrated into policy discussions as well as regulatory measures (Goldman, 2011). This includes recognizing the contribution of climate change to the impacts on the availability of water, as well as the necessity of multistakeholder management that includes stakeholders from various sectors. These approaches can mitigate the adverse impacts of climate change while promoting green strategies that harmonize environmental protection with economic development. By answering these regulatory challenges, policymakers can build a more sustainable future on both the basis of environmental health and community resilience (Figure 15.16).

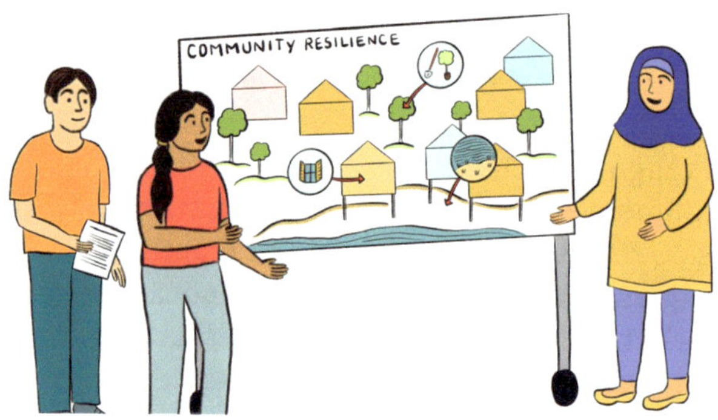

Figure 15.16. Advance community resilience.

Source: https://external-content.duckduckgo.com/iu/?u=https%3A%2F%2Fwww.noaa.gov%2Fsites%2Fdefault%2Ffiles%2Fstyles%2Flandscape_width_1275%2Fpublic%2F2021-09%2FCP%25206-16b.png%3Fh%3D014ef245%26itok%3DZxK3GTJ6&f=1&nofb=1&ipt=8f530b1a370cfc05d79476f2fd509854fef4d1ce26da29f68268fa865c904457.

15.6.3. Social and Cultural Resistance

Social and cultural resistance is vital in the formation of sustainable development, particularly in mobilizing communities to advocate for their environmental health. Resistance often stems from local knowledge systems that challenge hegemonic discourses promoted by global institutions and corporations. For instance, small-scale farmers of sub-Saharan West Africa, who hugely depend on local means, embody this kind of resistance by embracing traditional farming methods that give more emphasis to ecological balance than industrial ones. Their reliance on local knowledge emphasizes the importance of combining localized decision-making with sustainability initiatives, as noted in the research coordination activities in Mali, Burkina Faso, and Benin, where comparisons between agricultural systems noted food security and climate change resilience (Fliessbach et al., 2012). Thus, the cultural frameworks under which these communities live not only give rise to a sense of identity but also drive innovation and critical responses to external pressures. When rural development schemes are examined, the shortcomings of conventional analysis methods underscore the necessity of embracing social and cultural resistance. The EU Commission's Common Monitoring and Evaluation Framework, while purposed to quantify program impact through measurable indicators, has a tendency to overlook the richness of local dynamics and the transformative power of local agency. It overlooks the influence of the way social innovation based on collaborative action among local actors has the ability to bring about far-reaching changes in sustainability behaviors. This demand for more comprehensiveness reflects the importance of building in variability within local contexts in assessing program success. Through the recognition of social innovation processes, rural development initiatives may be reimagined to address the values and realities of the very people they aim to serve, making sustainability not merely a goal but a shared process (Balázs et al., 2013). Furthermore, social and cultural resistance in sustainable development frameworks encourages a paradigm shift in environmental health intervention. Such people resist unsustainable behaviors not necessarily due to lack, but also as an expression of agency against external economic forces that aim to undermine their existence. Such resistance comes through various mechanisms, including grassroots mobilization, agitations for policy change, and conservation of local ecosystems. Through the creation of an environment where local values and priorities are prioritized, stakeholders are in a position to develop resilience against environmentally degrading practices fostered by broader market pressures. The intersection of social and cultural resistance and sustainable development actually enhances the capacity of communities to decide for themselves about resources and their own futures, thereby affirming the critical role of people and communities in the greater endeavor of sustainability.

CLOSER LOOK

FUTURE FOR SUSTAINABLE DEVELOPMENT

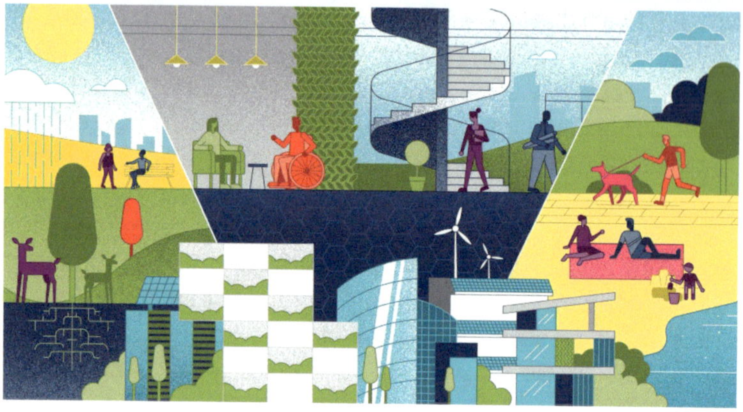

Figure 15.17. Illustration showcasing elements of sustainable urban design, including green architecture, renewable energy, and inclusive public spaces.

Source: https://external-content.duckduckgo.com/iu/?u=https%3A%2F%2Fhga.com%2Fwp-content%2Fuploads%2F2021%2F04%2FHGA-Sustainable-Design-1.jpg&f=1&nofb=1&ipt=d18cf1c3ee8db11f6857360cadc970ab74667c750c279eb31b2b476639d554c0.

The paths of future sustainable development rely in great part on the coming together of advanced technologies aimed at enhancing environmental health. While the urban and rural landscapes are facing growing challenges of pollution, resource depletion, and climate change, advanced solutions like Internet of Things (IoT) solutions are leading the way as tools that are necessary. Especially, safeguarding sensitive information, such as health information, through advanced encryption methods may support individual privacy and further the broader mission of sustainability. Protecting health information is necessary and aligns with the broader objective of creating sustainable communities where individuals are safe and invested. Besides, good simulations that show how technology can help guarantee data integrity through encryption point towards the future in which technology will lead to sustainable development, particularly in managing health, hence gaining confidence among human beings in the systems that control their environmental well-being. An important step in advancing sustainable development is establishing community engagement and education in environmental health. By making individuals and communities understand and manage issues of sustainability effectively, a major leap forward is observed in urban and rural development. For instance, problem-based learning (PBL) has been identified to enhance employees' conflict resolution ability and other soft skills in various industries. Adapted to community learning, PBL strategies can make it possible to better understand the disciplines of sustainability to help residents become empowered stakeholders in their environments. This localizing of knowledge not only builds community resilience but also fosters collaborative strategies towards sustainable practices that account for the unique needs and challenges of a given community. As sustainable development grows, it is evident that multi-disciplinary actions have an important role in tackling intricate environmental health problems. Future development should concentrate on inter-sector alliances among the government, private sectors, and non-governmental organizations. Inter-sector alliances can develop holistic frameworks for sustainable activities, which can effectively merge diverse perspectives and experiences. For instance, integrating data-driven decision-making processes can effectively allocate resources through city and rural communities. Involvement of all stakeholders in the development of sustainable infrastructure and service systems acknowledges the dynamic interdependence among ecological, social, and economic factors. Collective action based on shared goals for sustainability will highlight corridors for short-term and long-term progress toward realizing the ultimate goal of better environmental health and community well-being.

SUMMARY

The peak of the debate on sustainable development and ecological health is that effective solutions will hinge on blending in harmony sustainable operations in urban and rural settings equally. As environmental issues and their sophistication grow, stakeholders ranging from local governments to individual citizens will have to play active roles in coming up with and implementing strategies that ensure sustainability. Moreover, the value of gender equality cannot be overlooked; as studies have proven, equal access and control by women over resources not only enhances people's and households' welfare but also contributes to broader environmental sustainability (Herklotz et al., 2012). Accordingly, the integrated approach consisting of more than one perspective and experience is a principal support for achieving sustainable development. Critical analysis of environmental health points to a necessity of pragmatically reorienting policy and practices that address regional disparities, particularly those of rural water and sanitation services. While past experience has paid dividends in some measure, there remains much to be done, including long-term sustainability of the services (Pearce-Oroz, 2011). This entails revisiting existing municipal arrangements to re-establish strong local governance and accountability. Interestingly, these drivers need to be integrated with community engagement. That will enable citizens to take responsibility for their health environment since they will drive sustainable action. That will address their unique needs and circumstances. Thus, bridging the policy gap and community engagement gaps is imperative towards achieving feasible and sustainable environmental health improvements. To conclude, the successful implementation of sustainable development policies depends on a comprehensive vision of environmental well-being and active involvement of all levels of society. Individuals and communities must play a continued role in promoting sustainable practice, with a cross-generational culture of custodianship. Equally important is continued debate amongst stakeholders, where shared knowledge drives concerted action towards sustainability. As research continues to shed more light on the interconnections between the various issues of sustainability, including urbanization, climate change, and resource availability, it is more imperative that the communities work together effectively. It is only through this type of concerted action that we can possibly create resilient environments that not only support current populations but also ensure the health and opportunity of future generations.

One of the secrets of sustainable development is the ability to provide effective water and sanitation approaches, particularly for developing nations. The US Agency for International Development's very first global Water and Development Strategy emphasizes sustainability by working through host country systems. Localized governance and capacity building are fostered through such an approach, which is necessary to guarantee the integrity of water programs. New technology and science are necessary to defeat the challenges of contemporary times in water management, as they enable new solutions tailored to the context. From learning through past experience, stakeholders can devise systems not only to provide the relief urgently but also to achieve long-term sustainability, hence guaranteeing the interdependence between environmental health and the impulse for development in urban and rural planning approaches (N/A, 2013). In rural sanitation, the progress seen in Latin America during the past decade represents achievements and areas of ongoing concern. Although achievements have been made, much still lags behind the Millennium Development Goals for sanitation service upgrades. Insufficient sustainable sanitation has the potential to undermine public health and welfare, and points to the importance of having comprehensive monitoring systems in place to assess resource management and efficiency.

Sustenance of such services in the long term requires proactive action from local governments, including the application of appropriate legal and financial regimes. Solving these problems not only enhances resilience at the community level but also establishes greater people-to-people, people-to-institutions, and institutions-to-aims-for-sustainability connections (Pearce-Oroz, 2011). Lastly, the engagement of individuals and communities towards promoting sustainability cannot be overlooked. By coordination at the grassroots level, individuals and communities can embrace environmental health programs and implement ecological harmony. Education and awareness are critical in motivating collective action, enabling individuals to recognize their contribution towards enhanced sustainable practices. These collaborations may lead to innovative local solutions, complementing the effectiveness of extensive sustainability policies. As such, enabling individuals and communities is critical to building an enduring commitment to sustainable development in reasserting the imperative that local participation is essential to achieving maximum outcomes in environmental health and planning (N/A, 2013; Pearce-Oroz, 2011).

REFERENCES

1. Adesina, A. A., Okwandu, A. C., & Nwokediegwu, Z. Q. S. (2024). Towards sustainable urban development: Conceptualizing green infrastructure and its impact on urban planning. *International Journal of Applied Research in Social Sciences*. https://www.semanticscholar.org/paper/05a3ecab56ff5908361400252e5da8069e035993 (accessed on 11th June 2025).
2. Akinyemi, A. D., Egogo-Stanley, A. O., Ibrahim, O. M., & Ezeamii, G. C. (2025). Assessing the role of topographical analysis in sustainable urban development: Insights from GIS-driven terrain studies. *EPRA International Journal of Economic Growth and Environmental Issues*. https://www.semanticscholar.org/paper/beb916ddee3c4f692972c7cf515f020defbc884a (accessed on 11th June 2025).
3. Allen, A., Corubolo, E., & da Silva, N. (1999). *Environmental Problems and Opportunities of The Peri-Urban Interface and Their Impact Upon the Poor*. https://core.ac.uk/download/1668830.pdf (accessed on 11th June 2025).
4. Alstäde, V., Berg, P. G., Berghauser Pont, M., & Haupt, P., et al. (2021). *Systematic Review and Comparison of Densification Effects and Planning Motivations*. https://core.ac.uk/download/535015141.pdf (accessed on 11th June 2025).
5. Ashley, R., Blackwood, D. J., Butler, D., Davies, J., et al. (2008). *Making Asset Investment Decisions for Wastewater Systems That Include Sustainability*. https://core.ac.uk/download/228177026.pdf (accessed on 11th June 2025).
6. Balázs, B., Nemes, G., & Tisenkopfs, T. (2013). *Urban Food Strategies in Central and Eastern Europe: What's Specific and What's at Stake?* https://core.ac.uk/download/18544754.pdf (accessed on 11th June 2025).
7. Bellon, S., Deverre, C., Geniaux, G., Powell, B., et al. (2025). *Sustainable Development Indicator Frameworks and Initiatives*. https://core.ac.uk/download/pdf/6517845.pdf (accessed on 11th June 2025).
8. Boso, D., Govan, H., & Schwarz, A. H. (2011). *Towards Integrated Island Management: Lessons from Lau, Malaita, For the Implementation of a National Approach to Resource Management in Solomon Islands: Final report*. https://core.ac.uk/download/11023158.pdf (accessed on 11th June 2025).
9. Davis, H., Fredericks, J., Foth, M., Caldwell, G., & Parker, C. (2025). The role of participatory planning and design in addressing the UN Sustainable Development Goals. *Urban Planning*. https://www.semanticscholar.org/paper/68f15b4007d9ebde9ac2a4e1edcc926e86886425 (accessed on 11th June 2025).
10. Deep, S. (2018). *The Role of Problem-Based Learning in Developing Communication Conflict Resolving Skills Among Selected Non-Government Organizations in Pakistan*. https://core.ac.uk/download/12005620.pdf (accessed on 11th June 2025).
11. Evans, B. E., Peal, A. J., & van der Voorden, C. (2010). *Hygiene and Sanitation Software: An Overview of Approaches*.
12. Fisher, A., Gottlieb, B., Winne, M., & Forster, T. (2001). *The Healthy Farms, Food and Communities Act: Policy Initiatives for the 2002 Farm Bill and the First Decade of the 21st Century*. https://core.ac.uk/download/71342204.pdf (accessed on 11th June 2025).

13. Fliessbach, A., & Nicolay, G. L. (2012). *Production of Innovations Within Farmer–Researcher Associations Applying Transdisciplinary Research Principles.* https://core.ac.uk/download/10932781.pdf (accessed on 11th June 2025).

14. Gann, G. D., McDonald, T., Walder, B., Aronson, J., Nelson, C. R., Jonson, J., Hallett, J. G., et al. (2019). International principles and standards for the practice of ecological restoration (Second edition). *Restoration Ecology, 27.* https://doi.org/10.1111/rec.13035 (accessed on 11th June 2025).

15. Goldman, R. (2011). *Fresh Water and Smarter Growth: Restoring Healthy Land–Water Connections.* https://core.ac.uk/download/141922946.pdf (accessed on 11th June 2025).

16. Gupta, N., Purohit, M. R., & Daiman, A. (2024). A comprehensive exploration of land use dynamics, NDVI trends, and stakeholder engagement for crafting sustainable green spaces. *National Geographical Journal of India.* https://www.semanticscholar.org/paper/3ce37a460 15d1c65437489c480337293670c4dac (accessed on 11th June 2025).

17. Hedström, E., Sundbye, C., & Urbanos, G. (2023). *SunCare Hub: A Solar-Powered Portable Basic Healthcare Facility for Rural Areas.* https://core.ac.uk/download/622424991.pdf (accessed on 11th June 2025).

18. Herklotz, A., Nayar, A., Agarwal, B., Archer, C., Tirado, C., Elson, D., Maceachern, D., et al. (2012). *Powerful Synergies: Gender Equality, Economic Development and Environmental Sustainability.* https://core.ac.uk/download/75779706.pdf (accessed on 11th June 2025).

19. Ismael, K. M. (2020). *IoT Data Encryption Algorithm for Security.* https://core.ac.uk/download/12005706.pdf (accessed on 11th June 2025).

20. McGranahan, G., & SHARE. (2013). *Community-Driven Sanitation Improvement in Deprived Urban Neighborhoods: Meeting the Challenges of Local Collective Action, Co-Production, Affordability and A Trans-Sectoral Approach.* https://core.ac.uk/download/17192940.pdf (accessed on 11th June 2025).

21. Pearce-Oroz, G. (2011). *Rural Water Supply and Sanitation Challenges in Latin America for The Next Decade.* https://core.ac.uk/download/71360151.pdf (accessed on 11th June 2025).

22. Scott, S., & Si, Z. (2016). *No. 02: Approaching Sustainable Urban Development in China Through a Food System Planning Lens.* https://core.ac.uk/download/157834981.pdf (accessed on 11th June 2025).

23. Yoshikawa, H., Wuermli, A. J., Rebello Britto, P., Dreyer, B. P., Leckman, J. F., Lye, S. J., Ponguta, L. A., et al. (2020). Effects of the global Coronavirus Disease-2019 pandemic on early childhood development: Short- and long-term risks and mitigating program and policy actions. *The Journal of Pediatrics, 223*, 188–193. https://doi.org/10.1016/j.jpeds.2020.05.020 (accessed on 11th June 2025).

INDEX

D

E

F

G

H

Q

R

S

W

Z